A.D.A.M. Student Atlas of Anatomy

This is the second edition of a volume renowned for its innovative approach to understanding the human body. It features full-color art throughout, using a three-dimensional approach to anatomic structure. The *A.D.A.M. Student Atlas of Anatomy* is an invaluable learning and review tool developed for medical, allied health, and human biology undergraduate and graduate students.

This new edition emphasizes surface anatomy and features unique additional views (posterior, medial, lateral) of important structures. It has extensive coverage of those areas, such as the perineum, head, and neck, that are often difficult for students to understand and appreciate.

Todd R. Olson is Professor of Anatomy and Structural Biology and Director of Clinical and Developmental Anatomy at the Albert Einstein College of Medicine, New York.

Wojciech Pawlina is Professor and Chair of the Department of Anatomy at the Mayo Medical School, College of Medicine, Mayo Clinic, Rochester, Minnesota.

A.D.A.M. Student Atlas of Anatomy

2nd Edition

Todd R. Olson, Ph.D.

Professor
Department of Anatomy & Structural Biology
Albert Einstein College of Medicine
Yeshiva University
Bronx, New York

Wojciech Pawlina, M.D.

Professor and Chair
Department of Anatomy
Mayo Medical School
College of Medicine, Mayo Clinic
Rochester, Minnesota

Illustrative Art
A.D.A.M.®, Inc.
Atlanta, Georgia

Cadaver Photographs
The Bassett Collection
Stanford University
School of Medicine
Stanford, California

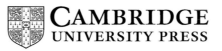

CAMBRIDGE
UNIVERSITY PRESS

CAMBRIDGE UNIVERSITY PRESS
Cambridge, New York, Melbourne, Madrid, Cape Town, Singapore, São Paolo, Delhi

Cambridge University Press
32 Avenue of the Americas, New York, NY 10013-2473, USA

www.cambridge.org
Information on this title: www.cambridge.org/9780521887564

First published 2008

Printed in Hong Kong by Golden Cup

A catalog record for this publication is available from the British Library.

Library of Congress Cataloging in Publication Data

Olson, Todd R.
    A.D.A.M. student atlas of anatomy / Todd R. Olson, Wojciech Pawlina.
– 2nd ed.
        p. ; cm.
    Includes bibliographical references and index.
    ISBN 978-0-521-88756-4 (hardback) – ISBN 978-0-521-71005-3
(paperback) 1. Human anatomy – Atlases. I. Pawlina, Wojciech.
II. Title.   III. Title: Student atlas of anatomy. IV. Title: ADAM student
atlas of anatomy.
    [DNLM: 1. Anatomy – Atlases. QS 17 O52a 2007]

    QM25.O47 2007
    611.0022′2–dc22   2007034103

ISBN 978-0-521-88756-4 hardback
ISBN 978-0-521-71005-3 paperback

Every effort has been made in preparing this publication to provide accurate and up-to-date information
that is in accord with accepted standards and practice at the time of publication. Nevertheless, the authors, editors, and publisher can make no warranties that the information contained herein is totally free
from error, not least because clinical standards are constantly changing through research and regulation.
The authors, editors, and publisher therefore disclaim all liability for direct or consequential damages re-
sulting from the use of material contained in this book. Readers are strongly advised to pay careful at-
tention to information provided by the manufacturer of any drugs or equipment that they plan to use.

Cambridge University Press has no responsibility for the persistence or accuracy of URLs for external or
third-party Internet Web sites referred to in this book and does not guarantee that any content on such
Web sites is, or will remain, accurate or appropriate.

To my mother and father
for the greatest of all contributions
to my existence, optimism, and ability to dream
and to my teachers, colleagues, and students
for their encouragement and contributions
to the realization of this dream.

Todd R. Olson

To my father, Dr. Kazimierz Pawlina,
who was my first anatomy teacher and
my inspiration to pursue an academic career.

Wojciech Pawlina

ACKNOWLEDGMENTS

I (TRO) must express my appreciation and gratitude to Prof. Wojciech Pawlina, M.D., for joining me as a co-author on this edition. Wojciech provided substantial help in the production of this work, and his presence as a co-author is a much-deserved recognition of the hours of work and creative input he contributed to the production of both editions of this atlas. We (TRO & WP) wish also to acknowledge the insightful changes introduced by Prof. Herbert Lippert in the German edition—some of which have been incorporated here—and the helpful comments of Prof. Christian Fontaine, who produced the French translation of the first edition. We also wish to acknowledge and express our gratitude to our colleagues, **Dr. Nirusha Lachman** at the Mayo Clinic and **Dr. Sherry A. Downie** at Albert Einstein, for their invaluable help, suggestions, and support in the production of this new edition.

The second edition of the *A.D.A.M. Student Atlas of Anatomy* is truly the product of a major collaborative effort. The authors wish to extend our appreciation to all individuals who worked on this project and, in particular, to six people whose contribution to this edition were most noteworthy. At Cambridge University Press, **Marc Strauss,** who had the determination and skill to assemble the talent needed to undertake the production of a second edition of this work, and **Nat Russo,** who had the conviction to push for its publication. At A.D.A.M., **Meredith Nienkamp** for her work in championing the second edition and **Lisa Higginbotham,** who worked tirelessly to produce the new artwork for this edition. **Robert A. Chase** at Stanford University School of Medicine for allowing us to include photographs from the David L. Bassett anatomical collection. And **Matthew Byrd** and his superb team at Aptara, Inc., for their excellent work in laying out and producing this book. The dedication to every detail of Matt's team elevated the content and quality of this edition well beyond what was originally perceived by the authors. Thank you!

The talent, dedication, and professionalism of all those at A.D.A.M. who were responsible for the artwork—both in this work and in the A.D.A.M. Interactive Anatomy products—are clearly visible on every page of this atlas. Their efforts and commitment to making this book a learning resource will benefit students everywhere.

A.D.A.M. Anatomical Illustration Team:
Meredith Nienkamp, VP of Production/Medical Illustrator
Mike Gleason, Medical Illustrator
Lisa Higginbotham, Medical Illustrator
Dan Johnson, Medical Illustrator
Kyle McNeir, VP of Production & Internet Design/Medical Illustrator

Prior edition contributions made by:
Mary Beth Clough, Medical Illustrator
Ron Collins, Medical Illustrator
Eric D. Grafman, Medical Illustrator
Lynda Leigh Levy, Medical Illustrator
Virginia Sue Mabry, Illustrator
Dee Mustafa-Bowne, Illustrator
Ed M. Stewart, Medical Illustrator
Gregory M. Swayne, Medical Illustrator
Lelayne Weiss, Illustrator

The authors and A.D.A.M., Inc., wish to thank all of the individuals at Cambridge University Press whose expertise, enthusiasm, and commitment to quality have been at the heart of this project from the beginning: Marc Strauss, Nat Russo, Cathy Felgar, Jennifer Bossert, and Carlos Aguirre. In particular, we wish to thank Marc Strauss for the kindness, patience within limits, and the good humor he displayed in performing his role as the drill sergeant for this entire effort. Finally, we wish to extend our appreciation to Lisa Adamitis, who designed the cover.

Todd R. Olson
Wojciech Pawlina
A.D.A.M., Inc.

PREFACE

Although our knowledge of human anatomy has changed relatively little in the past hundred years, the teaching of anatomy in all health science professions has changed profoundly. During most of the 20th century, gross human anatomy was the principle course in the first year of medical school. Today, one hundred years later, the importance of anatomy within the curriculum has been reduced in pedagogic and temporal significance to the degree that first-year medical students spend two to three times more time studying cellular, subcellular, molecular, and biochemical processes than they do the gross structure of the human body. The major reason for this de-emphasis has been the spectacular development of bioscience technology and the resultant explosion in clinically relevant knowledge that has been incorporated into basic medical education.

Anatomists successfully responded to the challenges created by this reduction in curricular importance and time in three ways. First, and most significantly, we have largely reduced the body of knowledge covered in our courses to those aspects of anatomy that are clinically relevant and therefore of greatest potential value to the student's future clinical practice. Second, we have sifted the body of anatomical knowledge to winnow out the specialist details that must now be taught in postgraduate programs, leaving the anatomical essentials that are fundamental to the basic clinical education of every health sciences and medical student. And third, we have expanded our teaching into the later years of the medical curriculum, introduced specialty and subspecialty focused elective courses for students prior to graduation, and greatly expanded our participation in graduate and continuing education courses. The vertical expansion of anatomical education into these new venues, beyond the traditional first-year course, has allowed a more effective and focused delivery of appropriate anatomical detail to students and graduated physicians who have a direct and specific need to know this information.

All three of these new pedagogic frontiers are critical components in the anatomical education of our future healthcare professionals. The purpose of this work is to focus on the initial phase of this educational process in which it is increasingly necessary to distill the voluminous details present in gross anatomy to their fundamental essentials. While there are an ever-growing number of gross anatomy textbooks that have adopted an "essentials" perspective, we have long thought it remarkable that no one has successfully incorporated this perspective into an anatomy atlas for beginning students. This all changed ten years ago when the first edition of the *A.D.A.M. Student Atlas of Anatomy* was published. From its inception in 1994, we have viewed the *A.D.A.M. Student Atlas* as, first and foremost, a visual guide and interactive learning resource to be used along with a clinical anatomy textbook. In the organization and content of the *A.D.A.M. Student Atlas*, our goal has been and remains to emphasize those parts of the body and structures that are fundamental to the clinical education of every medical and health sciences student.

To accomplish our goal, we decided to include more images of fewer structures and, in particular, more images of those parts of the body that present the beginning student with the greatest difficulties to comprehend and appreciate. We expect and fully hope that most students who use this book will soon become aware of both this distinctive emphasis and limited scope, as well as their own need to consult a more comprehensive atlas as their study of human anatomy matures. *Our primary design concept in support of our goal was neither to duplicate the efforts seen in existing comprehensive atlases, which fully display every named feature in the human body, nor to create an atlas to accompany and guide dissection.*

Nowhere in the *A.D.A.M. Student Atlas* is the emphasis on essentials of the most difficult regions of the body more evident than in Chapter 4 ("Pelvis and Perineum"), which is substantially longer than normally found in traditional atlases. There were two reasons why this chapter was created in this expanded form: First, there is a clear need to know the basic anatomy of the pelvis and perineum in the major clerkship of obstetrics and gynecology, and it is only slightly less important in urology; second, experience indicates that this region is possibly the most difficult for first time students to understand. The pelvis and perineum present unique problems of spatial and surface relationships, which are compounded by the fact that dissection of the pelvis only partially reveals its contents *in situ* and the perineum dissection is difficult and time-consuming, even for an experienced dissector working on an ideal specimen. In contrast to Chapter 4, the preceding chapter on the abdominal contents and their peritoneal relationships is relatively short because the beginning student generally finds them easier to dissect and identify their important anatomical structures and relationships.

All of the atlas's chapters, except the cranial nerves, are topographically/regionally arranged and organized to begin with surface anatomy and to end with the traditional sequences of superficial-to-deep images that the student will see when dissecting. Another innovation that we have included in the *A.D.A.M. Student*

Atlas is the lengthy systemic sections found at the beginning of the chapters on the trunk, limbs, and head and neck. Systemic descriptions were not included in Chapters 2 and 3, the thoracic and abdominal contents, respectively, because the systemic anatomy of the body walls of these regions is covered extensively in Chapter 1 on the trunk, and the distribution and pattern of deeper neurovasculature structures can be clearly appreciated in the sequence of dissection images within each of these two chapters.

While it is ultimately the objective in teaching patient-oriented anatomy to provide the student with an understanding of the composite anatomy of all or selected regions of the body, experience has convinced us that many, or even most, students initially find it easier to organize information by systems. The addition of these extensive systemic sections should not only make the *A.D.A.M. Student Atlas* a more useful book for beginning students but also make it a valuable resource for allied health students whose courses are usually systemically taught but who have never had access to a regional atlas that also emphasized this arrangement.

Another distinctive innovation of the *A.D.A.M. Student Atlas* is the placement of photographs of dissected or osteological specimens adjacent to newly rendered A.D.A.M. images. The rationale for this arrangement and the way we have chosen to label them is based upon the experience we have had with many first year medical students who purchase an expensive photographic atlas that is then used for a short period of time prior to laboratory practical exams. These atlases are helpful because students can test their knowledge on the pictures, which more closely approximate what they will see on the practical exam.

In structuring the *A.D.A.M. Student Atlas*, we have selected and arranged the cadaveric photographs to provide beginning students with an overview of the more important dissections that she/he will see in the lab. Also, by placing them adjacent to similar A.D.A.M. images, the student gains the benefit of seeing a detailed artistic image (as opposed to a highly simplified schematic drawing) that enhances and highlights what is most important in this view.

While an appreciation of both cross-sectional and radiographic anatomy is important in many areas of basic clinical work, it was impossible, within the scope of this atlas, to incorporate more than a limited number into each chapter. The cross-sections and radiographs that do appear have been included because they either best display the distribution of prominent structures, e.g., peritoneum, or provide another means of visualizing the relationships within a region. The limited use of these important visual methods and modalities reflects the physical restrictions of the book and does not imply that they are unimportant or should not be part of a course in clinical anatomy.

TRO & WP

CONTENTS

CHAPTER 1
TRUNK: BODY WALL AND SPINE 1

CHAPTER 2
THORAX 65

CHAPTER 3
ABDOMEN 109

CHAPTER 4
PELVIS AND PERINEUM 149

CHAPTER 5
LOWER LIMB 209

CHAPTER 6
UPPER LIMB 277

CHAPTER 7
HEAD AND NECK 347

CHAPTER 8
CRANIAL AND AUTONOMIC NERVES 445

INDEX 471

The *A.D.A.M. Student Atlas of Anatomy* was designed to be an interactive pictorial guide for the beginning student to master human anatomic methodology and basic terminology as well as the three-dimensional relationships of the body's constituent parts. The next few pages explain how to use the illustrations and special features of the atlas to their fullest advantage.

Three-Dimensional Anatomy

Among the problems faced by the beginning anatomy student, none is more universally perplexing than acquiring an appreciation of the three-dimensional relationships within the human body. Recent anatomy books have addressed this problem largely through the inclusion of cross-sections, CT, and MRI scans. Typically, anatomical atlases and textbooks illustrate an area or region from only one of the four traditional vertical perspectives (i.e., anterior, posterior, medial, or lateral), and students are left to extrapolate the anatomy of the third dimensional from a two-dimensional picture.

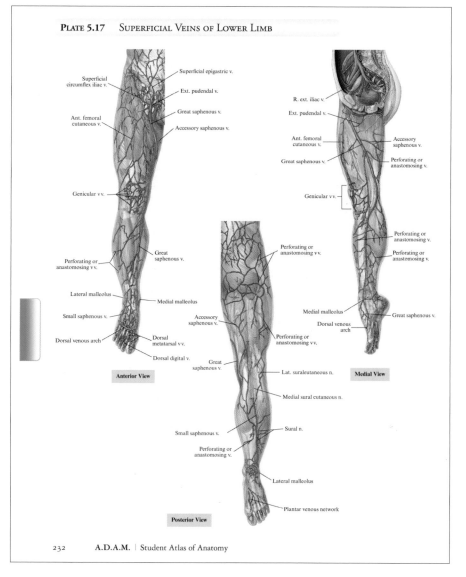

PLATE 5.17   SUPERFICIAL VEINS OF LOWER LIMB

Superficial circumflex iliac v.
Superficial epigastric v.
Superficial epigastric v.
Ext. pudendal v.
Great saphenous v.
Accessory saphenous v.
Ant. femoral cutaneous v.
R. ext. iliac v.
Ext. pudendal v.
Ant. femoral cutaneous v.
Accessory saphenous v.
Great saphenous v.
Perforating or anastomosing v.
Genicular v v.
Genicular v v.
Perforating or anastomosing v v.
Perforating or anastomosing v.
Perforating or anastomosing v.
Great saphenous v.
Perforating or anastomosing v v.
Lateral malleolus
Medial malleolus
Small saphenous v.
Accessory saphenous v.
Medial malleolus
Great saphenous v.
Dorsal venous arch
Dorsal venous arch
Perforating or anastomosing v v.
Dorsal metatarsal v v.
Dorsal digital v.
Great saphenous v.
Lat. suraleutaneous n.
Medial View
Anterior View
Medial sural cutaneous n.
Sural n.
Small saphenous v.
Perforating or anastomosing v.
Lateral malleolus
Plantar venous network
Posterior View

One of the most effective ways of overcoming this problem is to illustrate the region from an orientation that is at right angles to the view in question. Using A.D.A.M. Interactive Anatomy's distinctive ability to view the body from any one of the four vertical perspectives, figures on many plates depict at least two, and sometime more, orientations. For example, the anterior, medial, and posterior views of the leg in Plate 5.17 make visualizing the location, distribution, and relationships of the superficial veins, especially the clinically important saphenous vein, and cutaneous nerves of the lower limb much easier. The extensive use of these multiple views is one of the most striking and valuable characteristics of the *A.D.A.M. Student Atlas of Anatomy*.

Illustrations and Cadaver Photographs

The two figures here in Plate 1.48 illustrate how A.D.A.M. illustrations have been paired with photographs taken from Stanford University's Bassett Collection and intended use in the atlas.

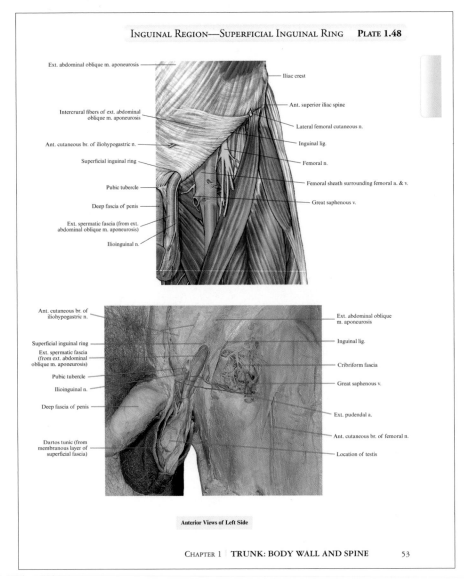

INGUINAL REGION—SUPERFICIAL INGUINAL RING   PLATE 1.48

Anterior Views of Left Side

CHAPTER 1 | TRUNK: BODY WALL AND SPINE   53

In structuring the *A.D.A.M. Student Atlas*, we have selected and arranged the cadaveric photographs to provide an overview of the more important dissections. By associating these photographs with adjacent A.D.A.M. images that depict similar but not identical anatomy, the student gains the benefit of seeing a detailed artistic image (as opposed to a highly simplified schematic drawing) to enhance and highlight what is most important to be seen in the photograph of the dissected specimen.

Joint Motion and Segmentary Nerve Supply

Motions in a single plane at each joint are typically initiated by motor neurons found in four successive spinal cord segments and their spinal nerves. The cranial pair of neurons innervate the muscles that produce movement in one direction and the caudal two innervate the muscles that produce the opposite motion. An appreciation of the actions, especially in the limbs, and their innervation is basic clinical knowledge that has practical value to a wide variety of health care professionals. The atlas includes tables that list the muscles and the nerve(s) that innervate them. The segmentary origin of each nerve is also listed. In those cases where a specific segmentary level is primarily associated with the supply of the muscle, the level is printed in **BOLD**. In addition, information about segmentary innervation is provided in illustrations showing how different spinal levels control antagonistic movements in the upper and lower limb.

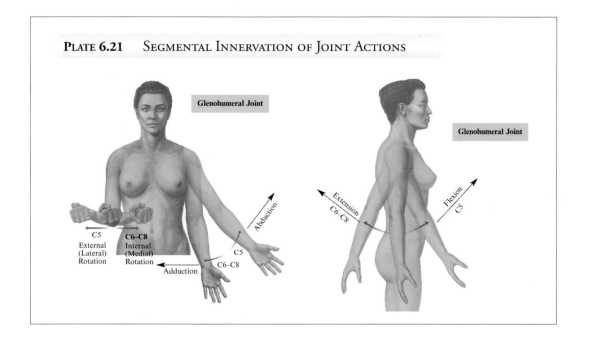

PLATE 6.21   SEGMENTAL INNERVATION OF JOINT ACTIONS

Anatomical Terminology

The anglicized and classical terminology used in the *A.D.A.M Student Atlas* follows the recent edition of the Terminologica *Anatomica*. In some case, the use of square [ ] and parentheses ( ) has formal meaning in the internationally recognized code of anatomical nomenclature.

> **[Square] brackets** signify:
> 1. An officially recognized alternative name or synonym.
>   > Fibularis [Peroneus] longus m.
>   > L. vagus n. [CN X], where CN refers to a cranial nerve
>   > L. gastro-omental [gastroepiploic] v.
>
> 2. An equivalent anatomical name for this structure.
>   > Subcostal n. [T12], where T12 = 12th thoracic spinal n.
>   > C1 [Atlas]
>
> **(Round) brackets** identify:
> 1. An official name of *inconsistent* structures.
>   > (Accessory parotid gland)
>   > (Frontal suture)
>
> 2. Eponyms and alternative names that are not officially recognized as appropriate in contemporary usage.
>   > Omental foramen (f. of Winslow)
>   > L. colic (splenic) flexure
>   > Costoaxillary (ext. mammary) v.
>   > Hepatopancreatic ampulla (of Vater)

3. Additional components of a name that are usually omitted that have been added for clarification or that are supplemental to the name.

> Greater tuberosity (of humerus)
> Acromion (process of scapula)
> Posterior basal bronchopulmonary segment (S10)

4. Motor and sensory segmental and spinal nerve levels of a peripheral nerve.

> Femoral n. (L2-L4)
> Lat. femoral cutaneous n. (L2,L3)
> Middle cluneal nn. (dorsal rami of S1-S3)

For TWO adjacent spinal nn., they are separated by a comma; however, when more than two spinal nn. are involved, only the cranial and caudal-most are listed, separated by a hyphen.

5. Conditions specific or unique to the image or dissection.

> L. rectus abdominis m. (reflected medially)
> R. primary bronchus (pulled to L.)

Hyphenated names. Hyphens appear in a name to:

1. More specifically identify a constituent part of a larger complex structure.

> Triceps brachii m. - long head
> Pectoralis major m. - sternal head

2. Separate the parts of compound name where the same vowel is found at the end of the first name and beginning of the second.

> Gastro-omental [gastroepiploic] v.
> Atlanto-occipital joint

Abbreviations

The following abbreviations are used in the atlas. **Bold** entries are abbreviated everywhere they appear, other entries are sometimes abbreviated in order to save space.

&	**= and**	inf.	= inferior	nn.	= nerves
a.	**= artery**	int.	= internal	port.	= portion
aa.	**= arteries**	**L.**	**= Left**	post.	= posterior
ant.	= anterior	lat.	= lateral	proc.	= process
asc.	= ascending	**lig.**	**= ligament**	pt.	= part
br.	**= branch**	**ligg.**	**= ligaments**	**R.**	**= Right**
brr.	**= branches**	**m.**	**= muscle**	sup.	= superior
comm.	**= communicating**	**mm.**	**= muscles**	trib.	= tributary
desc.	= descending	med.	= medial	**v.**	**= vein**
ext.	= external	**n.**	**= nerve**	**vv.**	**= veins**

Another system of abbreviation is typically used when segmental structures (i.e., vertebrae, spinal or intercostal nerves, ribs) are superimposed on or immediately adjacent to the structure. Thus, **C6** on or next to a vertebra identifies the sixth cervical vertebrae; the "C" distinguishes the vertebral type and the number its segmental location. Abbreviations used in this way are:

> C = Cervical
> Cc = Coccygeal
> L = Lumbar
> R = Rib
> S = Sacral
> T = Thoracic

1

TRUNK: BODY WALL AND SPINE

SURFACE ANATOMY

SKELETON

JOINTS & LIGAMENTS

MUSCLES

VASCULATURE

NERVES

SPINAL CORD & VERTEBRAL CANAL

ANTERIOR BODY WALL & MAMMARY GLAND

LATERAL BODY WALL

INGUINAL REGION

SUPERFICIAL BACK

DEEP BACK

SUBOCCIPITAL REGION

PLATE 1.1   SURFACE ANATOMY

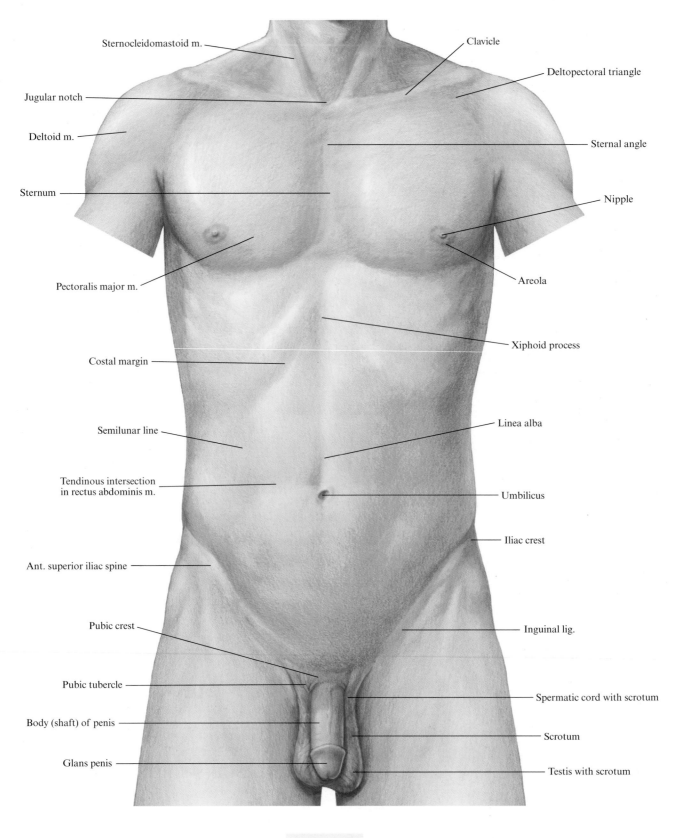

Sternocleidomastoid m.

Clavicle

Deltopectoral triangle

Jugular notch

Deltoid m.

Sternal angle

Sternum

Nipple

Pectoralis major m.

Areola

Xiphoid process

Costal margin

Linea alba

Semilunar line

Tendinous intersection
in rectus abdominis m.

Umbilicus

Iliac crest

Ant. superior iliac spine

Pubic crest

Inguinal lig.

Pubic tubercle

Spermatic cord with scrotum

Body (shaft) of penis

Scrotum

Glans penis

Testis with scrotum

Anterior View

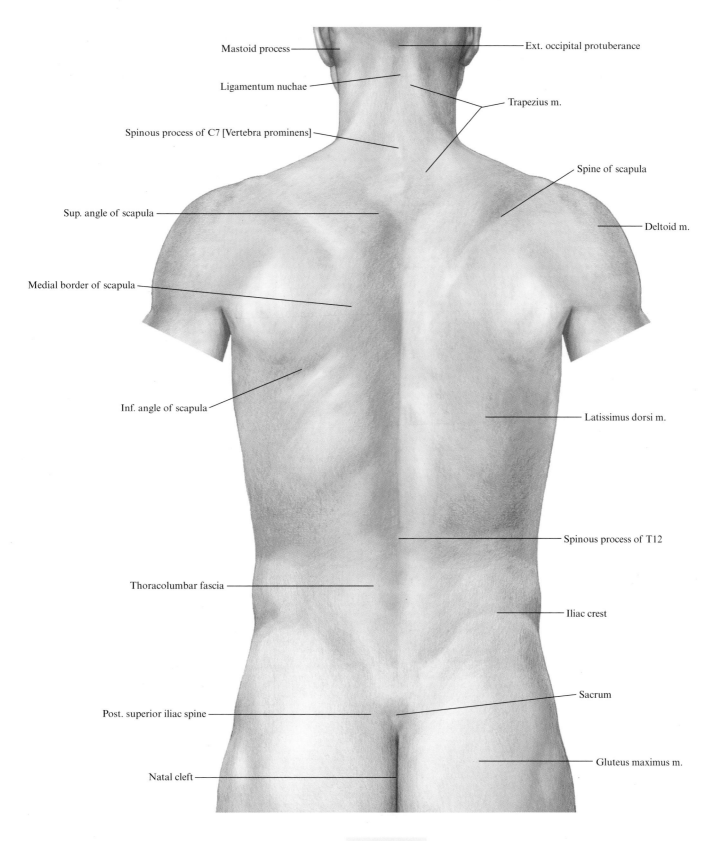

Mastoid process

Ext. occipital protuberance

Ligamentum nuchae

Trapezius m.

Spinous process of C7 [Vertebra prominens]

Spine of scapula

Sup. angle of scapula

Deltoid m.

Medial border of scapula

Inf. angle of scapula

Latissimus dorsi m.

Spinous process of T12

Thoracolumbar fascia

Iliac crest

Sacrum

Post. superior iliac spine

Natal cleft

Gluteus maximus m.

Posterior View

CHAPTER 1 │ **TRUNK: BODY WALL AND SPINE**

PLATE 1.3   SKELETON—MUSCLE ATTACHMENTS

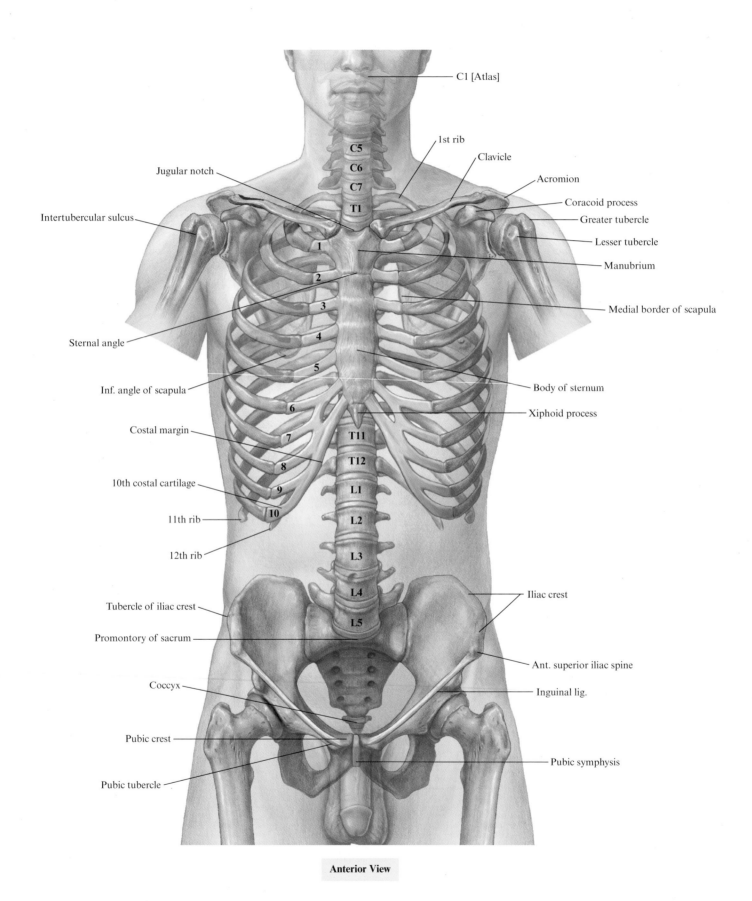

C1 [Atlas]

1st rib

Clavicle

Jugular notch

Acromion

Coracoid process

Intertubercular sulcus

Greater tubercle

Lesser tubercle

Manubrium

Medial border of scapula

Sternal angle

Body of sternum

Inf. angle of scapula

Xiphoid process

Costal margin

10th costal cartilage

11th rib

12th rib

Tubercle of iliac crest

Iliac crest

Promontory of sacrum

Ant. superior iliac spine

Coccyx

Inguinal lig.

Pubic crest

Pubic symphysis

Pubic tubercle

C5
C6
C7
T1

T11
T12
L1
L2
L3
L4
L5

1
2
3
4
5
6
7
8
9
10

Anterior View

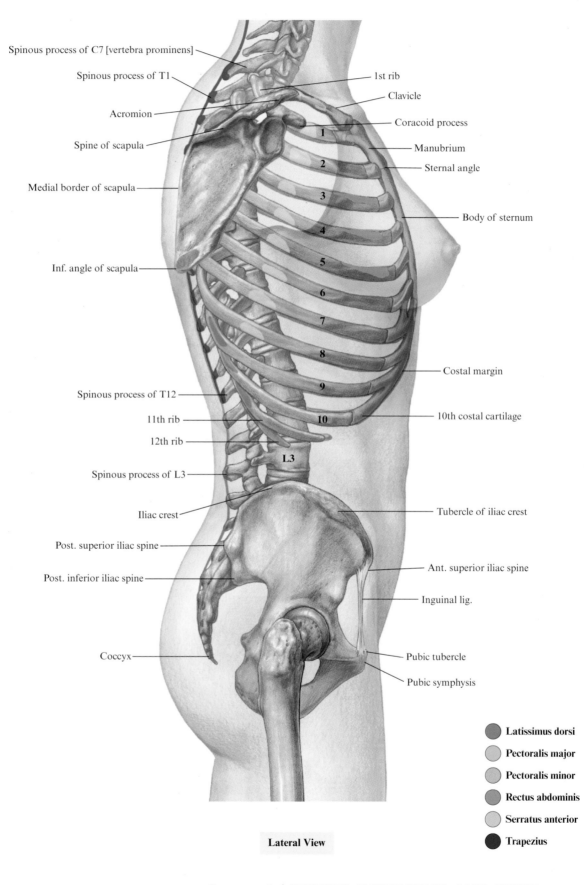

Spinous process of C7 [vertebra prominens]

Spinous process of T1

Acromion

Spine of scapula

Medial border of scapula

Inf. angle of scapula

Spinous process of T12

11th rib

12th rib

Spinous process of L3

Iliac crest

Post. superior iliac spine

Post. inferior iliac spine

Coccyx

1st rib

Clavicle

Coracoid process

Manubrium

Sternal angle

Body of sternum

Costal margin

10th costal cartilage

Tubercle of iliac crest

Ant. superior iliac spine

Inguinal lig.

Pubic tubercle

Pubic symphysis

1
2
3
4
5
6
7
8
9
10

L3

Lateral View

● **Latissimus dorsi**
○ **Pectoralis major**
○ **Pectoralis minor**
● **Rectus abdominis**
○ **Serratus anterior**
● **Trapezius**

CHAPTER 1 | **TRUNK: BODY WALL AND SPINE**

PLATE 1.5   SKELETON—MUSCLE ATTACHMENTS

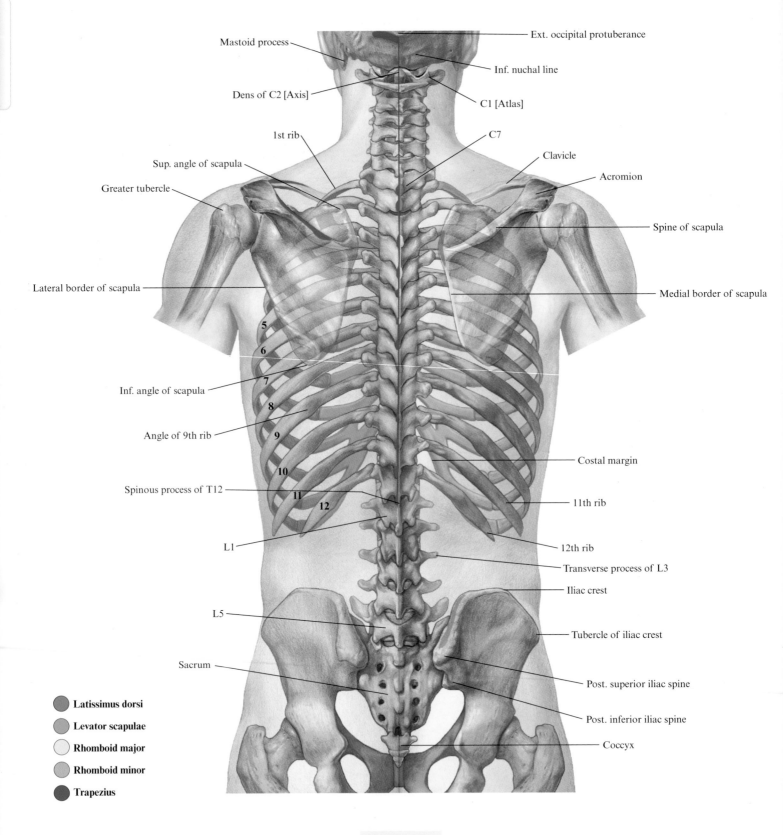

Mastoid process

Ext. occipital protuberance

Inf. nuchal line

Dens of C2 [Axis]

C1 [Atlas]

1st rib

C7

Sup. angle of scapula

Clavicle

Greater tubercle

Acromion

Spine of scapula

Lateral border of scapula

Medial border of scapula

5
6
7

Inf. angle of scapula

8

Angle of 9th rib

9

10

Costal margin

Spinous process of T12

11

12

11th rib

L1

12th rib

Transverse process of L3

Iliac crest

L5

Tubercle of iliac crest

Sacrum

Post. superior iliac spine

Post. inferior iliac spine

Coccyx

- ● **Latissimus dorsi**
- ● **Levator scapulae**
- ○ **Rhomboid major**
- ● **Rhomboid minor**
- ● **Trapezius**

Posterior View

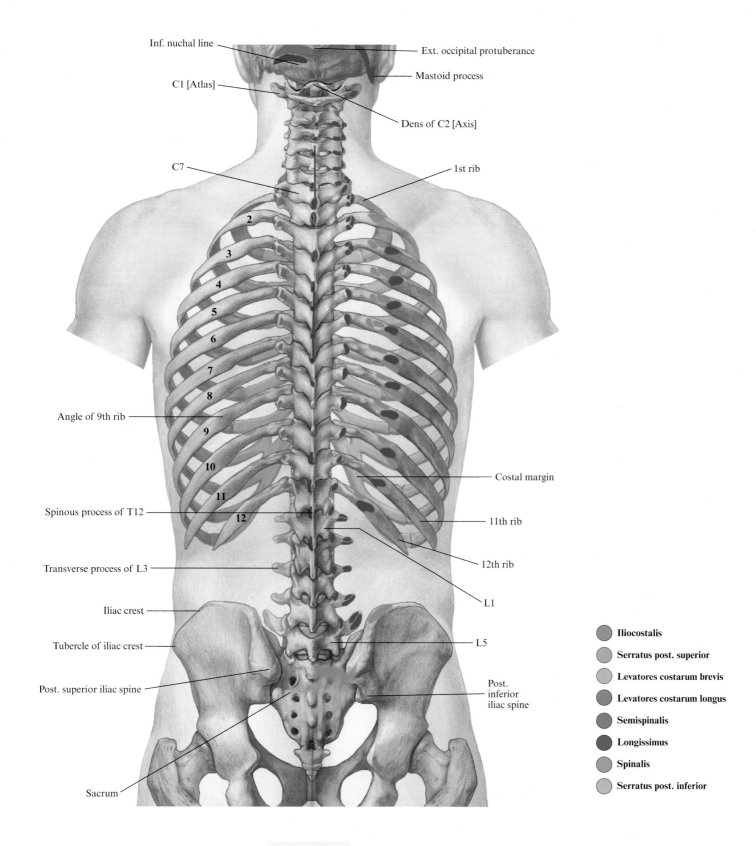

Inf. nuchal line

Ext. occipital protuberance

C1 [Atlas]

Mastoid process

Dens of C2 [Axis]

C7

1st rib

2

3

4

5

6

7

8

Angle of 9th rib

9

10

Costal margin

11

Spinous process of T12

12

11th rib

12th rib

Transverse process of L3

L1

Iliac crest

Tubercle of iliac crest

L5

Post. superior iliac spine

Post. inferior iliac spine

Sacrum

Iliocostalis

Serratus post. superior

Levatores costarum brevis

Levatores costarum longus

Semispinalis

Longissimus

Spinalis

Serratus post. inferior

Posterior View

PLATE 1.7   SKELETON—SPINE

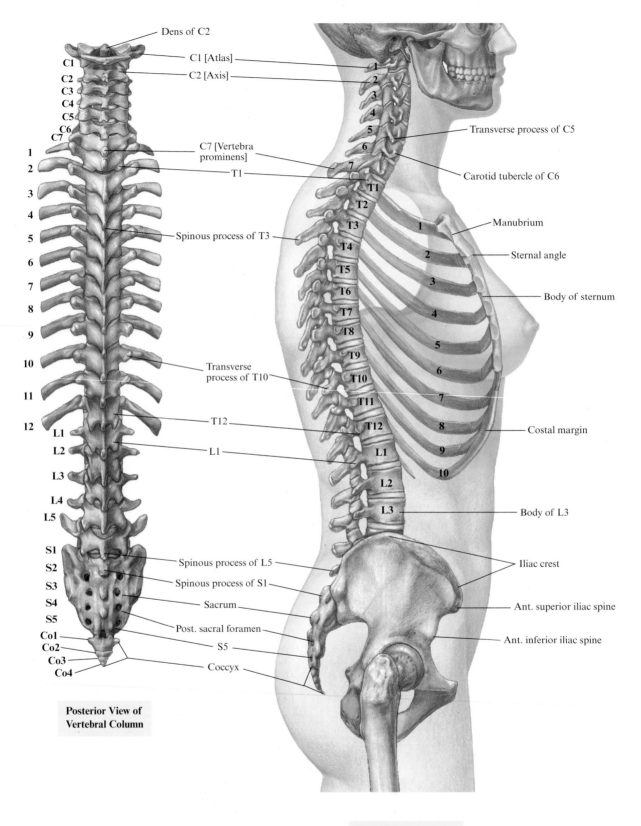

Dens of C2

C1 [Atlas]

C2 [Axis]

C1
C2
C3
C4
C5
C6
C7

Transverse process of C5

Carotid tubercle of C6

C7 [Vertebra prominens]

T1

Manubrium

Sternal angle

Spinous process of T3

Body of sternum

Transverse process of T10

Costal margin

T12

L1

Body of L3

Spinous process of L5

Spinous process of S1

Iliac crest

Sacrum

Ant. superior iliac spine

Post. sacral foramen

Ant. inferior iliac spine

S5

Coccyx

**Posterior View of
Vertebral Column**

**Lateral View of Right
Half of Skeleton**

T1
T2
T3
T4
T5
T6
T7
T8
T9
T10
T11
T12
L1
L2
L3

S1
S2
S3
S4
S5
Co1
Co2
Co3
Co4

L1
L2
L3
L4
L5

A.D.A.M. | Student Atlas of Anatomy

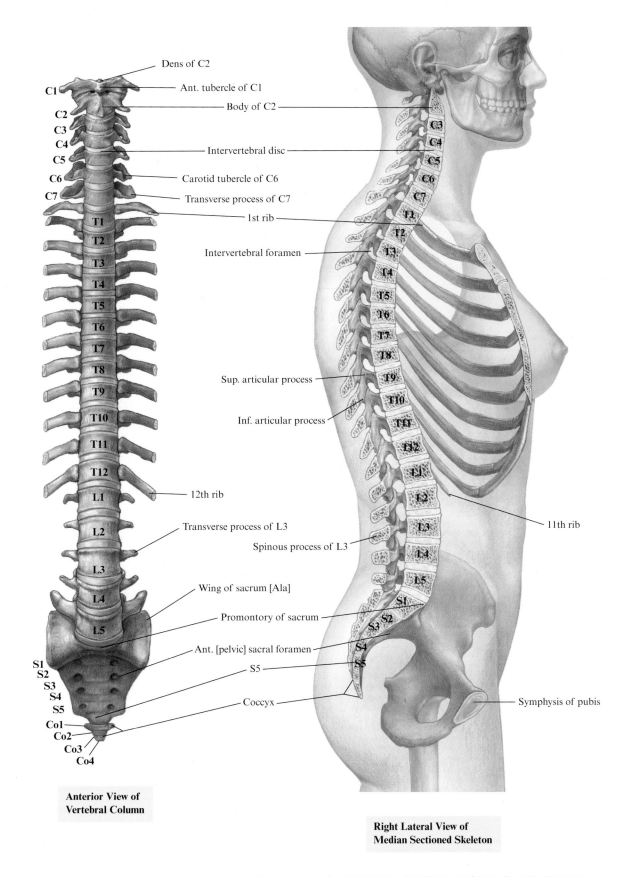

Dens of C2

Ant. tubercle of C1

Body of C2

Intervertebral disc

Carotid tubercle of C6

Transverse process of C7

1st rib

Intervertebral foramen

Sup. articular process

Inf. articular process

12th rib

Transverse process of L3

Spinous process of L3

Wing of sacrum [Ala]

Promontory of sacrum

Ant. [pelvic] sacral foramen

S5

Coccyx

11th rib

Symphysis of pubis

**Anterior View of
Vertebral Column**

**Right Lateral View of
Median Sectioned Skeleton**

CHAPTER 1 | **TRUNK: BODY WALL AND SPINE**   9

PLATE 1.9   CERVICAL VERTEBRAE

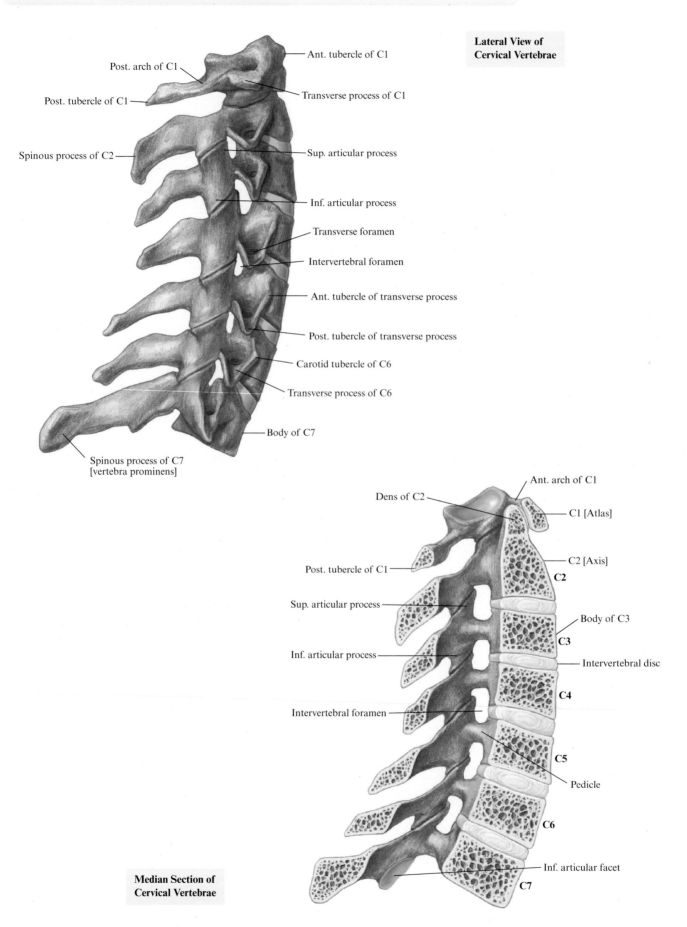

Lateral View of Cervical Vertebrae

Ant. tubercle of C1

Post. arch of C1

Transverse process of C1

Post. tubercle of C1

Spinous process of C2

Sup. articular process

Inf. articular process

Transverse foramen

Intervertebral foramen

Ant. tubercle of transverse process

Post. tubercle of transverse process

Carotid tubercle of C6

Transverse process of C6

Body of C7

Spinous process of C7 [vertebra prominens]

Ant. arch of C1

Dens of C2

C1 [Atlas]

C2 [Axis]

Post. tubercle of C1

C2

Sup. articular process

Body of C3

C3

Inf. articular process

Intervertebral disc

C4

Intervertebral foramen

C5

Pedicle

C6

Inf. articular facet

C7

Median Section of Cervical Vertebrae

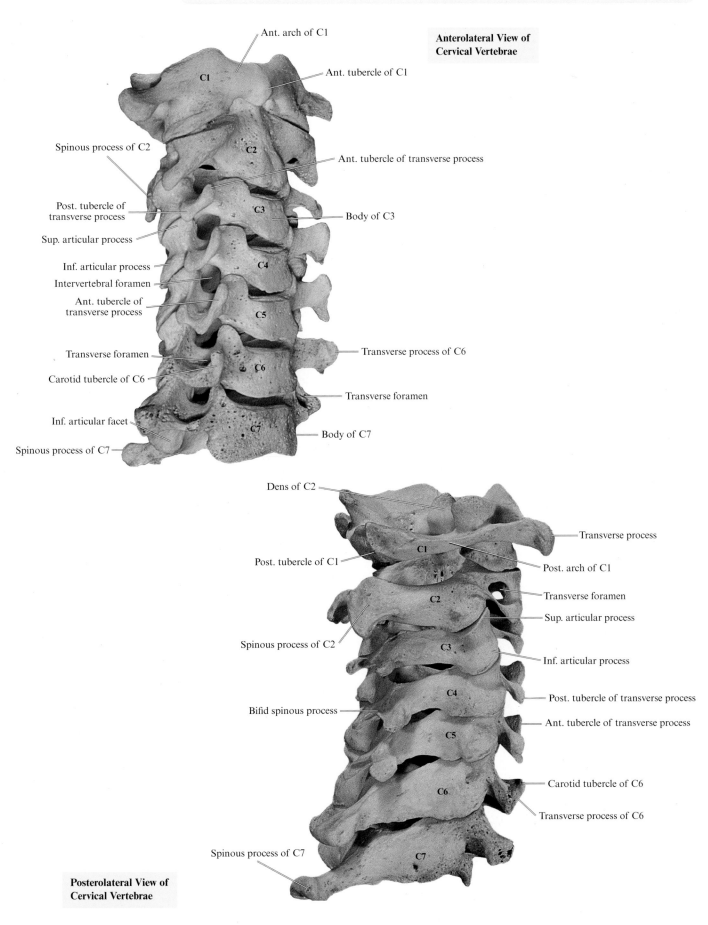

Anterolateral View of Cervical Vertebrae

Ant. arch of C1

C1

Ant. tubercle of C1

Spinous process of C2

C2

Ant. tubercle of transverse process

Post. tubercle of transverse process

C3

Body of C3

Sup. articular process

Inf. articular process

C4

Intervertebral foramen

Ant. tubercle of transverse process

C5

Transverse foramen

Transverse process of C6

Carotid tubercle of C6

C6

Transverse foramen

Inf. articular facet

C7

Body of C7

Spinous process of C7

Dens of C2

Transverse process

C1

Post. tubercle of C1

Post. arch of C1

C2

Transverse foramen

Sup. articular process

Spinous process of C2

C3

Inf. articular process

C4

Post. tubercle of transverse process

Bifid spinous process

Ant. tubercle of transverse process

C5

Carotid tubercle of C6

C6

Transverse process of C6

Spinous process of C7

C7

Posterolateral View of Cervical Vertebrae

CHAPTER 1 | **TRUNK: BODY WALL AND SPINE**

11

PLATE 1.11   THORACIC VERTEBRAE

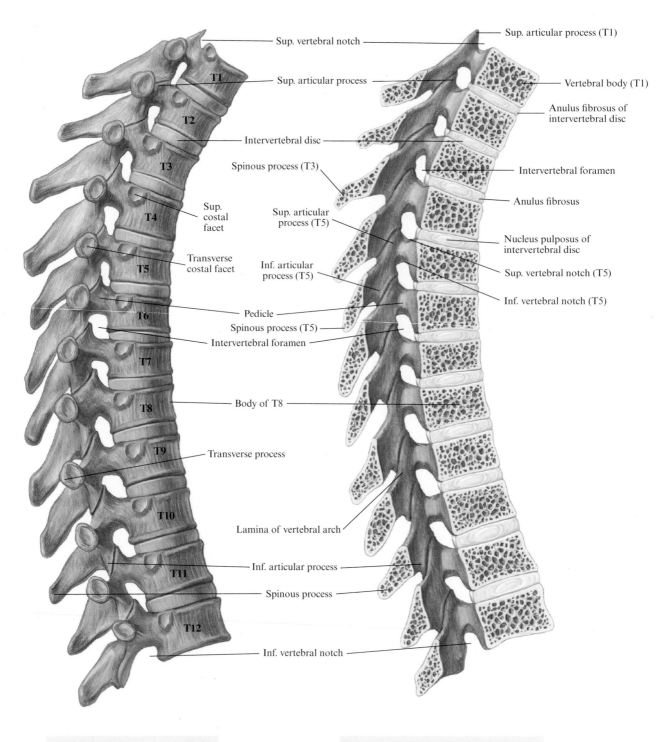

Sup. vertebral notch

T1

Sup. articular process

T2

Intervertebral disc

T3

Spinous process (T3)

Sup. costal facet

T4

Sup. articular process (T5)

Transverse costal facet

T5

Inf. articular process (T5)

Pedicle

T6

Spinous process (T5)

Intervertebral foramen

T7

Body of T8

T8

Transverse process

T9

T10

Lamina of vertebral arch

Inf. articular process

T11

Spinous process

T12

Inf. vertebral notch

Sup. articular process (T1)

Vertebral body (T1)

Anulus fibrosus of intervertebral disc

Intervertebral foramen

Anulus fibrosus

Nucleus pulposus of intervertebral disc

Sup. vertebral notch (T5)

Inf. vertebral notch (T5)

Lateral View of Thoracic Vertebrae

Midsagittal Section of Thoracic Vertebrae

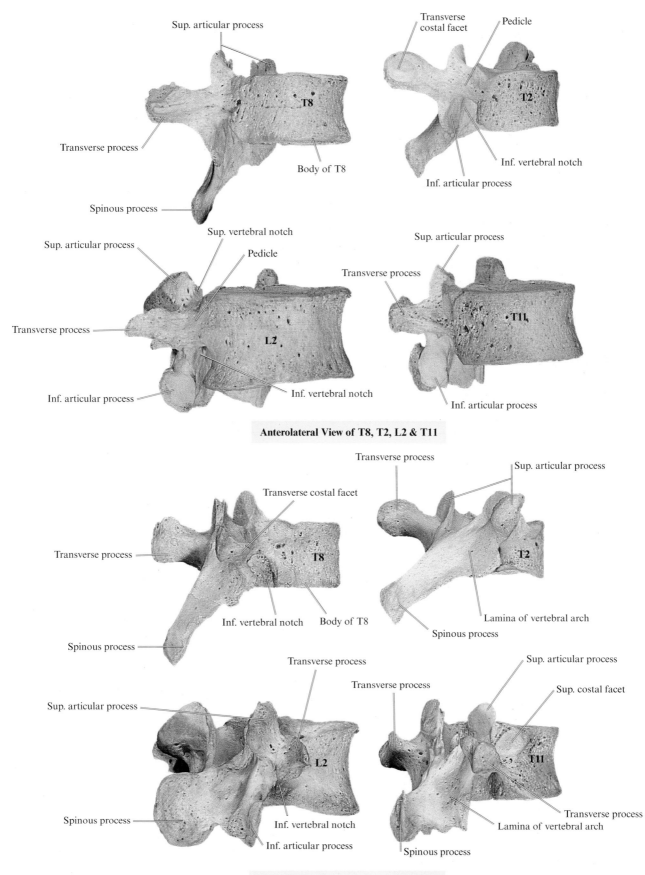

Sup. articular process

Transverse process

Spinous process

T8

Body of T8

Transverse costal facet

Pedicle

T2

Inf. vertebral notch

Inf. articular process

Sup. articular process

Sup. vertebral notch

Pedicle

Transverse process

L2

Inf. articular process

Inf. vertebral notch

Sup. articular process

Transverse process

T11

Inf. articular process

Anterolateral View of T8, T2, L2 & T11

Transverse process

Transverse costal facet

Transverse process

T8

Inf. vertebral notch

Body of T8

Spinous process

Transverse process

Sup. articular process

T2

Lamina of vertebral arch

Spinous process

Sup. articular process

Transverse process

Transverse process

Sup. articular process

Sup. costal facet

L2

T11

Spinous process

Inf. vertebral notch

Inf. articular process

Transverse process

Lamina of vertebral arch

Spinous process

Posterolateral View of T8, T2, L2 & T11

PLATE 1.13   LUMBAR VERTEBRAE

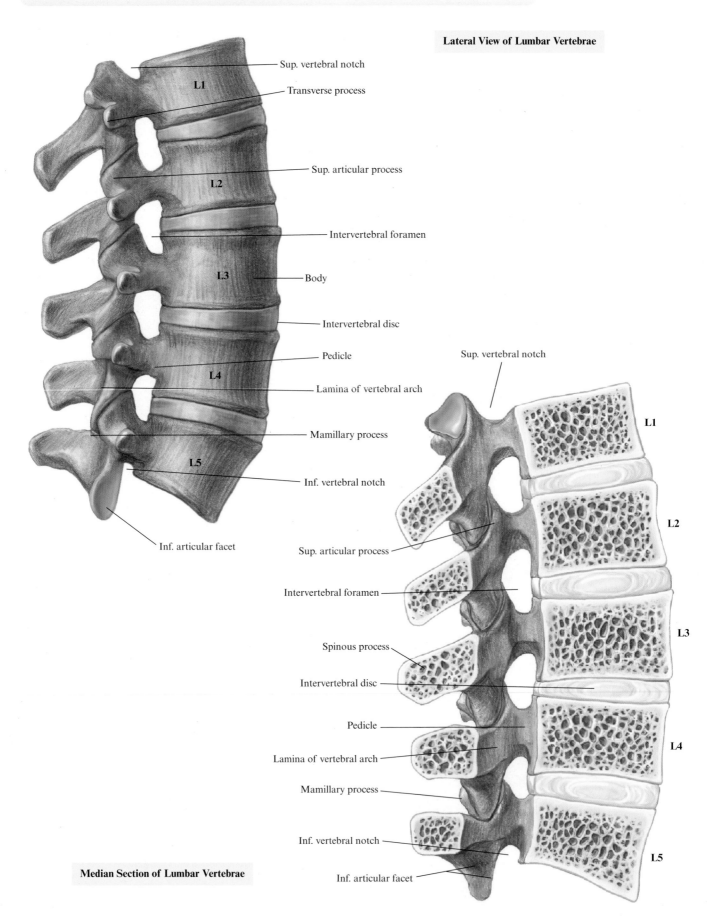

Lateral View of Lumbar Vertebrae

Sup. vertebral notch

L1

Transverse process

Sup. articular process

L2

Intervertebral foramen

L3

Body

Intervertebral disc

Pedicle

L4

Lamina of vertebral arch

Mamillary process

L5

Inf. vertebral notch

Inf. articular facet

Sup. vertebral notch

L1

L2

L3

Sup. articular process

Intervertebral foramen

Spinous process

Intervertebral disc

L4

Pedicle

Lamina of vertebral arch

Mamillary process

L5

Inf. vertebral notch

Inf. articular facet

Median Section of Lumbar Vertebrae

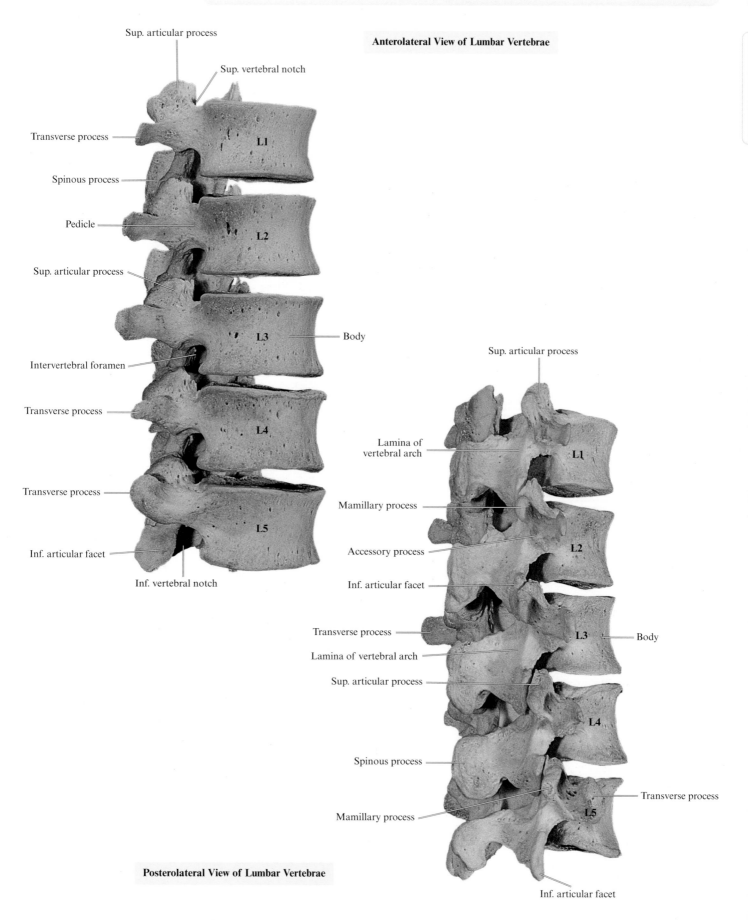

Anterolateral View of Lumbar Vertebrae

Sup. articular process

Sup. vertebral notch

Transverse process

L1

Spinous process

Pedicle

L2

Sup. articular process

L3

Body

Intervertebral foramen

Transverse process

L4

Sup. articular process

Transverse process

L5

Inf. articular facet

Inf. vertebral notch

Lamina of
vertebral arch

L1

Mamillary process

Accessory process

L2

Inf. articular facet

Transverse process

L3

Body

Lamina of vertebral arch

Sup. articular process

L4

Spinous process

Transverse process

Mamillary process

L5

Posterolateral View of Lumbar Vertebrae

Inf. articular facet

PLATE **1.15** SACRUM

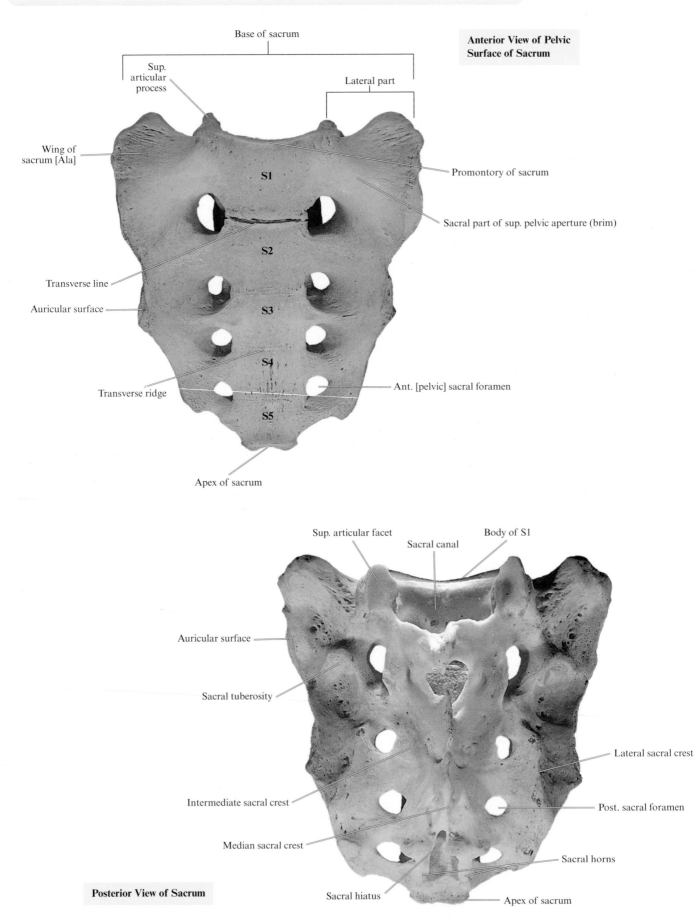

Base of sacrum

**Anterior View of Pelvic
Surface of Sacrum**

Sup. articular process

Lateral part

Wing of sacrum [Ala]

Promontory of sacrum

S1

Sacral part of sup. pelvic aperture (brim)

S2

Transverse line

Auricular surface

S3

S4

Ant. [pelvic] sacral foramen

Transverse ridge

S5

Apex of sacrum

Sup. articular facet

Sacral canal

Body of S1

Auricular surface

Sacral tuberosity

Lateral sacral crest

Intermediate sacral crest

Post. sacral foramen

Median sacral crest

Sacral horns

Posterior View of Sacrum

Sacral hiatus

Apex of sacrum

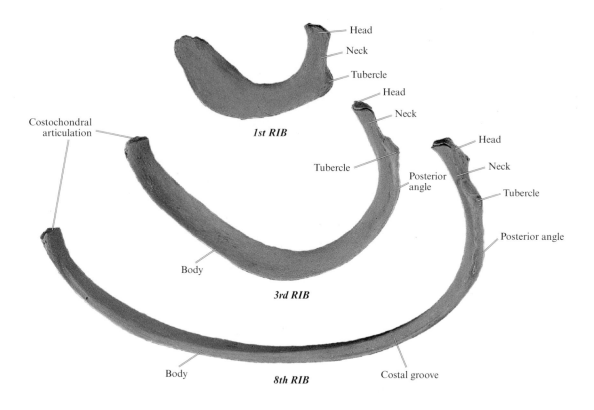

Head
Neck
Tubercle

1st RIB

Head
Neck

Costochondral
articulation

Tubercle
Posterior
angle

Head
Neck
Tubercle

Posterior angle

Body

3rd RIB

Body

8th RIB

Costal groove

Inferior View of Right Ribs 1, 3 & 8 (Right Side)

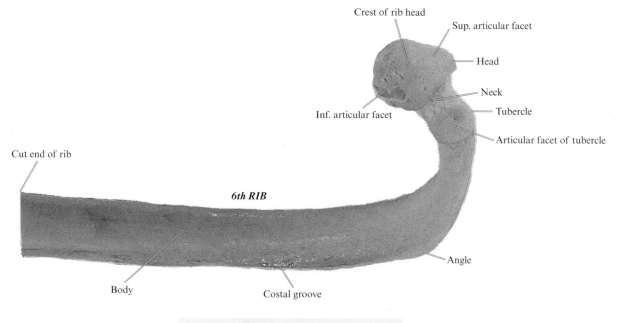

Crest of rib head
Sup. articular facet
Head
Neck
Tubercle
Articular facet of tubercle

Inf. articular facet

Cut end of rib

6th RIB

Angle

Body

Costal groove

Medial View of Proximal End of Right 6th Rib

PLATE 1.17 JOINTS & LIGAMENTS

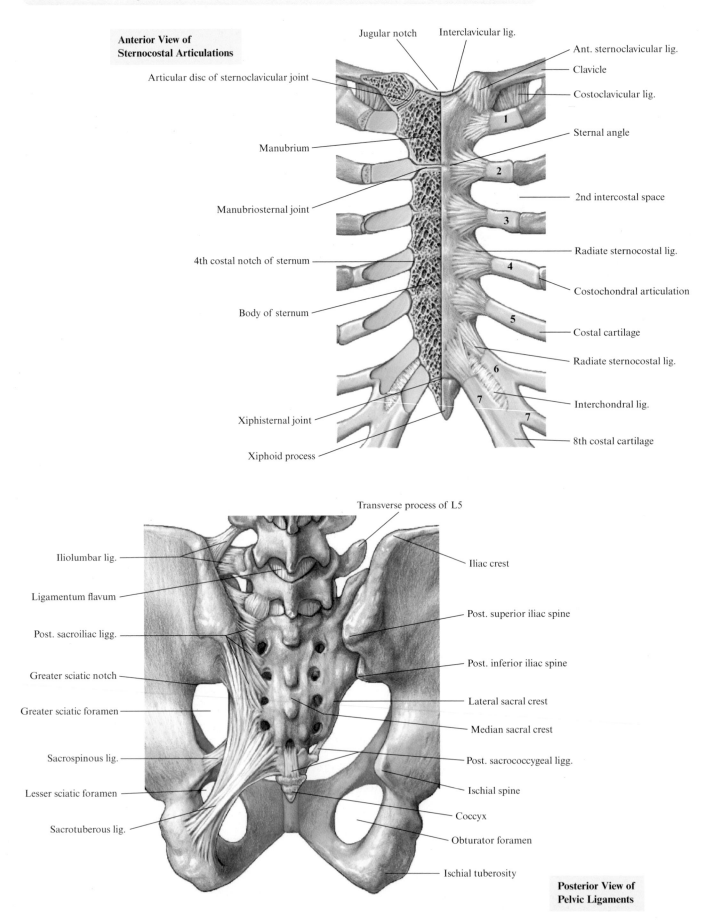

Anterior View of Sternocostal Articulations

Jugular notch

Interclavicular lig.

Ant. sternoclavicular lig.

Clavicle

Costoclavicular lig.

Articular disc of sternoclavicular joint

Manubrium

Sternal angle

1

2

2nd intercostal space

Manubriosternal joint

3

4th costal notch of sternum

Radiate sternocostal lig.

4

Costochondral articulation

Body of sternum

5

Costal cartilage

Radiate sternocostal lig.

6

Interchondral lig.

7

Xiphisternal joint

7

7

8th costal cartilage

Xiphoid process

Transverse process of L5

Iliolumbar lig.

Iliac crest

Ligamentum flavum

Post. sacroiliac ligg.

Post. superior iliac spine

Greater sciatic notch

Post. inferior iliac spine

Greater sciatic foramen

Lateral sacral crest

Median sacral crest

Sacrospinous lig.

Post. sacrococcygeal ligg.

Lesser sciatic foramen

Ischial spine

Sacrotuberous lig.

Coccyx

Obturator foramen

Ischial tuberosity

Posterior View of Pelvic Ligaments

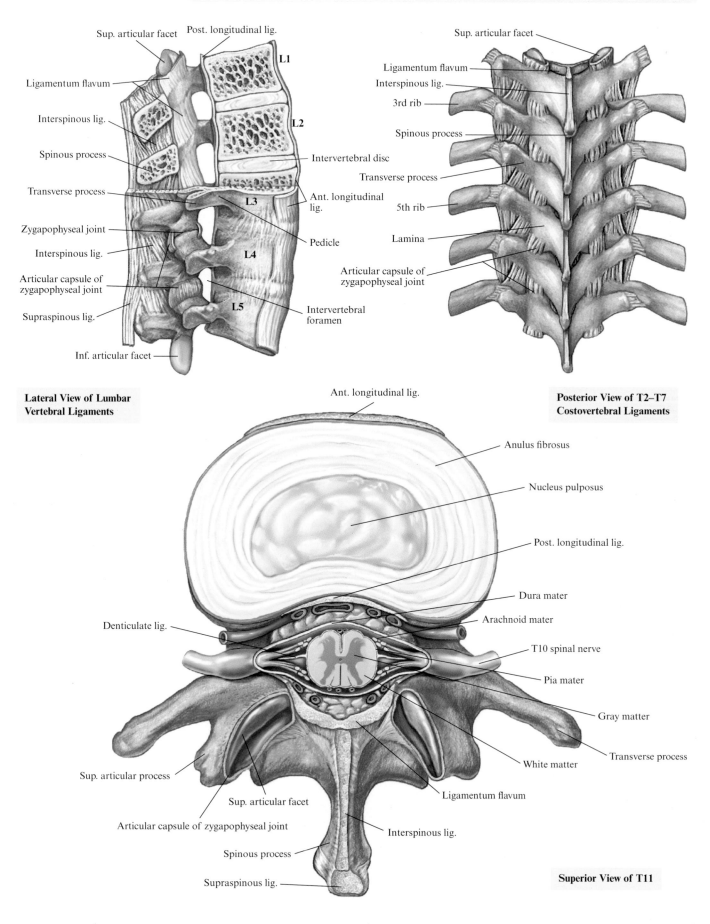

Sup. articular facet

Post. longitudinal lig.

Ligamentum flavum

Interspinous lig.

Spinous process

Transverse process

Zygapophyseal joint

Interspinous lig.

Articular capsule of zygapophyseal joint

Supraspinous lig.

Inf. articular facet

L1

L2

L3

L4

L5

Intervertebral disc

Ant. longitudinal lig.

Pedicle

Intervertebral foramen

Lateral View of Lumbar Vertebral Ligaments

Sup. articular facet

Ligamentum flavum

Interspinous lig.

3rd rib

Spinous process

Transverse process

5th rib

Lamina

Articular capsule of zygapophyseal joint

Posterior View of T2–T7 Costovertebral Ligaments

Ant. longitudinal lig.

Anulus fibrosus

Nucleus pulposus

Post. longitudinal lig.

Dura mater

Denticulate lig.

Arachnoid mater

T10 spinal nerve

Pia mater

Gray matter

Transverse process

White matter

Sup. articular process

Ligamentum flavum

Sup. articular facet

Articular capsule of zygapophyseal joint

Interspinous lig.

Spinous process

Supraspinous lig.

Superior View of T11

CHAPTER 1 | **TRUNK: BODY WALL AND SPINE**   19

TABLE 1.1   MUSCLES—THORACIC WALL

Muscle	Superior or Medial Attachment	Inferior or Lateral Attachment	Innervation	Action(s)
External intercostal	Inf. border of rib that bounds intercostal space cranially	Sup. border of rib bounding intercostal space caudally, muscular from costal tubercle to end of rib with membranous connection to sternum	1st to 11th intercostal nn. & subcostal n.	Elevate ribs in inspiration
Internal intercostal		Sup. border of rib bounding intercostal space caudally, muscular from angle to sternum		
Innermost intercostal		Separated from int. intercostal mm. only by neurovascular bundle		
Subcostal	Inf. border lateral to angle of rib that bounds intercostal space cranially	Int. surface near angle of rib that bounds intercostal space caudally, best developed between ribs 6 & 12, may cross 2 intercostal spaces		Depress ribs in expiration
Transversus thoracis	Int. surface of body & xiphoid of sternum	Inf. border of 2nd to 6th costal cartilages	2nd to 6th intercostal nn.	Depress costal cartilages in expiration
Levatores costarum *L. c. brevis m.* *L. c. longus m.*	Transverse processes of C7 to T11	Between tubercle & angle on ext. surface of rib caudal to vertebral attachment	Dorsal primary rami of C8 & T1 to T11 spinal nn.	Elevate ribs in inspiration; laterally flex spine
Serratus posterior superior	Inf. part of ligamentum nuchae & spinous process from C7 to T2/T3	Sup. border of 2nd to 5th ribs just lateral to angles	2nd to 5th intercostal nn.	Elevate ribs in inspiration
Serratus posterior inferior	Spinous processes & thoracolumbar fascia from T11/T12 to L3	Inf. border of 9th/10th to 12th ribs just lateral to angles	9th to 11th intercostal nn. & subcostal n.	Depress ribs in expiration

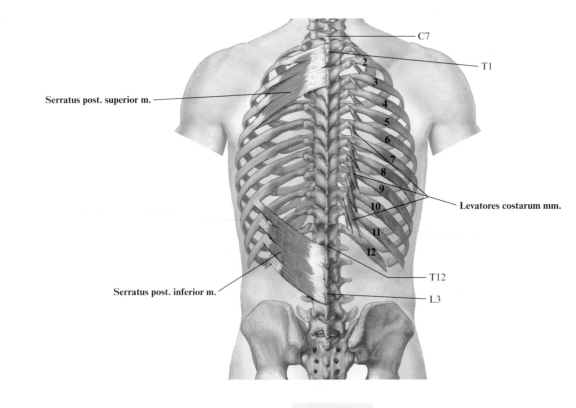

Posterior View

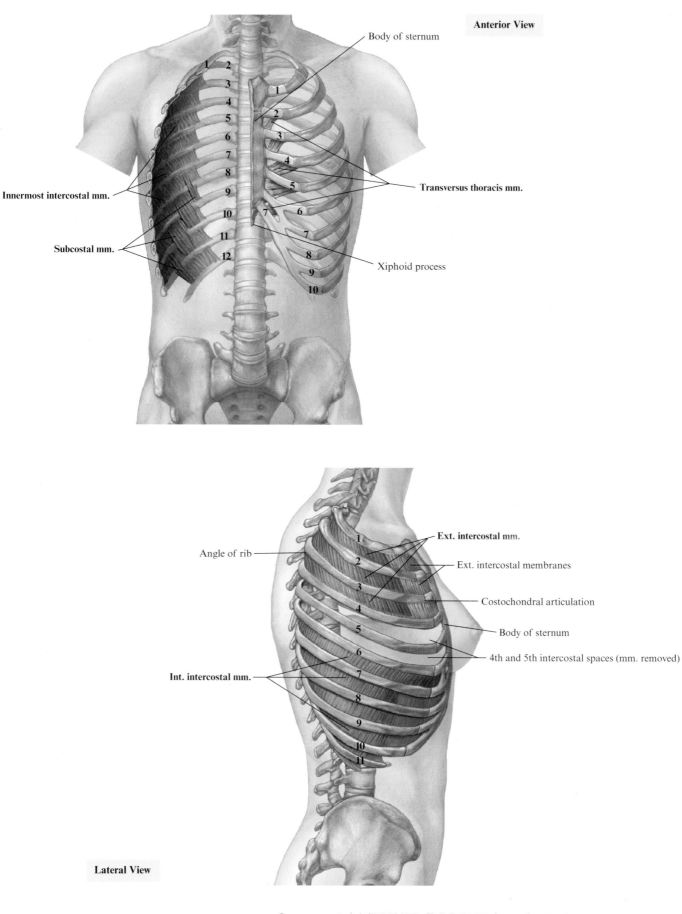

Anterior View

Body of sternum

1 2 3 4 5 6 7 8 9 10 11 12

1 2 3 4 5 6 7

Innermost intercostal mm.

Subcostal mm.

Transversus thoracis mm.

Xiphoid process

6 7 8 9 10

Lateral View

Ext. intercostal mm.

Angle of rib

Ext. intercostal membranes

Costochondral articulation

Body of sternum

4th and 5th intercostal spaces (mm. removed)

Int. intercostal mm.

1 2 3 4 5 6 7 8 9 10 11

TABLE 1.2   MUSCLES—ABDOMINAL WALL

Muscle	Lateral or Superior Attachment	Medial or Inferior Attachment	Innervation	Action(s)
External oblique	Ext. surfaces of 5th to 12th ribs	Linea alba, pubic tubercle & ant. half of iliac crest	Inf. six thoracic nn. & subcostal n.	Compress & support abdominal viscera; flex & rotate tunk
Internal oblique	Thoracolumbar fascia, ant. two-thirds of iliac crest & lateral half of inguinal lig.	Inf. borders of 10th to 12th ribs, linea alba & pubis via the conjoint tendon	Ventral rami of T6 to L1	
Transversus abdominis	Int. surfaces of 7th to 12th costal cartilages, thoracolumbar fascia, iliac crest & lateral third of inguinal lig.	Linea alba with aponeurosis of int. oblique, pubic crest & pecten pubis via conjoint tendon		Compress & support abdominal viscera
Rectus abdominis	Xiphoid process & 5th to 7th costal cartilages	Pubic symphysis & pubic crest	Ventral rami of inf. six thoracic nn.	Flex trunk & compress abdominal viscera
Quadratus lumborum	Medial half of inf. border of 12th rib & tips of lumbar transverse processes	Iliolumbar lig. & int. lip of iliac crest	Ventral rami of T12 & L1 to L4	Extend & laterally fixes the vertebral column; flex 12th rib during inspiration
Cremaster	Inf. edge of int. abdominal oblique, inguinal lig., pubic tubercle & pubic crest	Invest spermatic cord and testis	Genital br. of genitofemoral n. (L1 & L2)	Retract testis

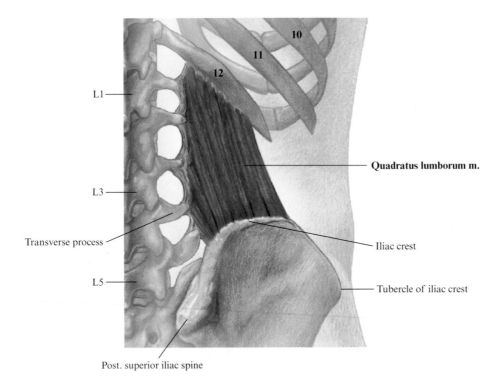

Posterior View

Body of sternum

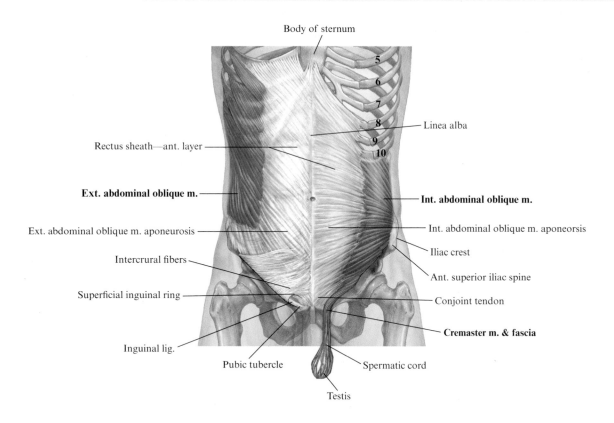

5
6
7
8 — Linea alba
9
10

Rectus sheath—ant. layer

Ext. abdominal oblique m.

Int. abdominal oblique m.

Ext. abdominal oblique m. aponeurosis

Int. abdominal oblique m. aponeorsis

Iliac crest

Intercrural fibers

Ant. superior iliac spine

Superficial inguinal ring

Conjoint tendon

Cremaster m. & fascia

Inguinal lig.

Pubic tubercle

Spermatic cord

Testis

Anterior Views

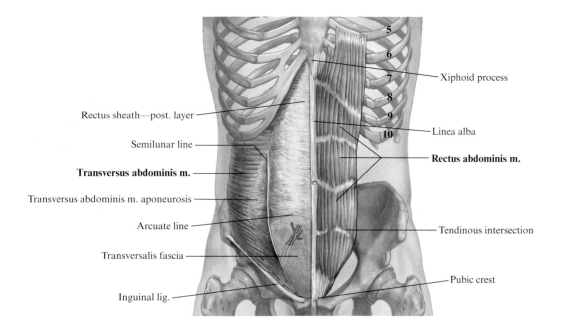

5
6
7 — Xiphoid process
8
9
10 — Linea alba

Rectus sheath—post. layer

Rectus abdominis m.

Semilunar line

Transversus abdominis m.

Transversus abdominis m. aponeurosis

Arcuate line

Tendinous intersection

Transversalis fascia

Inguinal lig.

Pubic crest

TABLE 1.3   INTRINSIC MUSCLES OF THE BACK

Intrinsic Muscles of the Back[a]

Muscle	Inferior or Medial Attachment	Superior or Lateral Attachment	Innervation	Action(s)
SUPERFICIAL LAYER—SPINOTRANSVERSE GROUP				
Splenius capitis	Inf. half of ligamentum nuchae, spinous processes of C7 to T3/T4	Mastoid process, lateral third of the sup. nuchal line	Dorsal primary rami of middle cervical spinal nn.	Unilaterally, rotate & laterally flex neck to same side, bilaterally, extend the neck & head
Splenius cervicis	Spinous processes of T3/T4 to T6	Post. tubercles of transverse processes of C1 to C3	Dorsal primary rami of lower cervical spinal nn.	
INTERMEDIATE LAYER—ERECTOR SPINAE GROUP				
Iliocostalis m. *I. cervicis* *I. thoracis* *I. lumborum*	Sacrum, medial part of iliac crest, 12th to 3rd ribs	Angles of all ribs, transverse processes of C7 to C4		Unilaterally, flex vertebral column to same side; bilaterally, extend vertebral column; important in maintaining erect posture while standing or walking
Longissimus m. *L. capitis* *L. cervicis* *L. thoracis*	Sacrum, transverse processes of all vertebrae from L5 to C7, transverse & articular processes of C6 to C4	Transverse processes of all vertebrae from T12 to C2, angles of all ribs, mastoid process	Dorsal primary rami of all cervical, thoracic & lumbar spinal nn.	
Spinalis m. *S. capitis* *S. cervicis* *S. thoracis*	Spinous processes of L2/L3 to T11, ligamentum nuchae & spinous processes of T2 to C7, transverse processes of C7/C6 to C2, articular processes of C6 to C4	Spinous processes from T9/T8 to C7/C6, spinous processes of C3/C4 & C2, occipital bone between sup. & inf. nuchal lines with semispinalis m.		
DEEP LAYER—TRANSVERSOSPINAL GROUP				
Semispinalis m. *S. capitis* *S. cervicis* *S. thoracis*	Transverse processes of all vertebrae from T10 to C3, articular processes of C6 to C4	Spinous processes from T4 to C2, occipital bone between sup. & inf. nuchal lines; usually includes spinalis capitis m.	Dorsal primary rami of T6 T1, all cervical spinal nn.	Unilaterally, lateral flex and/or rotate vertebral column & head to opposite side; bilaterally, extend vertebral column & head
Multifidus	All lamina from S4 to C2 transverse processes L5 to T1, articular processes C7 to C3	Spinous process of all vertebrae; spans 1 to 3 vertebrae	Dorsal primary rami of T6 to C1 spinal nn.	Unilaterally, lateral flex and/or rotate vertebral column to opposite side; bilaterally, extend or stabilize vertebral column
Rotatores	Transverse processes of all vertebrae L5 to T2	Lamina & roots of spinous process of next vertebra superiorly; best developed in thoracic region	Dorsal primary rami of L4 to T1 spinal nn.	

[a]The most superficial layer also includes the trapezius, latissimus dorsi, levator scapulae & rhomboid muscles which move the upper limb. The intermediate layer is formed by the serratus posterior muscles. The muscles of both of these layers are considered extrinsic to the back. The intrinsic muscles of the back form the deepest three muscle layers of the back.

A.D.A.M. | Student Atlas of Anatomy

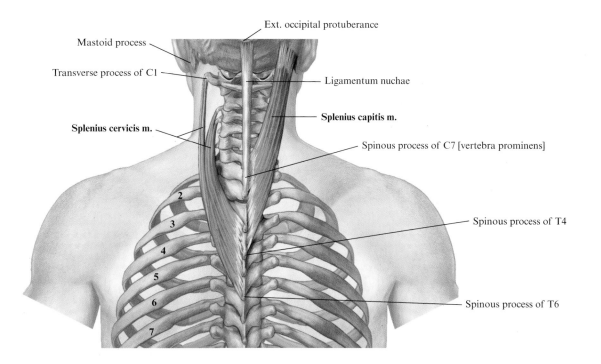

Ext. occipital protuberance

Mastoid process

Transverse process of C1

Ligamentum nuchae

Splenius cervicis m.

Splenius capitis m.

Spinous process of C7 [vertebra prominens]

2

3

Spinous process of T4

4

5

6

Spinous process of T6

7

Posterior Views

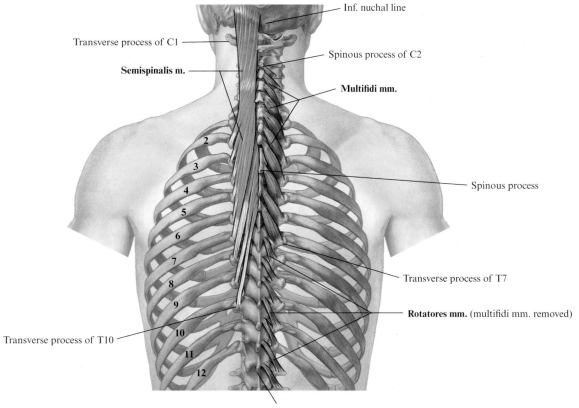

Inf. nuchal line

Transverse process of C1

Spinous process of C2

Semispinalis m.

Multifidi mm.

2

3

Spinous process

4

5

6

7

Transverse process of T7

8

9

Rotatores mm. (multifidi mm. removed)

10

Transverse process of T10

11

12

Spinous process of T12

PLATE 1.22   MUSCLES—ERECTOR SPINAE

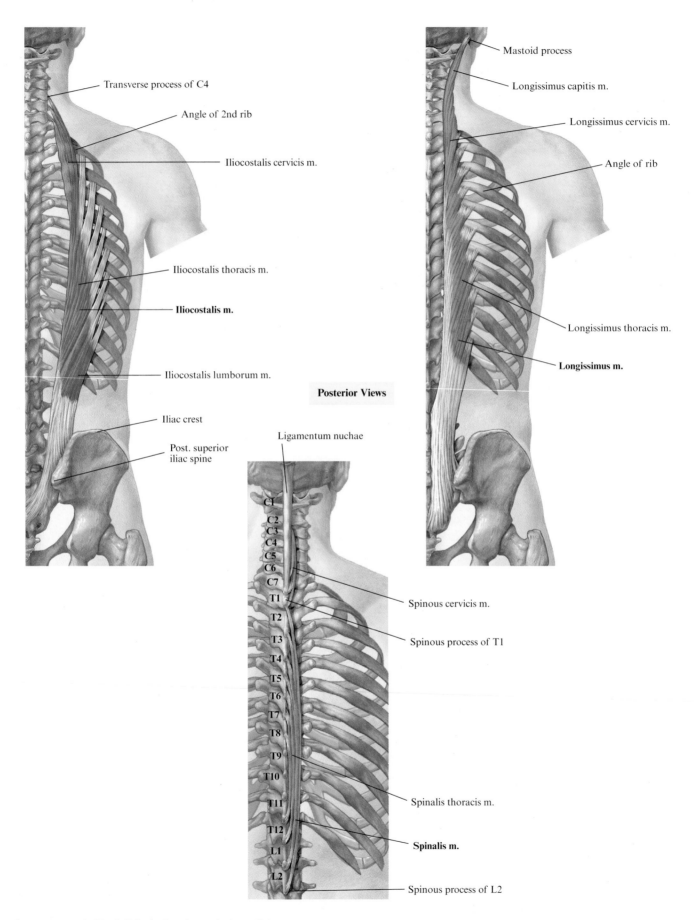

Transverse process of C4

Angle of 2nd rib

Iliocostalis cervicis m.

Iliocostalis thoracis m.

Iliocostalis m.

Iliocostalis lumborum m.

Iliac crest

Post. superior
iliac spine

Mastoid process

Longissimus capitis m.

Longissimus cervicis m.

Angle of rib

Longissimus thoracis m.

Longissimus m.

Posterior Views

Ligamentum nuchae

C1
C2
C3
C4
C5
C6
C7
T1
T2
T3
T4
T5
T6
T7
T8
T9
T10
T11
T12
L1
L2

Spinous cervicis m.

Spinous process of T1

Spinalis thoracis m.

Spinalis m.

Spinous process of L2

Muscle	Inferior or Medial Attachment	Superior or Lateral Attachment	Innervation	Action(s)
DEEP LAYER—SUBOCCIPITAL GROUP				
Rectus capitis posterior major	Spinous process of C2	Lateral part of inf. nuchal line	Dorsal primary ramus of C1 [suboccipital] n.	Unilaterally, rotate head to same side; bilaterally, extend head at atlanto-occipital joint
Rectus capitis posterior minor	Post. tubercle of C1	Medial part of inf. nuchal line		
Obliquus capitis superior	Transverse process of C1	Sup. to inf. nuchal line		Unilaterally, rotate C1 & head to same side around odontoid process; bilaterally, extend head at atlanto-axial joint
Obliquus capitis inferior	Spinous process of C2	Transverse process of C1		

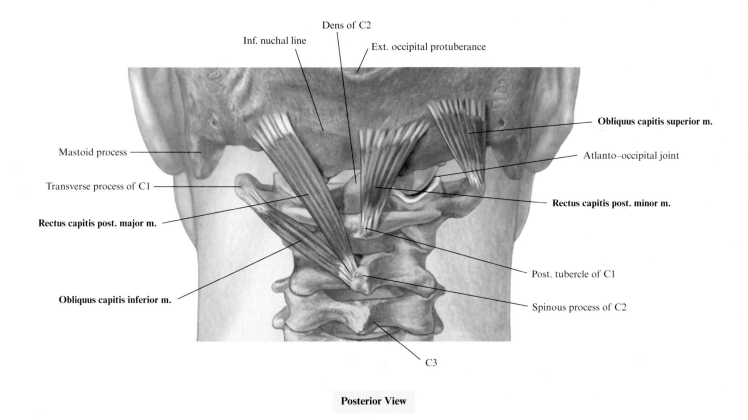

Posterior View

PLATE 1.23   VASCULATURE—ARTERIES

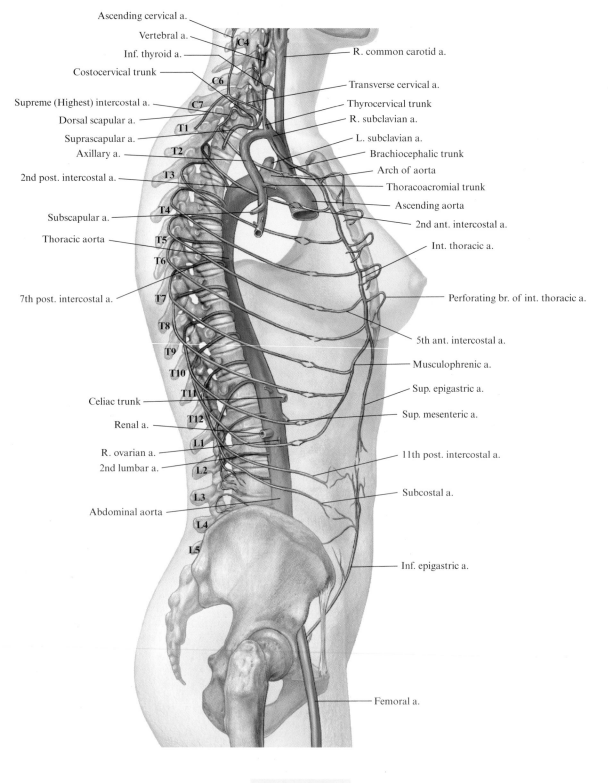

Ascending cervical a.
Vertebral a.
Inf. thyroid a.
Costocervical trunk
Supreme (Highest) intercostal a.
Dorsal scapular a.
Suprascapular a.
Axillary a.
2nd post. intercostal a.
Subscapular a.
Thoracic aorta
7th post. intercostal a.

C4
C6
C7
T1
T2
T3
T4
T5
T6
T7
T8
T9
T10
T11
T12
L1
L2
L3
L4
L5

R. common carotid a.
Transverse cervical a.
Thyrocervical trunk
R. subclavian a.
L. subclavian a.
Brachiocephalic trunk
Arch of aorta
Thoracoacromial trunk
Ascending aorta
2nd ant. intercostal a.
Int. thoracic a.
Perforating br. of int. thoracic a.
5th ant. intercostal a.
Musculophrenic a.
Sup. epigastric a.
Sup. mesenteric a.
11th post. intercostal a.
Subcostal a.
Inf. epigastric a.
Femoral a.

Celiac trunk
Renal a.
R. ovarian a.
2nd lumbar a.
Abdominal aorta

Right Lateral View

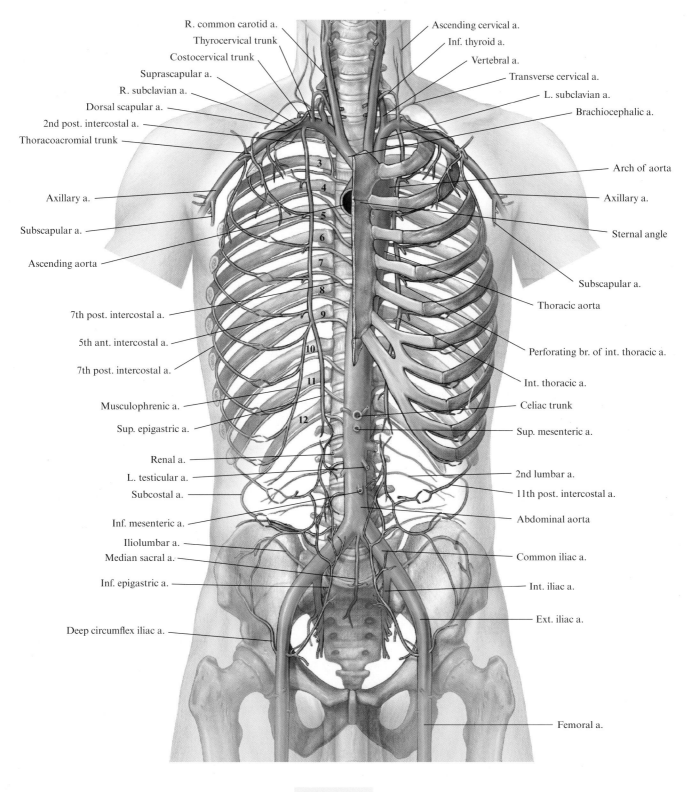

R. common carotid a.

Thyrocervical trunk

Costocervical trunk

Suprascapular a.

R. subclavian a.

Dorsal scapular a.

2nd post. intercostal a.

Thoracoacromial trunk

Axillary a.

Subscapular a.

Ascending aorta

7th post. intercostal a.

5th ant. intercostal a.

7th post. intercostal a.

Musculophrenic a.

Sup. epigastric a.

Renal a.

L. testicular a.

Subcostal a.

Inf. mesenteric a.

Iliolumbar a.

Median sacral a.

Inf. epigastric a.

Deep circumflex iliac a.

Ascending cervical a.

Inf. thyroid a.

Vertebral a.

Transverse cervical a.

L. subclavian a.

Brachiocephalic a.

Arch of aorta

Axillary a.

Sternal angle

Subscapular a.

Thoracic aorta

Perforating br. of int. thoracic a.

Int. thoracic a.

Celiac trunk

Sup. mesenteric a.

2nd lumbar a.

11th post. intercostal a.

Abdominal aorta

Common iliac a.

Int. iliac a.

Ext. iliac a.

Femoral a.

Anterior View

PLATE 1.25 **VASCULATURE—VEINS**

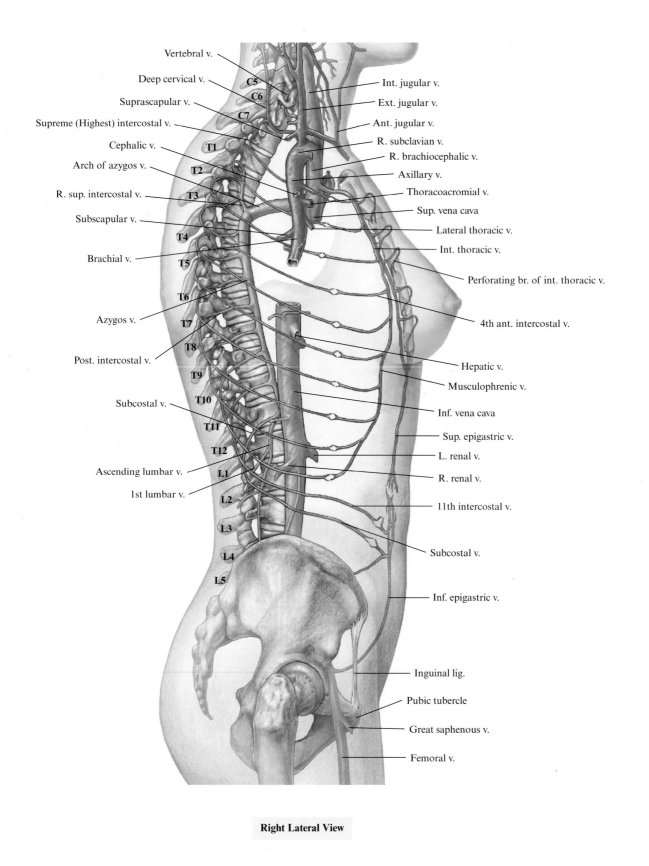

Vertebral v.

Deep cervical v.

C5

C6

Suprascapular v.

C7

Supreme (Highest) intercostal v.

Cephalic v.

T1

Arch of azygos v.

T2

R. sup. intercostal v.

T3

Subscapular v.

T4

Brachial v.

T5

T6

Azygos v.

T7

T8

Post. intercostal v.

T9

Subcostal v.

T10

T11

T12

Ascending lumbar v.

L1

1st lumbar v.

L2

L3

L4

L5

Int. jugular v.

Ext. jugular v.

Ant. jugular v.

R. subclavian v.

R. brachiocephalic v.

Axillary v.

Thoracoacromial v.

Sup. vena cava

Lateral thoracic v.

Int. thoracic v.

Perforating br. of int. thoracic v.

4th ant. intercostal v.

Hepatic v.

Musculophrenic v.

Inf. vena cava

Sup. epigastric v.

L. renal v.

R. renal v.

11th intercostal v.

Subcostal v.

Inf. epigastric v.

Inguinal lig.

Pubic tubercle

Great saphenous v.

Femoral v.

Right Lateral View

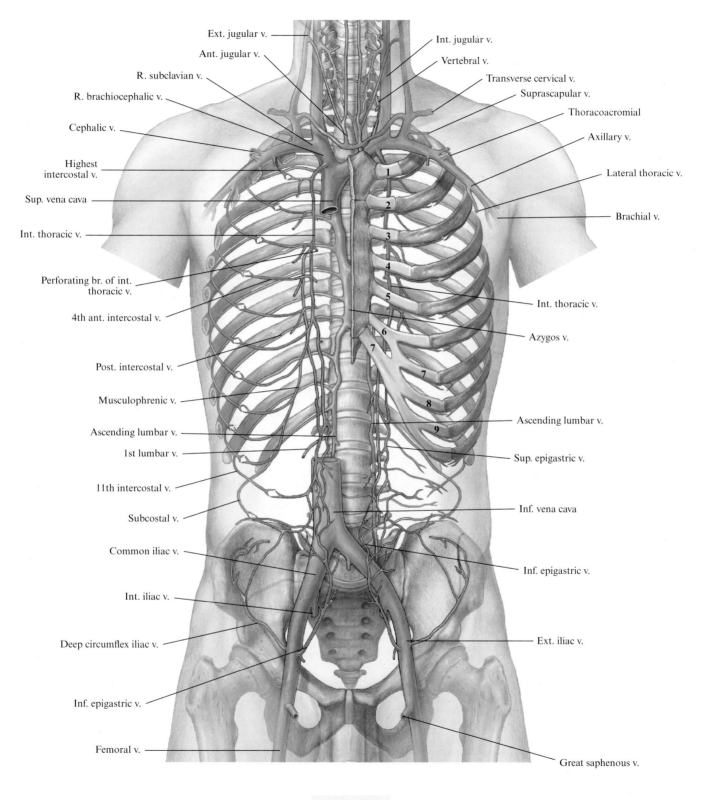

Ext. jugular v.

Ant. jugular v.

R. subclavian v.

R. brachiocephalic v.

Cephalic v.

Highest intercostal v.

Sup. vena cava

Int. thoracic v.

Perforating br. of int. thoracic v.

4th ant. intercostal v.

Post. intercostal v.

Musculophrenic v.

Ascending lumbar v.

1st lumbar v.

11th intercostal v.

Subcostal v.

Common iliac v.

Int. iliac v.

Deep circumflex iliac v.

Inf. epigastric v.

Femoral v.

Int. jugular v.

Vertebral v.

Transverse cervical v.

Suprascapular v.

Thoracoacromial

Axillary v.

Lateral thoracic v.

Brachial v.

Int. thoracic v.

Azygos v.

Ascending lumbar v.

Sup. epigastric v.

Inf. vena cava

Inf. epigastric v.

Ext. iliac v.

Great saphenous v.

1
2
3
4
5
6
7
7
8
9

Anterior View

PLATE 1.27   AZYGOS, HEMIAZYGOS & LUMBAR VEINS

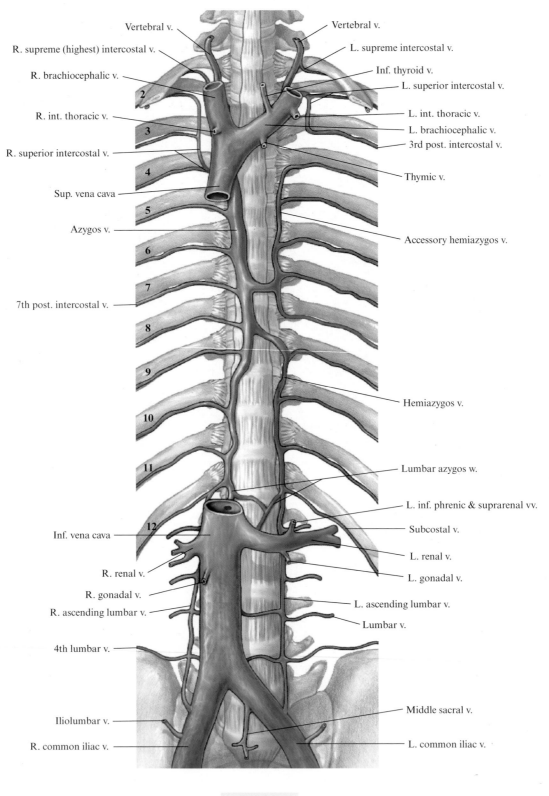

Vertebral v.

R. supreme (highest) intercostal v.

R. brachiocephalic v.

R. int. thoracic v.

R. superior intercostal v.

Sup. vena cava

Azygos v.

7th post. intercostal v.

Inf. vena cava

R. renal v.

R. gonadal v.

R. ascending lumbar v.

4th lumbar v.

Iliolumbar v.

R. common iliac v.

Vertebral v.

L. supreme intercostal v.

Inf. thyroid v.

L. superior intercostal v.

L. int. thoracic v.

L. brachiocephalic v.

3rd post. intercostal v.

Thymic v.

Accessory hemiazygos v.

Hemiazygos v.

Lumbar azygos vv.

L. inf. phrenic & suprarenal vv.

Subcostal v.

L. renal v.

L. gonadal v.

L. ascending lumbar v.

Lumbar v.

Middle sacral v.

L. common iliac v.

2
3
4
5
6
7
8
9
10
11
12

Anterior View

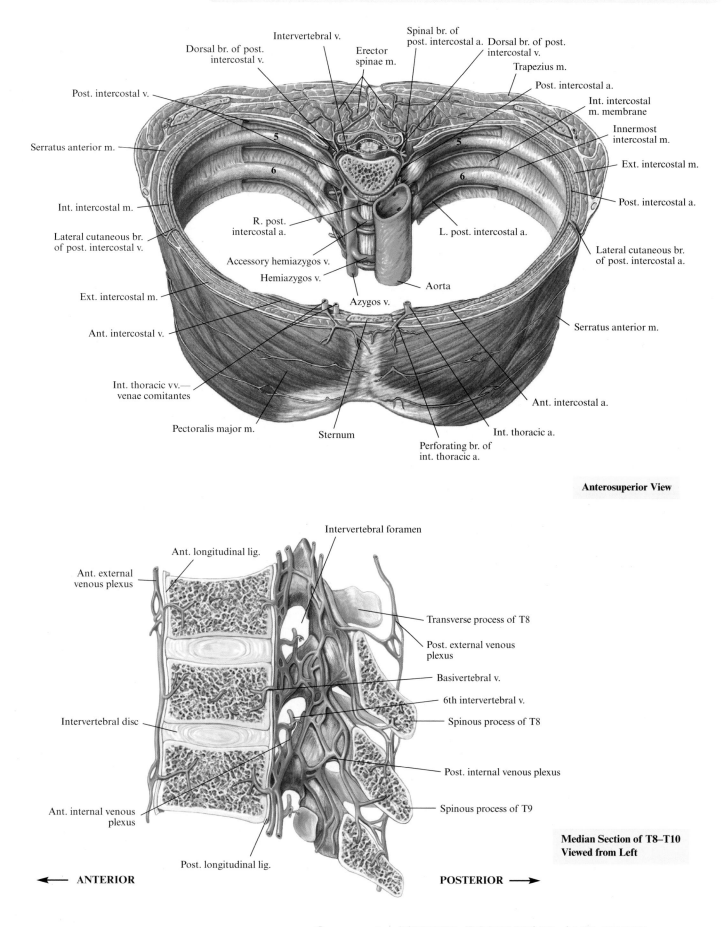

Intervertebral v.

Dorsal br. of post.
intercostal v.

Spinal br. of
post. intercostal a. Dorsal br. of post.
intercostal v.

Erector
spinae m.

Trapezius m.

Post. intercostal v.

Post. intercostal a.

Int. intercostal
m. membrane

Innermost
intercostal m.

Serratus anterior m.

5

5

6

6

Ext. intercostal m.

Int. intercostal m.

Post. intercostal a.

Lateral cutaneous br.
of post. intercostal v.

R. post.
intercostal a.

L. post. intercostal a.

Lateral cutaneous br.
of post. intercostal a.

Accessory hemiazygos v.

Hemiazygos v.

Ext. intercostal m.

Aorta

Azygos v.

Ant. intercostal v.

Serratus anterior m.

Int. thoracic vv.—
venae comitantes

Ant. intercostal a.

Pectoralis major m.

Sternum

Int. thoracic a.

Perforating br. of
int. thoracic a.

Anterosuperior View

Intervertebral foramen

Ant. longitudinal lig.

Ant. external
venous plexus

Transverse process of T8

Post. external venous
plexus

Basivertebral v.

6th intervertebral v.

Intervertebral disc

Spinous process of T8

Post. internal venous plexus

Ant. internal venous
plexus

Spinous process of T9

Post. longitudinal lig.

**Median Section of T8–T10
Viewed from Left**

← **ANTERIOR**

POSTERIOR →

PLATE 1.29   SPINAL CORD VASCULATURE

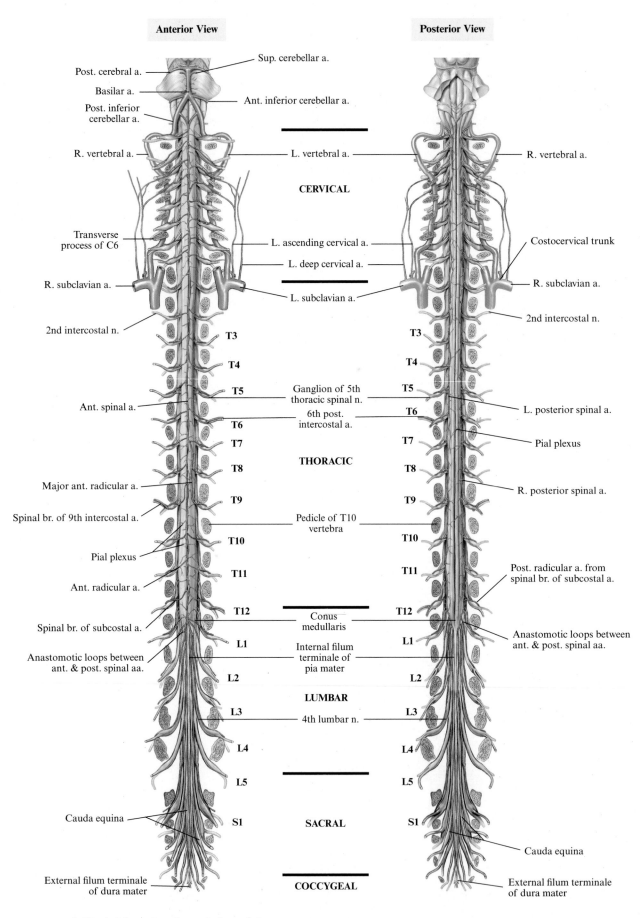

Anterior View

Posterior View

Sup. cerebellar a.

Post. cerebral a.

Basilar a.

Ant. inferior cerebellar a.

Post. inferior
cerebellar a.

R. vertebral a.

L. vertebral a.

R. vertebral a.

CERVICAL

Transverse
process of C6

L. ascending cervical a.

Costocervical trunk

L. deep cervical a.

R. subclavian a.

R. subclavian a.

L. subclavian a.

2nd intercostal n.

2nd intercostal n.

T3

T3

T4

T4

T5

T5

Ganglion of 5th
thoracic spinal n.

Ant. spinal a.

L. posterior spinal a.

6th post.
intercostal a.

T6

T6

T7

T7

Pial plexus

THORACIC

T8

T8

Major ant. radicular a.

R. posterior spinal a.

T9

T9

Spinal br. of 9th intercostal a.

Pedicle of T10
vertebra

T10

T10

Pial plexus

T11

T11

Post. radicular a. from
spinal br. of subcostal a.

Ant. radicular a.

T12

Conus
medullaris

T12

Spinal br. of subcostal a.

Anastomotic loops between
ant. & post. spinal aa.

L1

Internal filum
terminale of
pia mater

L1

Anastomotic loops between
ant. & post. spinal aa.

L2

L2

LUMBAR

L3

4th lumbar n.

L3

L4

L4

L5

L5

Cauda equina

S1

SACRAL

S1

Cauda equina

External filum terminale
of dura mater

COCCYGEAL

External filum terminale
of dura mater

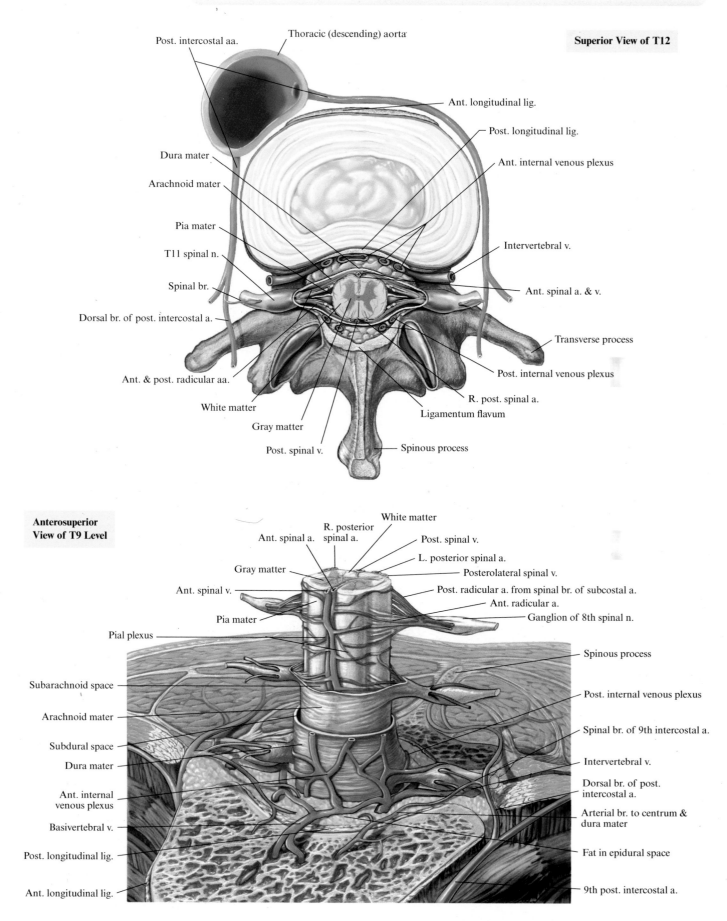

Post. intercostal aa.

Thoracic (descending) aorta

Superior View of T12

Ant. longitudinal lig.

Post. longitudinal lig.

Ant. internal venous plexus

Dura mater

Arachnoid mater

Pia mater

T11 spinal n.

Intervertebral v.

Spinal br.

Ant. spinal a. & v.

Dorsal br. of post. intercostal a.

Transverse process

Ant. & post. radicular aa.

Post. internal venous plexus

White matter

R. post. spinal a.

Gray matter

Ligamentum flavum

Post. spinal v.

Spinous process

Anterosuperior
View of T9 Level

White matter

R. posterior
spinal a.

Ant. spinal a.

Post. spinal v.

L. posterior spinal a.

Gray matter

Posterolateral spinal v.

Ant. spinal v.

Post. radicular a. from spinal br. of subcostal a.

Pia mater

Ant. radicular a.

Ganglion of 8th spinal n.

Pial plexus

Spinous process

Subarachnoid space

Post. internal venous plexus

Arachnoid mater

Spinal br. of 9th intercostal a.

Subdural space

Intervertebral v.

Dura mater

Dorsal br. of post.
intercostal a.

Ant. internal
venous plexus

Arterial br. to centrum &
dura mater

Basivertebral v.

Fat in epidural space

Post. longitudinal lig.

Ant. longitudinal lig.

9th post. intercostal a.

PLATE 1.31   DERMATOMES & CUTANEOUS INNERVATION

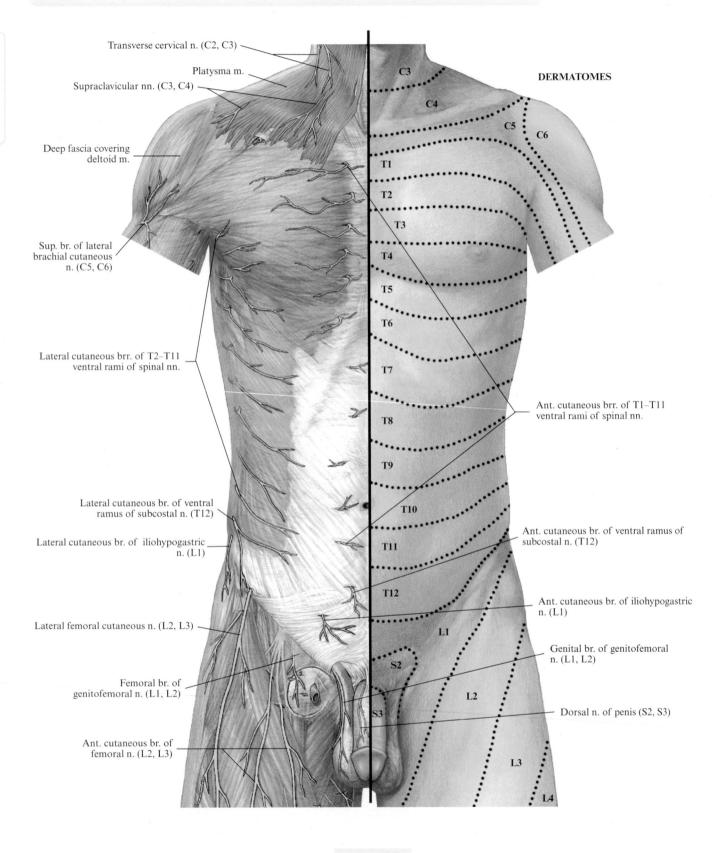

Transverse cervical n. (C2, C3)

Platysma m.

Supraclavicular nn. (C3, C4)

Deep fascia covering deltoid m.

Sup. br. of lateral brachial cutaneous n. (C5, C6)

Lateral cutaneous brr. of T2–T11 ventral rami of spinal nn.

Lateral cutaneous br. of ventral ramus of subcostal n. (T12)

Lateral cutaneous br. of iliohypogastric n. (L1)

Lateral femoral cutaneous n. (L2, L3)

Femoral br. of genitofemoral n. (L1, L2)

Ant. cutaneous br. of femoral n. (L2, L3)

DERMATOMES

C3
C4
C5
C6
T1
T2
T3
T4
T5
T6
T7
T8
T9
T10
T11
T12
L1
S2
L2
S3
L3
L4

Ant. cutaneous brr. of T1–T11 ventral rami of spinal nn.

Ant. cutaneous br. of ventral ramus of subcostal n. (T12)

Ant. cutaneous br. of iliohypogastric n. (L1)

Genital br. of genitofemoral n. (L1, L2)

Dorsal n. of penis (S2, S3)

Anterior View

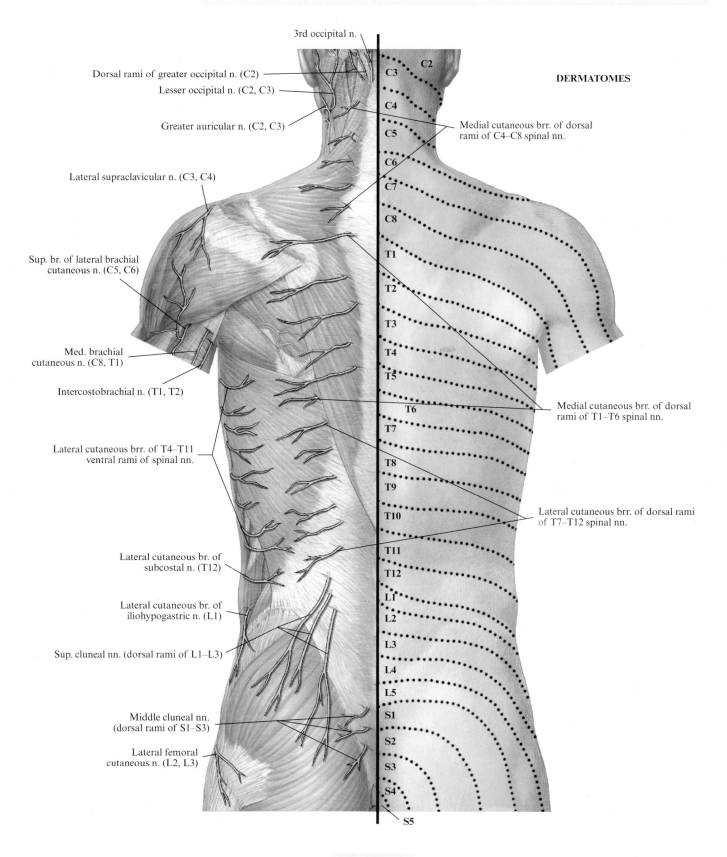

3rd occipital n.

Dorsal rami of greater occipital n. (C2)

Lesser occipital n. (C2, C3)

Greater auricular n. (C2, C3)

Lateral supraclavicular n. (C3, C4)

Sup. br. of lateral brachial cutaneous n. (C5, C6)

Med. brachial cutaneous n. (C8, T1)

Intercostobrachial n. (T1, T2)

Lateral cutaneous brr. of T4–T11 ventral rami of spinal nn.

Lateral cutaneous br. of subcostal n. (T12)

Lateral cutaneous br. of iliohypogastric n. (L1)

Sup. cluneal nn. (dorsal rami of L1–L3)

Middle cluneal nn. (dorsal rami of S1–S3)

Lateral femoral cutaneous n. (L2, L3)

DERMATOMES

Medial cutaneous brr. of dorsal rami of C4–C8 spinal nn.

Medial cutaneous brr. of dorsal rami of T1–T6 spinal nn.

Lateral cutaneous brr. of dorsal rami of T7–T12 spinal nn.

C2
C3
C4
C5
C6
C7
C8
T1
T2
T3
T4
T5
T6
T7
T8
T9
T10
T11
T12
L1
L2
L3
L4
L5
S1
S2
S3
S4
S5

Posterior View

PLATE 1.33   NERVES

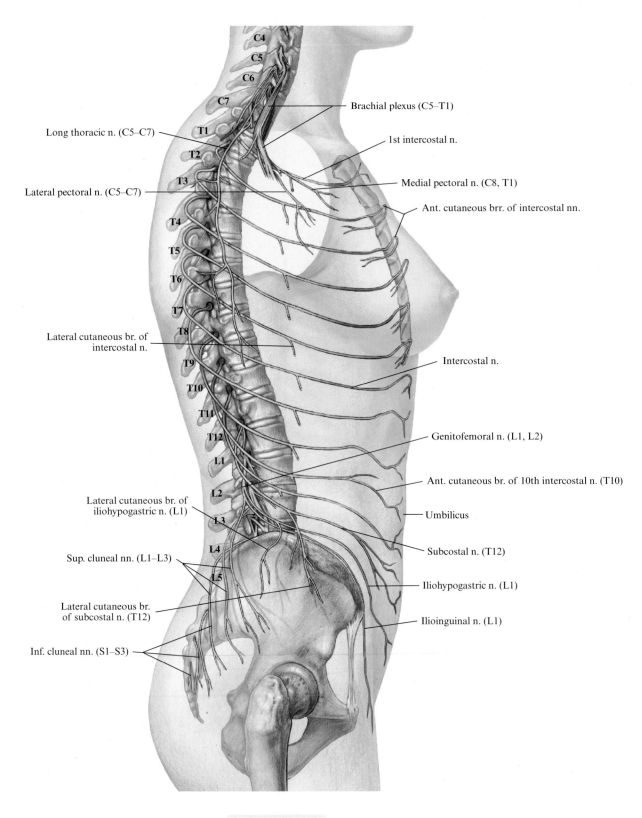

Brachial plexus (C5–T1)

Long thoracic n. (C5–C7)

1st intercostal n.

Medial pectoral n. (C8, T1)

Lateral pectoral n. (C5–C7)

Ant. cutaneous brr. of intercostal nn.

Lateral cutaneous br. of intercostal n.

Intercostal n.

Genitofemoral n. (L1, L2)

Ant. cutaneous br. of 10th intercostal n. (T10)

Lateral cutaneous br. of iliohypogastric n. (L1)

Umbilicus

Subcostal n. (T12)

Sup. cluneal nn. (L1–L3)

Iliohypogastric n. (L1)

Lateral cutaneous br. of subcostal n. (T12)

Ilioinguinal n. (L1)

Inf. cluneal nn. (S1–S3)

C4
C5
C6
C7
T1
T2
T3
T4
T5
T6
T7
T8
T9
T10
T11
T12
L1
L2
L3
L4
L5

Right Lateral View

A.D.A.M. Student Atlas of Anatomy

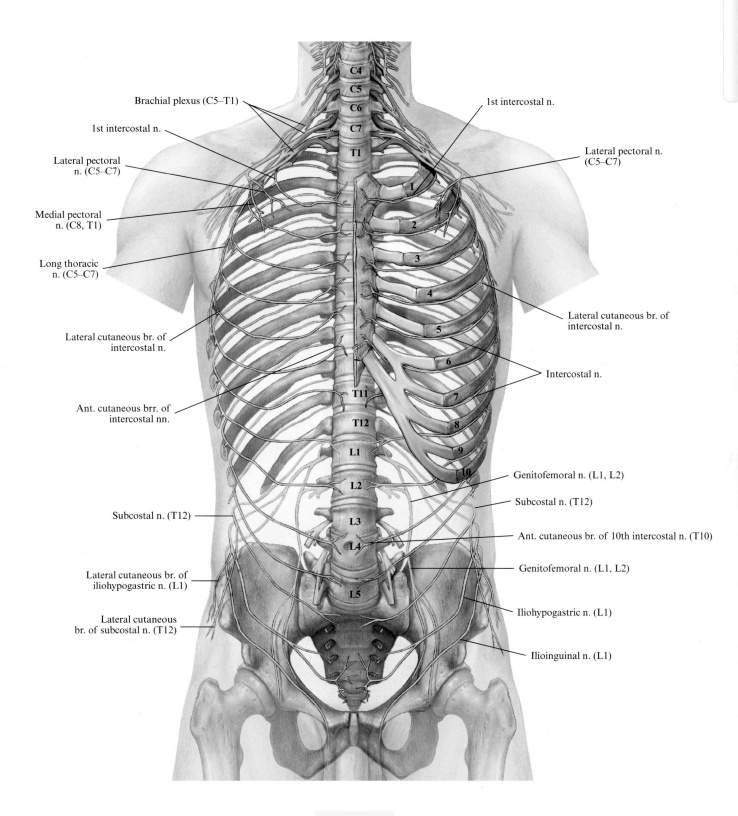

Brachial plexus (C5–T1)

1st intercostal n.

Lateral pectoral n. (C5–C7)

Medial pectoral n. (C8, T1)

Long thoracic n. (C5–C7)

Lateral cutaneous br. of intercostal n.

Ant. cutaneous brr. of intercostal nn.

Subcostal n. (T12)

Lateral cutaneous br. of iliohypogastric n. (L1)

Lateral cutaneous br. of subcostal n. (T12)

1st intercostal n.

Lateral pectoral n. (C5–C7)

Lateral cutaneous br. of intercostal n.

Intercostal n.

Genitofemoral n. (L1, L2)

Subcostal n. (T12)

Ant. cutaneous br. of 10th intercostal n. (T10)

Genitofemoral n. (L1, L2)

Iliohypogastric n. (L1)

Ilioinguinal n. (L1)

C4
C5
C6
C7
T1

T11
T12
L1
L2
L3
L4
L5

Anterior View

PLATE 1.35   **INTERCOSTAL NERVES**

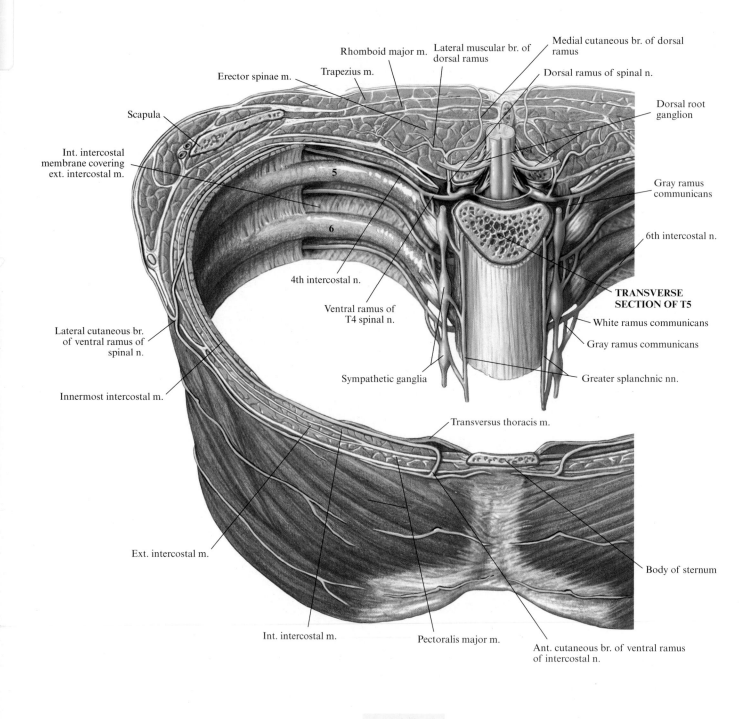

Rhomboid major m.

Erector spinae m.

Trapezius m.

Lateral muscular br. of dorsal ramus

Medial cutaneous br. of dorsal ramus

Dorsal ramus of spinal n.

Scapula

Dorsal root ganglion

Int. intercostal membrane covering ext. intercostal m.

Gray ramus communicans

5

6

6th intercostal n.

4th intercostal n.

Ventral ramus of T4 spinal n.

TRANSVERSE SECTION OF T5

White ramus communicans

Gray ramus communicans

Lateral cutaneous br. of ventral ramus of spinal n.

Sympathetic ganglia

Greater splanchnic nn.

Innermost intercostal m.

Transversus thoracis m.

Body of sternum

Ext. intercostal m.

Int. intercostal m.

Pectoralis major m.

Ant. cutaneous br. of ventral ramus of intercostal n.

Anterosuperior

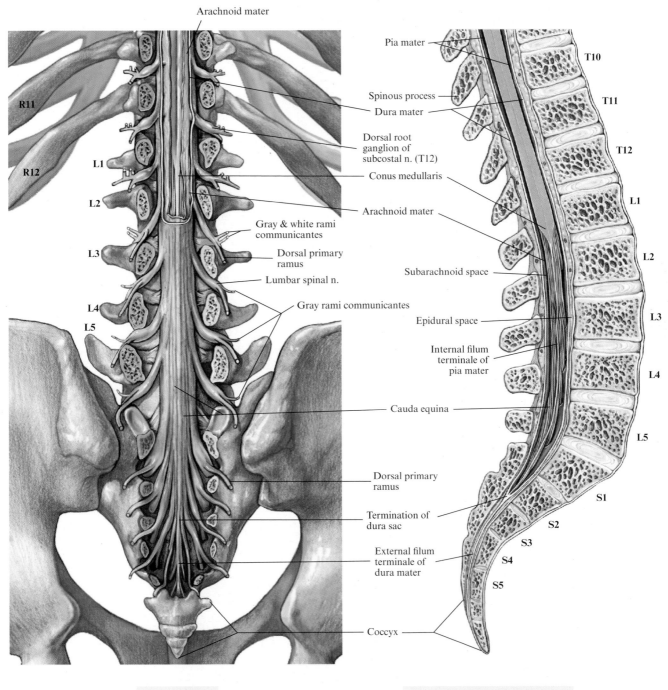

Arachnoid mater

R11

R12

L1

L2

L3

L4

L5

Gray & white rami
communicantes

Dorsal primary
ramus

Lumbar spinal n.

Gray rami communicantes

Dorsal primary
ramus

Termination of
dura sac

External filum
terminale of
dura mater

Coccyx

Pia mater

Spinous process

Dura mater

Dorsal root
ganglion of
subcostal n. (T12)

Conus medullaris

Arachnoid mater

Subarachnoid space

Epidural space

Internal filum
terminale of
pia mater

Cauda equina

T10

T11

T12

L1

L2

L3

L4

L5

S1

S2

S3

S4

S5

Posterior View

Median Section Viewed from Right

PLATE 1.37   ANTERIOR BODY WALL—SUPERFICIAL

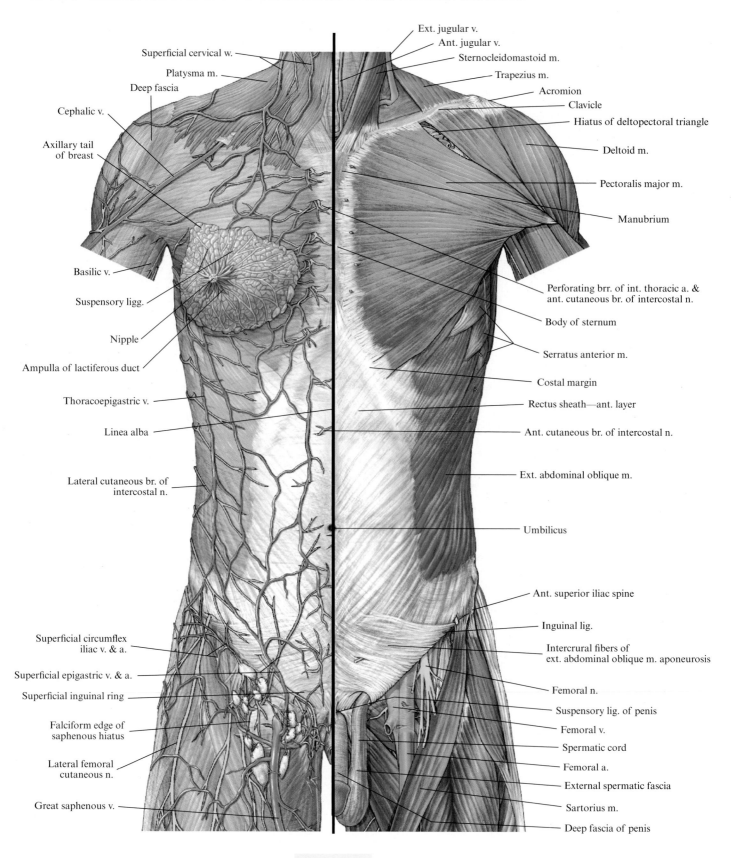

Ext. jugular v.

Ant. jugular v.

Superficial cervical w.

Sternocleidomastoid m.

Platysma m.

Trapezius m.

Deep fascia

Acromion

Cephalic v.

Clavicle

Hiatus of deltopectoral triangle

Axillary tail
of breast

Deltoid m.

Pectoralis major m.

Manubrium

Basilic v.

Perforating brr. of int. thoracic a. &
ant. cutaneous br. of intercostal n.

Suspensory ligg.

Body of sternum

Nipple

Serratus anterior m.

Ampulla of lactiferous duct

Costal margin

Thoracoepigastric v.

Rectus sheath—ant. layer

Linea alba

Ant. cutaneous br. of intercostal n.

Ext. abdominal oblique m.

Lateral cutaneous br. of
intercostal n.

Umbilicus

Ant. superior iliac spine

Inguinal lig.

Superficial circumflex
iliac v. & a.

Intercrural fibers of
ext. abdominal oblique m. aponeurosis

Superficial epigastric v. & a.

Femoral n.

Superficial inguinal ring

Suspensory lig. of penis

Falciform edge of
saphenous hiatus

Femoral v.

Spermatic cord

Lateral femoral
cutaneous n.

Femoral a.

External spermatic fascia

Great saphenous v.

Sartorius m.

Deep fascia of penis

Anterior View

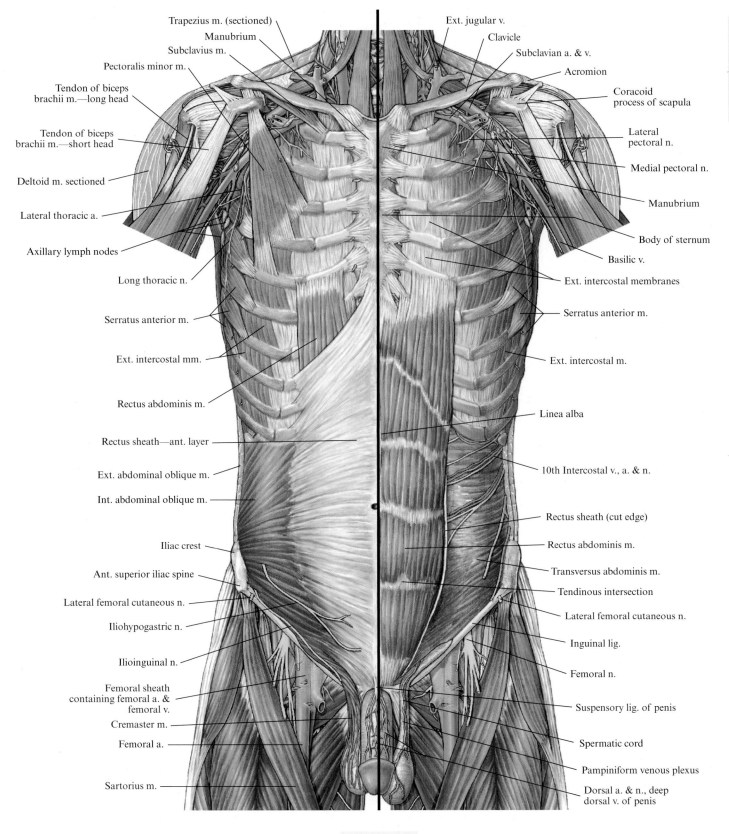

Trapezius m. (sectioned)
Manubrium
Subclavius m.
Pectoralis minor m.
Tendon of biceps brachii m.—long head
Tendon of biceps brachii m.—short head
Deltoid m. sectioned
Lateral thoracic a.
Axillary lymph nodes
Long thoracic n.
Serratus anterior m.
Ext. intercostal mm.
Rectus abdominis m.
Rectus sheath—ant. layer
Ext. abdominal oblique m.
Int. abdominal oblique m.
Iliac crest
Ant. superior iliac spine
Lateral femoral cutaneous n.
Iliohypogastric n.
Ilioinguinal n.
Femoral sheath containing femoral a. & femoral v.
Cremaster m.
Femoral a.
Sartorius m.

Ext. jugular v.
Clavicle
Subclavian a. & v.
Acromion
Coracoid process of scapula
Lateral pectoral n.
Medial pectoral n.
Manubrium
Body of sternum
Basilic v.
Ext. intercostal membranes
Serratus anterior m.
Ext. intercostal m.
Linea alba
10th Intercostal v., a. & n.
Rectus sheath (cut edge)
Rectus abdominis m.
Transversus abdominis m.
Tendinous intersection
Lateral femoral cutaneous n.
Inguinal lig.
Femoral n.
Suspensory lig. of penis
Spermatic cord
Pampiniform venous plexus
Dorsal a. & n., deep dorsal v. of penis

Anterior View

PLATE 1.39   ANTERIOR BODY WALL—DEEP

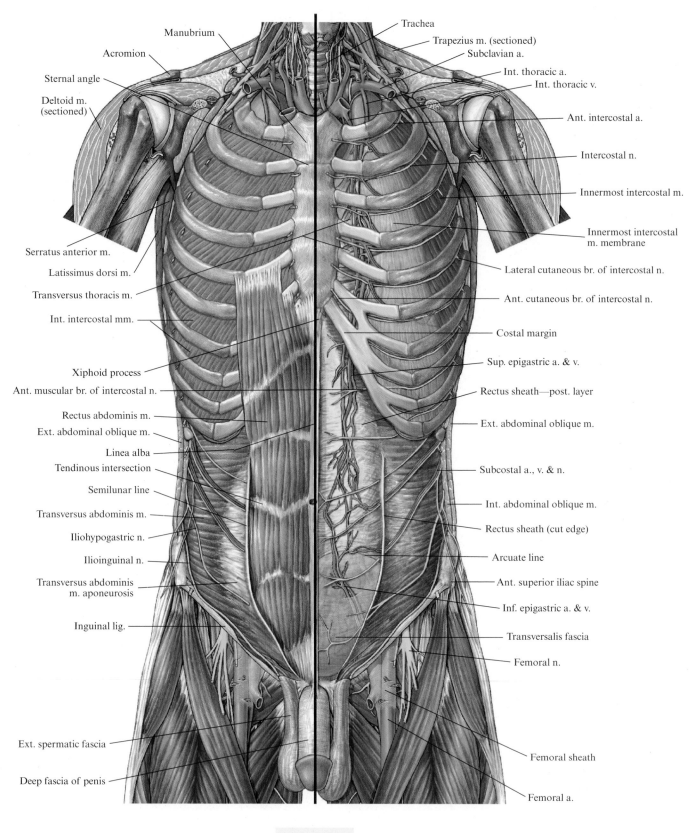

Manubrium

Acromion

Sternal angle

Deltoid m. (sectioned)

Serratus anterior m.

Latissimus dorsi m.

Transversus thoracis m.

Int. intercostal mm.

Xiphoid process

Ant. muscular br. of intercostal n.

Rectus abdominis m.

Ext. abdominal oblique m.

Linea alba

Tendinous intersection

Semilunar line

Transversus abdominis m.

Iliohypogastric n.

Ilioinguinal n.

Transversus abdominis m. aponeurosis

Inguinal lig.

Ext. spermatic fascia

Deep fascia of penis

Trachea

Trapezius m. (sectioned)

Subclavian a.

Int. thoracic a.

Int. thoracic v.

Ant. intercostal a.

Intercostal n.

Innermost intercostal m.

Innermost intercostal m. membrane

Lateral cutaneous br. of intercostal n.

Ant. cutaneous br. of intercostal n.

Costal margin

Sup. epigastric a. & v.

Rectus sheath—post. layer

Ext. abdominal oblique m.

Subcostal a., v. & n.

Int. abdominal oblique m.

Rectus sheath (cut edge)

Arcuate line

Ant. superior iliac spine

Inf. epigastric a. & v.

Transversalis fascia

Femoral n.

Femoral sheath

Femoral a.

Anterior View

A.D.A.M. | Student Atlas of Anatomy

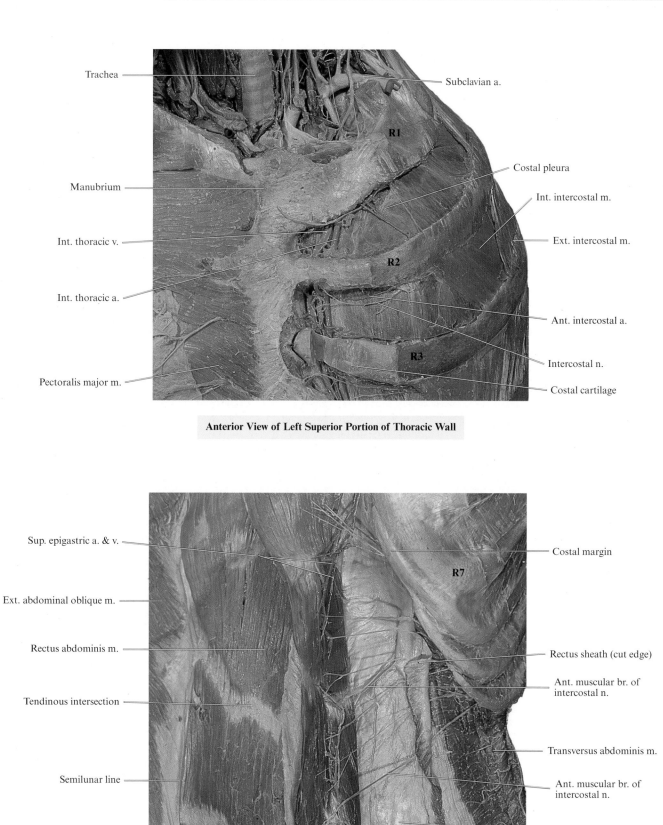

Trachea

Subclavian a.

R1

Costal pleura

Manubrium

Int. intercostal m.

Int. thoracic v.

Ext. intercostal m.

R2

Int. thoracic a.

Ant. intercostal a.

R3

Intercostal n.

Pectoralis major m.

Costal cartilage

Anterior View of Left Superior Portion of Thoracic Wall

Sup. epigastric a. & v.

Costal margin

R7

Ext. abdominal oblique m.

Rectus abdominis m.

Rectus sheath (cut edge)

Ant. muscular br. of
intercostal n.

Tendinous intersection

Transversus abdominis m.

Semilunar line

Ant. muscular br. of
intercostal n.

L. rectus abdominis m.
(reflected medially)

Rectus sheath—post. layer

Anterior View of Subcostal Portion of Abdominal Wall

PLATE 1.41   ANTERIOR BODY WALL—MAMMARY GLAND

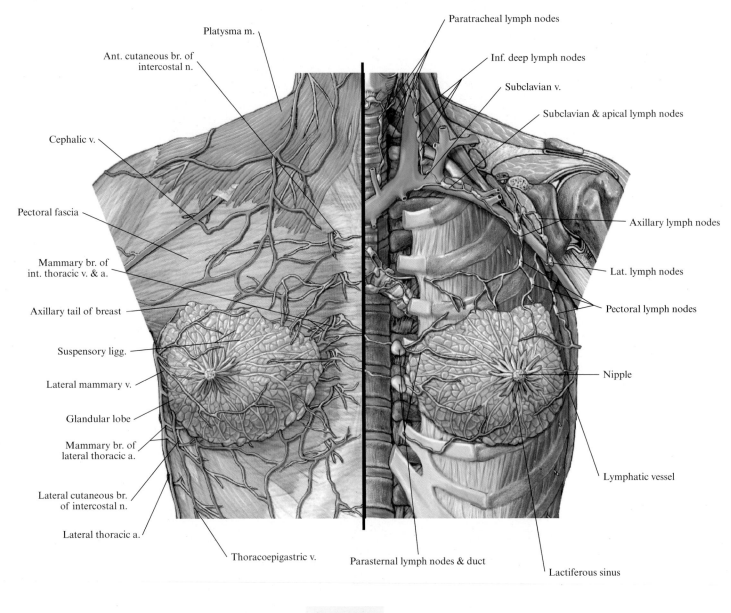

Platysma m.

Ant. cutaneous br. of
intercostal n.

Cephalic v.

Pectoral fascia

Mammary br. of
int. thoracic v. & a.

Axillary tail of breast

Suspensory ligg.

Lateral mammary v.

Glandular lobe

Mammary br. of
lateral thoracic a.

Lateral cutaneous br.
of intercostal n.

Lateral thoracic a.

Thoracoepigastric v.

Parasternal lymph nodes & duct

Paratracheal lymph nodes

Inf. deep lymph nodes

Subclavian v.

Subclavian & apical lymph nodes

Axillary lymph nodes

Lat. lymph nodes

Pectoral lymph nodes

Nipple

Lymphatic vessel

Lactiferous sinus

Anterior View

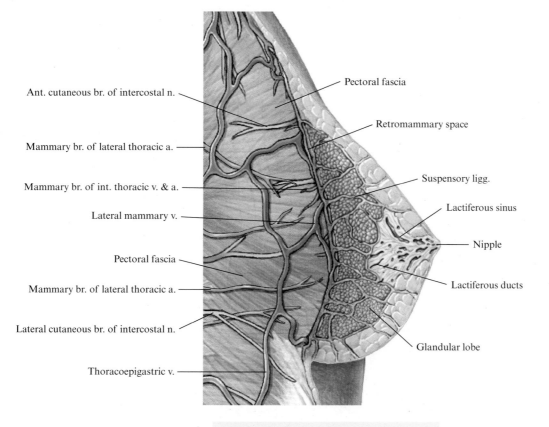

Ant. cutaneous br. of intercostal n.

Mammary br. of lateral thoracic a.

Mammary br. of int. thoracic v. & a.

Lateral mammary v.

Pectoral fascia

Mammary br. of lateral thoracic a.

Lateral cutaneous br. of intercostal n.

Thoracoepigastric v.

Pectoral fascia

Retromammary space

Suspensory ligg.

Lactiferous sinus

Nipple

Lactiferous ducts

Glandular lobe

Right Lateral View of Median Sectioned Breast

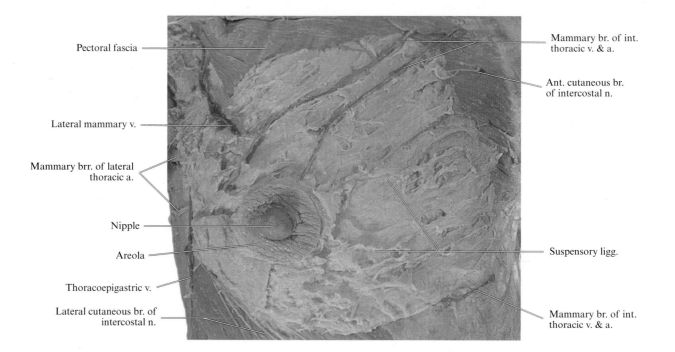

Pectoral fascia

Lateral mammary v.

Mammary brr. of lateral thoracic a.

Nipple

Areola

Thoracoepigastric v.

Lateral cutaneous br. of intercostal n.

Mammary br. of int. thoracic v. & a.

Ant. cutaneous br. of intercostal n.

Suspensory ligg.

Mammary br. of int. thoracic v. & a.

Anterior View of Right Breast

PLATE 1.43   ANTERIOR BODY WALL—INTERNAL SURFACE

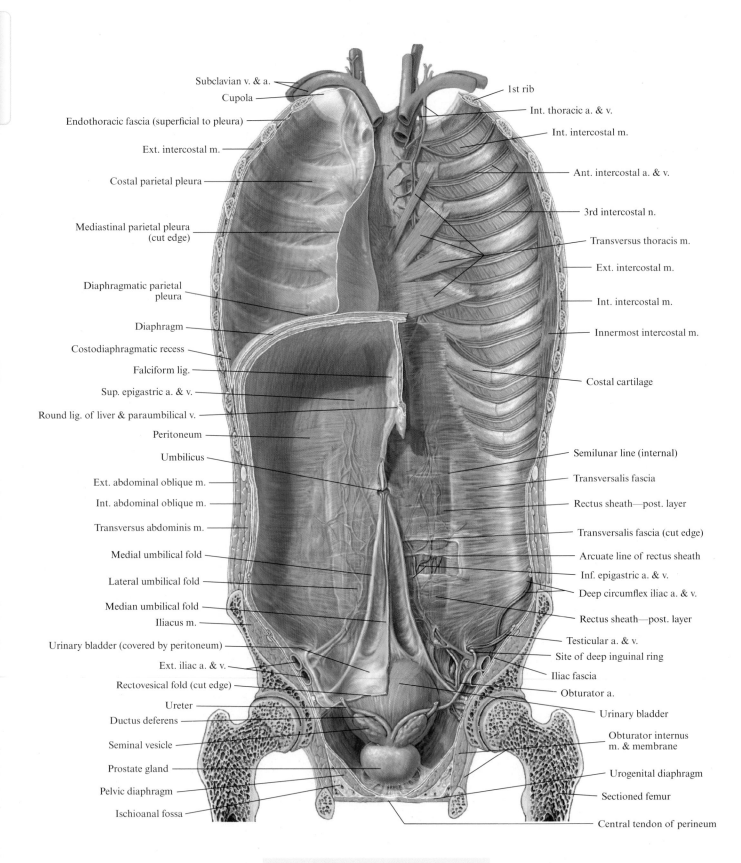

Subclavian v. & a.
Cupola
Endothoracic fascia (superficial to pleura)
Ext. intercostal m.
Costal parietal pleura
Mediastinal parietal pleura (cut edge)
Diaphragmatic parietal pleura
Diaphragm
Costodiaphragmatic recess
Falciform lig.
Sup. epigastric a. & v.
Round lig. of liver & paraumbilical v.
Peritoneum
Umbilicus
Ext. abdominal oblique m.
Int. abdominal oblique m.
Transversus abdominis m.
Medial umbilical fold
Lateral umbilical fold
Median umbilical fold
Iliacus m.
Urinary bladder (covered by peritoneum)
Ext. iliac a. & v.
Rectovesical fold (cut edge)
Ureter
Ductus deferens
Seminal vesicle
Prostate gland
Pelvic diaphragm
Ischioanal fossa

1st rib
Int. thoracic a. & v.
Int. intercostal m.
Ant. intercostal a. & v.
3rd intercostal n.
Transversus thoracis m.
Ext. intercostal m.
Int. intercostal m.
Innermost intercostal m.
Costal cartilage
Semilunar line (internal)
Transversalis fascia
Rectus sheath—post. layer
Transversalis fascia (cut edge)
Arcuate line of rectus sheath
Inf. epigastric a. & v.
Deep circumflex iliac a. & v.
Rectus sheath—post. layer
Testicular a. & v.
Site of deep inguinal ring
Iliac fascia
Obturator a.
Urinary bladder
Obturator internus m. & membrane
Urogenital diaphragm
Sectioned femur
Central tendon of perineum

Posterior (Internal) View of Anterior Body Wall

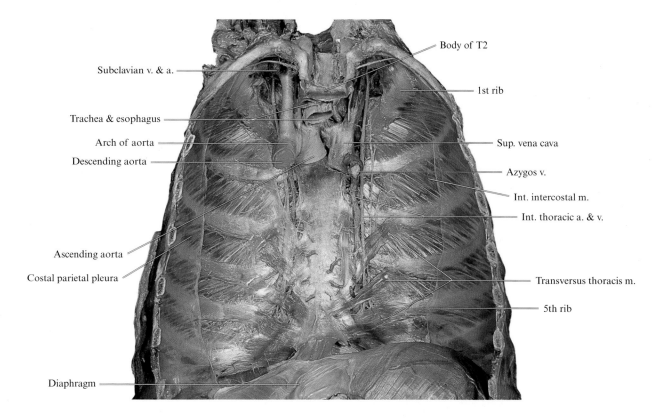

Subclavian v. & a.

Trachea & esophagus

Arch of aorta

Descending aorta

Ascending aorta

Costal parietal pleura

Diaphragm

Body of T2

1st rib

Sup. vena cava

Azygos v.

Int. intercostal m.

Int. thoracic a. & v.

Transversus thoracis m.

5th rib

Posterior (Internal) View of Anterior Thoracic Wall

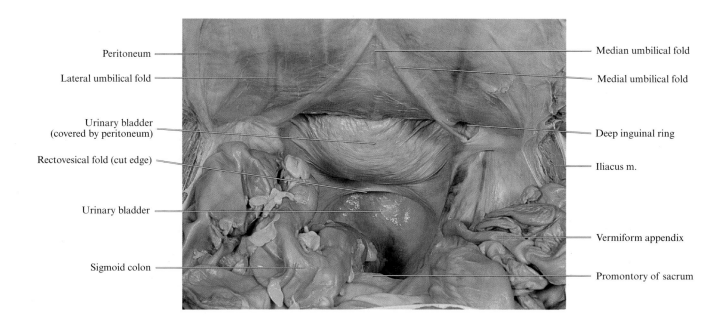

Peritoneum

Lateral umbilical fold

Urinary bladder
(covered by peritoneum)

Rectovesical fold (cut edge)

Urinary bladder

Sigmoid colon

Median umbilical fold

Medial umbilical fold

Deep inguinal ring

Iliacus m.

Vermiform appendix

Promontory of sacrum

Posterosuperior View of Anterior Abdominal Wall & Pelvic Contents

CHAPTER 1 TRUNK: BODY WALL AND SPINE

PLATE 1.45   LATERAL BODY WALL—SUPERFICIAL

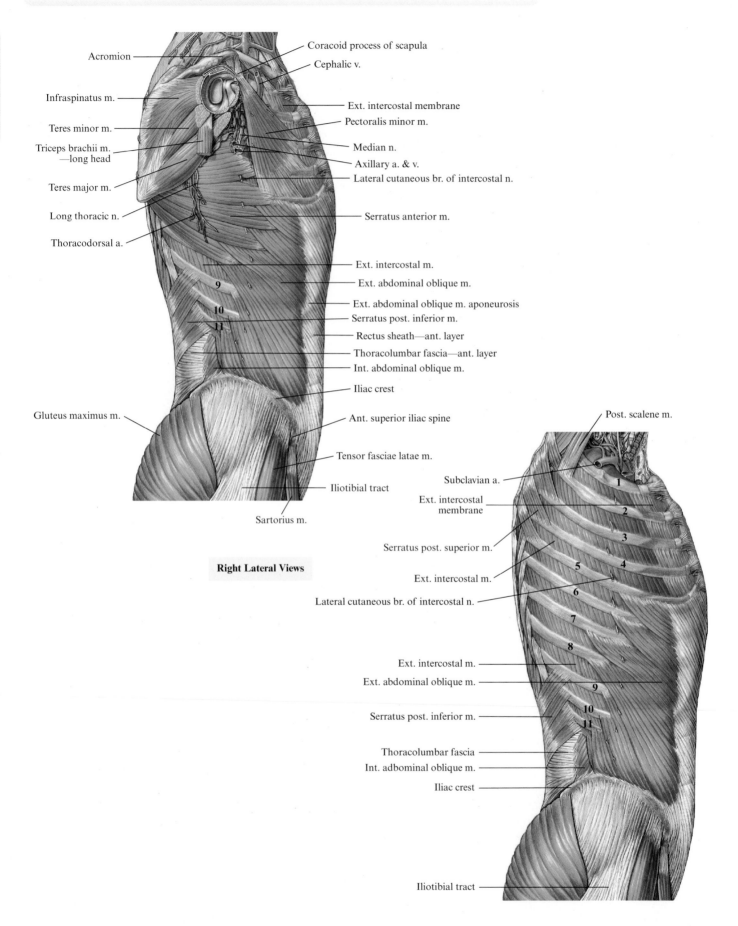

Acromion

Infraspinatus m.

Teres minor m.

Triceps brachii m.
—long head

Teres major m.

Long thoracic n.

Thoracodorsal a.

Coracoid process of scapula

Cephalic v.

Ext. intercostal membrane

Pectoralis minor m.

Median n.

Axillary a. & v.

Lateral cutaneous br. of intercostal n.

Serratus anterior m.

Ext. intercostal m.

Ext. abdominal oblique m.

Ext. abdominal oblique m. aponeurosis

Serratus post. inferior m.

Rectus sheath—ant. layer

Thoracolumbar fascia—ant. layer

Int. abdominal oblique m.

Iliac crest

Gluteus maximus m.

Ant. superior iliac spine

Tensor fasciae latae m.

Iliotibial tract

Sartorius m.

Right Lateral Views

Post. scalene m.

Subclavian a.

Ext. intercostal
membrane

Serratus post. superior m.

Ext. intercostal m.

Lateral cutaneous br. of intercostal n.

Ext. intercostal m.

Ext. abdominal oblique m.

Serratus post. inferior m.

Thoracolumbar fascia

Int. adbominal oblique m.

Iliac crest

Iliotibial tract

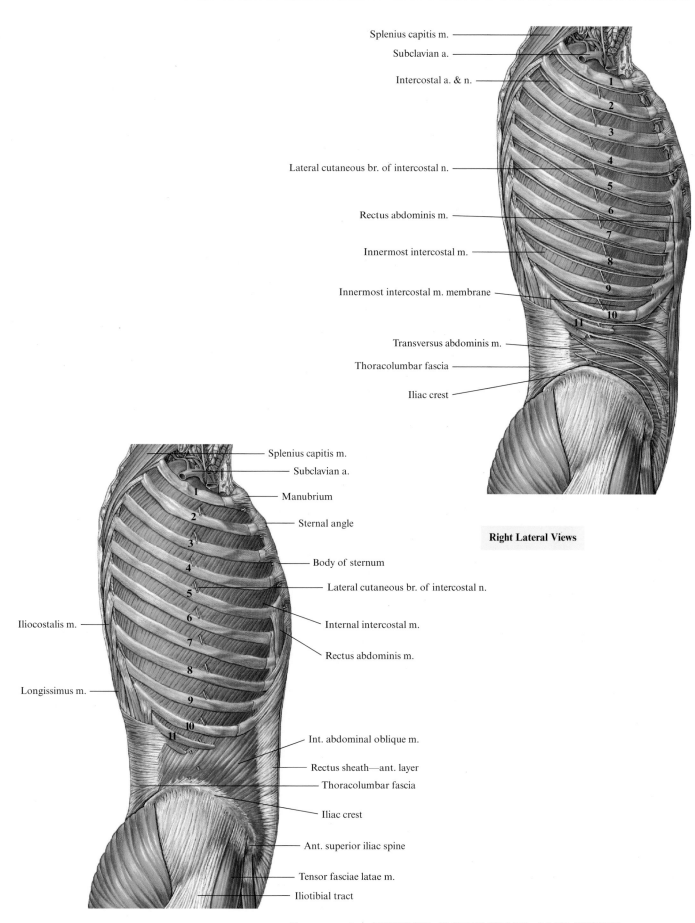

Splenius capitis m.

Subclavian a.

Intercostal a. & n.

Lateral cutaneous br. of intercostal n.

Rectus abdominis m.

Innermost intercostal m.

Innermost intercostal m. membrane

Transversus abdominis m.

Thoracolumbar fascia

Iliac crest

Right Lateral Views

Splenius capitis m.

Subclavian a.

Manubrium

Sternal angle

Body of sternum

Lateral cutaneous br. of intercostal n.

Internal intercostal m.

Rectus abdominis m.

Iliocostalis m.

Longissimus m.

Int. abdominal oblique m.

Rectus sheath—ant. layer

Thoracolumbar fascia

Iliac crest

Ant. superior iliac spine

Tensor fasciae latae m.

Iliotibial tract

CHAPTER 1   **TRUNK: BODY WALL AND SPINE**   51

PLATE 1.47   INGUINAL REGION—SUPERFICIAL FASCIA

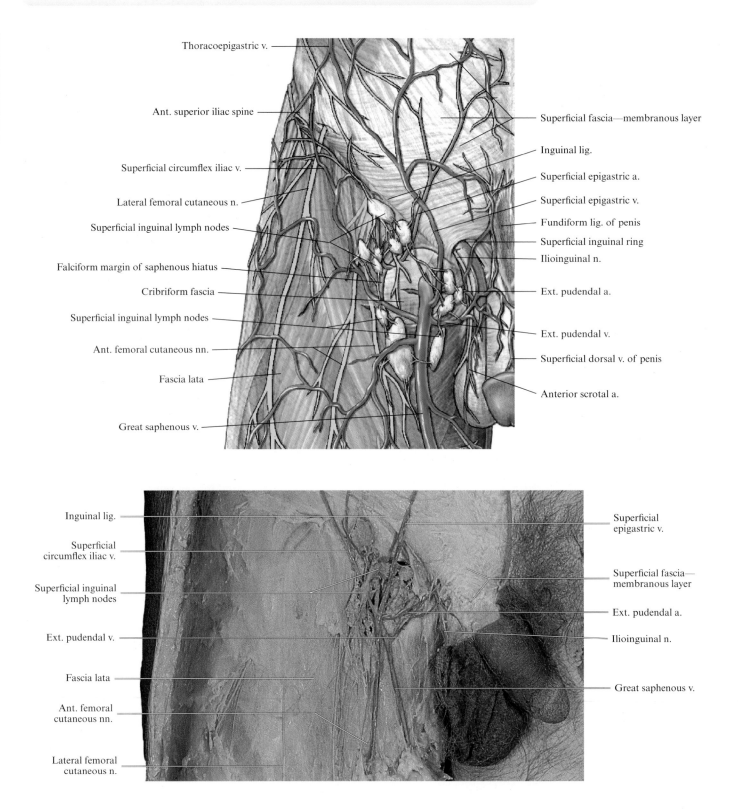

Thoracoepigastric v.

Ant. superior iliac spine

Superficial circumflex iliac v.

Lateral femoral cutaneous n.

Superficial inguinal lymph nodes

Falciform margin of saphenous hiatus

Cribriform fascia

Superficial inguinal lymph nodes

Ant. femoral cutaneous nn.

Fascia lata

Great saphenous v.

Superficial fascia—membranous layer

Inguinal lig.

Superficial epigastric a.

Superficial epigastric v.

Fundiform lig. of penis

Superficial inguinal ring

Ilioinguinal n.

Ext. pudendal a.

Ext. pudendal v.

Superficial dorsal v. of penis

Anterior scrotal a.

Inguinal lig.

Superficial circumflex iliac v.

Superficial inguinal lymph nodes

Ext. pudendal v.

Fascia lata

Ant. femoral cutaneous nn.

Lateral femoral cutaneous n.

Superficial epigastric v.

Superficial fascia—membranous layer

Ext. pudendal a.

Ilioinguinal n.

Great saphenous v.

Anterior Views of Right Side

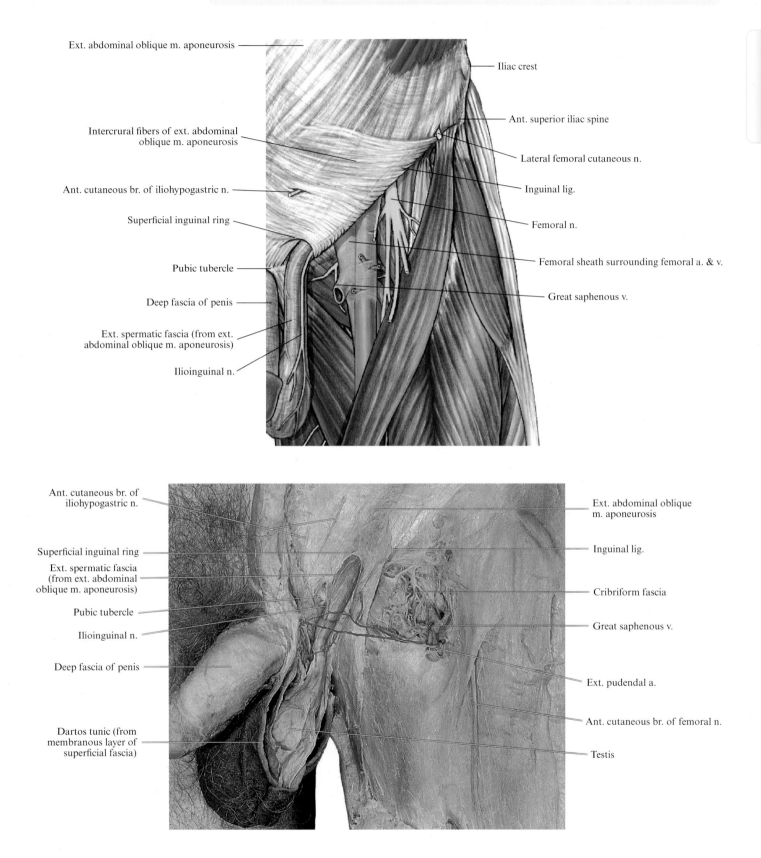

Ext. abdominal oblique m. aponeurosis

Intercrural fibers of ext. abdominal oblique m. aponeurosis

Ant. cutaneous br. of iliohypogastric n.

Superficial inguinal ring

Pubic tubercle

Deep fascia of penis

Ext. spermatic fascia (from ext. abdominal oblique m. aponeurosis)

Ilioinguinal n.

Iliac crest

Ant. superior iliac spine

Lateral femoral cutaneous n.

Inguinal lig.

Femoral n.

Femoral sheath surrounding femoral a. & v.

Great saphenous v.

Ant. cutaneous br. of iliohypogastric n.

Superficial inguinal ring

Ext. spermatic fascia (from ext. abdominal oblique m. aponeurosis)

Pubic tubercle

Ilioinguinal n.

Deep fascia of penis

Dartos tunic (from membranous layer of superficial fascia)

Ext. abdominal oblique m. aponeurosis

Inguinal lig.

Cribriform fascia

Great saphenous v.

Ext. pudendal a.

Ant. cutaneous br. of femoral n.

Testis

Anterior Views of Left Side

PLATE 1.49   INGUINAL REGION—EXTERNAL SPERMATIC FASCIA

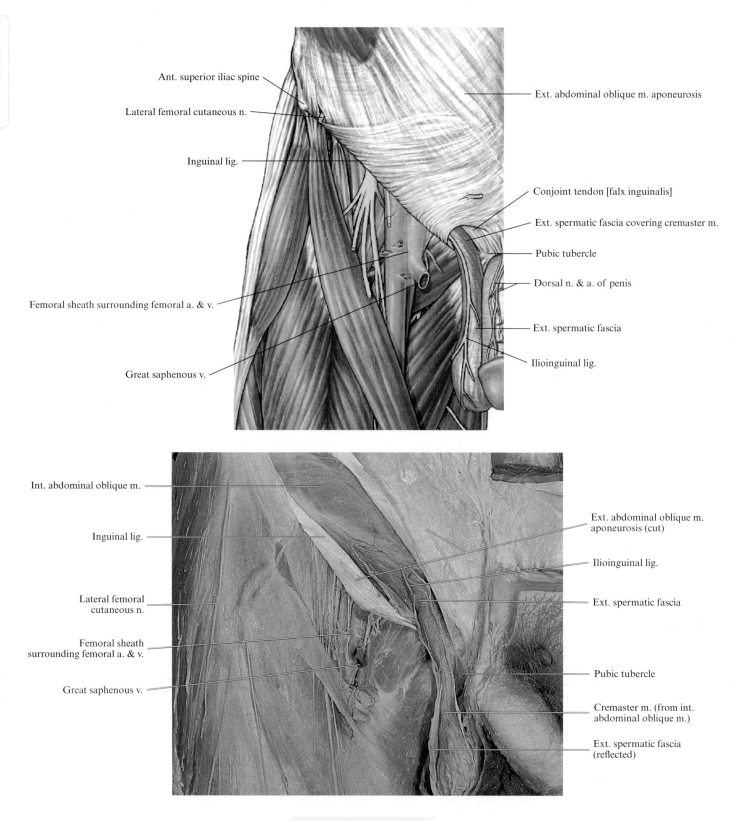

Ant. superior iliac spine

Lateral femoral cutaneous n.

Inguinal lig.

Ext. abdominal oblique m. aponeurosis

Conjoint tendon [falx inguinalis]

Ext. spermatic fascia covering cremaster m.

Pubic tubercle

Dorsal n. & a. of penis

Ext. spermatic fascia

Ilioinguinal lig.

Femoral sheath surrounding femoral a. & v.

Great saphenous v.

Int. abdominal oblique m.

Inguinal lig.

Lateral femoral cutaneous n.

Femoral sheath surrounding femoral a. & v.

Great saphenous v.

Ext. abdominal oblique m. aponeurosis (cut)

Ilioinguinal lig.

Ext. spermatic fascia

Pubic tubercle

Cremaster m. (from int. abdominal oblique m.)

Ext. spermatic fascia (reflected)

Anterior Views of Right Side

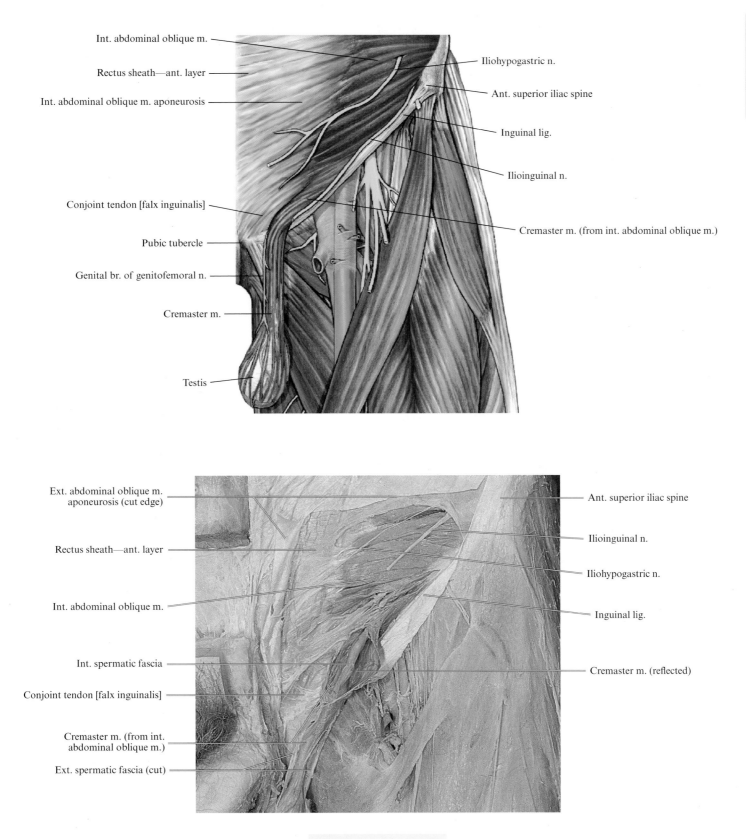

Int. abdominal oblique m.

Rectus sheath—ant. layer

Int. abdominal oblique m. aponeurosis

Conjoint tendon [falx inguinalis]

Pubic tubercle

Genital br. of genitofemoral n.

Cremaster m.

Testis

Iliohypogastric n.

Ant. superior iliac spine

Inguinal lig.

Ilioinguinal n.

Cremaster m. (from int. abdominal oblique m.)

Ext. abdominal oblique m. aponeurosis (cut edge)

Rectus sheath—ant. layer

Int. abdominal oblique m.

Int. spermatic fascia

Conjoint tendon [falx inguinalis]

Cremaster m. (from int. abdominal oblique m.)

Ext. spermatic fascia (cut)

Ant. superior iliac spine

Ilioinguinal n.

Iliohypogastric n.

Inguinal lig.

Cremaster m. (reflected)

Anterior Views of Left Side

PLATE 1.51   INGUINAL REGION—INTERNAL SPERMATIC FASCIA

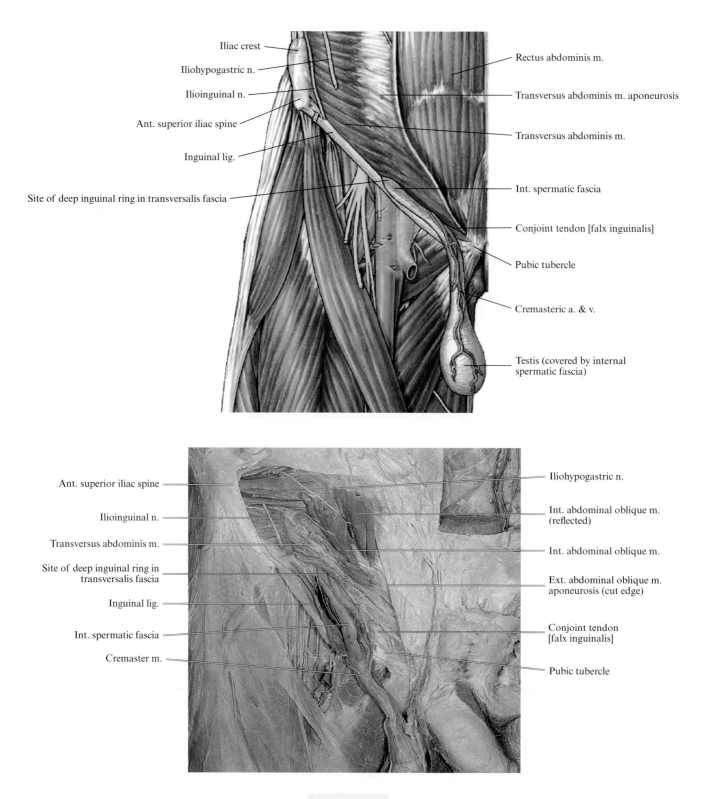

Iliac crest

Iliohypogastric n.

Ilioinguinal n.

Ant. superior iliac spine

Inguinal lig.

Site of deep inguinal ring in transversalis fascia

Rectus abdominis m.

Transversus abdominis m. aponeurosis

Transversus abdominis m.

Int. spermatic fascia

Conjoint tendon [falx inguinalis]

Pubic tubercle

Cremasteric a. & v.

Testis (covered by internal spermatic fascia)

Ant. superior iliac spine

Ilioinguinal n.

Transversus abdominis m.

Site of deep inguinal ring in transversalis fascia

Inguinal lig.

Int. spermatic fascia

Cremaster m.

Iliohypogastric n.

Int. abdominal oblique m. (reflected)

Int. abdominal oblique m.

Ext. abdominal oblique m. aponeurosis (cut edge)

Conjoint tendon [falx inguinalis]

Pubic tubercle

Anterior Views

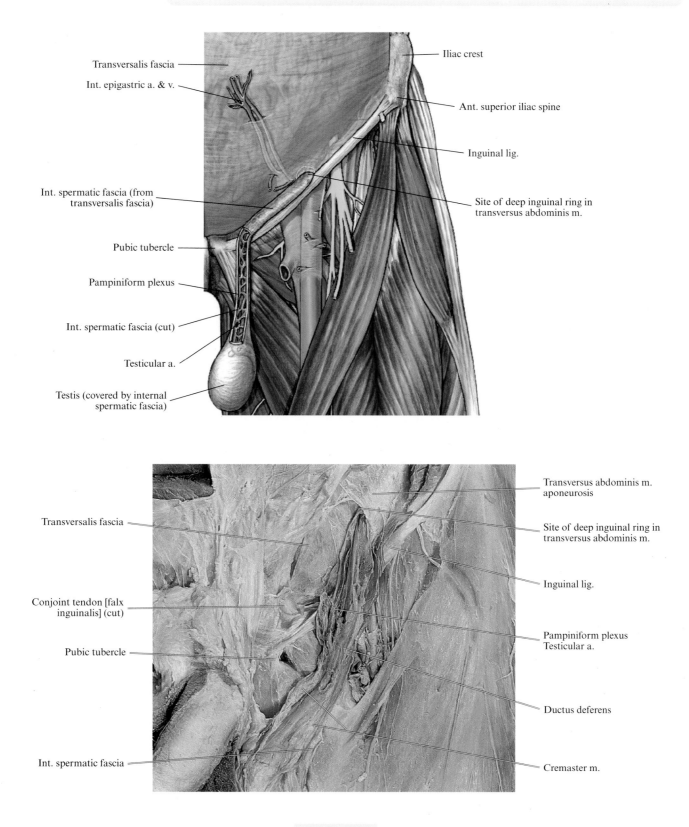

Transversalis fascia

Int. epigastric a. & v.

Int. spermatic fascia (from transversalis fascia)

Pubic tubercle

Pampiniform plexus

Int. spermatic fascia (cut)

Testicular a.

Testis (covered by internal spermatic fascia)

Iliac crest

Ant. superior iliac spine

Inguinal lig.

Site of deep inguinal ring in transversus abdominis m.

Transversalis fascia

Conjoint tendon [falx inguinalis] (cut)

Pubic tubercle

Int. spermatic fascia

Transversus abdominis m. aponeurosis

Site of deep inguinal ring in transversus abdominis m.

Inguinal lig.

Pampiniform plexus
Testicular a.

Ductus deferens

Cremaster m.

Anterior Views

PLATE 1.53   SUPERFICIAL BACK

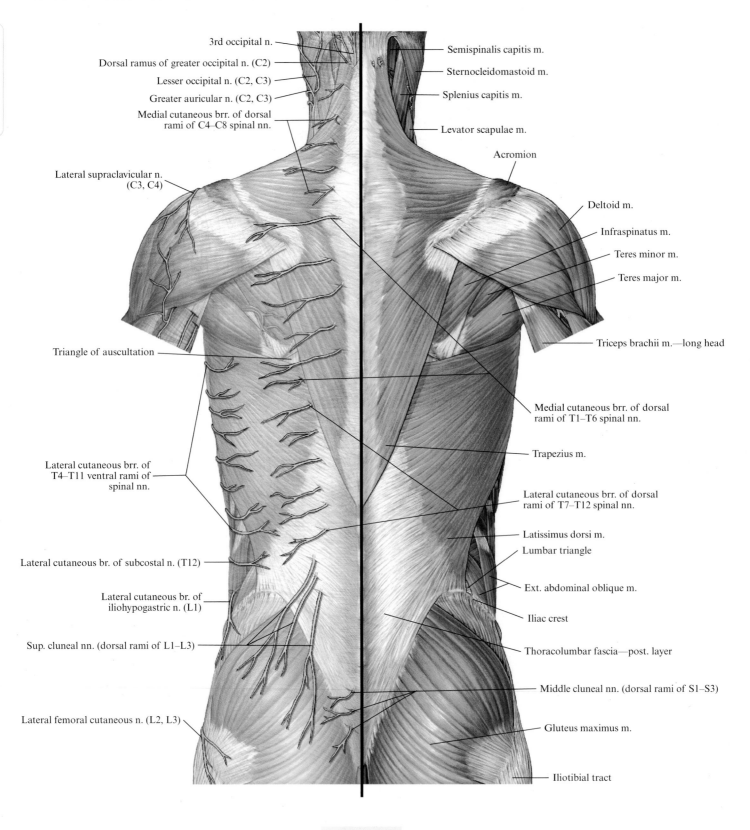

3rd occipital n.

Dorsal ramus of greater occipital n. (C2)

Lesser occipital n. (C2, C3)

Greater auricular n. (C2, C3)

Medial cutaneous brr. of dorsal rami of C4–C8 spinal nn.

Lateral supraclavicular n. (C3, C4)

Triangle of auscultation

Lateral cutaneous brr. of T4–T11 ventral rami of spinal nn.

Lateral cutaneous br. of subcostal n. (T12)

Lateral cutaneous br. of iliohypogastric n. (L1)

Sup. cluneal nn. (dorsal rami of L1–L3)

Lateral femoral cutaneous n. (L2, L3)

Semispinalis capitis m.

Sternocleidomastoid m.

Splenius capitis m.

Levator scapulae m.

Acromion

Deltoid m.

Infraspinatus m.

Teres minor m.

Teres major m.

Triceps brachii m.—long head

Medial cutaneous brr. of dorsal rami of T1–T6 spinal nn.

Trapezius m.

Lateral cutaneous brr. of dorsal rami of T7–T12 spinal nn.

Latissimus dorsi m.

Lumbar triangle

Ext. abdominal oblique m.

Iliac crest

Thoracolumbar fascia—post. layer

Middle cluneal nn. (dorsal rami of S1–S3)

Gluteus maximus m.

Iliotibial tract

Posterior View

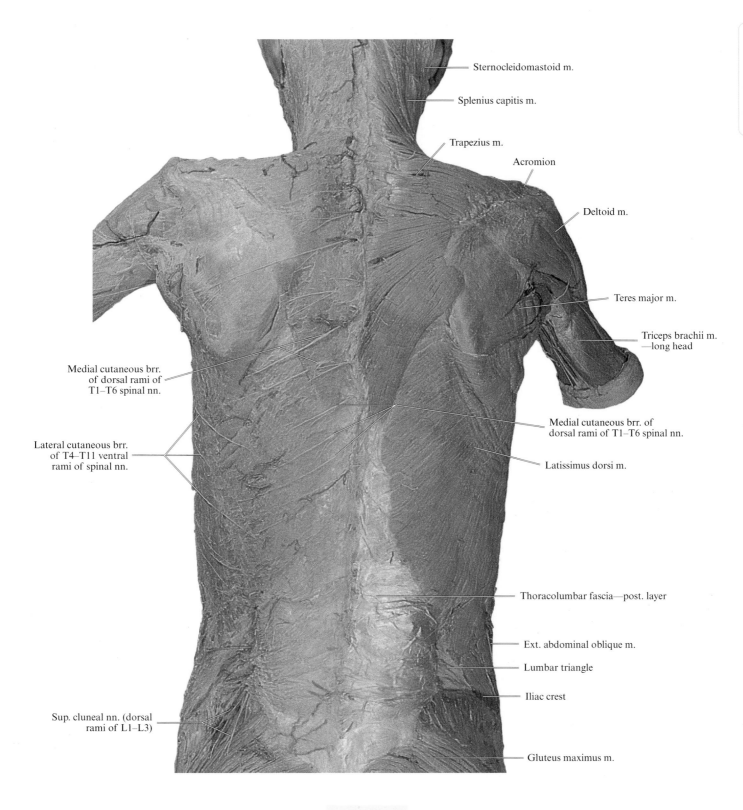

Sternocleidomastoid m.

Splenius capitis m.

Trapezius m.

Acromion

Deltoid m.

Teres major m.

Triceps brachii m.
—long head

Medial cutaneous brr.
of dorsal rami of
T1–T6 spinal nn.

Medial cutaneous brr. of
dorsal rami of T1–T6 spinal nn.

Lateral cutaneous brr.
of T4–T11 ventral
rami of spinal nn.

Latissimus dorsi m.

Thoracolumbar fascia—post. layer

Ext. abdominal oblique m.

Lumbar triangle

Iliac crest

Sup. cluneal nn. (dorsal
rami of L1–L3)

Gluteus maximus m.

Posterior View

PLATE 1.55 INTERMEDIATE BACK

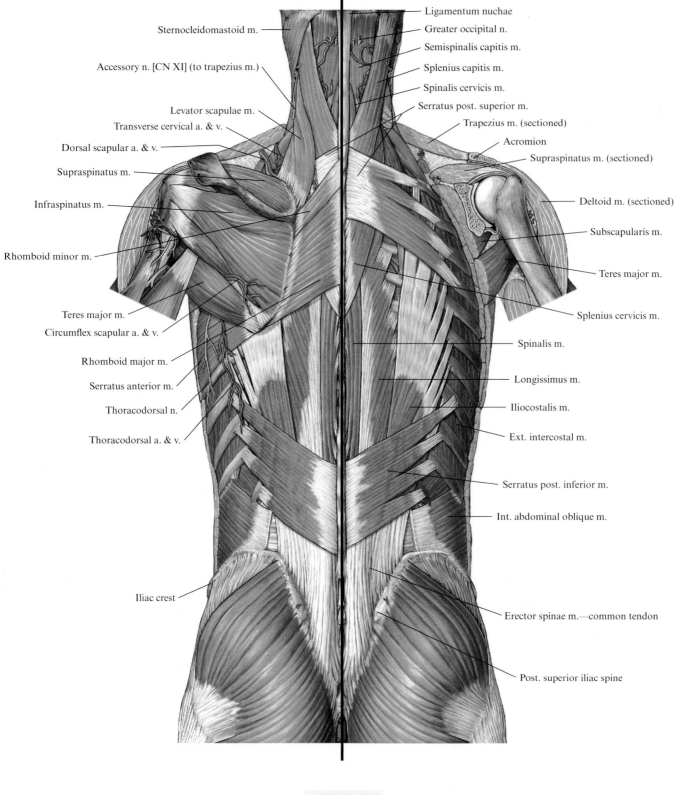

Sternocleidomastoid m.

Accessory n. [CN XI] (to trapezius m.)

Levator scapulae m.
Transverse cervical a. & v.

Dorsal scapular a. & v.

Supraspinatus m.

Infraspinatus m.

Rhomboid minor m.

Teres major m.
Circumflex scapular a. & v.

Rhomboid major m.

Serratus anterior m.

Thoracodorsal n.

Thoracodorsal a. & v.

Iliac crest

Ligamentum nuchae
Greater occipital n.
Semispinalis capitis m.
Splenius capitis m.
Spinalis cervicis m.
Serratus post. superior m.
Trapezius m. (sectioned)
Acromion
Supraspinatus m. (sectioned)

Deltoid m. (sectioned)

Subscapularis m.

Teres major m.

Splenius cervicis m.

Spinalis m.

Longissimus m.

Iliocostalis m.

Ext. intercostal m.

Serratus post. inferior m.

Int. abdominal oblique m.

Erector spinae m.—common tendon

Post. superior iliac spine

Posterior View

A.D.A.M. | Student Atlas of Anatomy

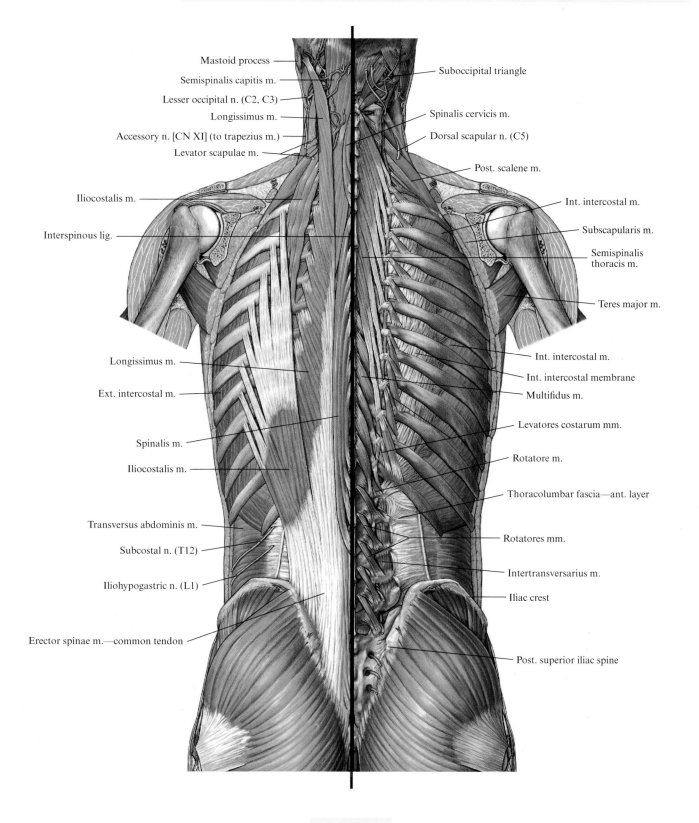

Mastoid process

Semispinalis capitis m.

Lesser occipital n. (C2, C3)

Longissimus m.

Accessory n. [CN XI] (to trapezius m.)

Levator scapulae m.

Iliocostalis m.

Interspinous lig.

Longissimus m.

Ext. intercostal m.

Spinalis m.

Iliocostalis m.

Transversus abdominis m.

Subcostal n. (T12)

Iliohypogastric n. (L1)

Erector spinae m.—common tendon

Suboccipital triangle

Spinalis cervicis m.

Dorsal scapular n. (C5)

Post. scalene m.

Int. intercostal m.

Subscapularis m.

Semispinalis thoracis m.

Teres major m.

Int. intercostal m.

Int. intercostal membrane

Multifidus m.

Levatores costarum mm.

Rotatore m.

Thoracolumbar fascia—ant. layer

Rotatores mm.

Intertransversarius m.

Iliac crest

Post. superior iliac spine

Posterior View

PLATE 1.57   SUBOCCIPITAL REGION

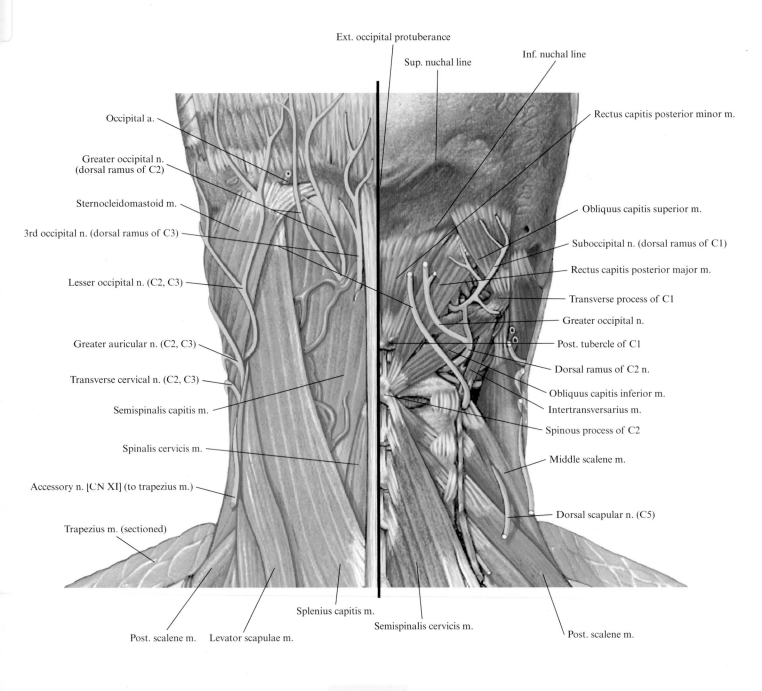

Ext. occipital protuberance

Sup. nuchal line

Inf. nuchal line

Occipital a.

Greater occipital n.
(dorsal ramus of C2)

Sternocleidomastoid m.

3rd occipital n. (dorsal ramus of C3)

Lesser occipital n. (C2, C3)

Greater auricular n. (C2, C3)

Transverse cervical n. (C2, C3)

Semispinalis capitis m.

Spinalis cervicis m.

Accessory n. [CN XI] (to trapezius m.)

Trapezius m. (sectioned)

Rectus capitis posterior minor m.

Obliquus capitis superior m.

Suboccipital n. (dorsal ramus of C1)

Rectus capitis posterior major m.

Transverse process of C1

Greater occipital n.

Post. tubercle of C1

Dorsal ramus of C2 n.

Obliquus capitis inferior m.

Intertransversarius m.

Spinous process of C2

Middle scalene m.

Dorsal scapular n. (C5)

Post. scalene m.   Levator scapulae m.   Splenius capitis m.

Semispinalis cervicis m.

Post. scalene m.

Posterior View

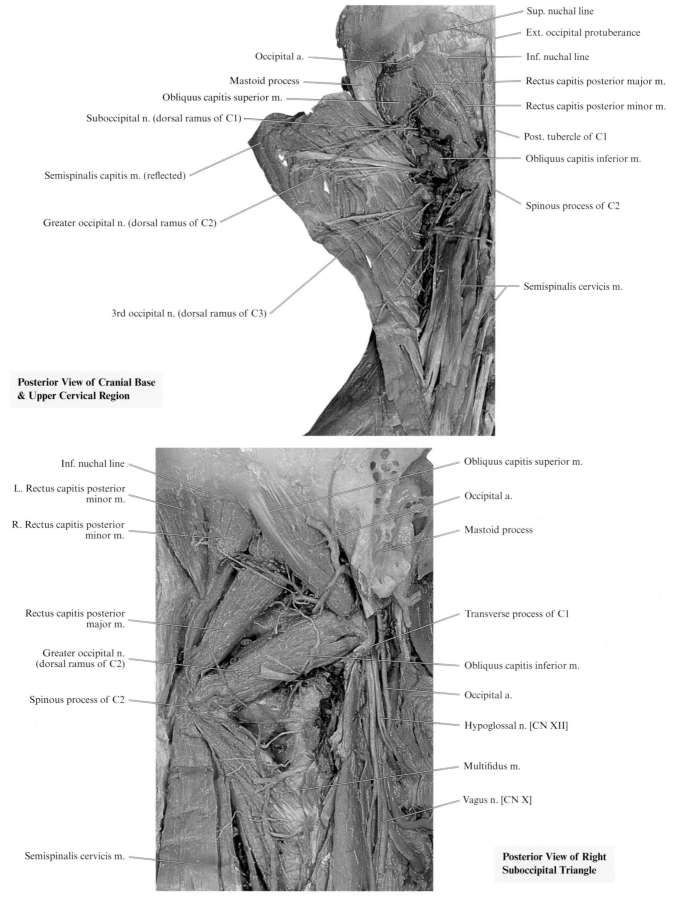

Sup. nuchal line

Ext. occipital protuberance

Occipital a.

Inf. nuchal line

Mastoid process

Rectus capitis posterior major m.

Obliquus capitis superior m.

Rectus capitis posterior minor m.

Suboccipital n. (dorsal ramus of C1)

Post. tubercle of C1

Obliquus capitis inferior m.

Semispinalis capitis m. (reflected)

Greater occipital n. (dorsal ramus of C2)

Spinous process of C2

Semispinalis cervicis m.

3rd occipital n. (dorsal ramus of C3)

**Posterior View of Cranial Base
& Upper Cervical Region**

Inf. nuchal line

Obliquus capitis superior m.

L. Rectus capitis posterior
minor m.

Occipital a.

R. Rectus capitis posterior
minor m.

Mastoid process

Rectus capitis posterior
major m.

Transverse process of C1

Greater occipital n.
(dorsal ramus of C2)

Obliquus capitis inferior m.

Spinous process of C2

Occipital a.

Hypoglossal n. [CN XII]

Multifidus m.

Vagus n. [CN X]

Semispinalis cervicis m.

**Posterior View of Right
Suboccipital Triangle**

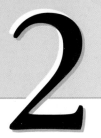

2 THORAX

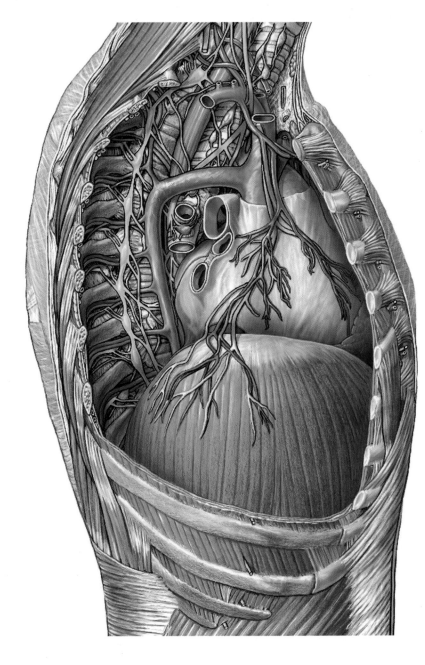

SURFACE ANATOMY

TOPOGRAPHY OF VISCERA

LUNGS, TRACHEA, & BRONCHI

PERICARDIUM & HEART

MEDIASTINUM

PARAVERTEBRAL STRUCTURES

ESOPHAGUS

SUPERIOR THORACIC APERTURE

DIAPHRAGM

PLATE 2.1   **SURFACE ANATOMY**

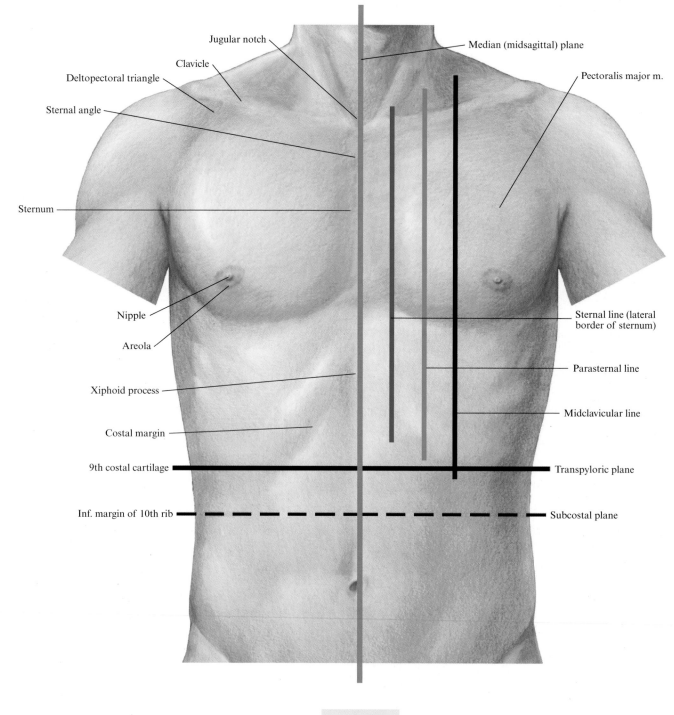

Jugular notch

Clavicle

Deltopectoral triangle

Sternal angle

Median (midsagittal) plane

Pectoralis major m.

Sternum

Nipple

Areola

Sternal line (lateral border of sternum)

Xiphoid process

Parasternal line

Costal margin

Midclavicular line

9th costal cartilage

Transpyloric plane

Inf. margin of 10th rib

Subcostal plane

Anterior View

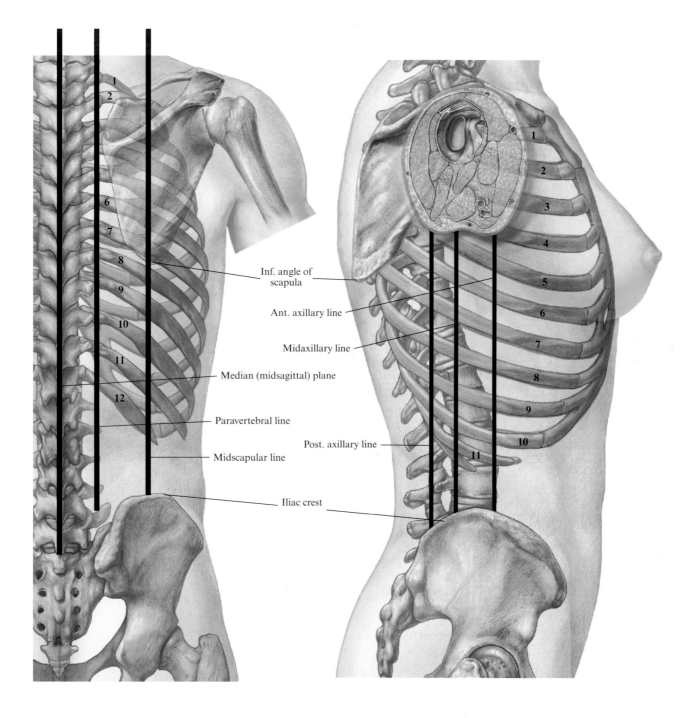

Inf. angle of
scapula

Ant. axillary line

Midaxillary line

Median (midsagittal) plane

Paravertebral line

Post. axillary line

Midscapular line

Iliac crest

Posterior View

Right Lateral View

PLATE 2.3   TOPOGRAPHY OF VISCERA

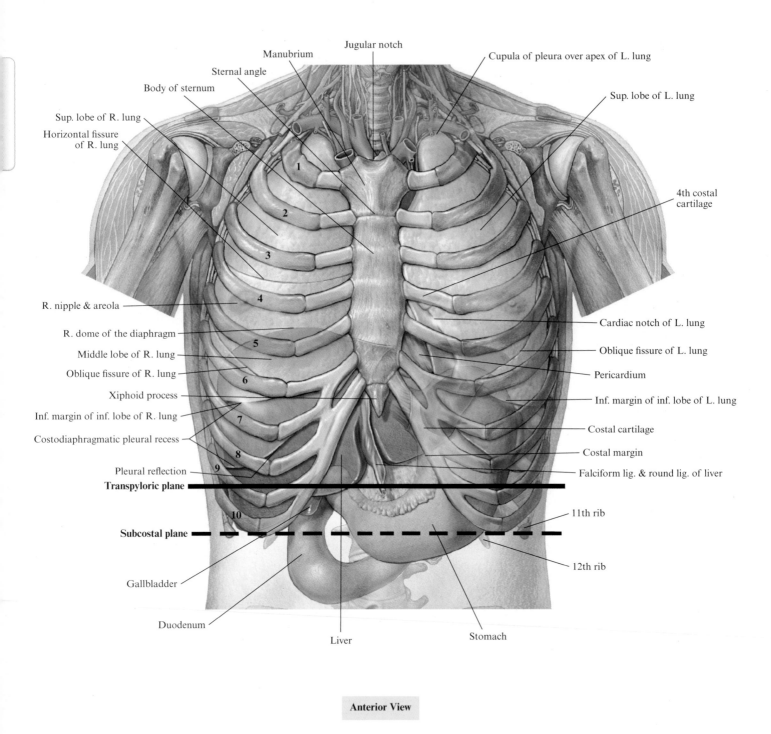

Jugular notch

Manubrium

Sternal angle

Body of sternum

Cupula of pleura over apex of L. lung

Sup. lobe of R. lung

Horizontal fissure of R. lung

Sup. lobe of L. lung

1

2

3

4

5

6

7

8

9

10

4th costal cartilage

R. nipple & areola

R. dome of the diaphragm

Middle lobe of R. lung

Oblique fissure of R. lung

Xiphoid process

Inf. margin of inf. lobe of R. lung

Costodiaphragmatic pleural recess

Pleural reflection

Transpyloric plane

Subcostal plane

Cardiac notch of L. lung

Oblique fissure of L. lung

Pericardium

Inf. margin of inf. lobe of L. lung

Costal cartilage

Costal margin

Falciform lig. & round lig. of liver

11th rib

12th rib

Gallbladder

Duodenum

Liver

Stomach

Anterior View

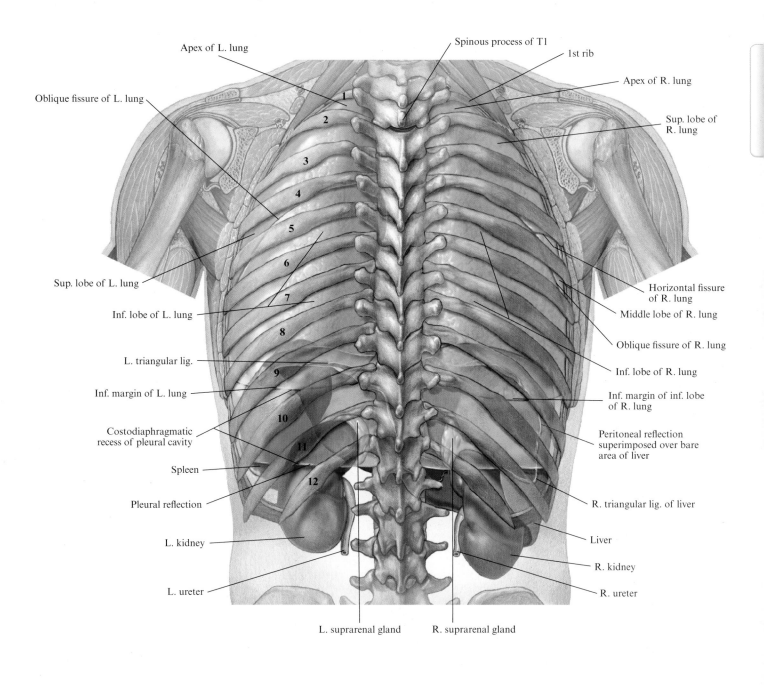

Apex of L. lung

Spinous process of T1

1st rib

Oblique fissure of L. lung

Apex of R. lung

Sup. lobe of R. lung

Sup. lobe of L. lung

Horizontal fissure of R. lung

Inf. lobe of L. lung

Middle lobe of R. lung

L. triangular lig.

Oblique fissure of R. lung

Inf. margin of L. lung

Inf. lobe of R. lung

Costodiaphragmatic recess of pleural cavity

Inf. margin of inf. lobe of R. lung

Spleen

Peritoneal reflection superimposed over bare area of liver

Pleural reflection

R. triangular lig. of liver

L. kidney

Liver

R. kidney

L. ureter

R. ureter

L. suprarenal gland

R. suprarenal gland

Posterior View

PLATE 2.5   TOPOGRAPHY OF VISCERA

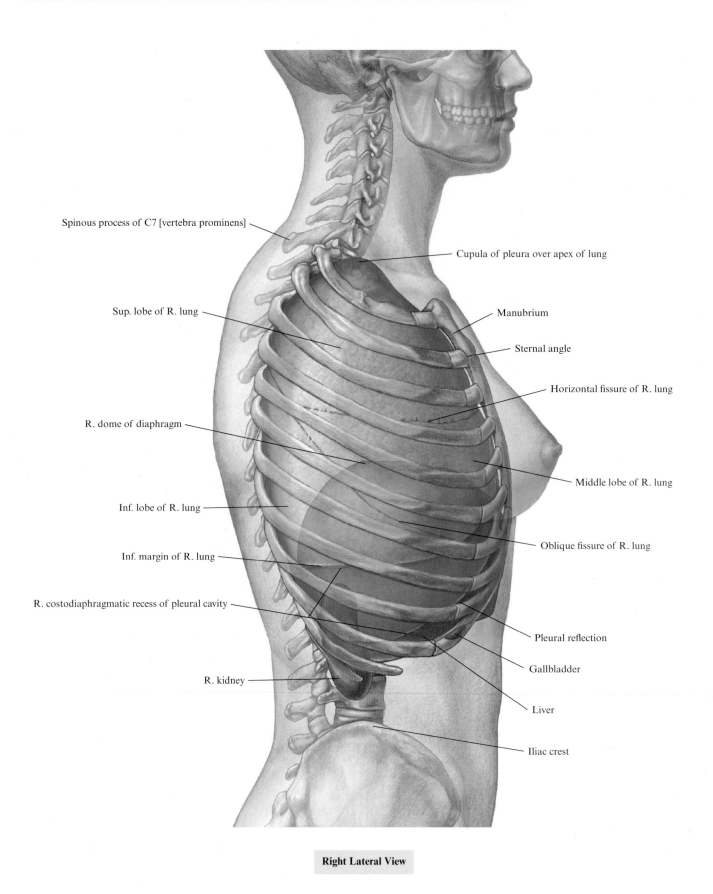

Spinous process of C7 [vertebra prominens]

Cupula of pleura over apex of lung

Sup. lobe of R. lung

Manubrium

Sternal angle

Horizontal fissure of R. lung

R. dome of diaphragm

Inf. lobe of R. lung

Middle lobe of R. lung

Inf. margin of R. lung

Oblique fissure of R. lung

R. costodiaphragmatic recess of pleural cavity

Pleural reflection

Gallbladder

R. kidney

Liver

Iliac crest

Right Lateral View

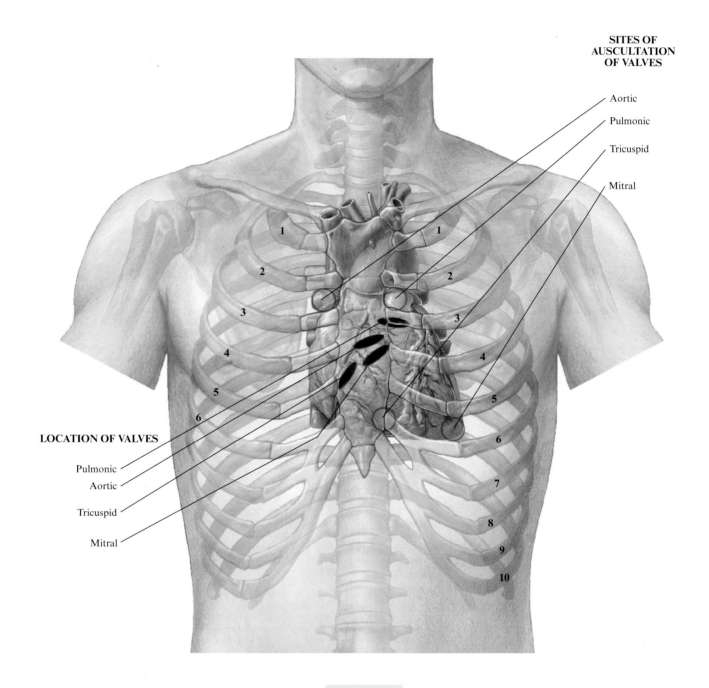

SITES OF
AUSCULTATION
OF VALVES

Aortic

Pulmonic

Tricuspid

Mitral

1

2

3

4

5

6

7

8

9

10

LOCATION OF VALVES

Pulmonic

Aortic

Tricuspid

Mitral

Anterior View

PLATE 2.7   THORACIC VISCERA IN SITU

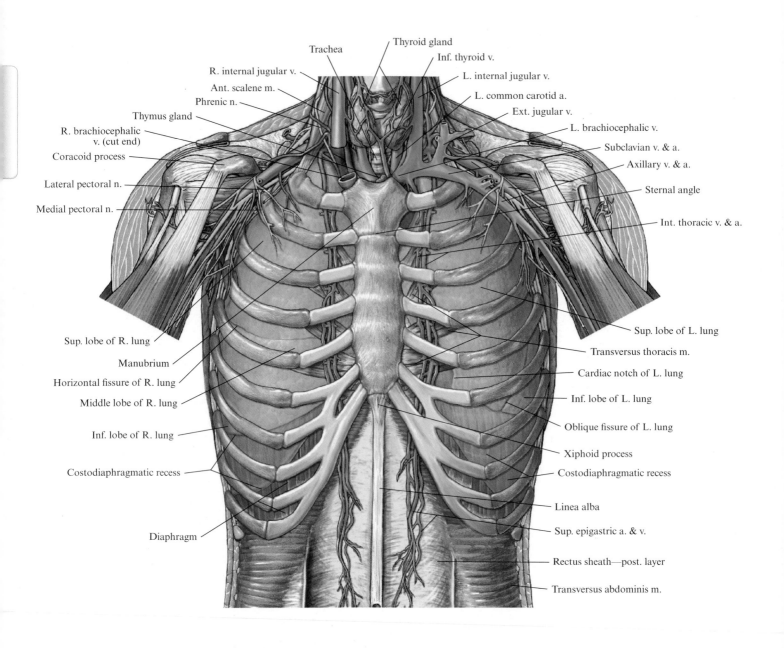

Trachea

Thyroid gland

Inf. thyroid v.

R. internal jugular v.

Ant. scalene m.

Phrenic n.

Thymus gland

R. brachiocephalic
v. (cut end)

Coracoid process

Lateral pectoral n.

Medial pectoral n.

L. internal jugular v.

L. common carotid a.

Ext. jugular v.

L. brachiocephalic v.

Subclavian v. & a.

Axillary v. & a.

Sternal angle

Int. thoracic v. & a.

Sup. lobe of R. lung

Manubrium

Horizontal fissure of R. lung

Middle lobe of R. lung

Inf. lobe of R. lung

Costodiaphragmatic recess

Diaphragm

Sup. lobe of L. lung

Transversus thoracis m.

Cardiac notch of L. lung

Inf. lobe of L. lung

Oblique fissure of L. lung

Xiphoid process

Costodiaphragmatic recess

Linea alba

Sup. epigastric a. & v.

Rectus sheath—post. layer

Transversus abdominis m.

Anterior View

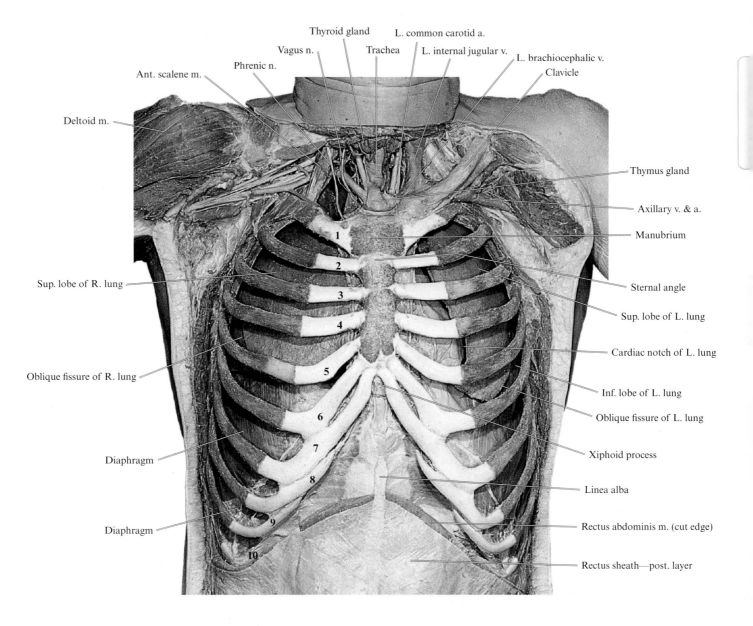

Thyroid gland

Vagus n.

L. common carotid a.

Trachea

L. internal jugular v.

Phrenic n.

L. brachiocephalic v.

Ant. scalene m.

Clavicle

Deltoid m.

Thymus gland

Axillary v. & a.

Manubrium

1

Sup. lobe of R. lung

2

Sternal angle

3

4

Sup. lobe of L. lung

Cardiac notch of L. lung

Oblique fissure of R. lung

5

Inf. lobe of L. lung

Oblique fissure of L. lung

6

7

Xiphoid process

8

Diaphragm

Linea alba

9

Diaphragm

Rectus abdominis m. (cut edge)

10

Rectus sheath—post. layer

Anterior View

PLATE 2.9   LUNGS—MEDIAL

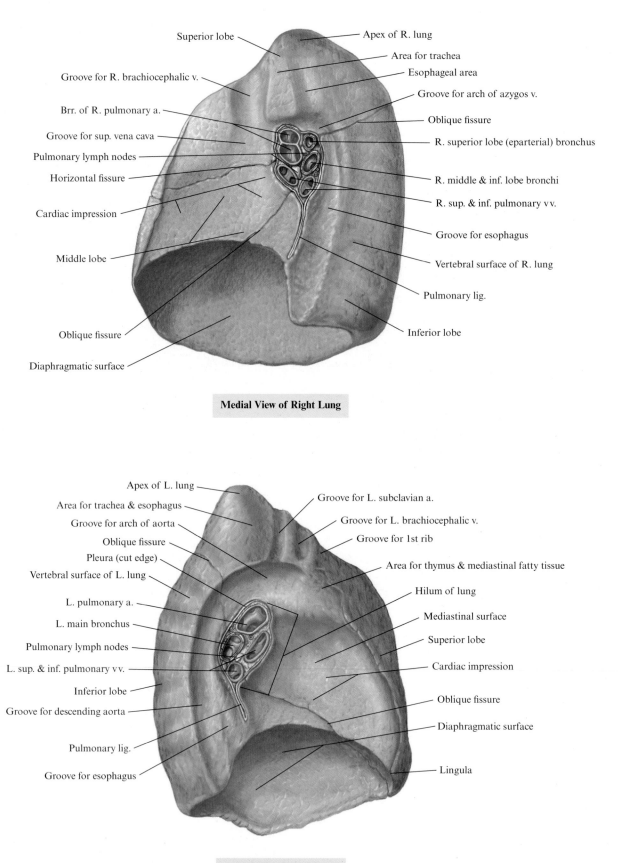

Superior lobe

Apex of R. lung

Area for trachea

Groove for R. brachiocephalic v.

Esophageal area

Groove for arch of azygos v.

Brr. of R. pulmonary a.

Oblique fissure

Groove for sup. vena cava

R. superior lobe (eparterial) bronchus

Pulmonary lymph nodes

Horizontal fissure

R. middle & inf. lobe bronchi

Cardiac impression

R. sup. & inf. pulmonary vv.

Groove for esophagus

Middle lobe

Vertebral surface of R. lung

Pulmonary lig.

Oblique fissure

Inferior lobe

Diaphragmatic surface

Medial View of Right Lung

Apex of L. lung

Groove for L. subclavian a.

Area for trachea & esophagus

Groove for L. brachiocephalic v.

Groove for arch of aorta

Groove for 1st rib

Oblique fissure

Pleura (cut edge)

Area for thymus & mediastinal fatty tissue

Vertebral surface of L. lung

Hilum of lung

L. pulmonary a.

Mediastinal surface

L. main bronchus

Superior lobe

Pulmonary lymph nodes

Cardiac impression

L. sup. & inf. pulmonary vv.

Inferior lobe

Oblique fissure

Groove for descending aorta

Diaphragmatic surface

Pulmonary lig.

Groove for esophagus

Lingula

Medial View of Left Lung

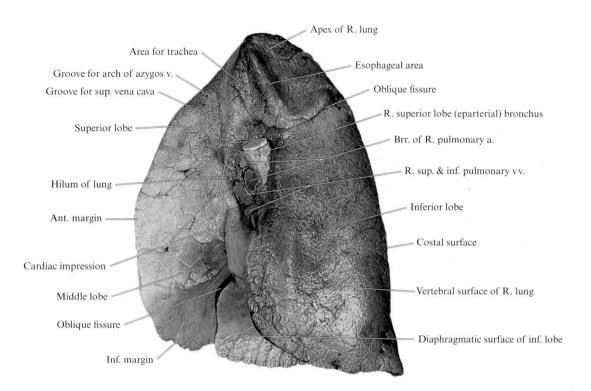

Apex of R. lung

Area for trachea

Esophageal area

Groove for arch of azygos v.

Oblique fissure

Groove for sup. vena cava

R. superior lobe (eparterial) bronchus

Superior lobe

Brr. of R. pulmonary a.

R. sup. & inf. pulmonary vv.

Hilum of lung

Inferior lobe

Ant. margin

Costal surface

Cardiac impression

Middle lobe

Vertebral surface of R. lung

Oblique fissure

Diaphragmatic surface of inf. lobe

Inf. margin

Posteromedial View of Right Lung

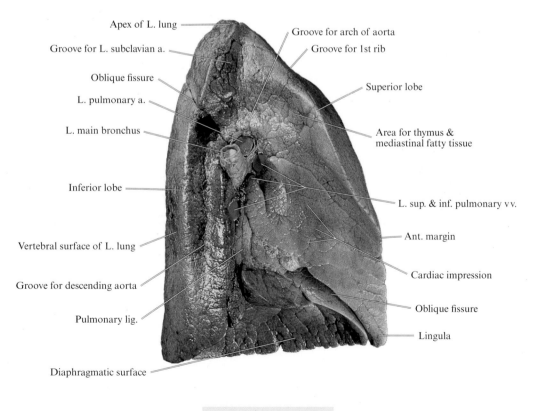

Apex of L. lung

Groove for arch of aorta

Groove for L. subclavian a.

Groove for 1st rib

Oblique fissure

Superior lobe

L. pulmonary a.

L. main bronchus

Area for thymus &
mediastinal fatty tissue

Inferior lobe

L. sup. & inf. pulmonary vv.

Vertebral surface of L. lung

Ant. margin

Groove for descending aorta

Cardiac impression

Pulmonary lig.

Oblique fissure

Lingula

Diaphragmatic surface

Medial View of Left Lung

PLATE 2.11   TRACHEA, BRONCHI & LUNGS

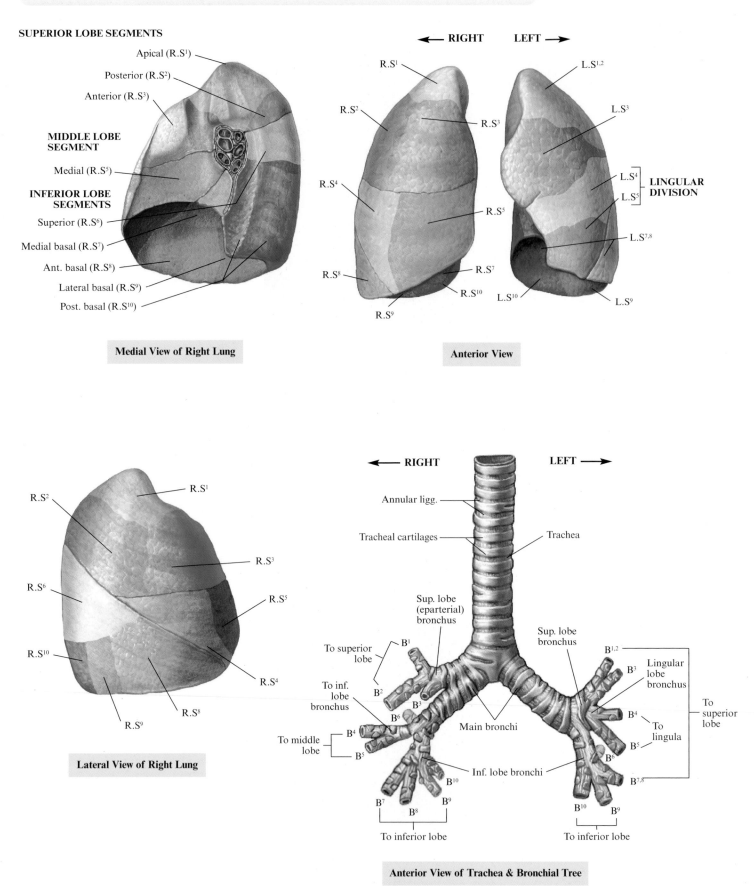

SUPERIOR LOBE SEGMENTS

Apical (R.S^1)

Posterior (R.S^2)

Anterior (R.S^3)

MIDDLE LOBE SEGMENT

Medial (R.S^5)

INFERIOR LOBE SEGMENTS

Superior (R.S^6)

Medial basal (R.S^7)

Ant. basal (R.S^8)

Lateral basal (R.S^9)

Post. basal (R.S^{10})

Medial View of Right Lung

← **RIGHT**   **LEFT** →

R.S^1 L.S^{1,2}

R.S^2 R.S^3 L.S^3

L.S^4 **LINGULAR DIVISION**

R.S^4 L.S^5

R.S^5 L.S^{7,8}

R.S^8 R.S^7 L.S^9

R.S^{10} L.S^{10}

R.S^9

Anterior View

R.S^1

R.S^2

R.S^3

R.S^6

R.S^5

R.S^{10}

R.S^4

R.S^8

R.S^9

Lateral View of Right Lung

← **RIGHT**   **LEFT** →

Annular ligg.

Tracheal cartilages

Trachea

Sup. lobe (eparterial) bronchus

Sup. lobe bronchus

To superior lobe

B^1 B^{1,2}

B^3 Lingular lobe bronchus

B^2

B^3 B^4

To inf. lobe bronchus

B^6 To lingula

Main bronchi   To superior lobe

To middle lobe   B^4 B^5

B^5 B^6

Inf. lobe bronchi   B^{7,8}

B^{10}

B^7 B^9 B^{10} B^9

B^8

To inferior lobe   To inferior lobe

Anterior View of Trachea & Bronchial Tree

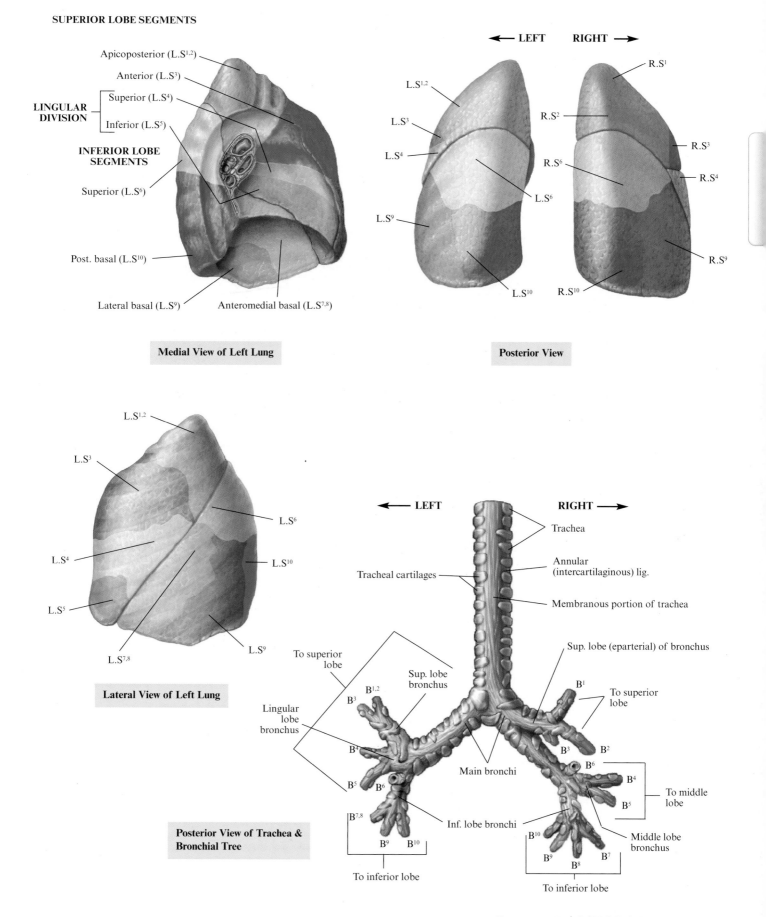

SUPERIOR LOBE SEGMENTS

Apicoposterior (L.S¹,²)

Anterior (L.S³)

Superior (L.S⁴)

LINGULAR DIVISION

Inferior (L.S⁵)

INFERIOR LOBE SEGMENTS

Superior (L.S⁶)

Post. basal (L.S¹⁰)

Lateral basal (L.S⁹)   Anteromedial basal (L.S⁷,⁸)

Medial View of Left Lung

← LEFT   RIGHT →

L.S¹,²

L.S³

L.S⁴

R.S¹

R.S²

R.S³

R.S⁶

R.S⁴

L.S⁶

L.S⁹

R.S⁹

L.S¹⁰   R.S¹⁰

Posterior View

L.S¹,²

L.S³

L.S⁴

L.S⁵

L.S⁶

L.S¹⁰

L.S⁷,⁸   L.S⁹

Lateral View of Left Lung

← LEFT   RIGHT →

Trachea

Annular (intercartilaginous) lig.

Tracheal cartilages

Membranous portion of trachea

Sup. lobe (eparterial) of bronchus

To superior lobe

Sup. lobe bronchus

B¹,²

B³

B¹

To superior lobe

Lingular lobe bronchus

B⁴

B³   B²

B⁶

B⁴

B⁵

B⁵   B⁶

Main bronchi

To middle lobe

Middle lobe bronchus

B⁷,⁸

Inf. lobe bronchi

B¹⁰

B⁹   B¹⁰

B⁹   B⁸   B⁷

Posterior View of Trachea & Bronchial Tree

To inferior lobe   To inferior lobe

PLATE 2.13   TRACHEA, BRONCHI & LUNGS—LYMPHATICS

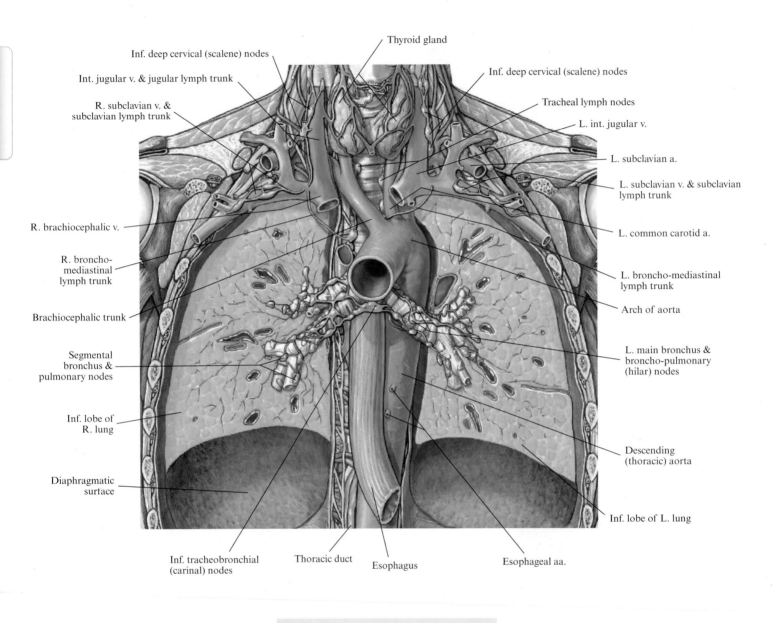

Inf. deep cervical (scalene) nodes

Thyroid gland

Int. jugular v. & jugular lymph trunk

Inf. deep cervical (scalene) nodes

R. subclavian v. &
subclavian lymph trunk

Tracheal lymph nodes

L. int. jugular v.

L. subclavian a.

L. subclavian v. & subclavian
lymph trunk

R. brachiocephalic v.

L. common carotid a.

R. broncho-
mediastinal
lymph trunk

L. broncho-mediastinal
lymph trunk

Brachiocephalic trunk

Arch of aorta

Segmental
bronchus &
pulmonary nodes

L. main bronchus &
broncho-pulmonary
(hilar) nodes

Inf. lobe of
R. lung

Diaphragmatic
surface

Descending
(thoracic) aorta

Inf. lobe of L. lung

Inf. tracheobronchial
(carinal) nodes

Thoracic duct   Esophagus

Esophageal aa.

Anterior View with Coronally Sectioned Lungs

A.D.A.M. | Student Atlas of Anatomy

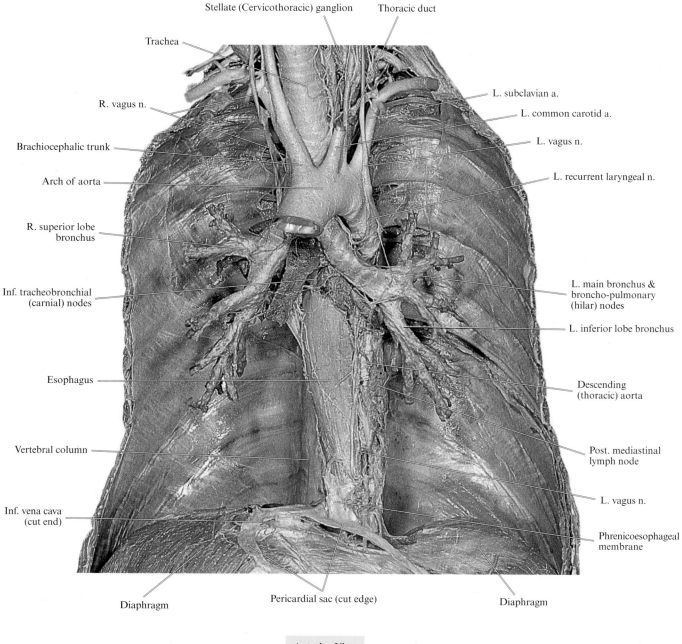

Stellate (Cervicothoracic) ganglion   Thoracic duct

Trachea

R. vagus n.

Brachiocephalic trunk

Arch of aorta

R. superior lobe
bronchus

Inf. tracheobronchial
(carnial) nodes

Esophagus

Vertebral column

Inf. vena cava
(cut end)

Diaphragm

L. subclavian a.

L. common carotid a.

L. vagus n.

L. recurrent laryngeal n.

L. main bronchus &
broncho-pulmonary
(hilar) nodes

L. inferior lobe bronchus

Descending
(thoracic) aorta

Post. mediastinal
lymph node

L. vagus n.

Phrenicoesophageal
membrane

Pericardial sac (cut edge)   Diaphragm

Anterior View

PLATE 2.15 LUNGS & HEART—CROSS SECTION

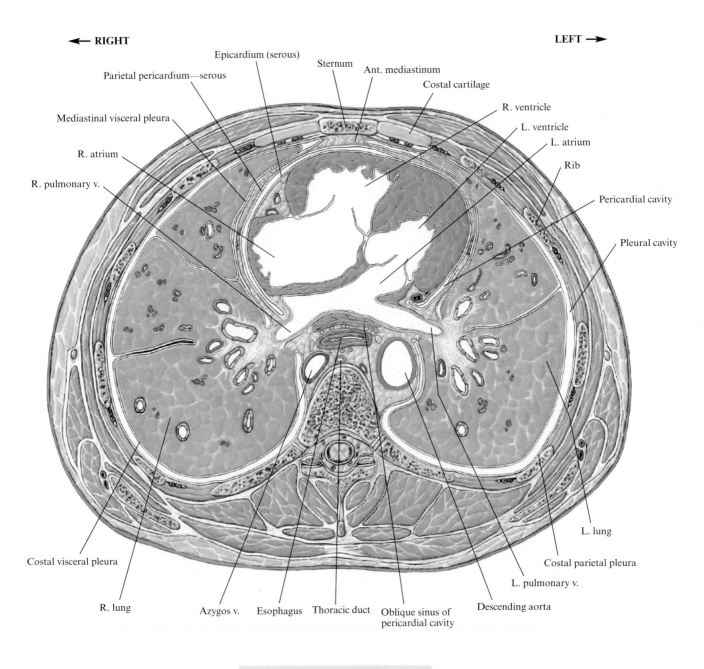

← RIGHT

LEFT →

Epicardium (serous)

Parietal pericardium—serous

Sternum

Ant. mediastinum

Costal cartilage

Mediastinal visceral pleura

R. ventricle

L. ventricle

R. atrium

L. atrium

R. pulmonary v.

Rib

Pericardial cavity

Pleural cavity

Costal visceral pleura

L. lung

Costal parietal pleura

R. lung

Azygos v.

Esophagus

Thoracic duct

Oblique sinus of pericardial cavity

L. pulmonary v.

Descending aorta

Transverse Section at T8—Inferior View

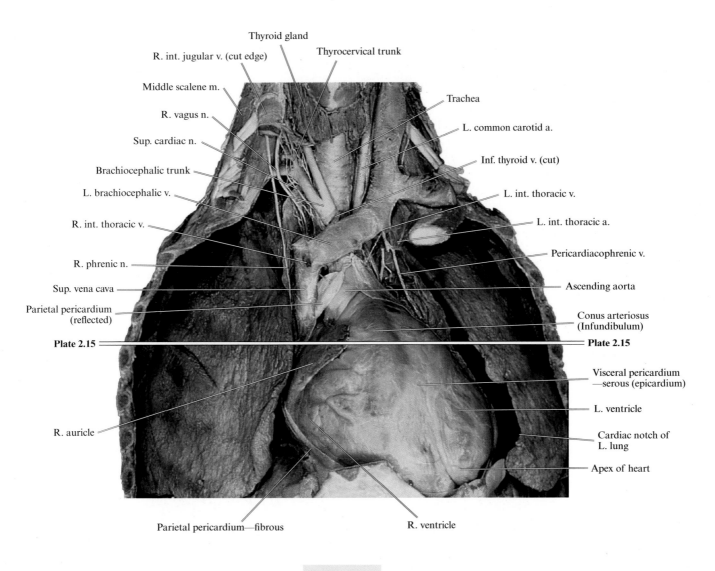

Thyroid gland

R. int. jugular v. (cut edge)

Thyrocervical trunk

Middle scalene m.

R. vagus n.

Sup. cardiac n.

Brachiocephalic trunk

L. brachiocephalic v.

R. int. thoracic v.

R. phrenic n.

Sup. vena cava

Parietal pericardium (reflected)

Plate 2.15

R. auricle

Trachea

L. common carotid a.

Inf. thyroid v. (cut)

L. int. thoracic v.

L. int. thoracic a.

Pericardiacophrenic v.

Ascending aorta

Conus arteriosus (Infundibulum)

Plate 2.15

Visceral pericardium —serous (epicardium)

L. ventricle

Cardiac notch of L. lung

Apex of heart

Parietal pericardium—fibrous

R. ventricle

Anterior View

PLATE 2.17   HEART & GREAT VESSELS—ANTERIOR

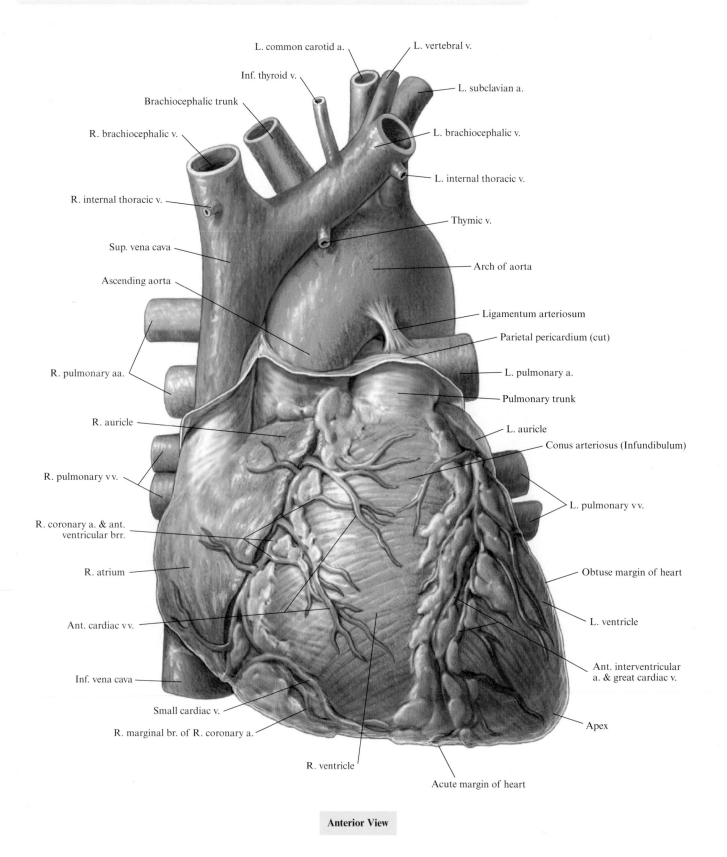

L. common carotid a.

L. vertebral v.

Inf. thyroid v.

L. subclavian a.

Brachiocephalic trunk

R. brachiocephalic v.

L. brachiocephalic v.

R. internal thoracic v.

L. internal thoracic v.

Thymic v.

Sup. vena cava

Arch of aorta

Ascending aorta

Ligamentum arteriosum

Parietal pericardium (cut)

R. pulmonary aa.

L. pulmonary a.

Pulmonary trunk

R. auricle

L. auricle

Conus arteriosus (Infundibulum)

R. pulmonary v v.

L. pulmonary v v.

R. coronary a. & ant.
ventricular brr.

R. atrium

Obtuse margin of heart

L. ventricle

Ant. cardiac v v.

Ant. interventricular
a. & great cardiac v.

Inf. vena cava

Small cardiac v.

R. marginal br. of R. coronary a.

Apex

R. ventricle

Acute margin of heart

Anterior View

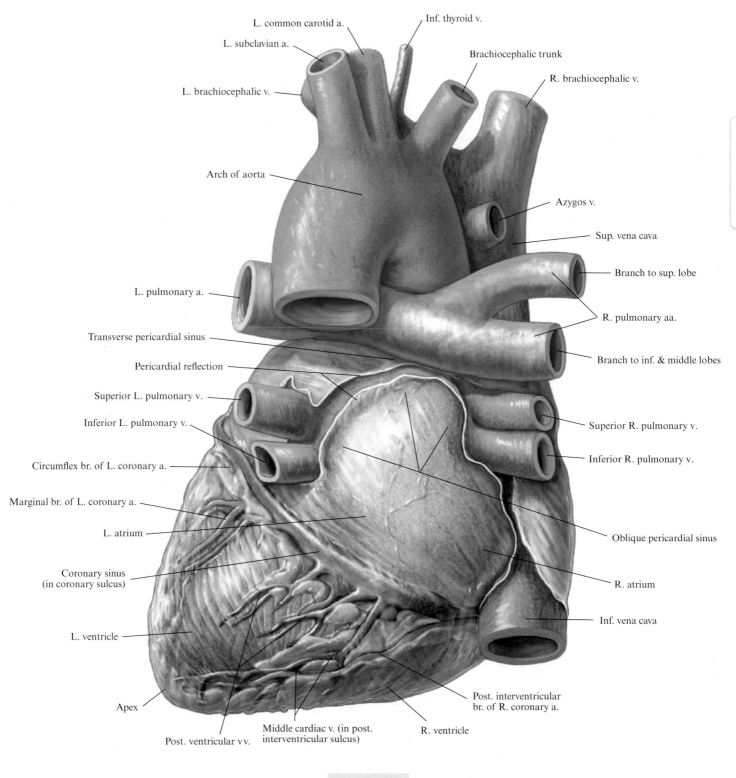

L. common carotid a.

Inf. thyroid v.

L. subclavian a.

Brachiocephalic trunk

L. brachiocephalic v.

R. brachiocephalic v.

Arch of aorta

Azygos v.

Sup. vena cava

Branch to sup. lobe

L. pulmonary a.

R. pulmonary aa.

Transverse pericardial sinus

Branch to inf. & middle lobes

Pericardial reflection

Superior L. pulmonary v.

Inferior L. pulmonary v.

Superior R. pulmonary v.

Circumflex br. of L. coronary a.

Inferior R. pulmonary v.

Marginal br. of L. coronary a.

L. atrium

Oblique pericardial sinus

Coronary sinus
(in coronary sulcus)

R. atrium

L. ventricle

Inf. vena cava

Apex

Post. interventricular
br. of R. coronary a.

Post. ventricular vv.

Middle cardiac v. (in post.
interventricular sulcus)

R. ventricle

Posterior View

PLATE 2.19   HEART IN SYSTOLE & DIASTOLE

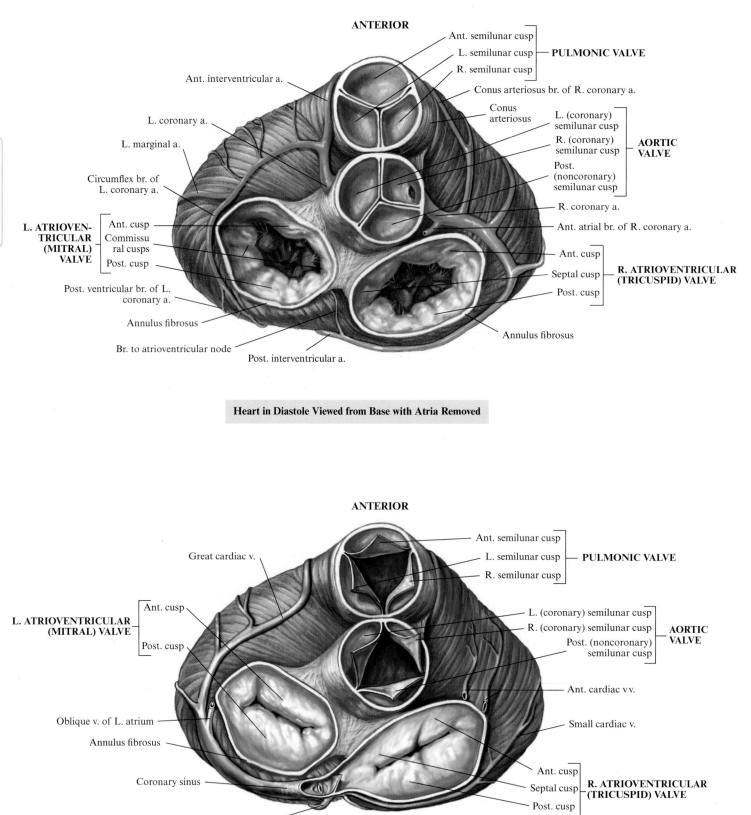

Heart in Diastole Viewed from Base with Atria Removed

Heart in Systole Viewed from Base with Atria Removed

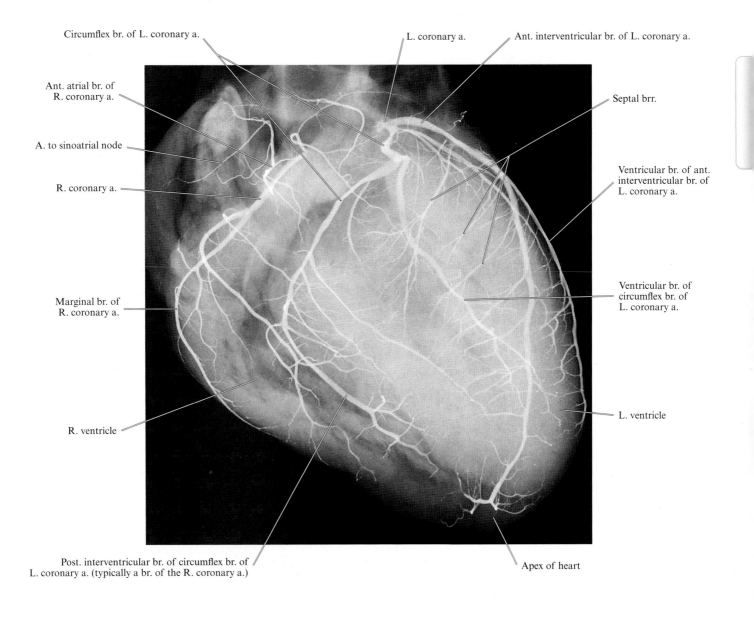

Circumflex br. of L. coronary a.

L. coronary a.

Ant. interventricular br. of L. coronary a.

Ant. atrial br. of
R. coronary a.

Septal brr.

A. to sinoatrial node

R. coronary a.

Ventricular br. of ant.
interventricular br. of
L. coronary a.

Marginal br. of
R. coronary a.

Ventricular br. of
circumflex br. of
L. coronary a.

L. ventricle

R. ventricle

Post. interventricular br. of circumflex br. of
L. coronary a. (typically a br. of the R. coronary a.)

Apex of heart

Anteroposterior View

PLATE 2.21   CORONARY ARTERIES

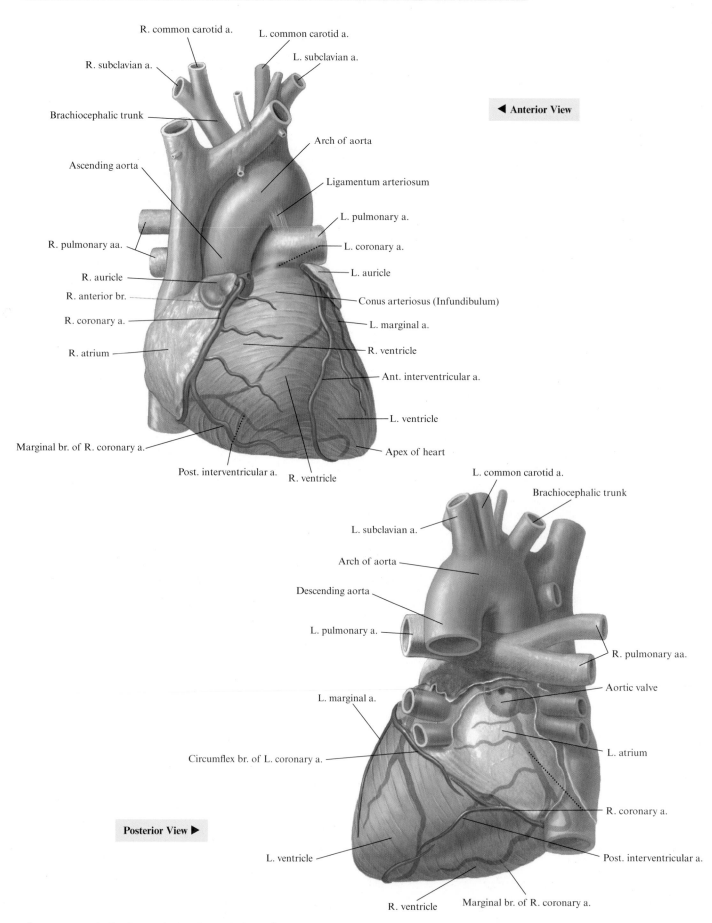

R. common carotid a.

L. common carotid a.

R. subclavian a.

L. subclavian a.

Brachiocephalic trunk

◀ Anterior View

Arch of aorta

Ascending aorta

Ligamentum arteriosum

L. pulmonary a.

R. pulmonary aa.

L. coronary a.

R. auricle

L. auricle

R. anterior br.

Conus arteriosus (Infundibulum)

R. coronary a.

L. marginal a.

R. atrium

R. ventricle

Ant. interventricular a.

L. ventricle

Marginal br. of R. coronary a.

Apex of heart

Post. interventricular a.   R. ventricle

L. common carotid a.

Brachiocephalic trunk

L. subclavian a.

Arch of aorta

Descending aorta

L. pulmonary a.

R. pulmonary aa.

Aortic valve

L. marginal a.

Circumflex br. of L. coronary a.

L. atrium

R. coronary a.

Posterior View ▶

L. ventricle

Post. interventricular a.

R. ventricle   Marginal br. of R. coronary a.

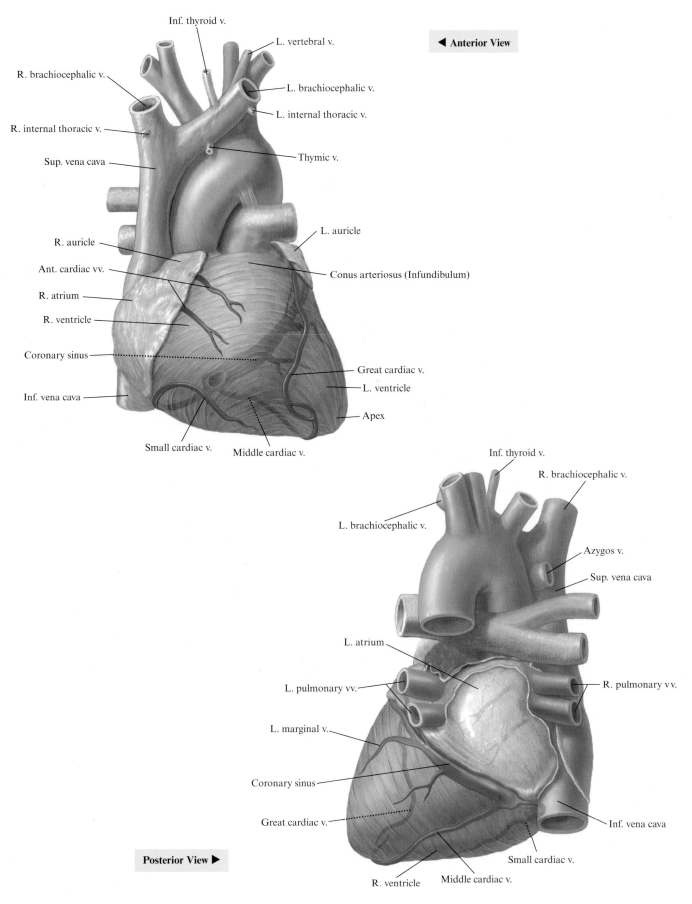

◀ Anterior View

Inf. thyroid v.

L. vertebral v.

R. brachiocephalic v.

L. brachiocephalic v.

L. internal thoracic v.

R. internal thoracic v.

Thymic v.

Sup. vena cava

L. auricle

R. auricle

Ant. cardiac vv.

Conus arteriosus (Infundibulum)

R. atrium

R. ventricle

Coronary sinus

Great cardiac v.

L. ventricle

Inf. vena cava

Apex

Small cardiac v.

Middle cardiac v.

Inf. thyroid v.

R. brachiocephalic v.

L. brachiocephalic v.

Azygos v.

Sup. vena cava

L. atrium

L. pulmonary vv.

R. pulmonary vv.

L. marginal v.

Coronary sinus

Great cardiac v.

Inf. vena cava

Small cardiac v.

Posterior View ▶

R. ventricle   Middle cardiac v.

PLATE 2.23   RIGHT ATRIUM

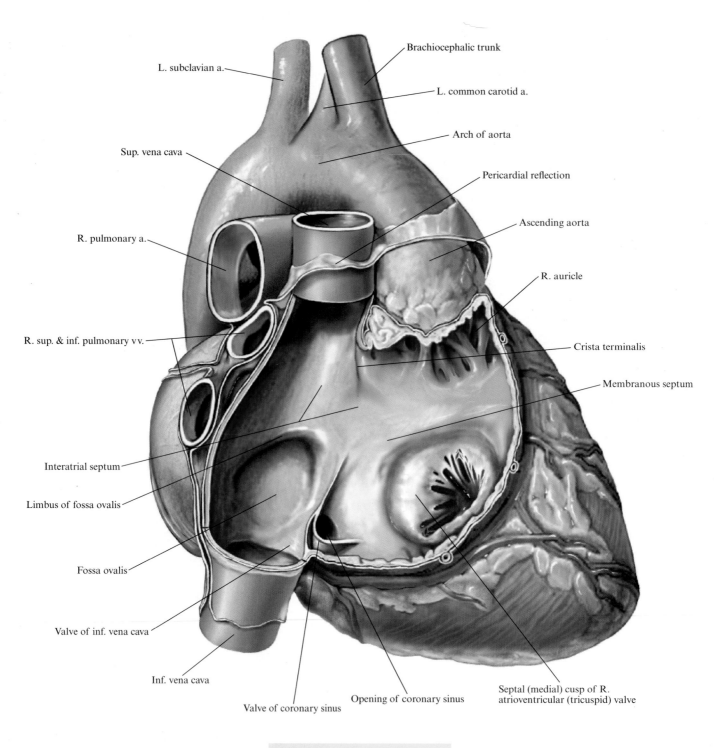

L. subclavian a.

Sup. vena cava

R. pulmonary a.

R. sup. & inf. pulmonary vv.

Interatrial septum

Limbus of fossa ovalis

Fossa ovalis

Valve of inf. vena cava

Inf. vena cava

Valve of coronary sinus

Brachiocephalic trunk

L. common carotid a.

Arch of aorta

Pericardial reflection

Ascending aorta

R. auricle

Crista terminalis

Membranous septum

Septal (medial) cusp of R. atrioventricular (tricuspid) valve

Opening of coronary sinus

Lateral View of Opened Right Atrium

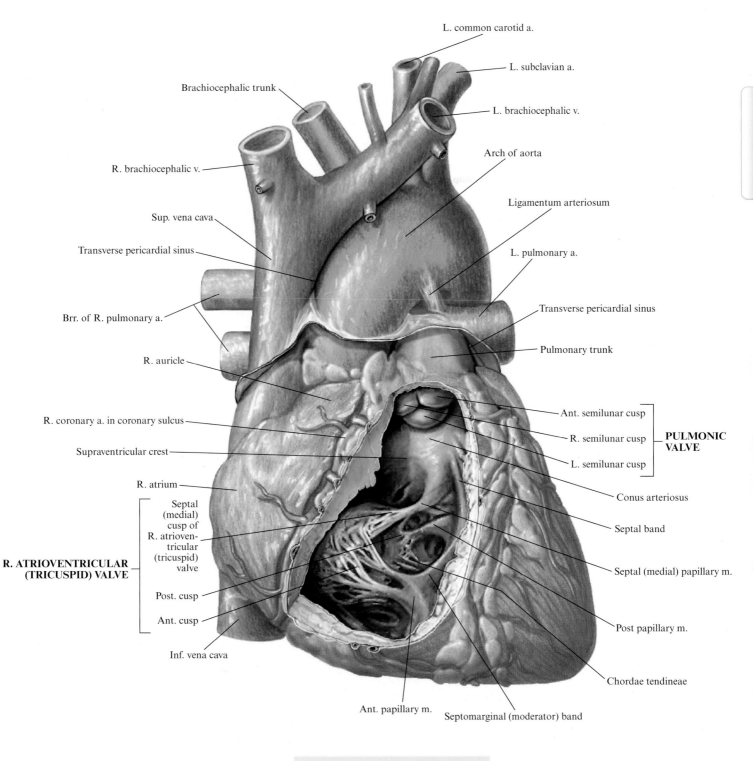

L. common carotid a.

L. subclavian a.

Brachiocephalic trunk

L. brachiocephalic v.

R. brachiocephalic v.

Arch of aorta

Sup. vena cava

Ligamentum arteriosum

Transverse pericardial sinus

L. pulmonary a.

Brr. of R. pulmonary a.

Transverse pericardial sinus

R. auricle

Pulmonary trunk

R. coronary a. in coronary sulcus

Ant. semilunar cusp

R. semilunar cusp

PULMONIC VALVE

Supraventricular crest

L. semilunar cusp

R. atrium

Conus arteriosus

Septal (medial) cusp of R. atrioventricular (tricuspid) valve

Septal band

R. ATRIOVENTRICULAR (TRICUSPID) VALVE

Septal (medial) papillary m.

Post. cusp

Ant. cusp

Post papillary m.

Inf. vena cava

Chordae tendineae

Ant. papillary m.   Septomarginal (moderator) band

Anterior View of Opened Right Ventricle

PLATE 2.25   LEFT ATRIUM & VENTRICLE

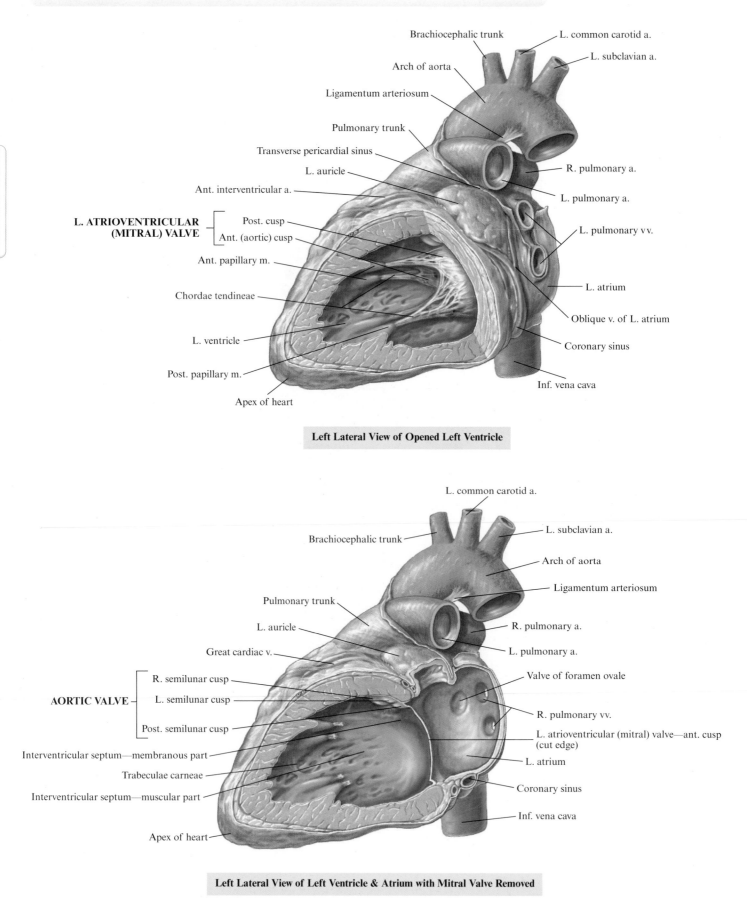

Brachiocephalic trunk

L. common carotid a.

L. subclavian a.

Arch of aorta

Ligamentum arteriosum

Pulmonary trunk

Transverse pericardial sinus

L. auricle

R. pulmonary a.

Ant. interventricular a.

L. pulmonary a.

L. ATRIOVENTRICULAR (MITRAL) VALVE { Post. cusp

Ant. (aortic) cusp

L. pulmonary vv.

Ant. papillary m.

Chordae tendineae

L. atrium

Oblique v. of L. atrium

L. ventricle

Coronary sinus

Post. papillary m.

Inf. vena cava

Apex of heart

Left Lateral View of Opened Left Ventricle

L. common carotid a.

L. subclavian a.

Brachiocephalic trunk

Arch of aorta

Ligamentum arteriosum

Pulmonary trunk

R. pulmonary a.

L. auricle

L. pulmonary a.

Great cardiac v.

Valve of foramen ovale

AORTIC VALVE { R. semilunar cusp

L. semilunar cusp

R. pulmonary vv.

Post. semilunar cusp

L. atrioventricular (mitral) valve—ant. cusp (cut edge)

Interventricular septum—membranous part

L. atrium

Trabeculae carneae

Coronary sinus

Interventricular septum—muscular part

Inf. vena cava

Apex of heart

Left Lateral View of Left Ventricle & Atrium with Mitral Valve Removed

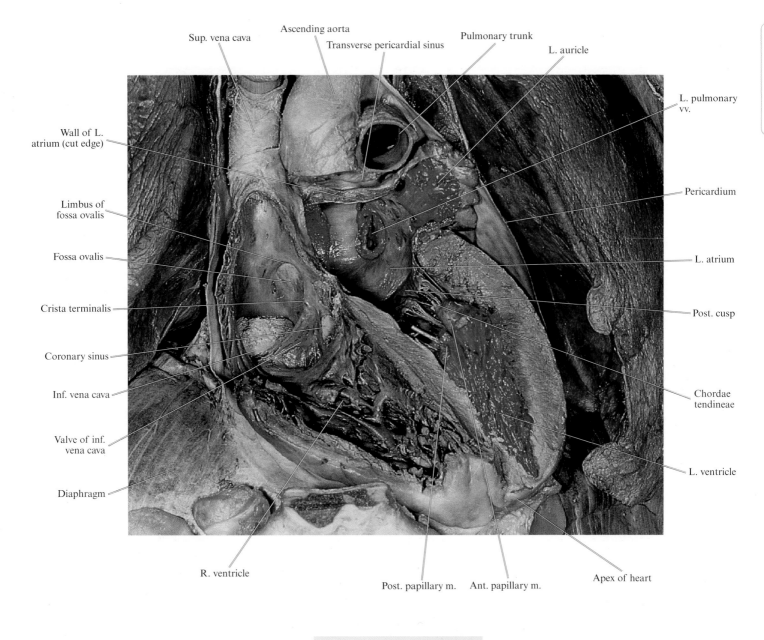

Sup. vena cava

Ascending aorta

Transverse pericardial sinus

Pulmonary trunk

L. auricle

L. pulmonary vv.

Wall of L. atrium (cut edge)

Pericardium

Limbus of fossa ovalis

Fossa ovalis

L. atrium

Crista terminalis

Post. cusp

Coronary sinus

Inf. vena cava

Chordae tendineae

Valve of inf. vena cava

L. ventricle

Diaphragm

R. ventricle

Post. papillary m.   Ant. papillary m.

Apex of heart

Interior of Anterior View of Heart

PLATE 2.27   PERICARDIAL CAVITY

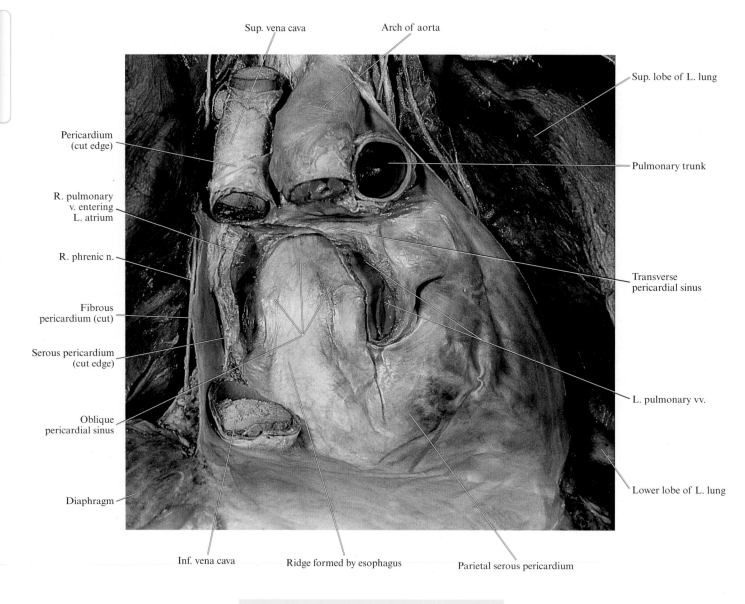

Sup. vena cava

Arch of aorta

Sup. lobe of L. lung

Pericardium
(cut edge)

Pulmonary trunk

R. pulmonary
v. entering
L. atrium

R. phrenic n.

Transverse
pericardial sinus

Fibrous
pericardium (cut)

Serous pericardium
(cut edge)

L. pulmonary vv.

Oblique
pericardial sinus

Lower lobe of L. lung

Diaphragm

Inf. vena cava

Ridge formed by esophagus

Parietal serous pericardium

Anterior View of Pericardial Cavity with Heart Removed

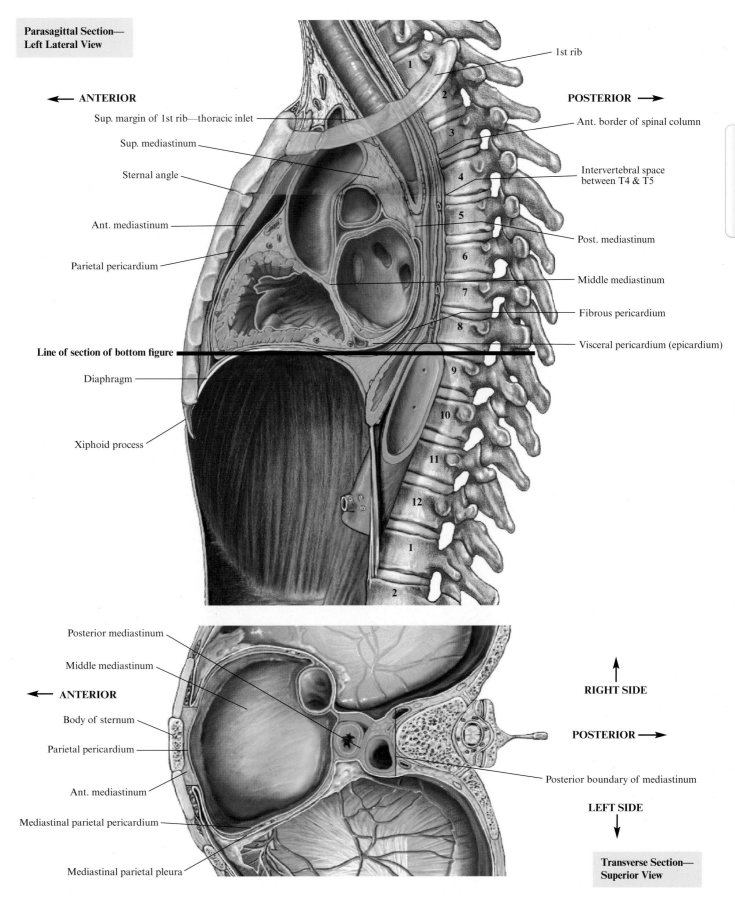

Parasagittal Section—
Left Lateral View

← ANTERIOR

Sup. margin of 1st rib—thoracic inlet

Sup. mediastinum

Sternal angle

Ant. mediastinum

Parietal pericardium

Line of section of bottom figure

Diaphragm

Xiphoid process

1st rib

POSTERIOR →

Ant. border of spinal column

Intervertebral space
between T4 & T5

Post. mediastinum

Middle mediastinum

Fibrous pericardium

Visceral pericardium (epicardium)

Posterior mediastinum

Middle mediastinum

← ANTERIOR

Body of sternum

Parietal pericardium

Ant. mediastinum

Mediastinal parietal pericardium

Mediastinal parietal pleura

RIGHT SIDE

POSTERIOR →

Posterior boundary of mediastinum

LEFT SIDE

Transverse Section—
Superior View

PLATE 2.29   MEDIASTINUM—LEFT LATERAL VIEW

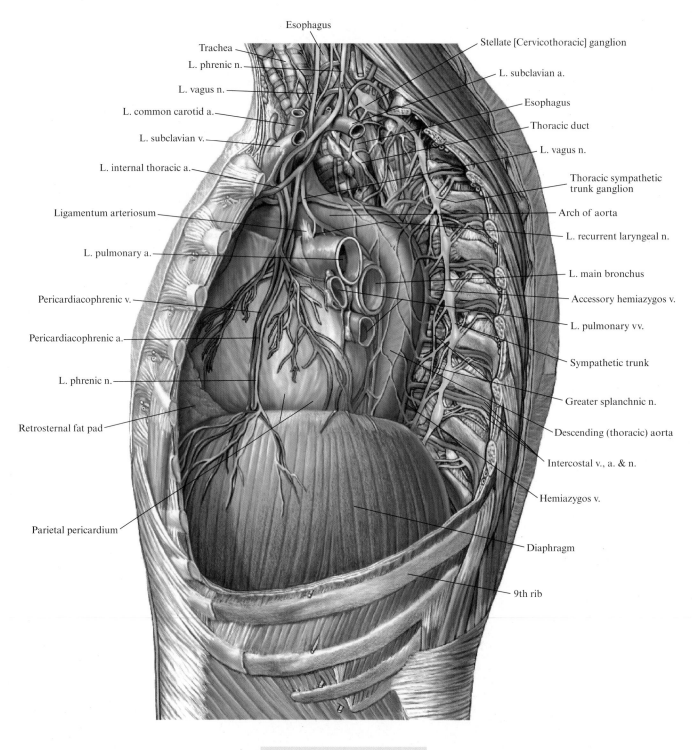

Esophagus

Trachea

L. phrenic n.

L. vagus n.

L. common carotid a.

L. subclavian v.

L. internal thoracic a.

Ligamentum arteriosum

L. pulmonary a.

Pericardiacophrenic v.

Pericardiacophrenic a.

L. phrenic n.

Retrosternal fat pad

Parietal pericardium

Stellate [Cervicothoracic] ganglion

L. subclavian a.

Esophagus

Thoracic duct

L. vagus n.

Thoracic sympathetic trunk ganglion

Arch of aorta

L. recurrent laryngeal n.

L. main bronchus

Accessory hemiazygos v.

L. pulmonary vv.

Sympathetic trunk

Greater splanchnic n.

Descending (thoracic) aorta

Intercostal v., a. & n.

Hemiazygos v.

Diaphragm

9th rib

Left Lateral View of Mediastinum

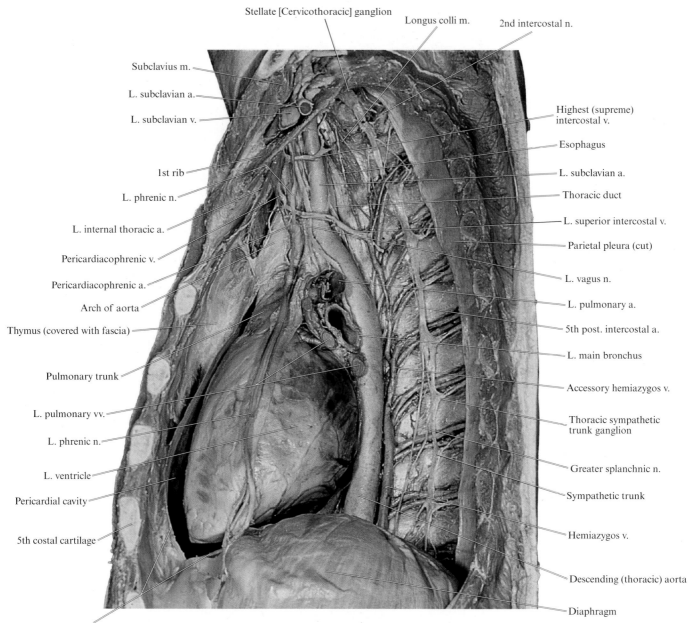

Stellate [Cervicothoracic] ganglion

Longus colli m.

2nd intercostal n.

Subclavius m.

L. subclavian a.

L. subclavian v.

Highest (supreme) intercostal v.

Esophagus

1st rib

L. subclavian a.

L. phrenic n.

Thoracic duct

L. internal thoracic a.

L. superior intercostal v.

Pericardiacophrenic v.

Parietal pleura (cut)

Pericardiacophrenic a.

L. vagus n.

Arch of aorta

L. pulmonary a.

Thymus (covered with fascia)

5th post. intercostal a.

L. main bronchus

Pulmonary trunk

Accessory hemiazygos v.

L. pulmonary vv.

Thoracic sympathetic trunk ganglion

L. phrenic n.

L. ventricle

Greater splanchnic n.

Pericardial cavity

Sympathetic trunk

5th costal cartilage

Hemiazygos v.

Descending (thoracic) aorta

Diaphragm

Parietal pericardium (cut edge)

Left Lateral View of Mediastinum

PLATE 2.31   MEDIASTINUM—RIGHT LATERAL VIEW

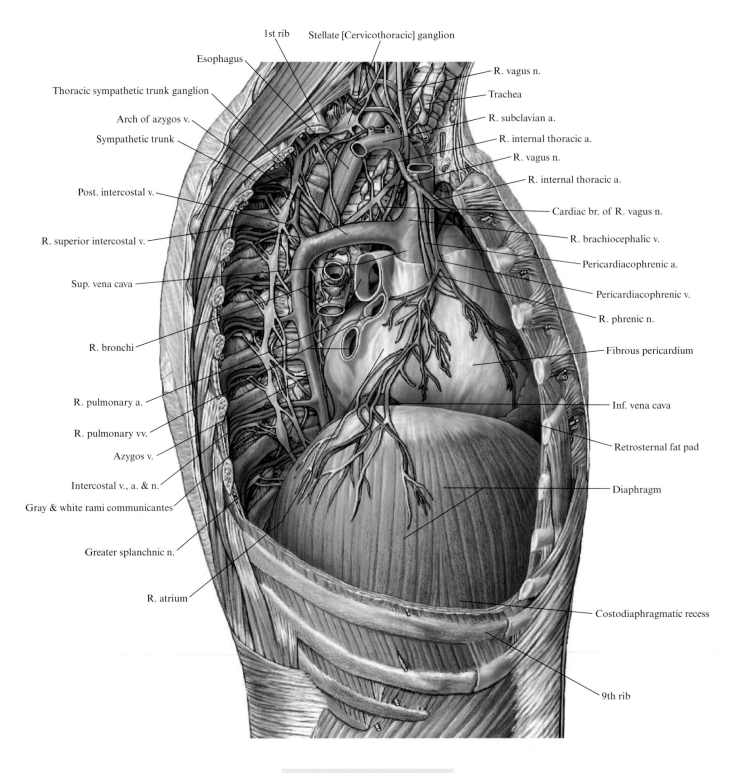

1st rib

Stellate [Cervicothoracic] ganglion

Esophagus

Thoracic sympathetic trunk ganglion

Arch of azygos v.

Sympathetic trunk

Post. intercostal v.

R. superior intercostal v.

Sup. vena cava

R. bronchi

R. pulmonary a.

R. pulmonary vv.

Azygos v.

Intercostal v., a. & n.

Gray & white rami communicantes

Greater splanchnic n.

R. atrium

R. vagus n.

Trachea

R. subclavian a.

R. internal thoracic a.

R. vagus n.

R. internal thoracic a.

Cardiac br. of R. vagus n.

R. brachiocephalic v.

Pericardiacophrenic a.

Pericardiacophrenic v.

R. phrenic n.

Fibrous pericardium

Inf. vena cava

Retrosternal fat pad

Diaphragm

Costodiaphragmatic recess

9th rib

Right Lateral View of Mediastinum

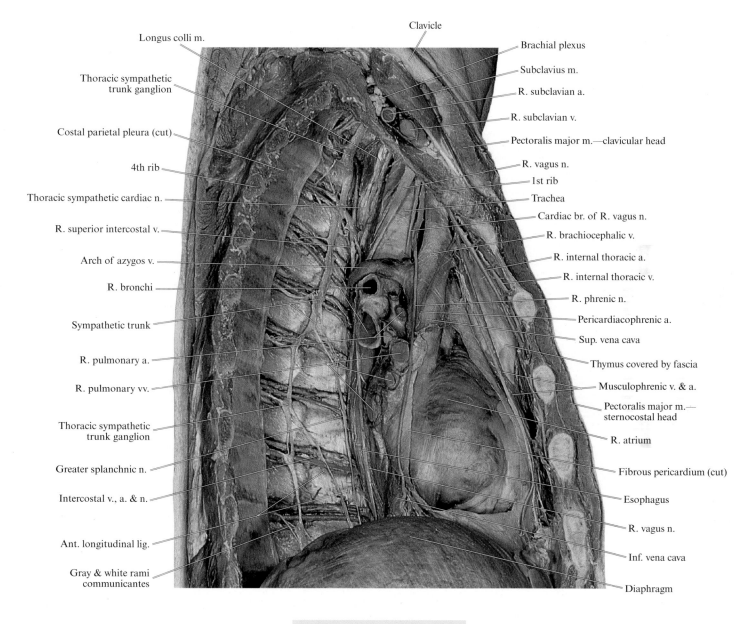

Clavicle

Longus colli m.

Thoracic sympathetic
trunk ganglion

Costal parietal pleura (cut)

4th rib

Thoracic sympathetic cardiac n.

R. superior intercostal v.

Arch of azygos v.

R. bronchi

Sympathetic trunk

R. pulmonary a.

R. pulmonary vv.

Thoracic sympathetic
trunk ganglion

Greater splanchnic n.

Intercostal v., a. & n.

Ant. longitudinal lig.

Gray & white rami
communicantes

Brachial plexus

Subclavius m.

R. subclavian a.

R. subclavian v.

Pectoralis major m.—clavicular head

R. vagus n.

1st rib

Trachea

Cardiac br. of R. vagus n.

R. brachiocephalic v.

R. internal thoracic a.

R. internal thoracic v.

R. phrenic n.

Pericardiacophrenic a.

Sup. vena cava

Thymus covered by fascia

Pectoralis major m.—
sternocostal head

R. atrium

Fibrous pericardium (cut)

Esophagus

R. vagus n.

Inf. vena cava

Diaphragm

Right Lateral View of Mediastinum

PLATE 2.33   PARAVERTEBRAL STRUCTURES—RIGHT

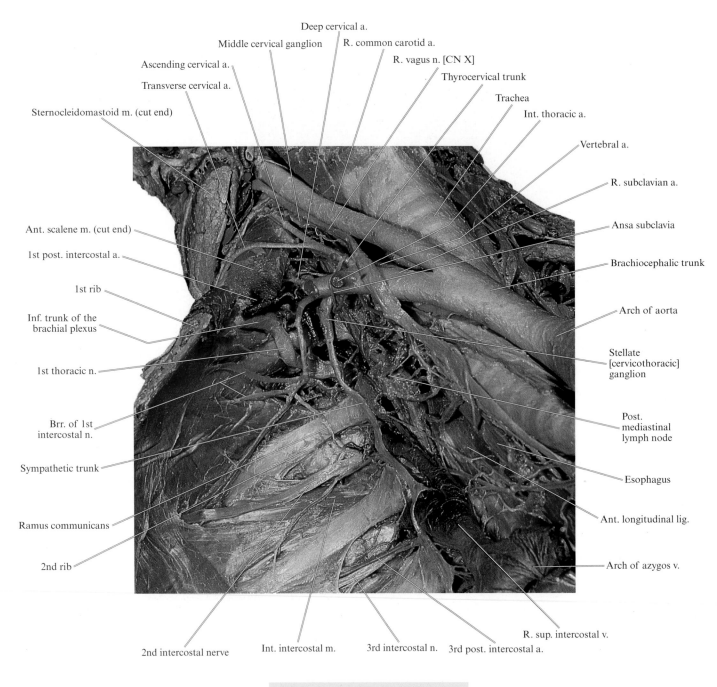

Deep cervical a.

Middle cervical ganglion

R. common carotid a.

Ascending cervical a.

R. vagus n. [CN X]

Transverse cervical a.

Thyrocervical trunk

Trachea

Sternocleidomastoid m. (cut end)

Int. thoracic a.

Vertebral a.

Ant. scalene m. (cut end)

R. subclavian a.

1st post. intercostal a.

Ansa subclavia

1st rib

Brachiocephalic trunk

Inf. trunk of the
brachial plexus

Arch of aorta

1st thoracic n.

Stellate
[cervicothoracic]
ganglion

Brr. of 1st
intercostal n.

Post.
mediastinal
lymph node

Sympathetic trunk

Esophagus

Ramus communicans

Ant. longitudinal lig.

2nd rib

Arch of azygos v.

R. sup. intercostal v.

2nd intercostal nerve   Int. intercostal m.   3rd intercostal n.   3rd post. intercostal a.

Right Anterolateral Inferior Oblique View

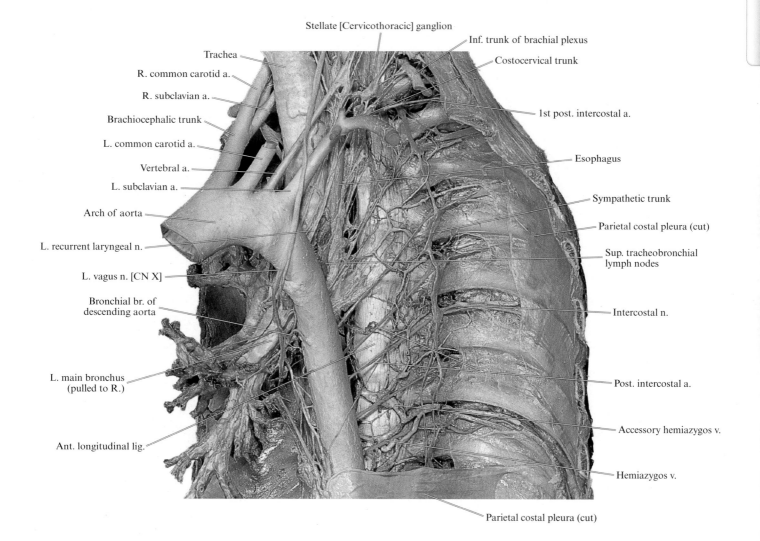

Stellate [Cervicothoracic] ganglion

Inf. trunk of brachial plexus

Trachea

Costocervical trunk

R. common carotid a.

R. subclavian a.

1st post. intercostal a.

Brachiocephalic trunk

L. common carotid a.

Esophagus

Vertebral a.

L. subclavian a.

Sympathetic trunk

Arch of aorta

Parietal costal pleura (cut)

L. recurrent laryngeal n.

Sup. tracheobronchial
lymph nodes

L. vagus n. [CN X]

Bronchial br. of
descending aorta

Intercostal n.

L. main bronchus
(pulled to R.)

Post. intercostal a.

Accessory hemiazygos v.

Ant. longitudinal lig.

Hemiazygos v.

Parietal costal pleura (cut)

Left Anterolateral View

PLATE 2.35   ESOPHAGUS

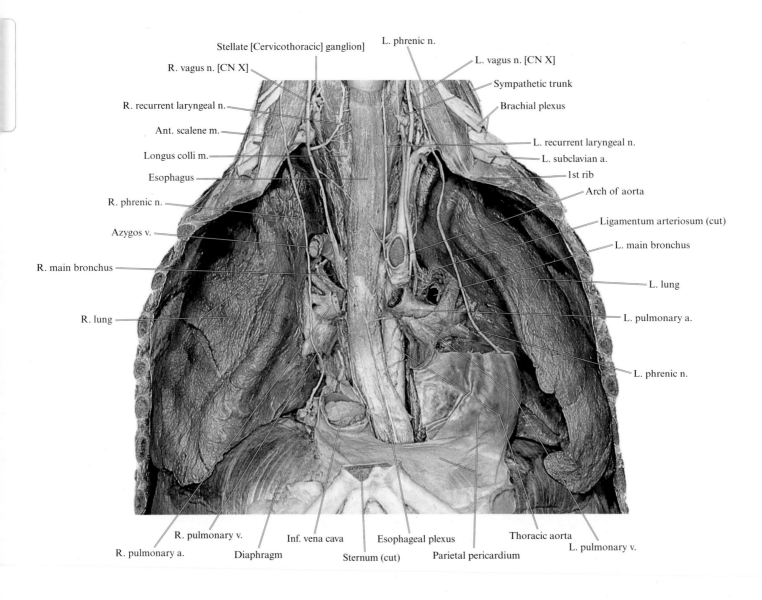

Stellate [Cervicothoracic] ganglion]

L. phrenic n.

R. vagus n. [CN X]

L. vagus n. [CN X]

R. recurrent laryngeal n.

Sympathetic trunk

Brachial plexus

Ant. scalene m.

L. recurrent laryngeal n.

Longus colli m.

L. subclavian a.

Esophagus

1st rib

R. phrenic n.

Arch of aorta

Azygos v.

Ligamentum arteriosum (cut)

L. main bronchus

R. main bronchus

L. lung

R. lung

L. pulmonary a.

L. phrenic n.

R. pulmonary v.

Inf. vena cava

Esophageal plexus

Thoracic aorta

L. pulmonary v.

R. pulmonary a.

Diaphragm

Sternum (cut)

Parietal pericardium

Anterior View of Posterior Mediastinal Structures

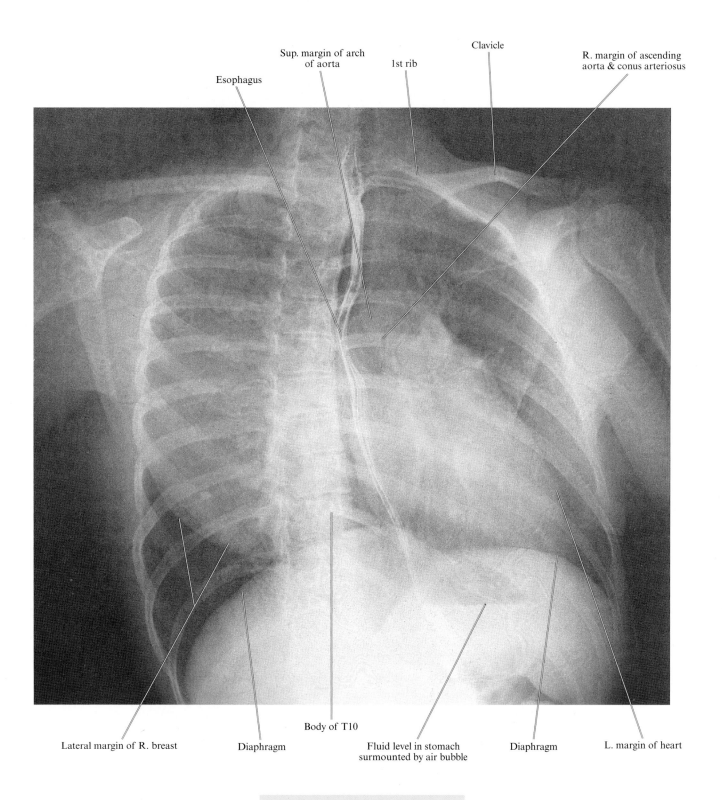

Esophagus

Sup. margin of arch of aorta

1st rib

Clavicle

R. margin of ascending aorta & conus arteriosus

Lateral margin of R. breast

Diaphragm

Body of T10

Fluid level in stomach surmounted by air bubble

Diaphragm

L. margin of heart

Right Anterior Oblique View of Esophagus

PLATE 2.37   SUPERIOR THORACIC APERTURE—LATERAL VIEWS

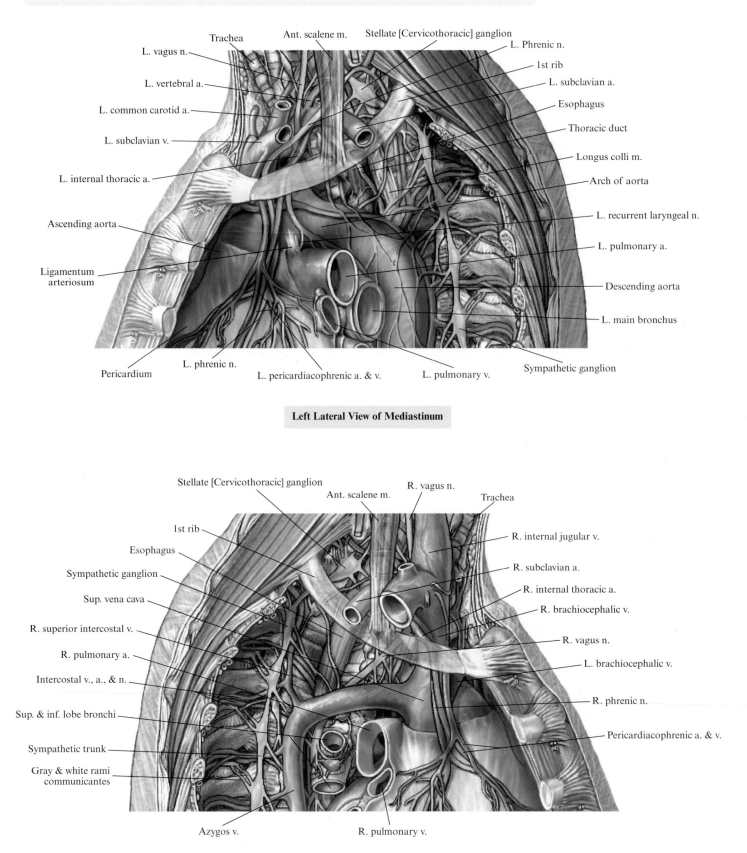

Left Lateral View of Mediastinum

Right Lateral View of Mediastinum

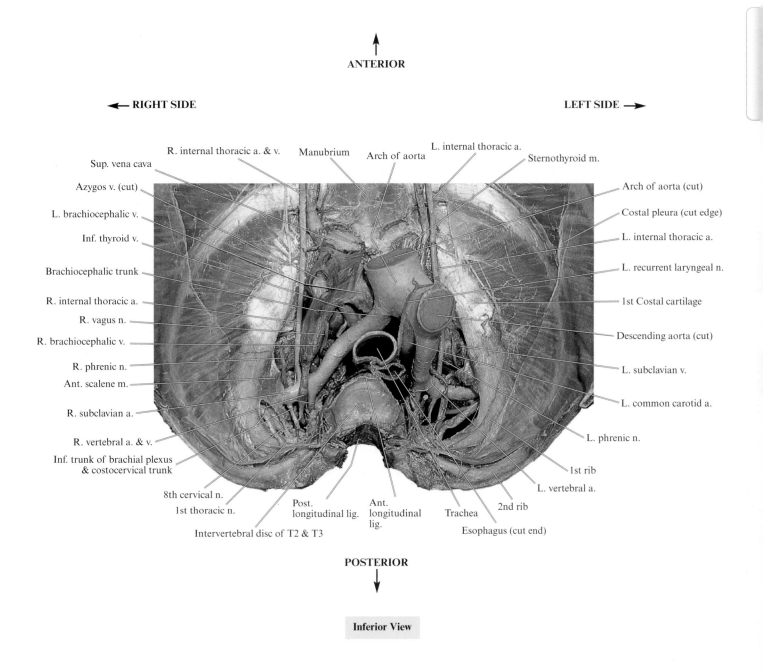

ANTERIOR

← RIGHT SIDE   LEFT SIDE →

R. internal thoracic a. & v.   Manubrium   Arch of aorta   L. internal thoracic a.

Sup. vena cava   Sternothyroid m.

Azygos v. (cut)   Arch of aorta (cut)

L. brachiocephalic v.   Costal pleura (cut edge)

Inf. thyroid v.   L. internal thoracic a.

Brachiocephalic trunk   L. recurrent laryngeal n.

R. internal thoracic a.   1st Costal cartilage

R. vagus n.   Descending aorta (cut)

R. brachiocephalic v.

R. phrenic n.   L. subclavian v.

Ant. scalene m.   L. common carotid a.

R. subclavian a.

R. vertebral a. & v.   L. phrenic n.

Inf. trunk of brachial plexus
& costocervical trunk   1st rib

8th cervical n.   L. vertebral a.

1st thoracic n.   Post.   Ant.   2nd rib
                         longitudinal lig. longitudinal   Trachea
                                            lig.
                                                           Esophagus (cut end)
Intervertebral disc of T2 & T3

POSTERIOR

Inferior View

PLATE 2.39   DIAPHRAGM

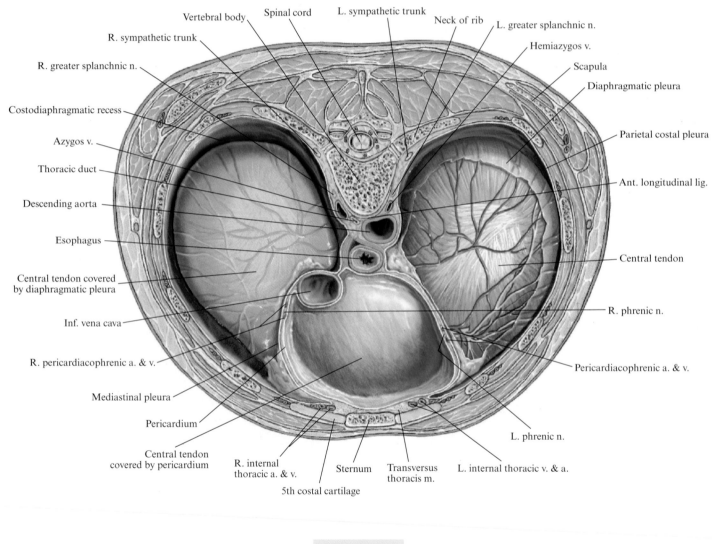

Vertebral body   Spinal cord   L. sympathetic trunk
                                              Neck of rib   L. greater splanchnic n.

R. sympathetic trunk

R. greater splanchnic n.

Hemiazygos v.

Scapula

Diaphragmatic pleura

Costodiaphragmatic recess

Parietal costal pleura

Azygos v.

Thoracic duct

Descending aorta

Ant. longitudinal lig.

Esophagus

Central tendon

Central tendon covered
by diaphragmatic pleura

Inf. vena cava

R. phrenic n.

R. pericardiacophrenic a. & v.

Pericardiacophrenic a. & v.

Mediastinal pleura

Pericardium

L. phrenic n.

Central tendon
covered by pericardium   R. internal
                           thoracic a. & v.   Sternum   Transversus   L. internal thoracic v. & a.
                                                        thoracis m.
                    5th costal cartilage

Superior Surface

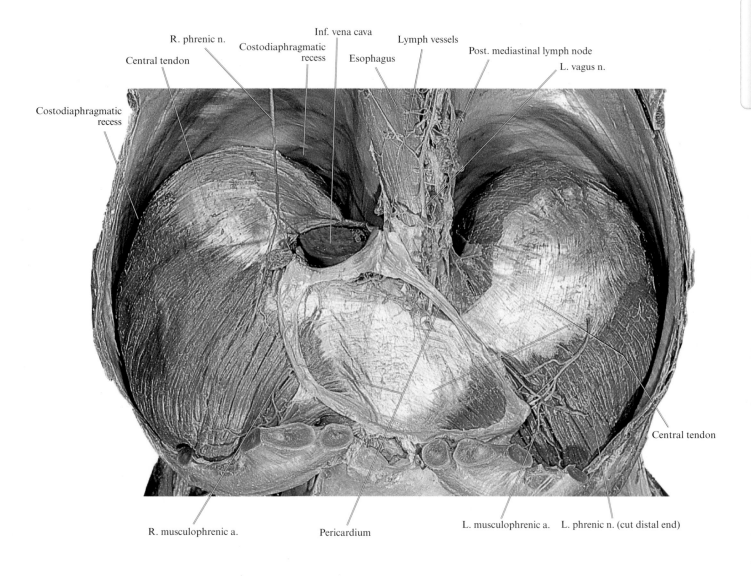

R. phrenic n.

Central tendon

Costodiaphragmatic recess

Costodiaphragmatic recess

Inf. vena cava

Esophagus

Lymph vessels

Post. mediastinal lymph node

L. vagus n.

Central tendon

R. musculophrenic a.

Pericardium

L. musculophrenic a.

L. phrenic n. (cut distal end)

Anterior Superior Oblique View of Superior Surface of Diaphragm

PLATE 2.41 DIAPHRAGM—ABDOMINAL SURFACE

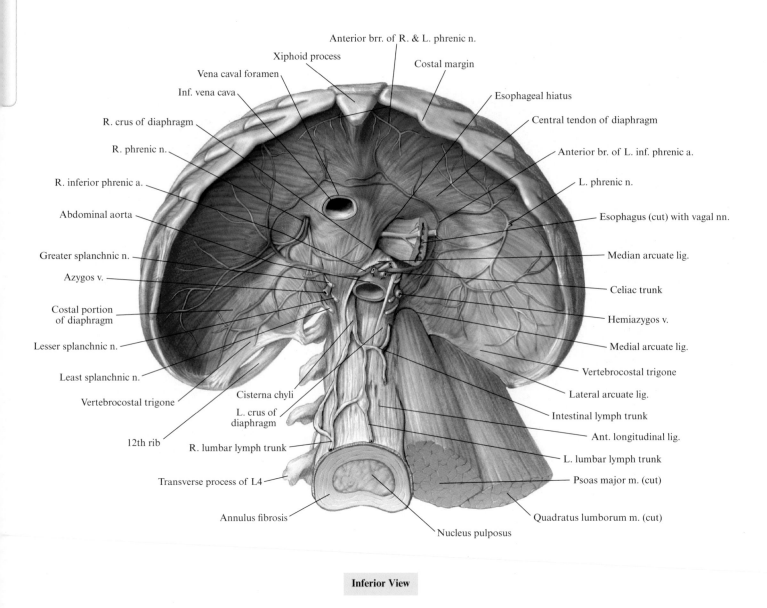

Anterior brr. of R. & L. phrenic n.

Xiphoid process

Vena caval foramen

Costal margin

Inf. vena cava

Esophageal hiatus

R. crus of diaphragm

Central tendon of diaphragm

R. phrenic n.

Anterior br. of L. inf. phrenic a.

R. inferior phrenic a.

L. phrenic n.

Abdominal aorta

Esophagus (cut) with vagal nn.

Greater splanchnic n.

Median arcuate lig.

Azygos v.

Celiac trunk

Costal portion of diaphragm

Hemiazygos v.

Lesser splanchnic n.

Medial arcuate lig.

Least splanchnic n.

Vertebrocostal trigone

Vertebrocostal trigone

Lateral arcuate lig.

Cisterna chyli

Intestinal lymph trunk

L. crus of diaphragm

Ant. longitudinal lig.

12th rib

R. lumbar lymph trunk

L. lumbar lymph trunk

Transverse process of L4

Psoas major m. (cut)

Annulus fibrosis

Quadratus lumborum m. (cut)

Nucleus pulposus

Inferior View

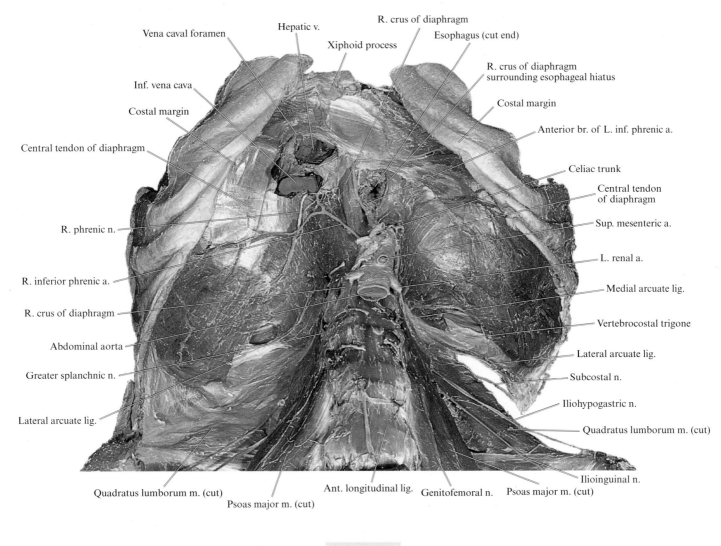

Vena caval foramen

Hepatic v.

R. crus of diaphragm

Xiphoid process

Esophagus (cut end)

Inf. vena cava

R. crus of diaphragm
surrounding esophageal hiatus

Costal margin

Costal margin

Central tendon of diaphragm

Anterior br. of L. inf. phrenic a.

Celiac trunk

Central tendon
of diaphragm

R. phrenic n.

Sup. mesenteric a.

R. inferior phrenic a.

L. renal a.

Medial arcuate lig.

R. crus of diaphragm

Vertebrocostal trigone

Abdominal aorta

Lateral arcuate lig.

Greater splanchnic n.

Subcostal n.

Iliohypogastric n.

Lateral arcuate lig.

Quadratus lumborum m. (cut)

Ilioinguinal n.

Quadratus lumborum m. (cut)

Psoas major m. (cut)

Ant. longitudinal lig.

Genitofemoral n.

Psoas major m. (cut)

Inferior View

3 ABDOMEN

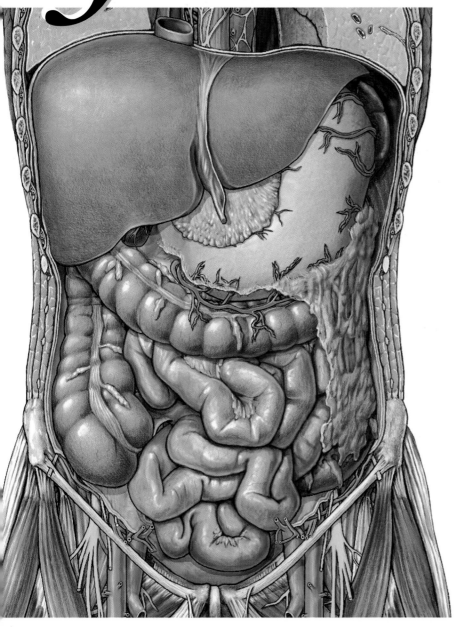

TOPOGRAPHY

PERITONEAL CAVITY

STOMACH

PANCREAS

GALLBLADDER &
DUCTS

LIVER

SMALL INTESTINES

LARGE INTESTINES

POSTERIOR ABDOMINAL
WALL

KIDNEYS &
SUPRARENAL GLANDS

PLATE 3.1   TOPOGRAPHY—ABDOMINAL PLANES & LINES

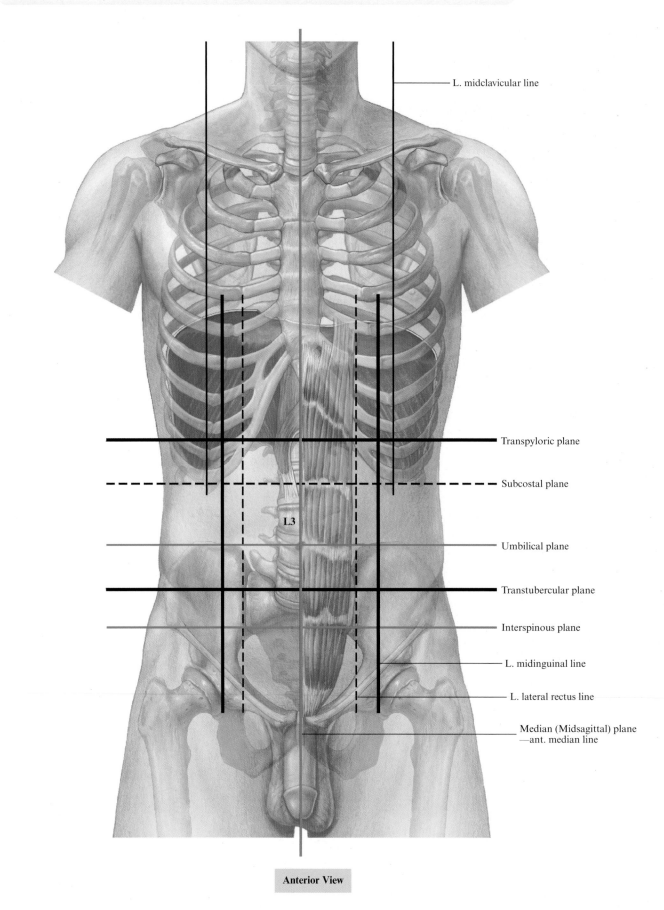

L. midclavicular line

Transpyloric plane

Subcostal plane

L3

Umbilical plane

Transtubercular plane

Interspinous plane

L. midinguinal line

L. lateral rectus line

Median (Midsagittal) plane
—ant. median line

Anterior View

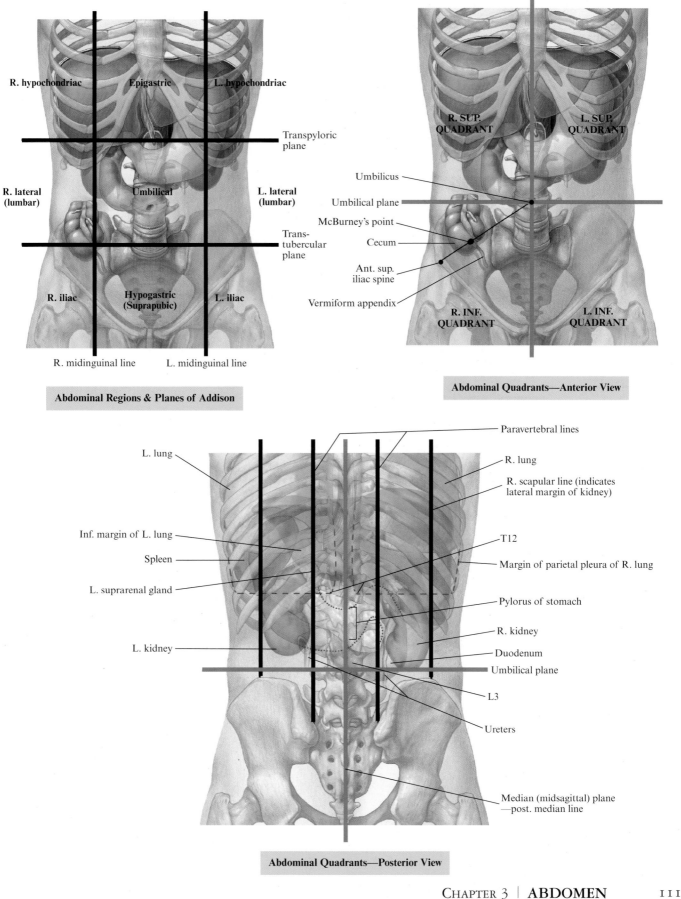

Median midsagittal plane

R. hypochondriac   **Epigastric**   **L. hypochondriac**

Transpyloric plane

R. lateral (lumbar)   **Umbilical**   **L. lateral (lumbar)**

Trans-tubercular plane

R. iliac   **Hypogastric (Suprapubic)**   **L. iliac**

R. midinguinal line   L. midinguinal line

Abdominal Regions & Planes of Addison

R. SUP. QUADRANT   **L. SUP. QUADRANT**

Umbilicus

Umbilical plane

McBurney's point

Cecum

Ant. sup. iliac spine

Vermiform appendix

R. INF. QUADRANT   **L. INF. QUADRANT**

Abdominal Quadrants—Anterior View

Paravertebral lines

L. lung

R. lung

R. scapular line (indicates lateral margin of kidney)

Inf. margin of L. lung

T12

Spleen

Margin of parietal pleura of R. lung

L. suprarenal gland

Pylorus of stomach

R. kidney

L. kidney

Duodenum

Umbilical plane

L3

Ureters

Median (midsagittal) plane —post. median line

Abdominal Quadrants—Posterior View

PLATE 3.3   PERITONEAL CAVITY

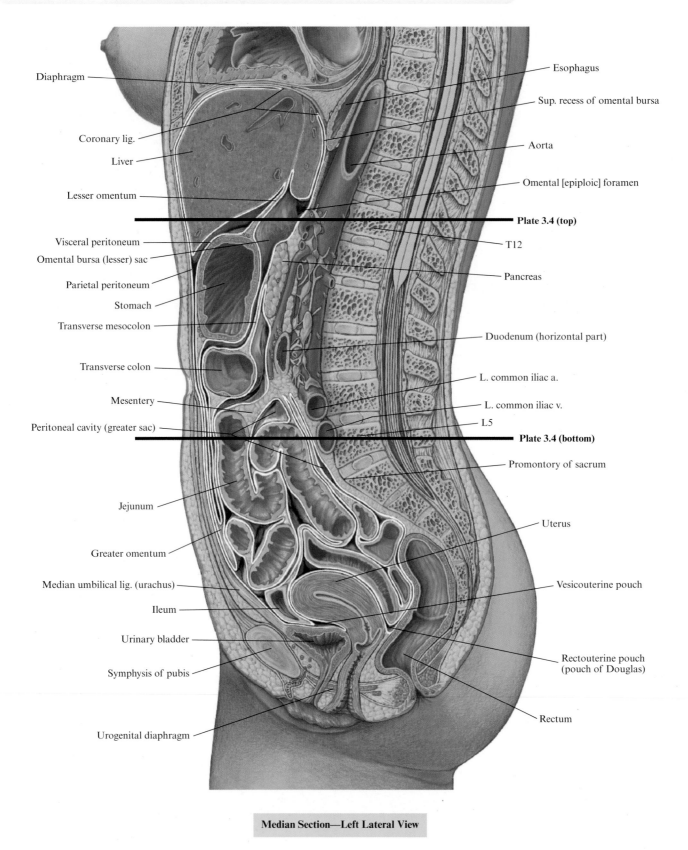

Diaphragm

Coronary lig.

Liver

Lesser omentum

Visceral peritoneum

Omental bursa (lesser) sac

Parietal peritoneum

Stomach

Transverse mesocolon

Transverse colon

Mesentery

Peritoneal cavity (greater sac)

Jejunum

Greater omentum

Median umbilical lig. (urachus)

Ileum

Urinary bladder

Symphysis of pubis

Urogenital diaphragm

Esophagus

Sup. recess of omental bursa

Aorta

Omental [epiploic] foramen

Plate 3.4 (top)

T12

Pancreas

Duodenum (horizontal part)

L. common iliac a.

L. common iliac v.

L5

Plate 3.4 (bottom)

Promontory of sacrum

Uterus

Vesicouterine pouch

Rectouterine pouch
(pouch of Douglas)

Rectum

Median Section—Left Lateral View

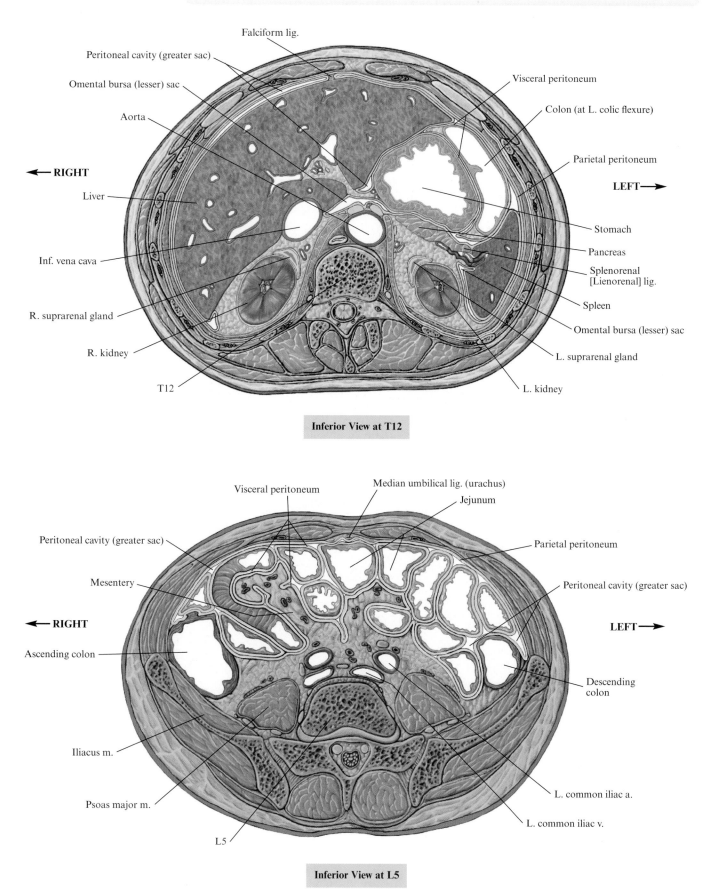

Falciform lig.

Peritoneal cavity (greater sac)

Omental bursa (lesser) sac

Aorta

Visceral peritoneum

Colon (at L. colic flexure)

Parietal peritoneum

←— RIGHT

LEFT —→

Liver

Stomach

Pancreas

Inf. vena cava

Splenorenal [Lienorenal] lig.

Spleen

R. suprarenal gland

Omental bursa (lesser) sac

R. kidney

L. suprarenal gland

T12

L. kidney

Inferior View at T12

Visceral peritoneum

Median umbilical lig. (urachus)

Jejunum

Peritoneal cavity (greater sac)

Parietal peritoneum

Mesentery

Peritoneal cavity (greater sac)

←— RIGHT

LEFT —→

Ascending colon

Descending colon

Iliacus m.

Psoas major m.

L. common iliac a.

L. common iliac v.

L5

Inferior View at L5

PLATE 3.5   PERITONEAL CAVITY—CONTENTS

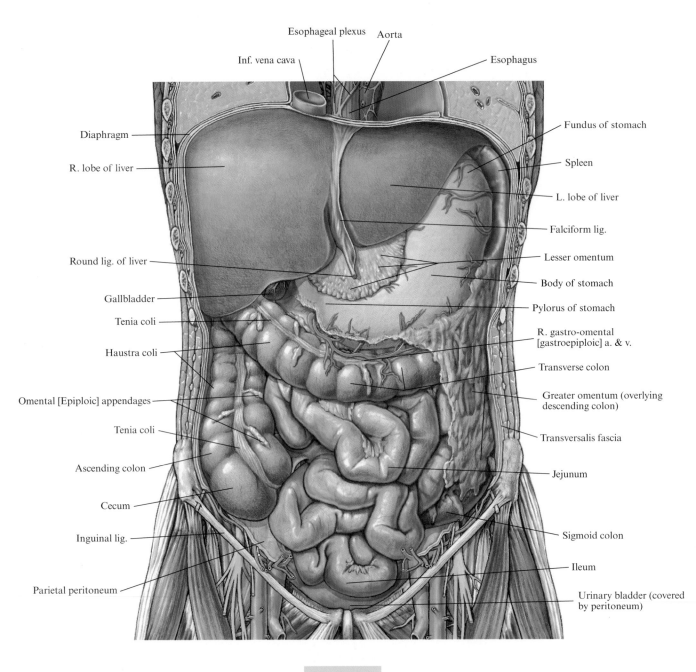

Esophageal plexus
Aorta
Inf. vena cava
Esophagus
Diaphragm
Fundus of stomach
R. lobe of liver
Spleen
L. lobe of liver
Falciform lig.
Round lig. of liver
Lesser omentum
Gallbladder
Body of stomach
Tenia coli
Pylorus of stomach
Haustra coli
R. gastro-omental [gastroepiploic] a. & v.
Transverse colon
Omental [Epiploic] appendages
Greater omentum (overlying descending colon)
Tenia coli
Transversalis fascia
Ascending colon
Cecum
Jejunum
Inguinal lig.
Sigmoid colon
Ileum
Parietal peritoneum
Urinary bladder (covered by peritoneum)

Anterior View

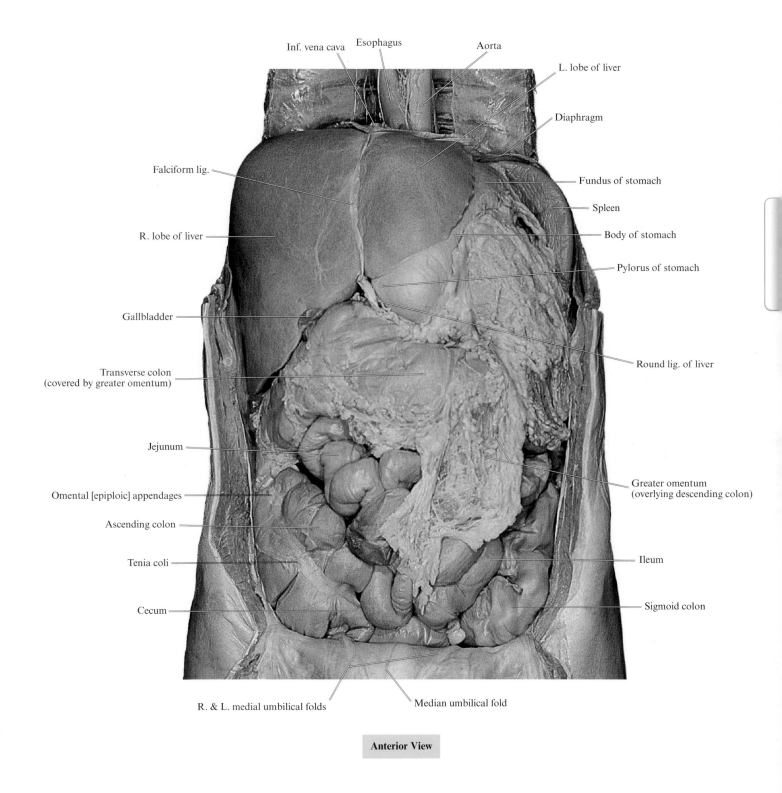

Inf. vena cava   Esophagus   Aorta

L. lobe of liver

Diaphragm

Falciform lig.

Fundus of stomach

Spleen

R. lobe of liver

Body of stomach

Pylorus of stomach

Gallbladder

Transverse colon
(covered by greater omentum)

Round lig. of liver

Jejunum

Omental [epiploic] appendages

Greater omentum
(overlying descending colon)

Ascending colon

Tenia coli

Ileum

Cecum

Sigmoid colon

R. & L. medial umbilical folds   Median umbilical fold

Anterior View

PLATE 3.7   PERITONEAL CAVITY—CONTENTS

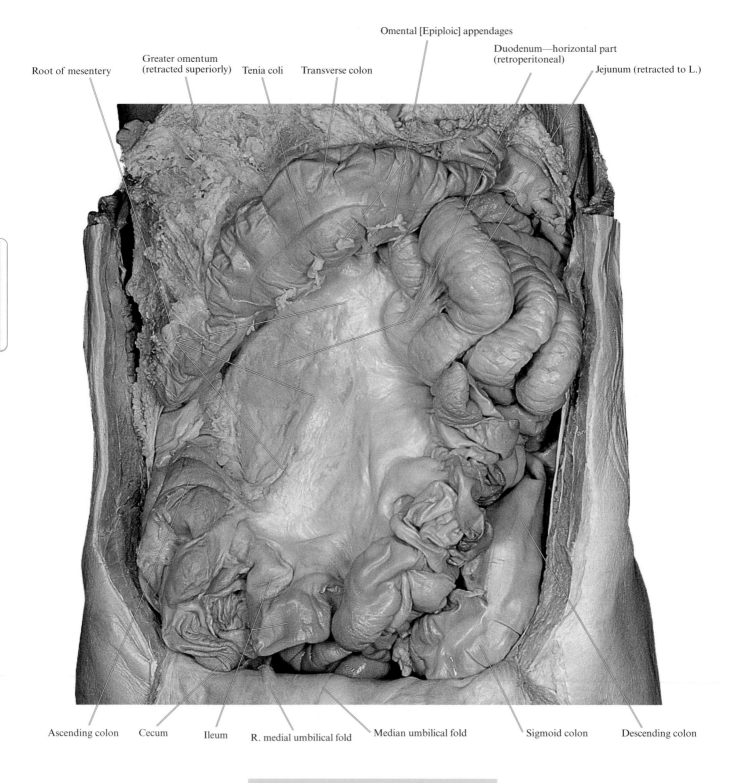

Omental [Epiploic] appendages

Duodenum—horizontal part
(retroperitoneal)

Root of mesentery   Greater omentum   Tenia coli   Transverse colon   Jejunum (retracted to L.)
(retracted superiorly)

Ascending colon   Cecum   Ileum   R. medial umbilical fold   Median umbilical fold   Sigmoid colon   Descending colon

Anterior View with Small Intestines Retracted to Left

Greater splanchnic n.

Hemiazygos v.

Fundus of stomach

Sympathetic
trunk

Spleen

Aorta

Intercostal v., a. & n.

Esophagus with esophageal plexus

Abdominal esophagus

Body of stomach

Coronary lig. of liver (cut)

L. lobe of liver
(retracted to R.)

Falciform lig.

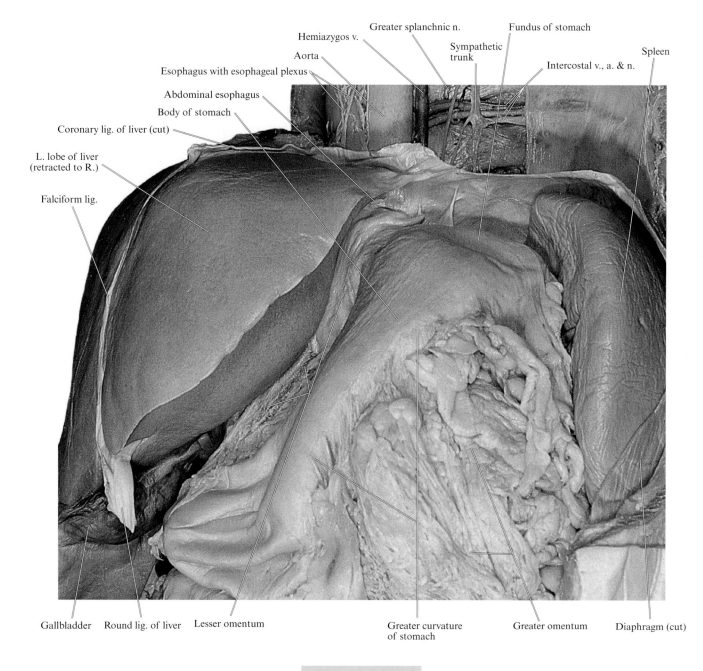

Gallbladder   Round lig. of liver   Lesser omentum

Greater curvature
of stomach

Greater omentum   Diaphragm (cut)

Left Anterolateral View

PLATE 3.9   STOMACH

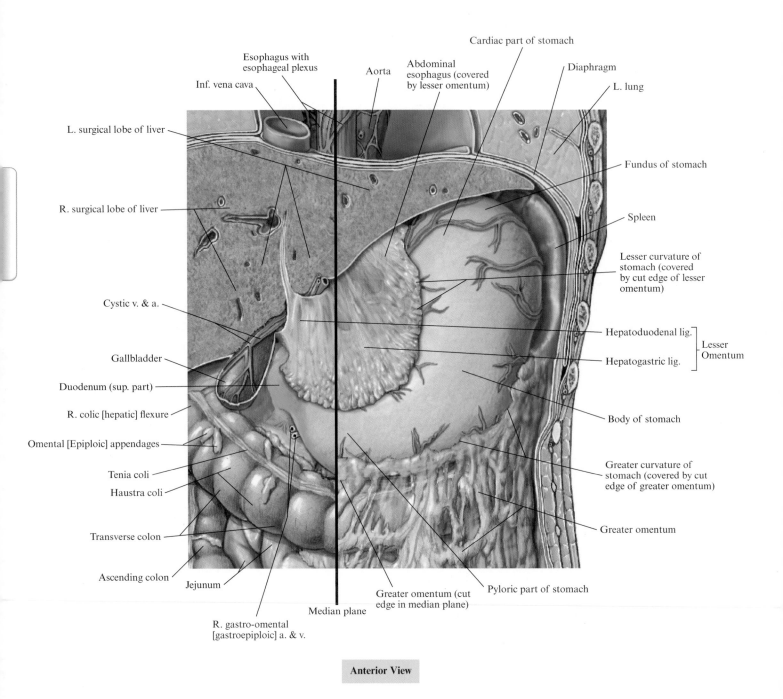

Cardiac part of stomach

Esophagus with
esophageal plexus

Aorta

Abdominal
esophagus (covered
by lesser omentum)

Diaphragm

Inf. vena cava

L. lung

L. surgical lobe of liver

Fundus of stomach

R. surgical lobe of liver

Spleen

Lesser curvature of
stomach (covered
by cut edge of lesser
omentum)

Cystic v. & a.

Hepatoduodenal lig.

Hepatogastric lig.

Lesser
Omentum

Gallbladder

Duodenum (sup. part)

Body of stomach

R. colic [hepatic] flexure

Omental [Epiploic] appendages

Tenia coli

Greater curvature of
stomach (covered by cut
edge of greater omentum)

Haustra coli

Transverse colon

Greater omentum

Ascending colon

Jejunum

Pyloric part of stomach

Median plane

Greater omentum (cut
edge in median plane)

R. gastro-omental
[gastroepiploic] a. & v.

Anterior View

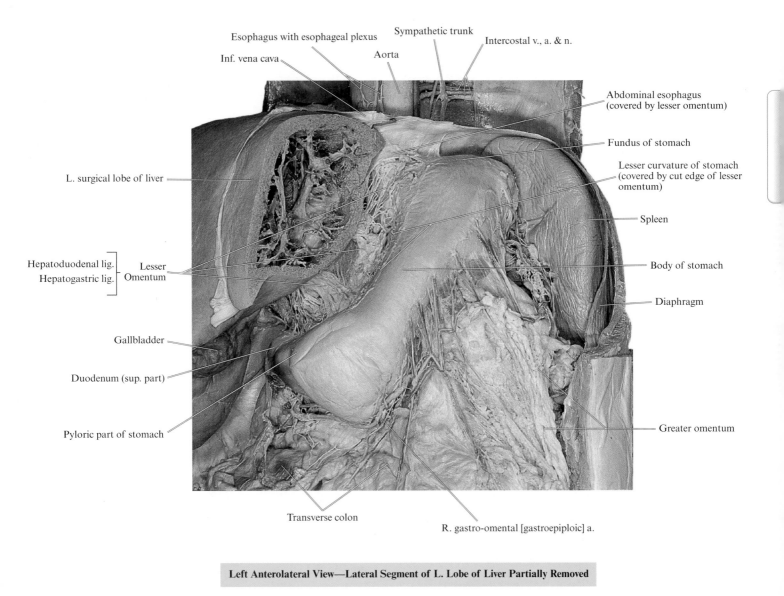

Esophagus with esophageal plexus

Inf. vena cava

Sympathetic trunk

Aorta

Intercostal v., a. & n.

Abdominal esophagus
(covered by lesser omentum)

Fundus of stomach

Lesser curvature of stomach
(covered by cut edge of lesser
omentum)

L. surgical lobe of liver

Spleen

Hepatoduodenal lig.
Hepatogastric lig.

Lesser
Omentum

Body of stomach

Diaphragm

Gallbladder

Duodenum (sup. part)

Pyloric part of stomach

Greater omentum

Transverse colon

R. gastro-omental [gastroepiploic] a.

Left Anterolateral View—Lateral Segment of L. Lobe of Liver Partially Removed

PLATE **3.11**   STOMACH

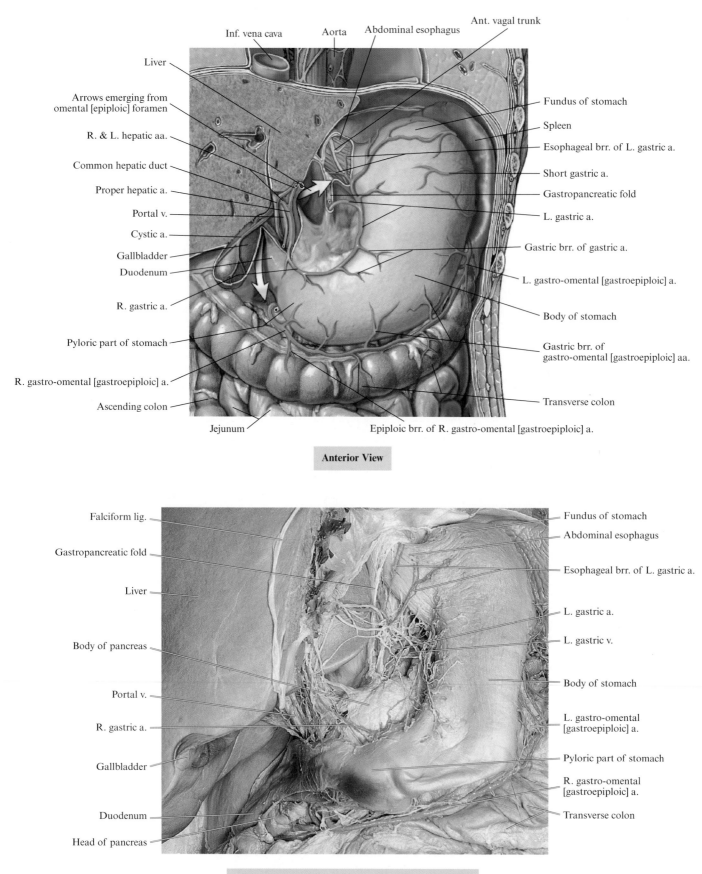

Inf. vena cava

Aorta

Abdominal esophagus

Ant. vagal trunk

Liver

Arrows emerging from omental [epiploic] foramen

R. & L. hepatic aa.

Common hepatic duct

Proper hepatic a.

Portal v.

Cystic a.

Gallbladder

Duodenum

R. gastric a.

Pyloric part of stomach

R. gastro-omental [gastroepiploic] a.

Ascending colon

Jejunum

Epiploic brr. of R. gastro-omental [gastroepiploic] a.

Fundus of stomach

Spleen

Esophageal brr. of L. gastric a.

Short gastric a.

Gastropancreatic fold

L. gastric a.

Gastric brr. of gastric a.

L. gastro-omental [gastroepiploic] a.

Body of stomach

Gastric brr. of gastro-omental [gastroepiploic] aa.

Transverse colon

Anterior View

Falciform lig.

Gastropancreatic fold

Liver

Body of pancreas

Portal v.

R. gastric a.

Gallbladder

Duodenum

Head of pancreas

Fundus of stomach

Abdominal esophagus

Esophageal brr. of L. gastric a.

L. gastric a.

L. gastric v.

Body of stomach

L. gastro-omental [gastroepiploic] a.

Pyloric part of stomach

R. gastro-omental [gastroepiploic] a.

Transverse colon

Anterior View—Liver Left of Falciform Lig. Removed

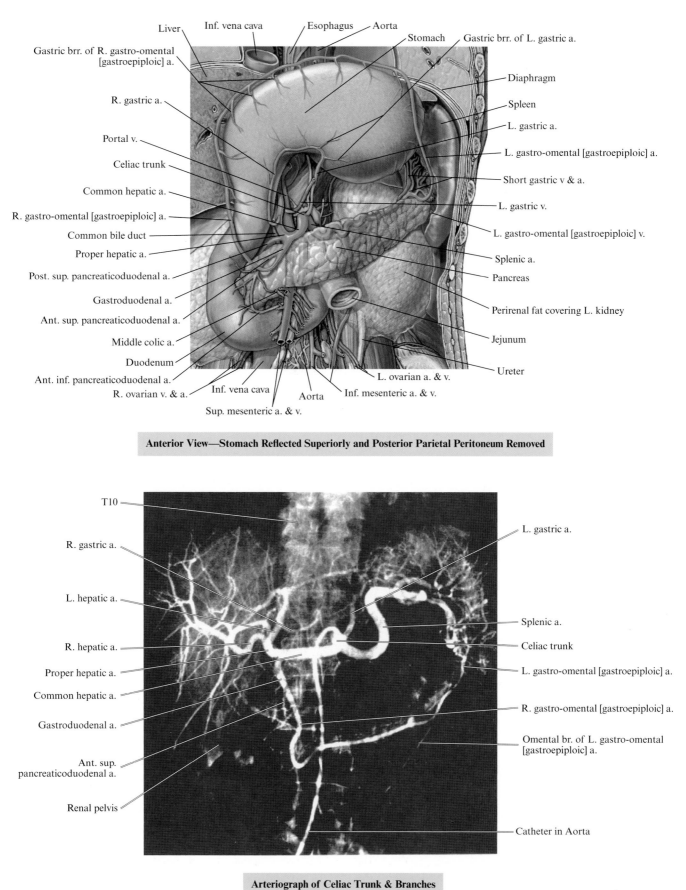

Liver — Inf. vena cava — Esophagus — Aorta
Stomach — Gastric brr. of L. gastric a.
Gastric brr. of R. gastro-omental [gastroepiploic] a.
Diaphragm
Spleen
R. gastric a.
L. gastric a.
L. gastro-omental [gastroepiploic] a.
Portal v.
Short gastric v & a.
Celiac trunk
Common hepatic a.
L. gastric v.
R. gastro-omental [gastroepiploic] a.
L. gastro-omental [gastroepiploic] v.
Common bile duct
Splenic a.
Proper hepatic a.
Pancreas
Post. sup. pancreaticoduodenal a.
Gastroduodenal a.
Perirenal fat covering L. kidney
Ant. sup. pancreaticoduodenal a.
Jejunum
Middle colic a.
Duodenum
Ureter
Ant. inf. pancreaticoduodenal a.
L. ovarian a. & v.
R. ovarian v. & a.   Inf. vena cava   Aorta   Inf. mesenteric a. & v.
Sup. mesenteric a. & v.

Anterior View—Stomach Reflected Superiorly and Posterior Parietal Peritoneum Removed

T10
L. gastric a.
R. gastric a.
L. hepatic a.
R. hepatic a.
Splenic a.
Proper hepatic a.
Celiac trunk
Common hepatic a.
L. gastro-omental [gastroepiploic] a.
Gastroduodenal a.
R. gastro-omental [gastroepiploic] a.
Omental br. of L. gastro-omental [gastroepiploic] a.
Ant. sup. pancreaticoduodenal a.
Renal pelvis
Catheter in Aorta

Arteriograph of Celiac Trunk & Branches

PLATE 3.13   PANCREAS

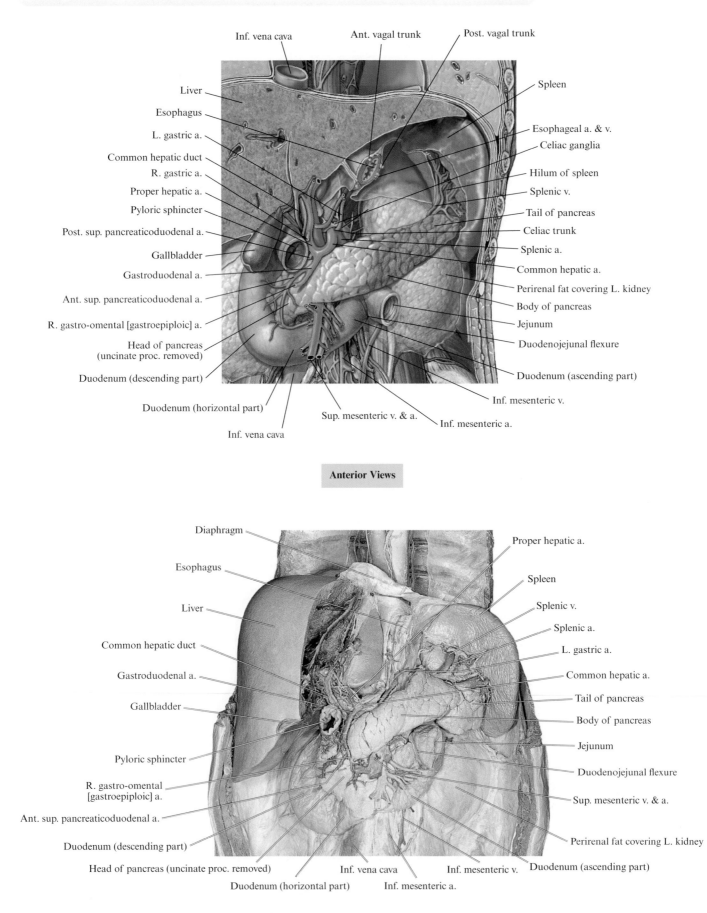

Inf. vena cava

Ant. vagal trunk

Post. vagal trunk

Liver

Esophagus

L. gastric a.

Common hepatic duct

R. gastric a.

Proper hepatic a.

Pyloric sphincter

Post. sup. pancreaticoduodenal a.

Gallbladder

Gastroduodenal a.

Ant. sup. pancreaticoduodenal a.

R. gastro-omental [gastroepiploic] a.

Head of pancreas
(uncinate proc. removed)

Duodenum (descending part)

Duodenum (horizontal part)

Inf. vena cava

Sup. mesenteric v. & a.

Inf. mesenteric a.

Inf. mesenteric v.

Duodenum (ascending part)

Duodenojejunal flexure

Jejunum

Body of pancreas

Perirenal fat covering L. kidney

Common hepatic a.

Splenic a.

Celiac trunk

Tail of pancreas

Splenic v.

Hilum of spleen

Celiac ganglia

Esophageal a. & v.

Spleen

Anterior Views

Diaphragm

Esophagus

Liver

Common hepatic duct

Gastroduodenal a.

Gallbladder

Pyloric sphincter

R. gastro-omental
[gastroepiploic] a.

Ant. sup. pancreaticoduodenal a.

Duodenum (descending part)

Head of pancreas (uncinate proc. removed)

Duodenum (horizontal part)

Inf. vena cava

Inf. mesenteric a.

Inf. mesenteric v.

Duodenum (ascending part)

Perirenal fat covering L. kidney

Sup. mesenteric v. & a.

Duodenojejunal flexure

Jejunum

Body of pancreas

Tail of pancreas

Common hepatic a.

L. gastric a.

Splenic a.

Splenic v.

Spleen

Proper hepatic a.

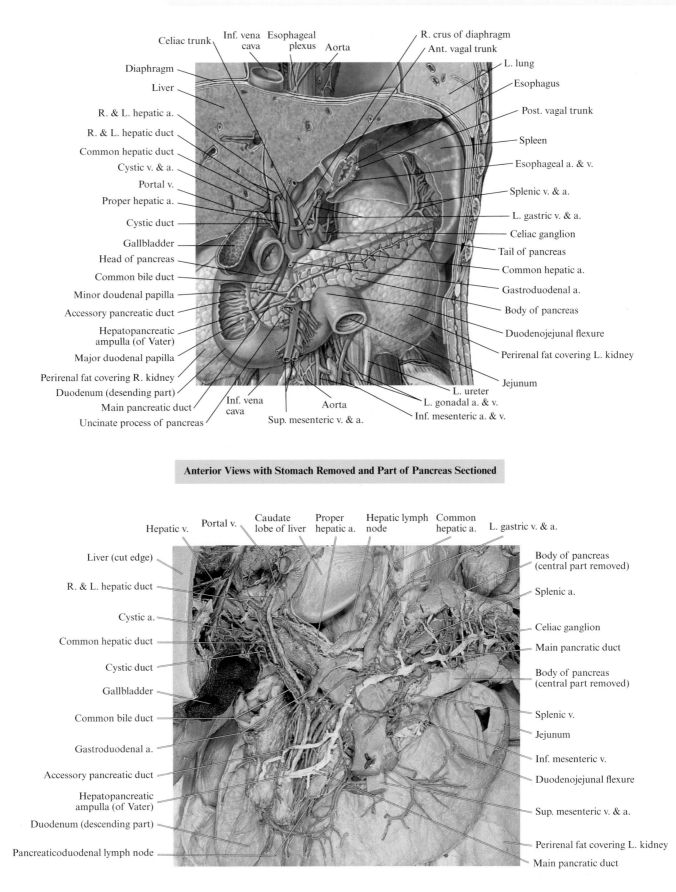

Celiac trunk

Inf. vena cava   Esophageal plexus   Aorta

R. crus of diaphragm

Ant. vagal trunk

Diaphragm

Liver

R. & L. hepatic a.

R. & L. hepatic duct

Common hepatic duct

Cystic v. & a.

Portal v.

Proper hepatic a.

Cystic duct

Gallbladder

Head of pancreas

Common bile duct

Minor doudenal papilla

Accessory pancreatic duct

Hepatopancreatic ampulla (of Vater)

Major duodenal papilla

Perirenal fat covering R. kidney

Duodenum (desending part)

Main pancreatic duct

Uncinate process of pancreas

Inf. vena cava

Aorta

Sup. mesenteric v. & a.

L. lung

Esophagus

Post. vagal trunk

Spleen

Esophageal a. & v.

Splenic v. & a.

L. gastric v. & a.

Celiac ganglion

Tail of pancreas

Common hepatic a.

Gastroduodenal a.

Body of pancreas

Duodenojejunal flexure

Perirenal fat covering L. kidney

Jejunum

L. ureter

L. gonadal a. & v.

Inf. mesenteric a. & v.

Anterior Views with Stomach Removed and Part of Pancreas Sectioned

Hepatic v.   Portal v.

Caudate lobe of liver

Proper hepatic a.

Hepatic lymph node

Common hepatic a.

L. gastric v. & a.

Liver (cut edge)

R. & L. hepatic duct

Cystic a.

Common hepatic duct

Cystic duct

Gallbladder

Common bile duct

Gastroduodenal a.

Accessory pancreatic duct

Hepatopancreatic ampulla (of Vater)

Duodenum (descending part)

Pancreaticoduodenal lymph node

Body of pancreas (central part removed)

Splenic a.

Celiac ganglion

Main pancratic duct

Body of pancreas (central part removed)

Splenic v.

Jejunum

Inf. mesenteric v.

Duodenojejunal flexure

Sup. mesenteric v. & a.

Perirenal fat covering L. kidney

Main pancratic duct

PLATE 3.15   PORTAL VEIN

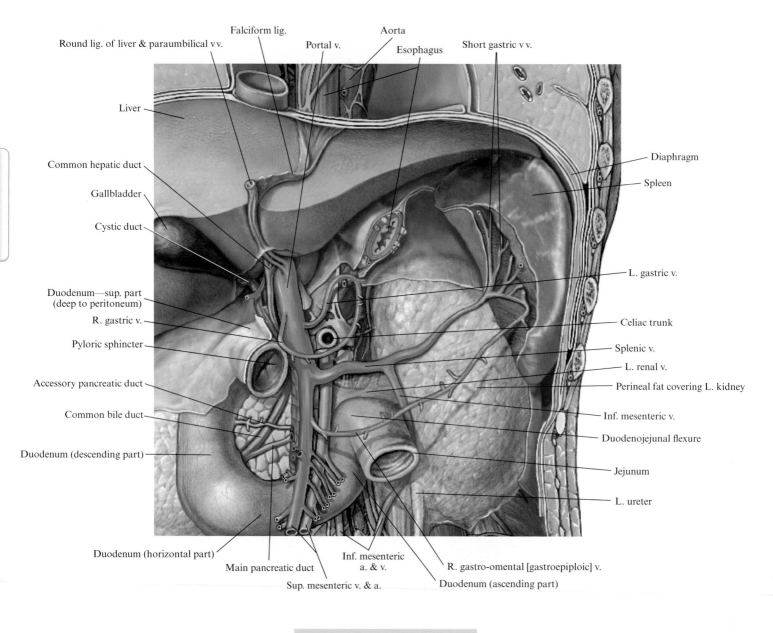

Round lig. of liver & paraumbilical vv.

Falciform lig.

Portal v.

Aorta

Esophagus

Short gastric vv.

Liver

Common hepatic duct

Gallbladder

Cystic duct

Duodenum—sup. part
(deep to peritoneum)

R. gastric v.

Pyloric sphincter

Accessory pancreatic duct

Common bile duct

Duodenum (descending part)

Duodenum (horizontal part)

Main pancreatic duct

Sup. mesenteric v. & a.

Inf. mesenteric
a. & v.

Duodenum (ascending part)

R. gastro-omental [gastroepiploic] v.

Diaphragm

Spleen

L. gastric v.

Celiac trunk

Splenic v.

L. renal v.

Perineal fat covering L. kidney

Inf. mesenteric v.

Duodenojejunal flexure

Jejunum

L. ureter

Anterior View with Stomach Removed

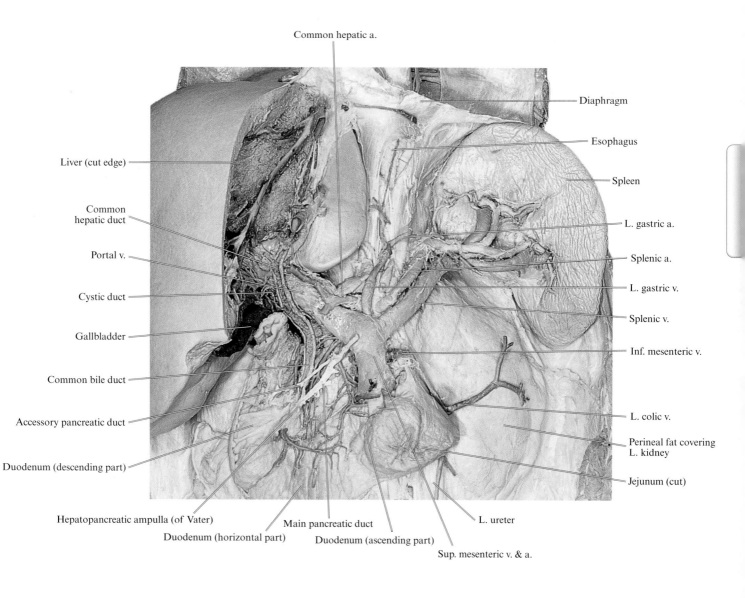

Common hepatic a.

Diaphragm

Esophagus

Liver (cut edge)

Spleen

Common hepatic duct

L. gastric a.

Splenic a.

Portal v.

L. gastric v.

Cystic duct

Splenic v.

Gallbladder

Inf. mesenteric v.

Common bile duct

Accessory pancreatic duct

L. colic v.

Perineal fat covering L. kidney

Duodenum (descending part)

Jejunum (cut)

Hepatopancreatic ampulla (of Vater)

Main pancreatic duct

L. ureter

Duodenum (horizontal part)

Duodenum (ascending part)

Sup. mesenteric v. & a.

Anterior View with Stomach, Left Half of Liver, and Pancreas Removed

PLATE **3.17**   LIVER

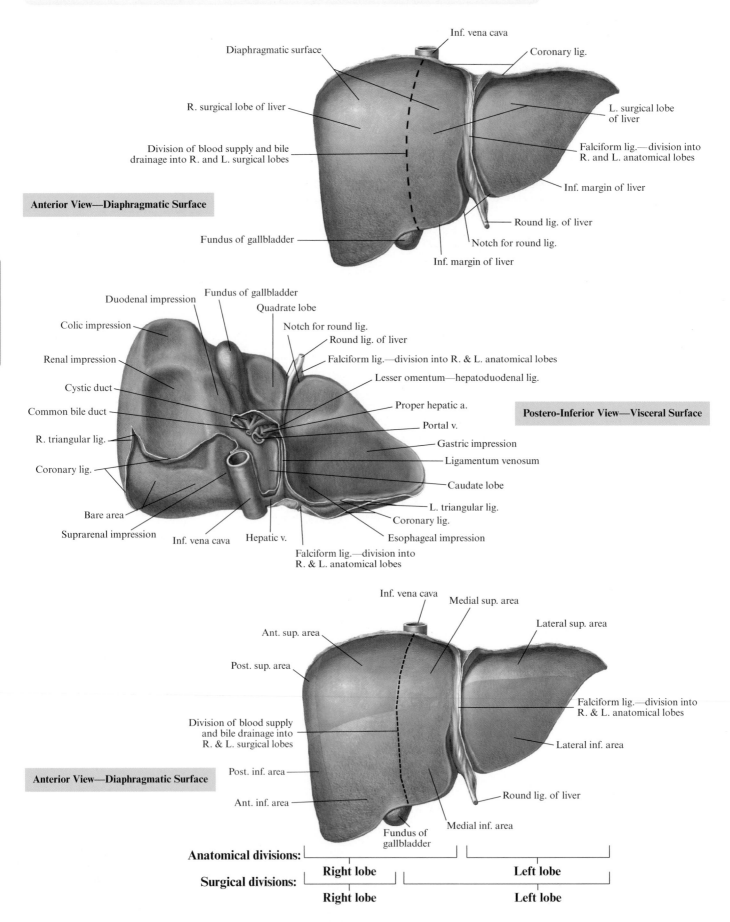

Inf. vena cava

Diaphragmatic surface

Coronary lig.

R. surgical lobe of liver

L. surgical lobe of liver

Division of blood supply and bile drainage into R. and L. surgical lobes

Falciform lig.—division into R. and L. anatomical lobes

Inf. margin of liver

Anterior View—Diaphragmatic Surface

Round lig. of liver

Fundus of gallbladder

Notch for round lig.

Inf. margin of liver

Duodenal impression

Fundus of gallbladder

Quadrate lobe

Colic impression

Notch for round lig.

Round lig. of liver

Renal impression

Falciform lig.—division into R. & L. anatomical lobes

Cystic duct

Lesser omentum—hepatoduodenal lig.

Common bile duct

Proper hepatic a.

R. triangular lig.

Portal v.

Postero-Inferior View—Visceral Surface

Gastric impression

Coronary lig.

Ligamentum venosum

Caudate lobe

L. triangular lig.

Bare area

Coronary lig.

Suprarenal impression

Inf. vena cava

Hepatic v.

Esophageal impression

Falciform lig.—division into
R. & L. anatomical lobes

Inf. vena cava

Medial sup. area

Ant. sup. area

Lateral sup. area

Post. sup. area

Falciform lig.—division into
R. & L. anatomical lobes

Division of blood supply
and bile drainage into
R. & L. surgical lobes

Lateral inf. area

Anterior View—Diaphragmatic Surface

Post. inf. area

Ant. inf. area

Round lig. of liver

Medial inf. area

Fundus of
gallbladder

Anatomical divisions: **Right lobe**   **Left lobe**

Surgical divisions: **Right lobe**   **Left lobe**

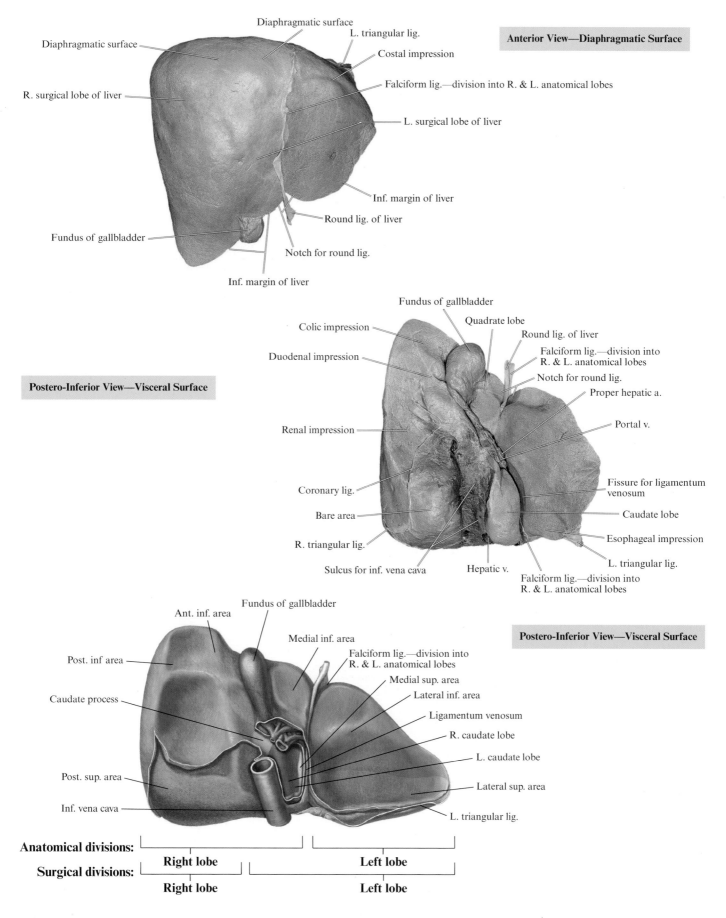

Diaphragmatic surface

Diaphragmatic surface

L. triangular lig.

Costal impression

Anterior View—Diaphragmatic Surface

R. surgical lobe of liver

Falciform lig.—division into R. & L. anatomical lobes

L. surgical lobe of liver

Inf. margin of liver

Round lig. of liver

Fundus of gallbladder

Notch for round lig.

Inf. margin of liver

Fundus of gallbladder

Quadrate lobe

Colic impression

Round lig. of liver

Duodenal impression

Falciform lig.—division into R. & L. anatomical lobes

Notch for round lig.

Postero-Inferior View—Visceral Surface

Proper hepatic a.

Renal impression

Portal v.

Coronary lig.

Fissure for ligamentum venosum

Caudate lobe

Bare area

Esophageal impression

R. triangular lig.

L. triangular lig.

Sulcus for inf. vena cava

Hepatic v.

Falciform lig.—division into R. & L. anatomical lobes

Ant. inf. area

Fundus of gallbladder

Medial inf. area

Post. inf area

Falciform lig.—division into R. & L. anatomical lobes

Postero-Inferior View—Visceral Surface

Medial sup. area

Caudate process

Lateral inf. area

Ligamentum venosum

R. caudate lobe

Post. sup. area

L. caudate lobe

Inf. vena cava

Lateral sup. area

L. triangular lig.

Anatomical divisions:

Surgical divisions:

Right lobe

Left lobe

Right lobe

Left lobe

PLATE 3.19   LIVER—PERITONEAL LIGAMENTS

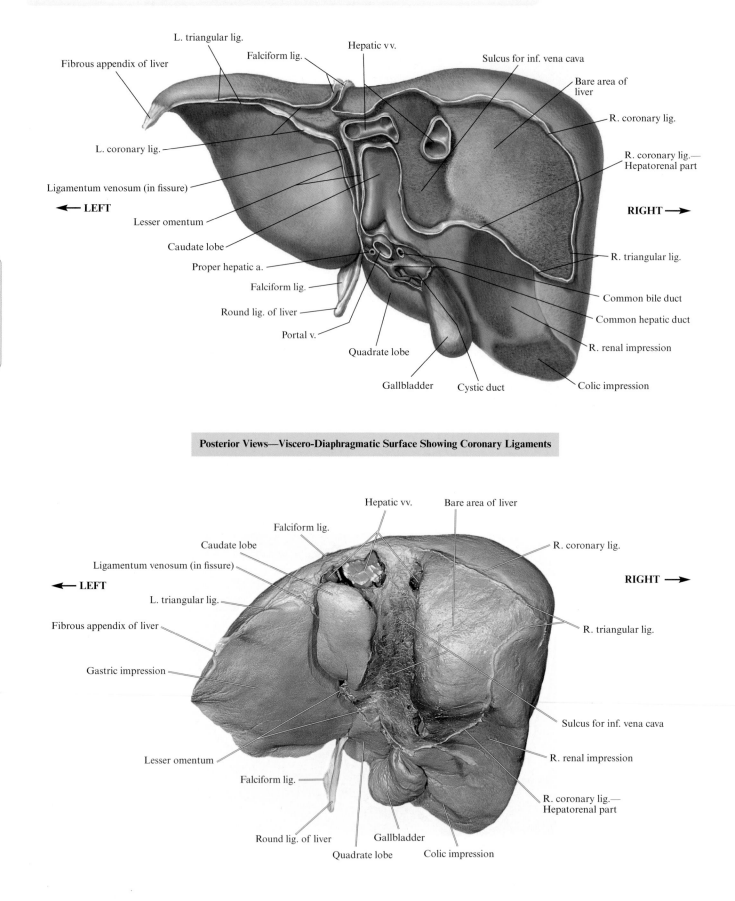

L. triangular lig.

Fibrous appendix of liver

Falciform lig.

Hepatic vv.

Sulcus for inf. vena cava

Bare area of liver

R. coronary lig.

L. coronary lig.

R. coronary lig.—
Hepatorenal part

Ligamentum venosum (in fissure)

◄— LEFT

RIGHT —►

Lesser omentum

Caudate lobe

R. triangular lig.

Proper hepatic a.

Falciform lig.

Common bile duct

Round lig. of liver

Common hepatic duct

Portal v.

R. renal impression

Quadrate lobe

Gallbladder   Cystic duct

Colic impression

Posterior Views—Viscero-Diaphragmatic Surface Showing Coronary Ligaments

Hepatic vv.   Bare area of liver

Falciform lig.

R. coronary lig.

Caudate lobe

Ligamentum venosum (in fissure)

◄— LEFT

RIGHT —►

L. triangular lig.

Fibrous appendix of liver

R. triangular lig.

Gastric impression

Sulcus for inf. vena cava

Lesser omentum

R. renal impression

Falciform lig.

R. coronary lig.—
Hepatorenal part

Round lig. of liver   Gallbladder

Quadrate lobe   Colic impression

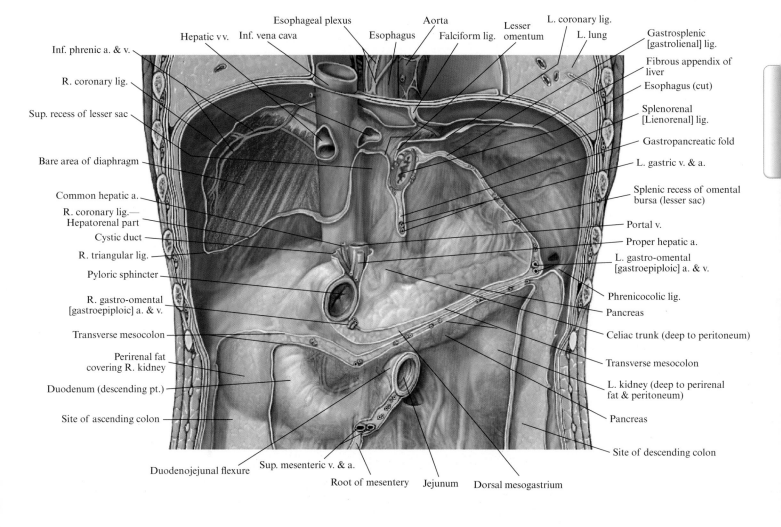

Esophageal plexus   Aorta   L. coronary lig.

Hepatic v v.   Inf. vena cava   Esophagus   Falciform lig.   Lesser omentum   L. lung   Gastrosplenic [gastrolienal] lig.

Inf. phrenic a. & v.

R. coronary lig.

Sup. recess of lesser sac

Bare area of diaphragm

Common hepatic a.

R. coronary lig.—
Hepatorenal part

Cystic duct

R. triangular lig.

Pyloric sphincter

R. gastro-omental
[gastroepiploic] a. & v.

Transverse mesocolon

Perirenal fat
covering R. kidney

Duodenum (descending pt.)

Site of ascending colon

Duodenojejunal flexure   Sup. mesenteric v. & a.

Root of mesentery   Jejunum   Dorsal mesogastrium

Fibrous appendix of liver

Esophagus (cut)

Splenorenal [Lienorenal] lig.

Gastropancreatic fold

L. gastric v. & a.

Splenic recess of omental bursa (lesser sac)

Portal v.

Proper hepatic a.

L. gastro-omental [gastroepiploic] a. & v.

Phrenicocolic lig.

Pancreas

Celiac trunk (deep to peritoneum)

Transverse mesocolon

L. kidney (deep to perirenal fat & peritoneum)

Pancreas

Site of descending colon

Anterior View—Posterior Abdominal Wall

PLATE 3.21   STOMACH & SMALL INTESTINES

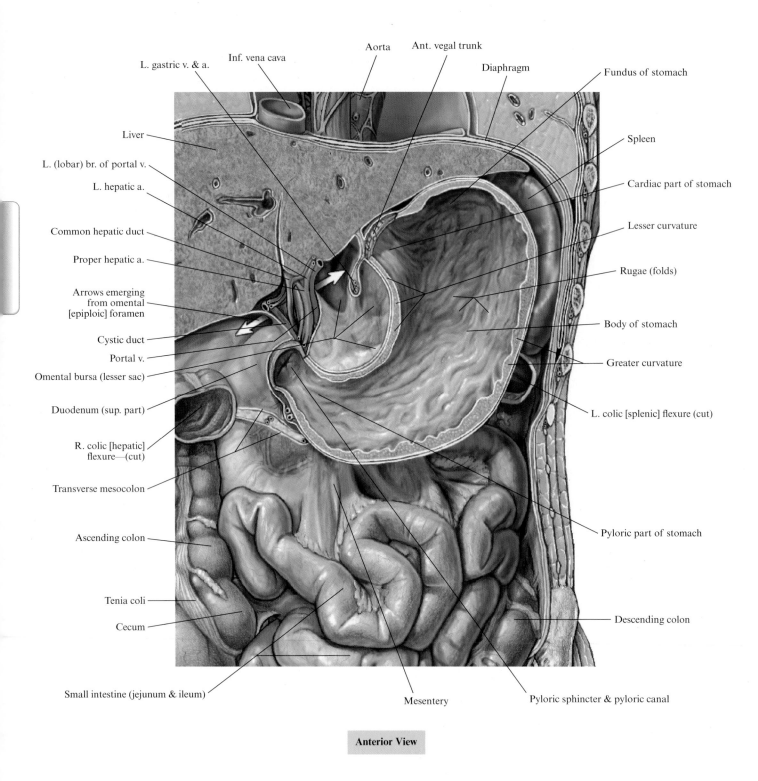

L. gastric v. & a.

Inf. vena cava

Aorta

Ant. vegal trunk

Diaphragm

Fundus of stomach

Liver

Spleen

L. (lobar) br. of portal v.

Cardiac part of stomach

L. hepatic a.

Lesser curvature

Common hepatic duct

Proper hepatic a.

Rugae (folds)

Arrows emerging
from omental
[epiploic] foramen

Body of stomach

Cystic duct

Portal v.

Greater curvature

Omental bursa (lesser sac)

Duodenum (sup. part)

L. colic [splenic] flexure (cut)

R. colic [hepatic]
flexure—(cut)

Transverse mesocolon

Ascending colon

Pyloric part of stomach

Tenia coli

Cecum

Descending colon

Small intestine (jejunum & ileum)

Mesentery

Pyloric sphincter & pyloric canal

Anterior View

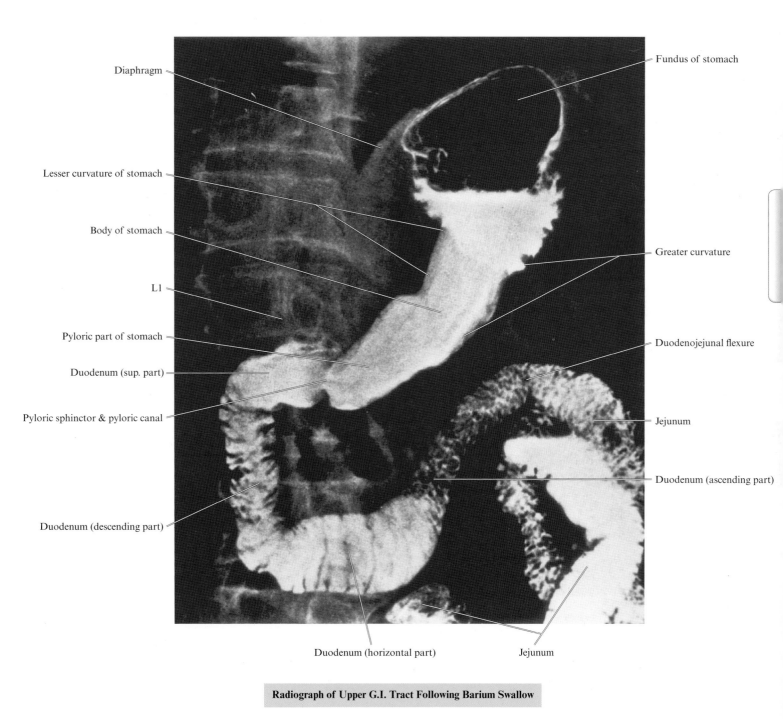

Diaphragm

Fundus of stomach

Lesser curvature of stomach

Body of stomach

Greater curvature

L1

Pyloric part of stomach

Duodenojejunal flexure

Duodenum (sup. part)

Pyloric sphincter & pyloric canal

Jejunum

Duodenum (ascending part)

Duodenum (descending part)

Duodenum (horizontal part)

Jejunum

Radiograph of Upper G.I. Tract Following Barium Swallow

PLATE 3.23   SMALL INTESTINES—VASCULATURE

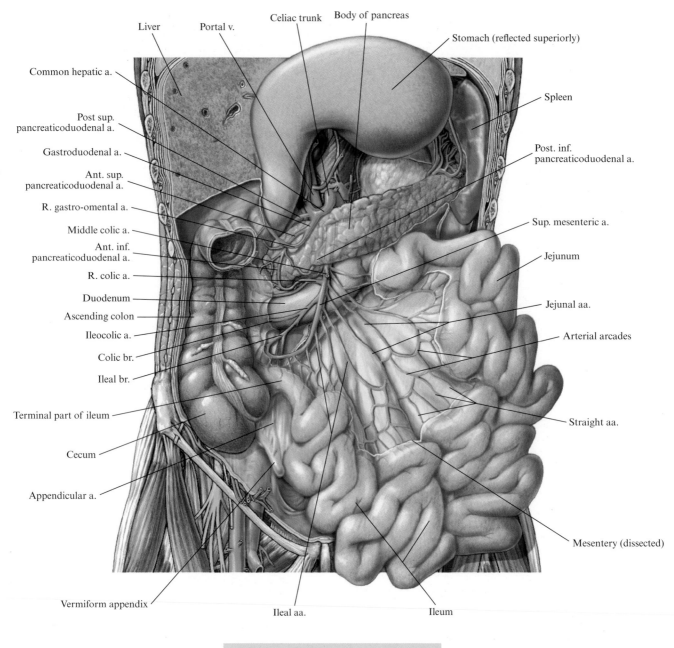

Liver   Portal v.   Celiac trunk   Body of pancreas

Common hepatic a.

Stomach (reflected superiorly)

Post sup. pancreaticoduodenal a.

Spleen

Gastroduodenal a.

Post. inf. pancreaticoduodenal a.

Ant. sup. pancreaticoduodenal a.

R. gastro-omental a.

Sup. mesenteric a.

Middle colic a.

Jejunum

Ant. inf. pancreaticoduodenal a.

R. colic a.

Jejunal aa.

Duodenum

Ascending colon

Arterial arcades

Ileocolic a.

Colic br.

Ileal br.

Straight aa.

Terminal part of ileum

Cecum

Appendicular a.

Mesentery (dissected)

Vermiform appendix   Ileal aa.   Ileum

Anterior View—Stomach Reflected Superiorly

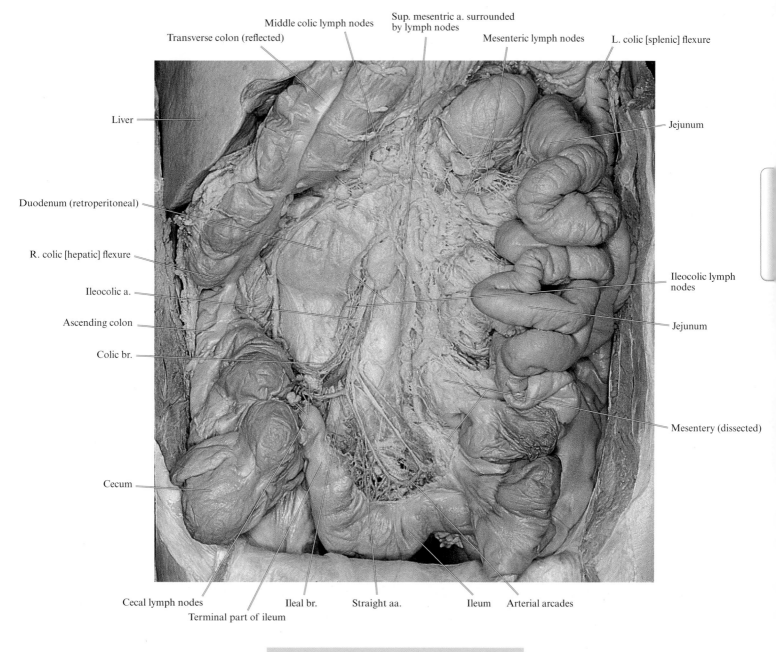

Middle colic lymph nodes

Sup. mesentric a. surrounded
by lymph nodes

Transverse colon (reflected)

Mesenteric lymph nodes

L. colic [splenic] flexure

Liver

Jejunum

Duodenum (retroperitoneal)

R. colic [hepatic] flexure

Ileocolic lymph
nodes

Ileocolic a.

Ascending colon

Jejunum

Colic br.

Cecum

Mesentery (dissected)

Cecal lymph nodes

Ileal br.

Straight aa.

Ileum

Arterial arcades

Terminal part of ileum

Anterior View—Transverse Colon Reflected Superiorly

PLATE 3.25 LARGE INTESTINES—VASCULATURE

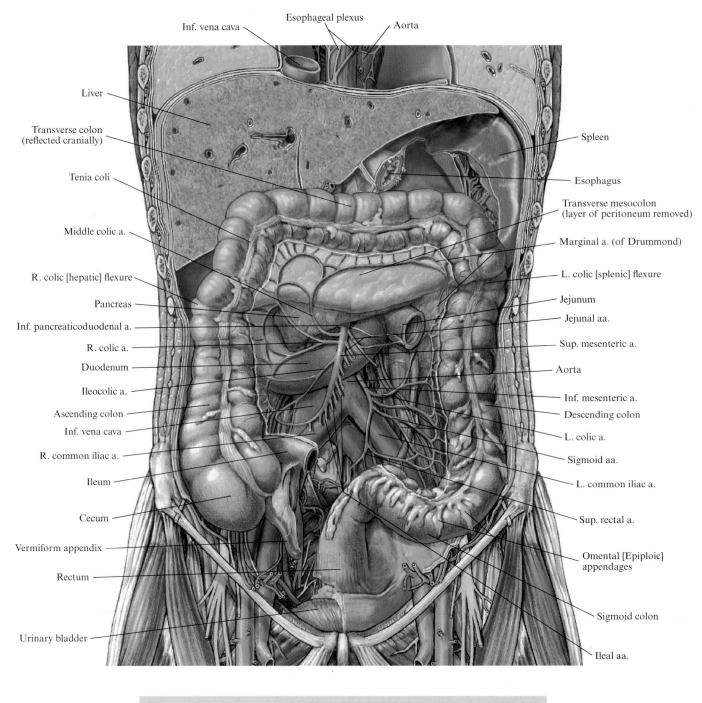

Inf. vena cava

Esophageal plexus

Aorta

Liver

Transverse colon
(reflected cranially)

Tenia coli

Middle colic a.

R. colic [hepatic] flexure

Pancreas

Inf. pancreaticoduodenal a.

R. colic a.

Duodenum

Ileocolic a.

Ascending colon

Inf. vena cava

R. common iliac a.

Ileum

Cecum

Vermiform appendix

Rectum

Urinary bladder

Spleen

Esophagus

Transverse mesocolon
(layer of peritoneum removed)

Marginal a. (of Drummond)

L. colic [splenic] flexure

Jejunum

Jejunal aa.

Sup. mesenteric a.

Aorta

Inf. mesenteric a.

Descending colon

L. colic a.

Sigmoid aa.

L. common iliac a.

Sup. rectal a.

Omental [Epiploic]
appendages

Sigmoid colon

Ileal aa.

Anterior View—Transverse Colon Reflected Superiorly & the Mesentery Proper Removed

T12

Sup. mesenteric a.

Middle colic a.

Jejunal aa.

R. colic a.

Arterial arcades

Sup. mesenteric a.

Ileocolic a.

Crest of ilium

Transverse process of L5

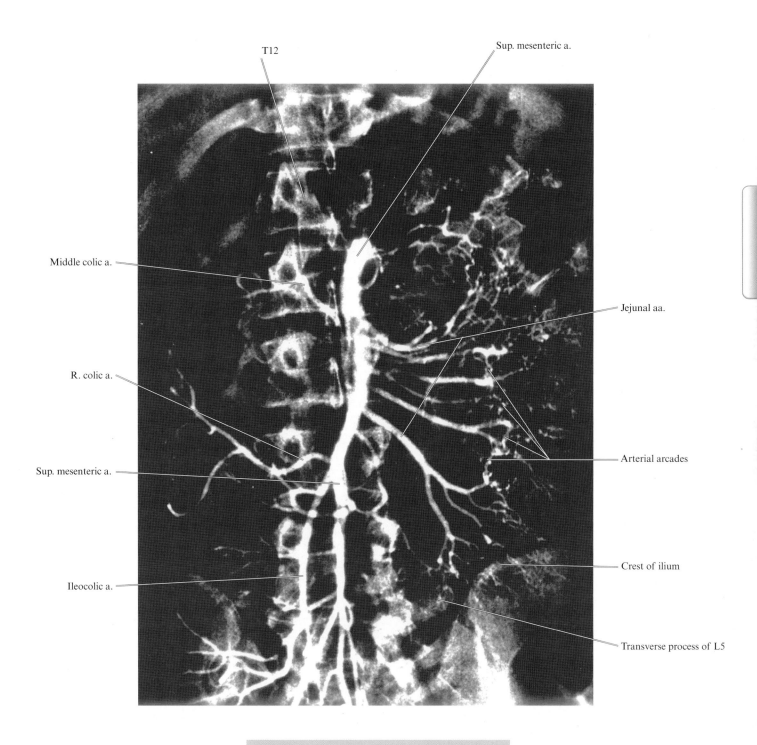

Arteriograph of Superior Mesenteric Artery & Branches

PLATE 3.27   LARGE INTESTINES

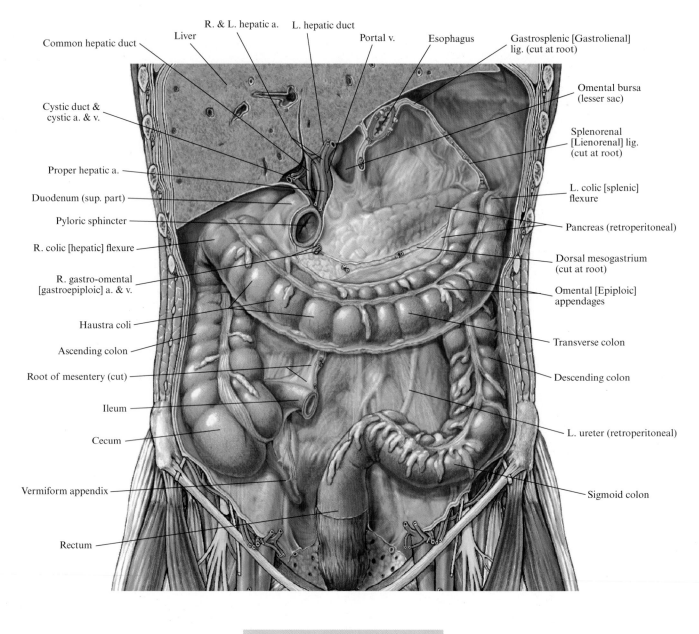

Common hepatic duct

R. & L. hepatic a.

Liver

L. hepatic duct

Portal v.

Esophagus

Gastrosplenic [Gastrolienal] lig. (cut at root)

Cystic duct & cystic a. & v.

Omental bursa (lesser sac)

Splenorenal [Lienorenal] lig. (cut at root)

Proper hepatic a.

L. colic [splenic] flexure

Duodenum (sup. part)

Pancreas (retroperitoneal)

Pyloric sphincter

R. colic [hepatic] flexure

Dorsal mesogastrium (cut at root)

R. gastro-omental [gastroepiploic] a. & v.

Omental [Epiploic] appendages

Haustra coli

Ascending colon

Transverse colon

Root of mesentery (cut)

Descending colon

Ileum

Cecum

L. ureter (retroperitoneal)

Vermiform appendix

Sigmoid colon

Rectum

Anterior View—Small Intestines Removed

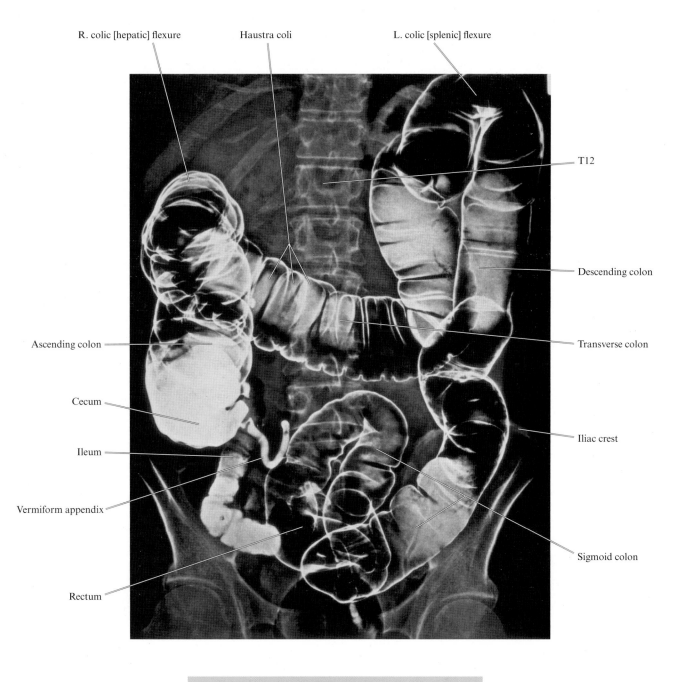

R. colic [hepatic] flexure

Haustra coli

L. colic [splenic] flexure

T12

Descending colon

Ascending colon

Transverse colon

Cecum

Ileum

Iliac crest

Vermiform appendix

Sigmoid colon

Rectum

Double Contrast (Air & Barium) Radiograph of Large Intestine

PLATE 3.29   LARGE INTESTINES—PORTAL VASCULATURE

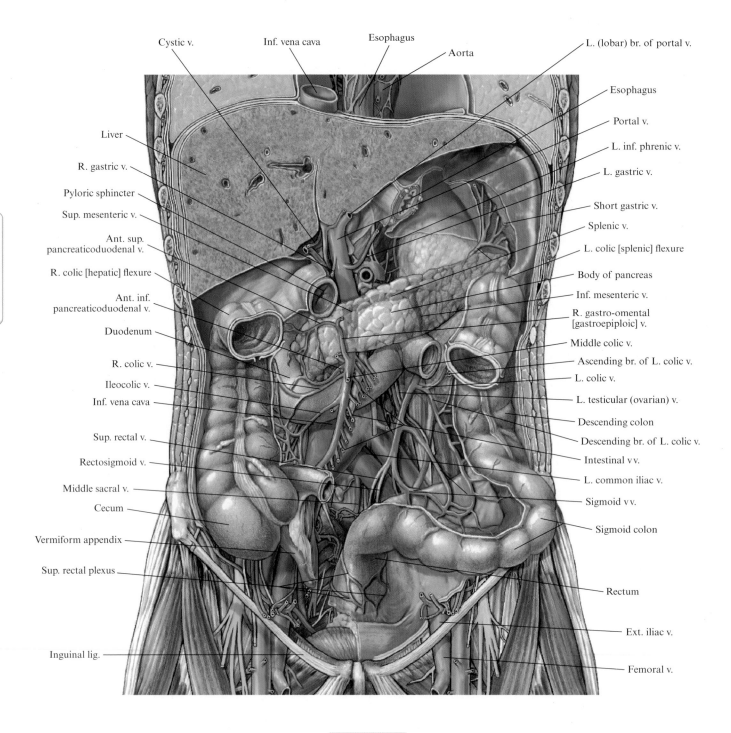

Cystic v.

Inf. vena cava

Esophagus

Aorta

L. (lobar) br. of portal v.

Esophagus

Liver

Portal v.

R. gastric v.

L. inf. phrenic v.

Pyloric sphincter

L. gastric v.

Sup. mesenteric v.

Short gastric v.

Ant. sup.
pancreaticoduodenal v.

Splenic v.

R. colic [hepatic] flexure

L. colic [splenic] flexure

Ant. inf.
pancreaticoduodenal v.

Body of pancreas

Duodenum

Inf. mesenteric v.

R. gastro-omental
[gastroepiploic] v.

R. colic v.

Middle colic v.

Ileocolic v.

Ascending br. of L. colic v.

Inf. vena cava

L. colic v.

Sup. rectal v.

L. testicular (ovarian) v.

Rectosigmoid v.

Descending colon

Middle sacral v.

Descending br. of L. colic v.

Cecum

Intestinal vv.

Vermiform appendix

L. common iliac v.

Sup. rectal plexus

Sigmoid vv.

Sigmoid colon

Inguinal lig.

Rectum

Ext. iliac v.

Femoral v.

Anterior View

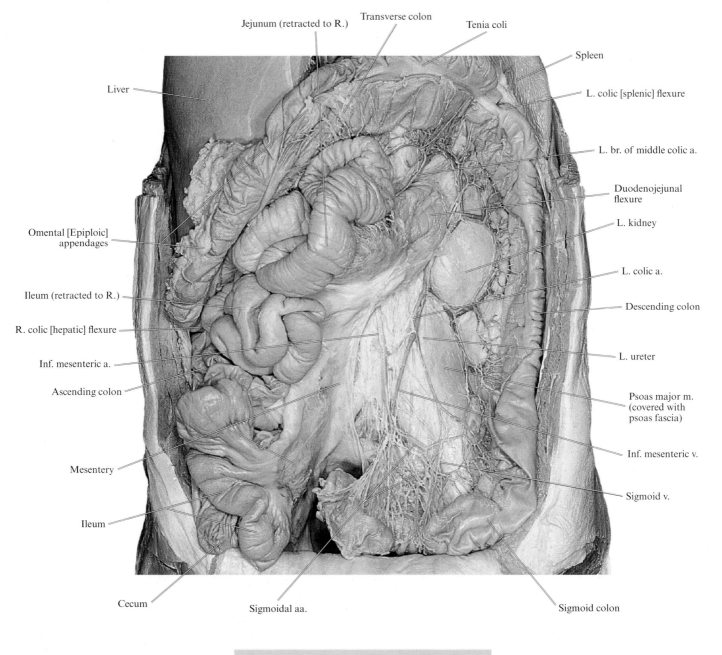

Jejunum (retracted to R.)   Transverse colon   Tenia coli

Spleen

Liver

L. colic [splenic] flexure

L. br. of middle colic a.

Duodenojejunal flexure

Omental [Epiploic] appendages

L. kidney

L. colic a.

Ileum (retracted to R.)

Descending colon

R. colic [hepatic] flexure

L. ureter

Inf. mesenteric a.

Ascending colon

Psoas major m. (covered with psoas fascia)

Inf. mesenteric v.

Mesentery

Sigmoid v.

Ileum

Cecum   Sigmoidal aa.   Sigmoid colon

Anterior View—Transverse Colon Reflected Superiorly

PLATE 3.31   POSTERIOR ABDOMINAL WALL

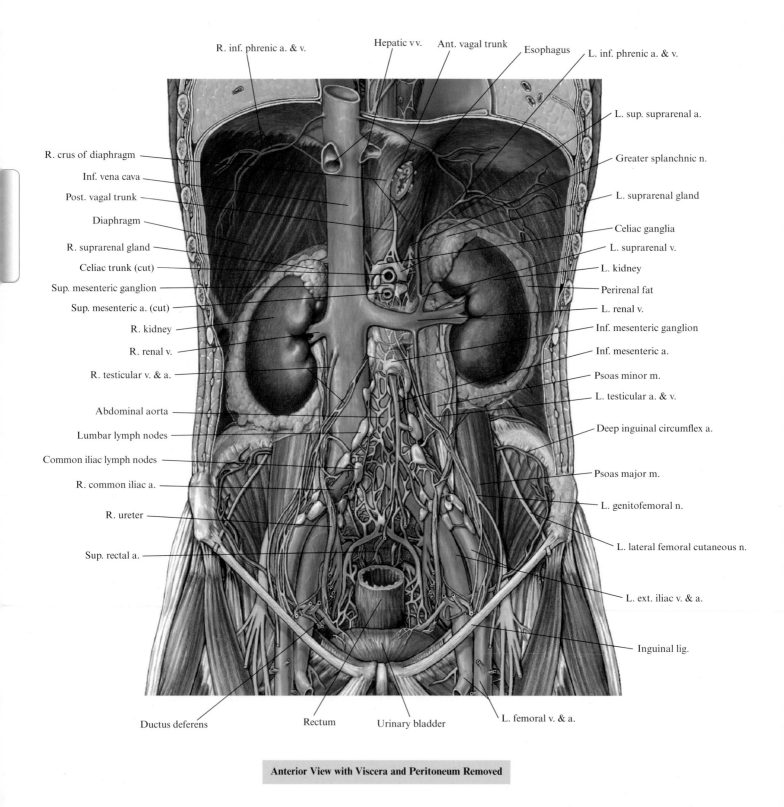

R. inf. phrenic a. & v.
Hepatic v v.
Ant. vagal trunk
Esophagus
L. inf. phrenic a. & v.

R. crus of diaphragm
Inf. vena cava
Post. vagal trunk
Diaphragm
R. suprarenal gland
Celiac trunk (cut)
Sup. mesenteric ganglion
Sup. mesenteric a. (cut)
R. kidney
R. renal v.
R. testicular v. & a.
Abdominal aorta
Lumbar lymph nodes
Common iliac lymph nodes
R. common iliac a.
R. ureter
Sup. rectal a.

L. sup. suprarenal a.
Greater splanchnic n.
L. suprarenal gland
Celiac ganglia
L. suprarenal v.
L. kidney
Perirenal fat
L. renal v.
Inf. mesenteric ganglion
Inf. mesenteric a.
Psoas minor m.
L. testicular a. & v.
Deep inguinal circumflex a.
Psoas major m.
L. genitofemoral n.
L. lateral femoral cutaneous n.
L. ext. iliac v. & a.
Inguinal lig.

Ductus deferens
Rectum
Urinary bladder
L. femoral v. & a.

Anterior View with Viscera and Peritoneum Removed

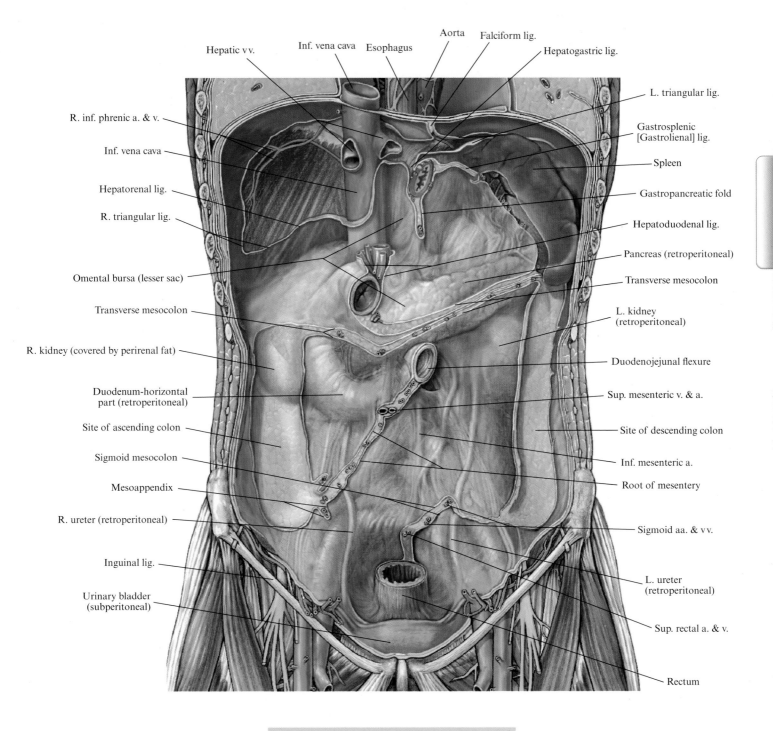

Hepatic v v.

Inf. vena cava

Esophagus

Aorta

Falciform lig.

Hepatogastric lig.

R. inf. phrenic a. & v.

Inf. vena cava

Hepatorenal lig.

R. triangular lig.

Omental bursa (lesser sac)

Transverse mesocolon

R. kidney (covered by perirenal fat)

Duodenum-horizontal part (retroperitoneal)

Site of ascending colon

Sigmoid mesocolon

Mesoappendix

R. ureter (retroperitoneal)

Inguinal lig.

Urinary bladder (subperitoneal)

L. triangular lig.

Gastrosplenic [Gastrolienal] lig.

Spleen

Gastropancreatic fold

Hepatoduodenal lig.

Pancreas (retroperitoneal)

Transverse mesocolon

L. kidney (retroperitoneal)

Duodenojejunal flexure

Sup. mesenteric v. & a.

Site of descending colon

Inf. mesenteric a.

Root of mesentery

Sigmoid aa. & v v.

L. ureter (retroperitoneal)

Sup. rectal a. & v.

Rectum

**Anterior View of Posterior Abdominal Wall Showing
Peritoneal Coverings and Mesentery Origins**

PLATE 3.33   POSTERIOR ABDOMINAL WALL

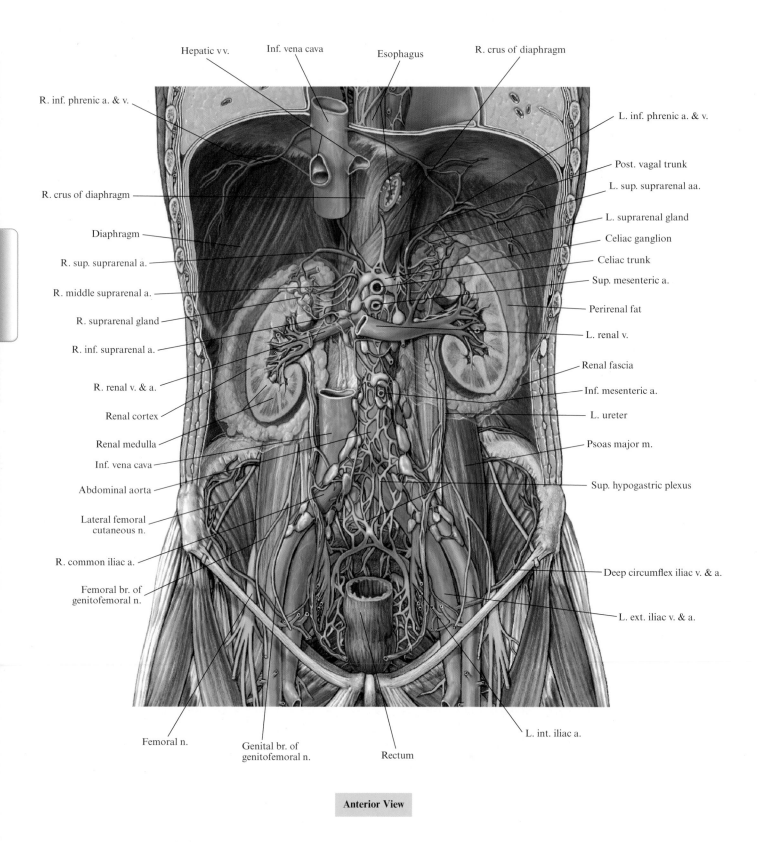

Hepatic v v.
Inf. vena cava
Esophagus
R. crus of diaphragm
R. inf. phrenic a. & v.
L. inf. phrenic a. & v.
Post. vagal trunk
R. crus of diaphragm
L. sup. suprarenal aa.
Diaphragm
L. suprarenal gland
R. sup. suprarenal a.
Celiac ganglion
Celiac trunk
R. middle suprarenal a.
Sup. mesenteric a.
R. suprarenal gland
Perirenal fat
R. inf. suprarenal a.
L. renal v.
R. renal v. & a.
Renal fascia
Renal cortex
Inf. mesenteric a.
Renal medulla
L. ureter
Inf. vena cava
Psoas major m.
Abdominal aorta
Sup. hypogastric plexus
Lateral femoral
cutaneous n.
R. common iliac a.
Deep circumflex iliac v. & a.
Femoral br. of
genitofemoral n.
L. ext. iliac v. & a.
Femoral n.
Genital br. of
genitofemoral n.
Rectum
L. int. iliac a.

Anterior View

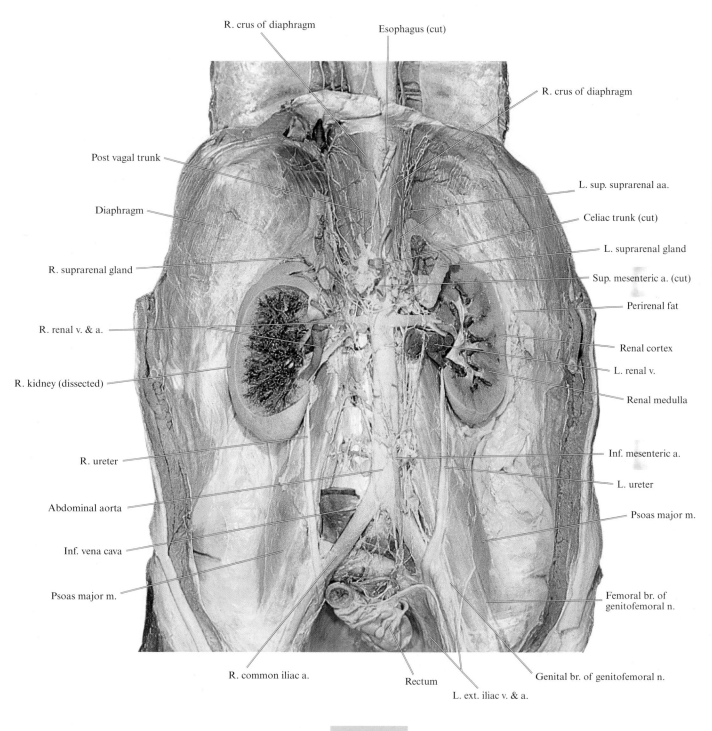

R. crus of diaphragm

Esophagus (cut)

R. crus of diaphragm

Post vagal trunk

L. sup. suprarenal aa.

Celiac trunk (cut)

Diaphragm

L. suprarenal gland

Sup. mesenteric a. (cut)

R. suprarenal gland

Perirenal fat

R. renal v. & a.

Renal cortex

L. renal v.

R. kidney (dissected)

Renal medulla

R. ureter

Inf. mesenteric a.

L. ureter

Abdominal aorta

Psoas major m.

Inf. vena cava

Psoas major m.

Femoral br. of
genitofemoral n.

R. common iliac a.

Rectum

Genital br. of genitofemoral n.

L. ext. iliac v. & a.

Anterior View

PLATE 3.35   KIDNEYS

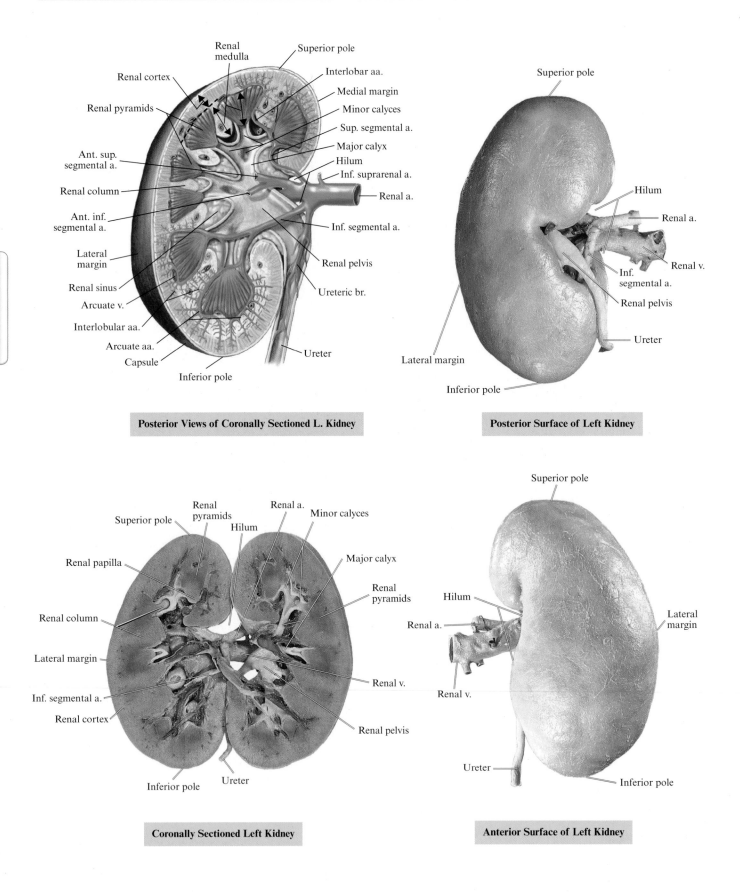

Posterior Views of Coronally Sectioned L. Kidney

Posterior Surface of Left Kidney

Coronally Sectioned Left Kidney

Anterior Surface of Left Kidney

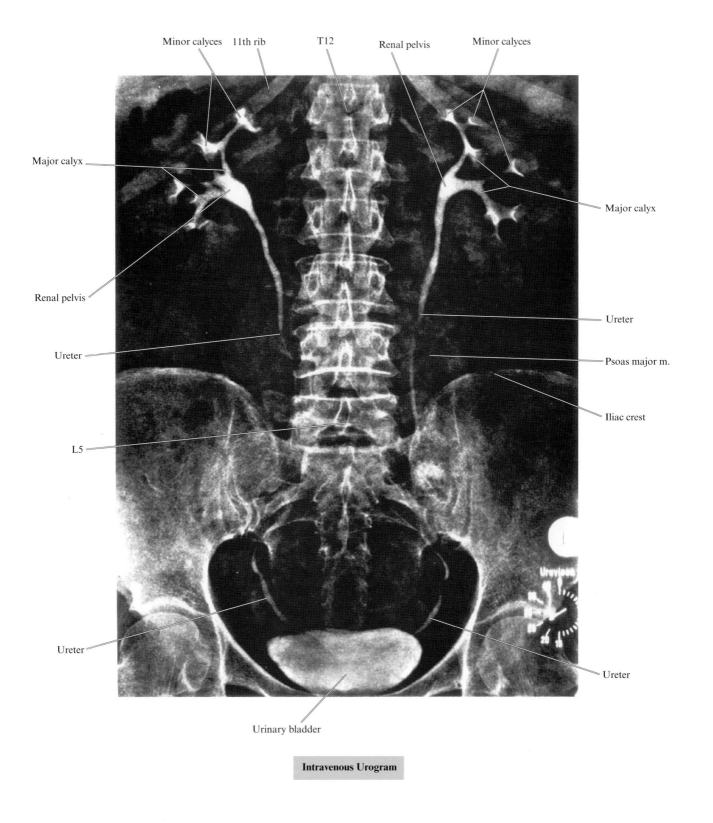

Minor calyces   11th rib   T12   Renal pelvis   Minor calyces

Major calyx

Renal pelvis

Ureter

L5

Ureter

Urinary bladder

Major calyx

Ureter

Psoas major m.

Iliac crest

Ureter

Intravenous Urogram

PLATE 3.37   SUPRARENAL GLANDS

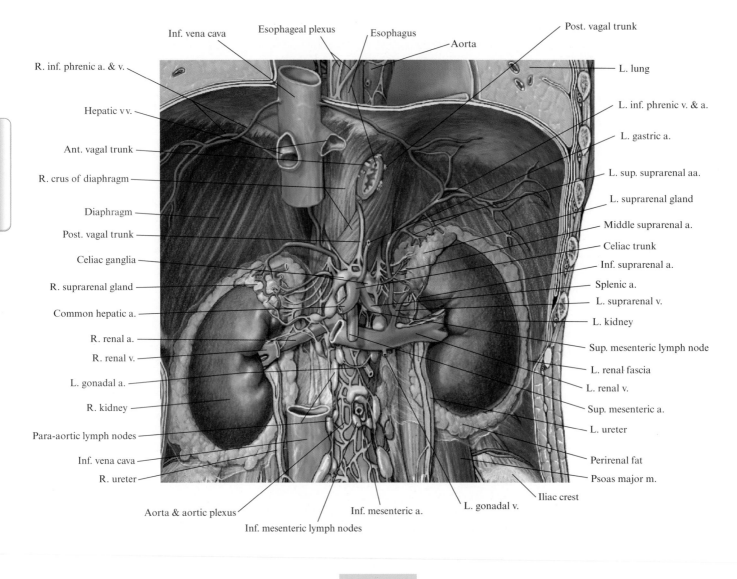

Inf. vena cava
Esophageal plexus
Esophagus
Aorta
Post. vagal trunk

R. inf. phrenic a. & v.
Hepatic v v.
Ant. vagal trunk
R. crus of diaphragm
Diaphragm
Post. vagal trunk
Celiac ganglia
R. suprarenal gland
Common hepatic a.
R. renal a.
R. renal v.
L. gonadal a.
R. kidney
Para-aortic lymph nodes
Inf. vena cava
R. ureter

L. lung
L. inf. phrenic v. & a.
L. gastric a.
L. sup. suprarenal aa.
L. suprarenal gland
Middle suprarenal a.
Celiac trunk
Inf. suprarenal a.
Splenic a.
L. suprarenal v.
L. kidney
Sup. mesenteric lymph node
L. renal fascia
L. renal v.
Sup. mesenteric a.
L. ureter
Perirenal fat
Psoas major m.
Iliac crest

Aorta & aortic plexus
Inf. mesenteric lymph nodes
Inf. mesenteric a.
L. gonadal v.

Anterior View

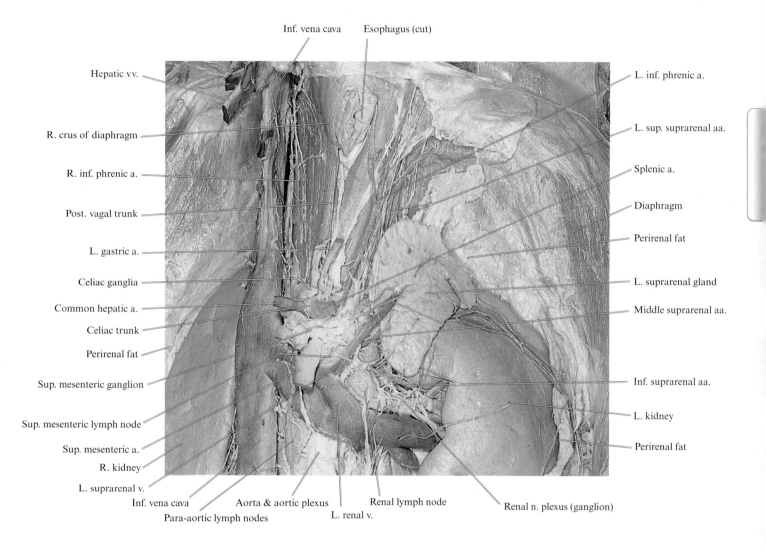

Inf. vena cava

Esophagus (cut)

Hepatic vv.

R. crus of diaphragm

R. inf. phrenic a.

Post. vagal trunk

L. gastric a.

Celiac ganglia

Common hepatic a.

Celiac trunk

Perirenal fat

Sup. mesenteric ganglion

Sup. mesenteric lymph node

Sup. mesenteric a.

R. kidney

L. suprarenal v.

Inf. vena cava

Para-aortic lymph nodes

Aorta & aortic plexus

L. renal v.

Renal lymph node

Renal n. plexus (ganglion)

L. inf. phrenic a.

L. sup. suprarenal aa.

Splenic a.

Diaphragm

Perirenal fat

L. suprarenal gland

Middle suprarenal aa.

Inf. suprarenal aa.

L. kidney

Perirenal fat

Anterior View of Superior Pole of L. Kidney

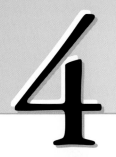

4 PELVIS AND PERINEUM

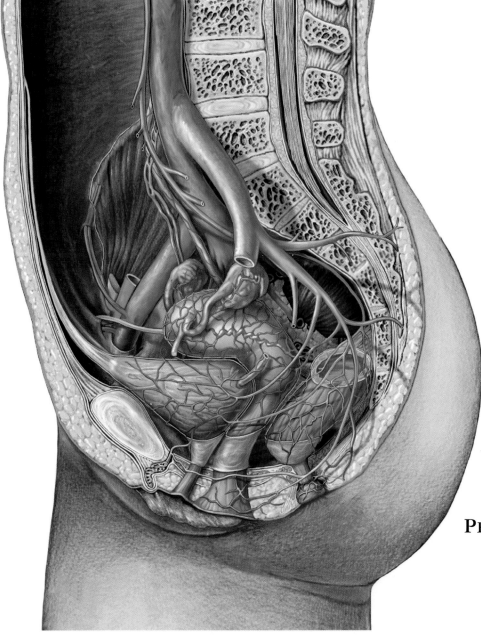

TOPOGRAPHY

SKELETON &
LIGAMENTS

MUSCLES

ARTERIES

VEINS

NERVES

LYMPHATICS

UROGENITAL
TRACTS

FEMALE PELVIC
CONTENTS

MALE PELVIC
CONTENTS

PERINEAL FASCIAE &
SPACES

FEMALE &
MALE PERINEUM

PUDENDAL
STRUCTURES

RECTUM &
ANAL CANAL

PLATE 4.1   TOPOGRAPHY—MALE

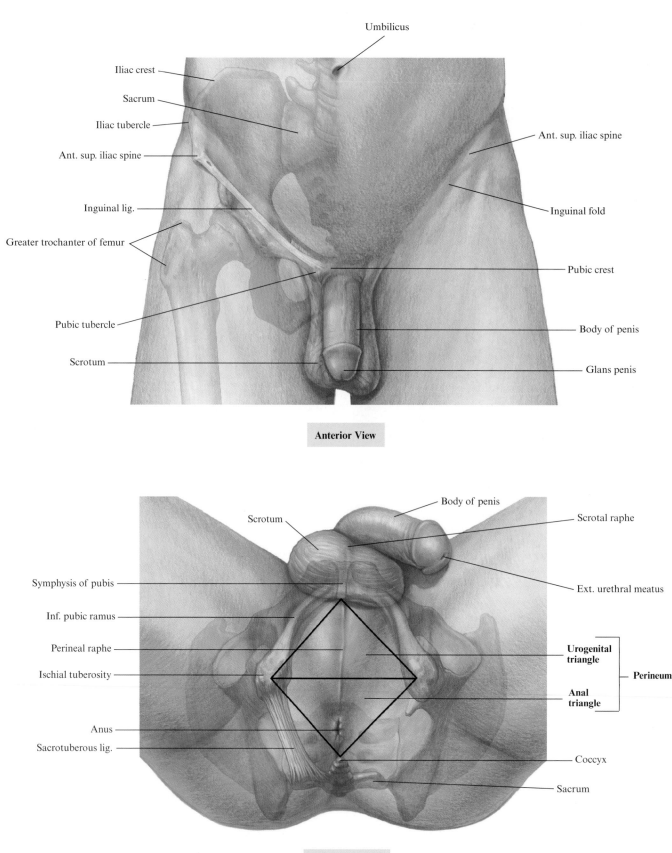

Umbilicus

Iliac crest

Sacrum

Iliac tubercle

Ant. sup. iliac spine

Ant. sup. iliac spine

Inguinal lig.

Inguinal fold

Greater trochanter of femur

Pubic crest

Pubic tubercle

Body of penis

Scrotum

Glans penis

Anterior View

Body of penis

Scrotum

Scrotal raphe

Symphysis of pubis

Ext. urethral meatus

Inf. pubic ramus

Perineal raphe

Urogenital triangle

Perineum

Ischial tuberosity

Anal triangle

Anus

Sacrotuberous lig.

Coccyx

Sacrum

Lithotomy View

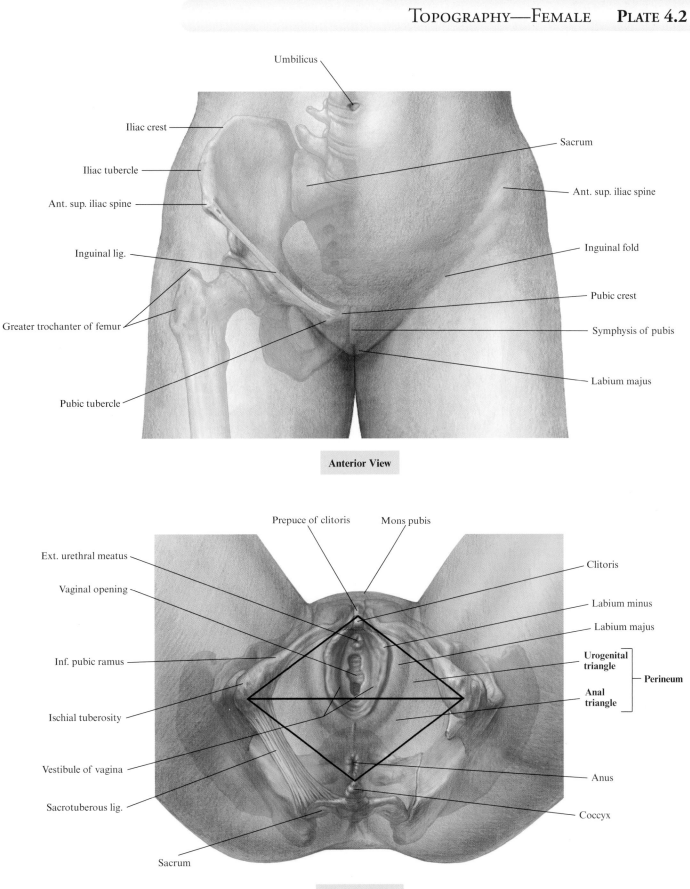

Umbilicus

Iliac crest

Iliac tubercle

Ant. sup. iliac spine

Inguinal lig.

Greater trochanter of femur

Pubic tubercle

Sacrum

Ant. sup. iliac spine

Inguinal fold

Pubic crest

Symphysis of pubis

Labium majus

Anterior View

Prepuce of clitoris   Mons pubis

Ext. urethral meatus

Vaginal opening

Inf. pubic ramus

Ischial tuberosity

Vestibule of vagina

Sacrotuberous lig.

Sacrum

Clitoris

Labium minus

Labium majus

Urogenital triangle

Perineum

Anal triangle

Anus

Coccyx

Lithotomy View

PLATE 4.3   SKELETON & LIGAMENTS

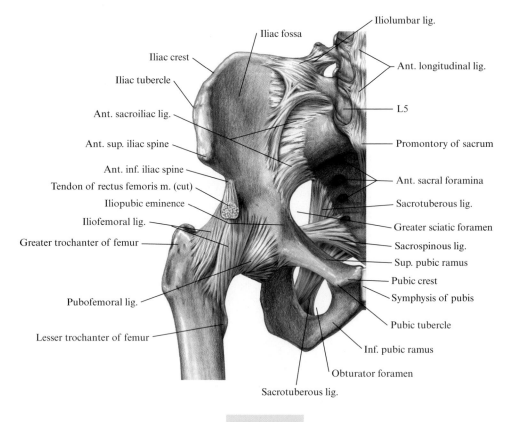

Iliac fossa

Iliolumbar lig.

Iliac crest

Ant. longitudinal lig.

Iliac tubercle

L5

Ant. sacroiliac lig.

Promontory of sacrum

Ant. sup. iliac spine

Ant. inf. iliac spine

Ant. sacral foramina

Tendon of rectus femoris m. (cut)

Sacrotuberous lig.

Iliopubic eminence

Greater sciatic foramen

Iliofemoral lig.

Sacrospinous lig.

Greater trochanter of femur

Sup. pubic ramus

Pubic crest

Pubofemoral lig.

Symphysis of pubis

Pubic tubercle

Lesser trochanter of femur

Inf. pubic ramus

Obturator foramen

Sacrotuberous lig.

Anterior View

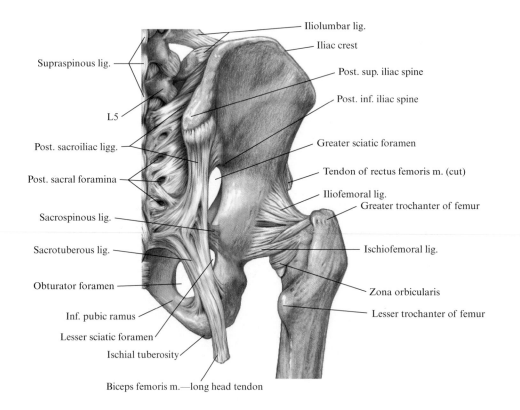

Iliolumbar lig.

Iliac crest

Supraspinous lig.

Post. sup. iliac spine

Post. inf. iliac spine

L5

Post. sacroiliac ligg.

Greater sciatic foramen

Post. sacral foramina

Tendon of rectus femoris m. (cut)

Iliofemoral lig.

Greater trochanter of femur

Sacrospinous lig.

Sacrotuberous lig.

Ischiofemoral lig.

Obturator foramen

Zona orbicularis

Inf. pubic ramus

Lesser trochanter of femur

Lesser sciatic foramen

Ischial tuberosity

Biceps femoris m.—long head tendon

Posterior View

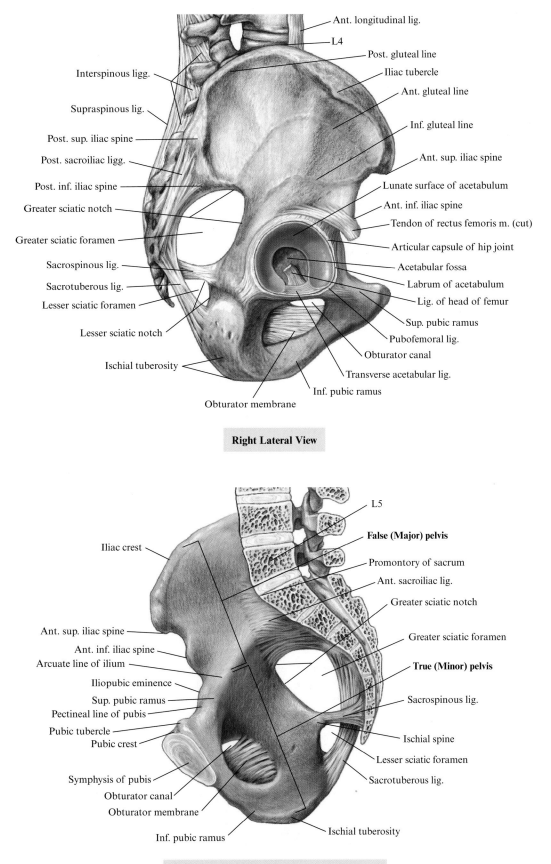

Ant. longitudinal lig.

L4

Post. gluteal line

Iliac tubercle

Ant. gluteal line

Inf. gluteal line

Ant. sup. iliac spine

Lunate surface of acetabulum

Ant. inf. iliac spine

Tendon of rectus femoris m. (cut)

Articular capsule of hip joint

Acetabular fossa

Labrum of acetabulum

Lig. of head of femur

Sup. pubic ramus

Pubofemoral lig.

Obturator canal

Transverse acetabular lig.

Inf. pubic ramus

Interspinous ligg.

Supraspinous lig.

Post. sup. iliac spine

Post. sacroiliac ligg.

Post. inf. iliac spine

Greater sciatic notch

Greater sciatic foramen

Sacrospinous lig.

Sacrotuberous lig.

Lesser sciatic foramen

Lesser sciatic notch

Ischial tuberosity

Obturator membrane

Right Lateral View

L5

False (Major) pelvis

Promontory of sacrum

Ant. sacroiliac lig.

Greater sciatic notch

Greater sciatic foramen

True (Minor) pelvis

Sacrospinous lig.

Ischial spine

Lesser sciatic foramen

Sacrotuberous lig.

Ischial tuberosity

Iliac crest

Ant. sup. iliac spine

Ant. inf. iliac spine

Arcuate line of ilium

Iliopubic eminence

Sup. pubic ramus

Pectineal line of pubis

Pubic tubercle

Pubic crest

Symphysis of pubis

Obturator canal

Obturator membrane

Inf. pubic ramus

Right Side of Hemisected Pelvis—Medial View

PLATE 4.5   BONY PELVIS—MALE

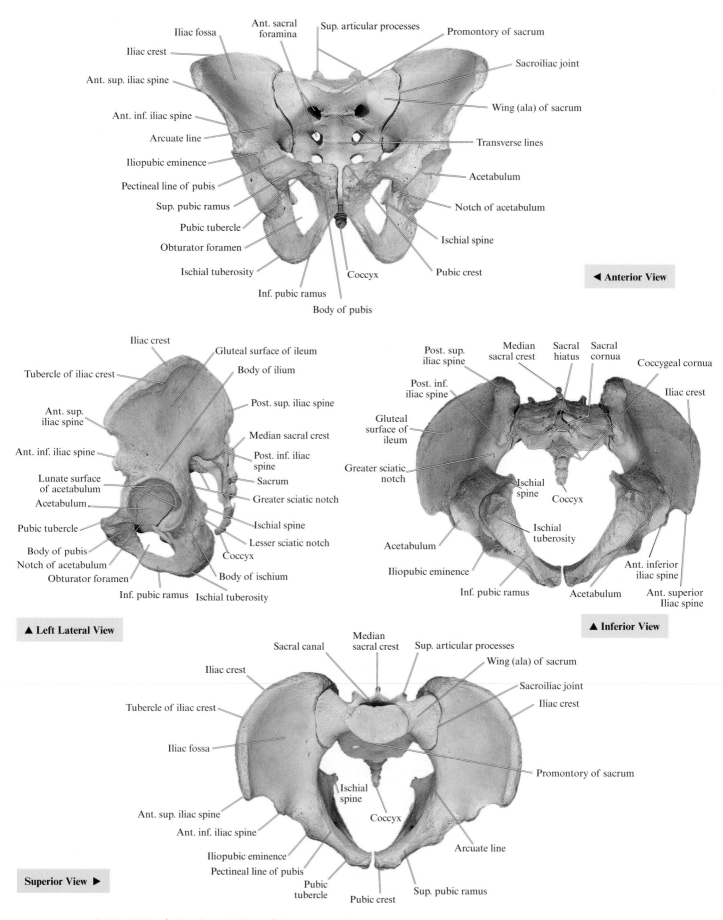

Iliac fossa

Ant. sacral foramina

Sup. articular processes

Promontory of sacrum

Iliac crest

Ant. sup. iliac spine

Ant. inf. iliac spine

Arcuate line

Iliopubic eminence

Pectineal line of pubis

Sup. pubic ramus

Pubic tubercle

Obturator foramen

Ischial tuberosity

Inf. pubic ramus

Body of pubis

Coccyx

Sacroiliac joint

Wing (ala) of sacrum

Transverse lines

Acetabulum

Notch of acetabulum

Ischial spine

Pubic crest

◀ **Anterior View**

Iliac crest

Tubercle of iliac crest

Ant. sup. iliac spine

Ant. inf. iliac spine

Lunate surface of acetabulum

Acetabulum

Pubic tubercle

Body of pubis

Notch of acetabulum

Obturator foramen

Inf. pubic ramus   Ischial tuberosity

Gluteal surface of ileum

Body of ilium

Post. sup. iliac spine

Median sacral crest

Post. inf. iliac spine

Sacrum

Greater sciatic notch

Ischial spine

Lesser sciatic notch

Coccyx

Body of ischium

▲ **Left Lateral View**

Post. sup. iliac spine

Post. inf. iliac spine

Gluteal surface of ileum

Greater sciatic notch

Acetabulum

Iliopubic eminence

Inf. pubic ramus

Median sacral crest

Sacral hiatus

Sacral cornua

Coccygeal cornua

Iliac crest

Ischial spine

Coccyx

Ischial tuberosity

Ant. inferior iliac spine

Acetabulum

Ant. superior Iliac spine

▲ **Inferior View**

Sacral canal

Median sacral crest

Sup. articular processes

Iliac crest

Tubercle of iliac crest

Iliac fossa

Ant. sup. iliac spine

Ant. inf. iliac spine

Iliopubic eminence

Pectineal line of pubis

Ischial spine

Coccyx

Pubic tubercle

Pubic crest

Sup. pubic ramus

Arcuate line

Promontory of sacrum

Iliac crest

Sacroiliac joint

Wing (ala) of sacrum

Superior View ▶

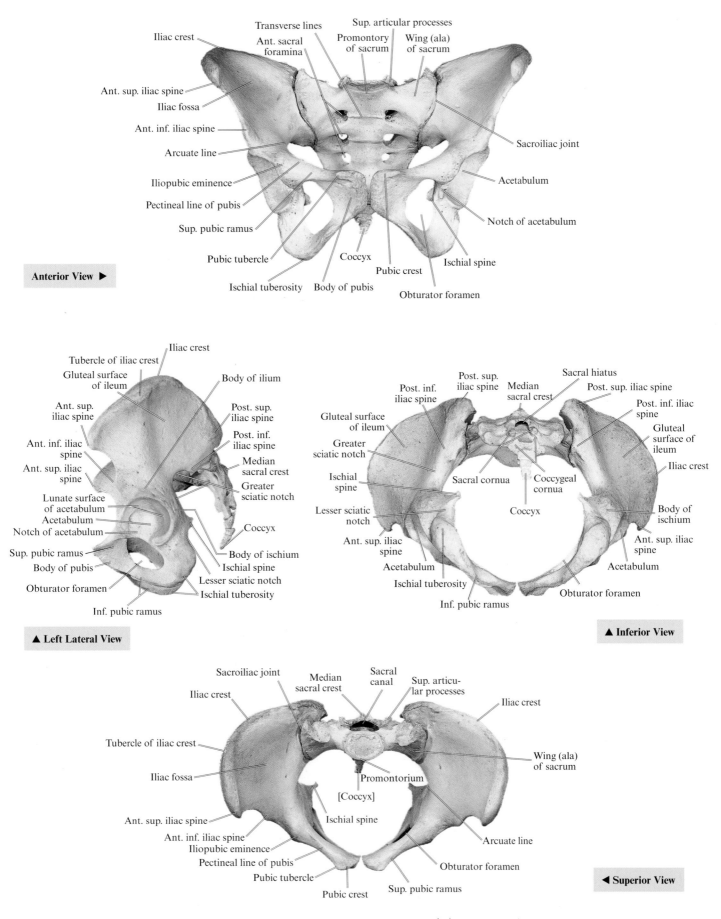

Anterior View ▶

Iliac crest

Transverse lines

Ant. sacral foramina

Sup. articular processes

Promontory of sacrum

Wing (ala) of sacrum

Ant. sup. iliac spine

Iliac fossa

Ant. inf. iliac spine

Arcuate line

Iliopubic eminence

Pectineal line of pubis

Sup. pubic ramus

Pubic tubercle

Coccyx

Ischial tuberosity

Body of pubis

Pubic crest

Ischial spine

Obturator foramen

Sacroiliac joint

Acetabulum

Notch of acetabulum

◀ Left Lateral View

Tubercle of iliac crest

Gluteal surface of ileum

Iliac crest

Body of ilium

Ant. sup. iliac spine

Post. sup. iliac spine

Post. inf. iliac spine

Ant. inf. iliac spine

Ant. sup. iliac spine

Median sacral crest

Greater sciatic notch

Lunate surface of acetabulum

Acetabulum

Notch of acetabulum

Coccyx

Sup. pubic ramus

Body of pubis

Body of ischium

Ischial spine

Lesser sciatic notch

Obturator foramen

Ischial tuberosity

Inf. pubic ramus

▲ Inferior View

Post. sup. iliac spine

Post. inf. iliac spine

Median sacral crest

Sacral hiatus

Post. sup. iliac spine

Post. inf. iliac spine

Gluteal surface of ileum

Greater sciatic notch

Ischial spine

Sacral cornua

Coccygeal cornua

Gluteal surface of ileum

Iliac crest

Lesser sciatic notch

Coccyx

Body of ischium

Ant. sup. iliac spine

Acetabulum

Ischial tuberosity

Ant. sup. iliac spine

Acetabulum

Inf. pubic ramus

Obturator foramen

◀ Superior View

Sacroiliac joint

Median sacral crest

Sacral canal

Sup. articular processes

Iliac crest

Iliac crest

Tubercle of iliac crest

Iliac fossa

Wing (ala) of sacrum

Promontorium

[Coccyx]

Ant. sup. iliac spine

Ischial spine

Ant. inf. iliac spine

Iliopubic eminence

Pectineal line of pubis

Pubic tubercle

Arcuate line

Obturator foramen

Pubic crest

Sup. pubic ramus

PLATE 4.7   PELVIC MUSCLES—SUPERFICIAL PERINEAL

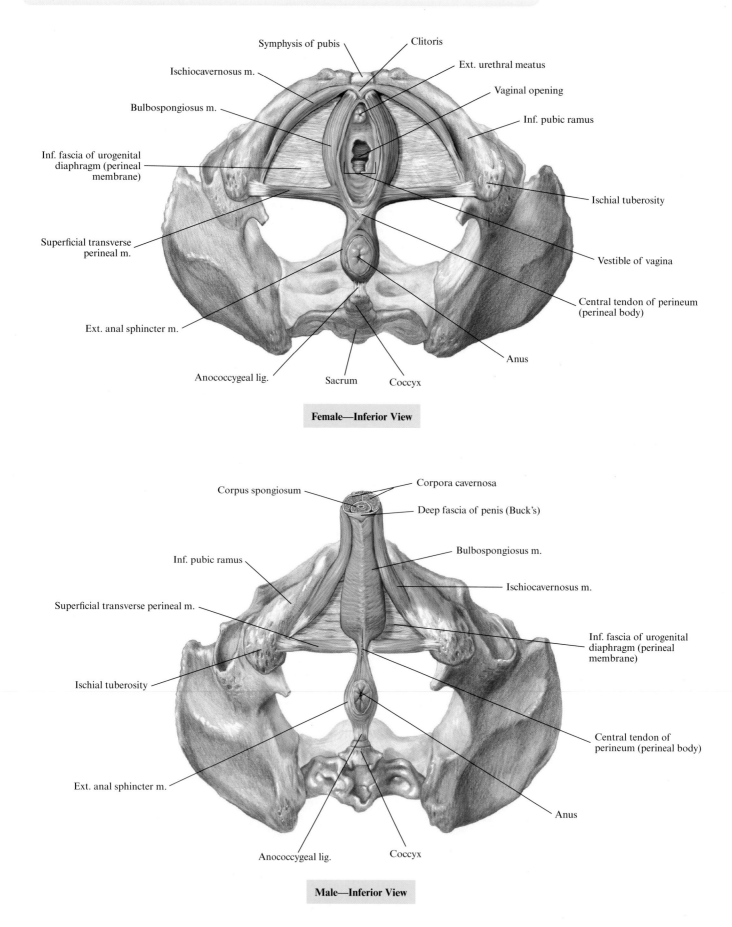

Female—Inferior View

Symphysis of pubis

Clitoris

Ischiocavernosus m.

Ext. urethral meatus

Bulbospongiosus m.

Vaginal opening

Inf. pubic ramus

Inf. fascia of urogenital diaphragm (perineal membrane)

Ischial tuberosity

Superficial transverse perineal m.

Vestible of vagina

Central tendon of perineum (perineal body)

Ext. anal sphincter m.

Anus

Anococcygeal lig.

Sacrum

Coccyx

Male—Inferior View

Corpus spongiosum

Corpora cavernosa

Inf. pubic ramus

Deep fascia of penis (Buck's)

Bulbospongiosus m.

Superficial transverse perineal m.

Ischiocavernosus m.

Inf. fascia of urogenital diaphragm (perineal membrane)

Ischial tuberosity

Central tendon of perineum (perineal body)

Ext. anal sphincter m.

Anus

Anococcygeal lig.

Coccyx

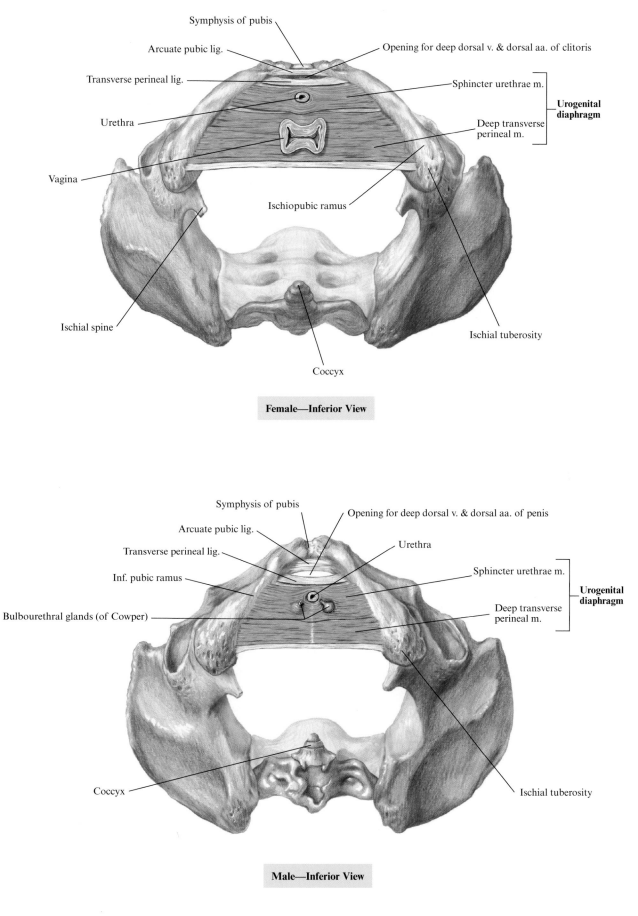

Symphysis of pubis

Arcuate pubic lig.

Opening for deep dorsal v. & dorsal aa. of clitoris

Transverse perineal lig.

Sphincter urethrae m.

Urogenital diaphragm

Urethra

Deep transverse perineal m.

Vagina

Ischiopubic ramus

Ischial spine

Ischial tuberosity

Coccyx

Female—Inferior View

Symphysis of pubis

Arcuate pubic lig.

Opening for deep dorsal v. & dorsal aa. of penis

Transverse perineal lig.

Urethra

Inf. pubic ramus

Sphincter urethrae m.

Urogenital diaphragm

Bulbourethral glands (of Cowper)

Deep transverse perineal m.

Coccyx

Ischial tuberosity

Male—Inferior View

PLATE 4.9   PELVIC MUSCLES—PELVIC DIAPHRAGM

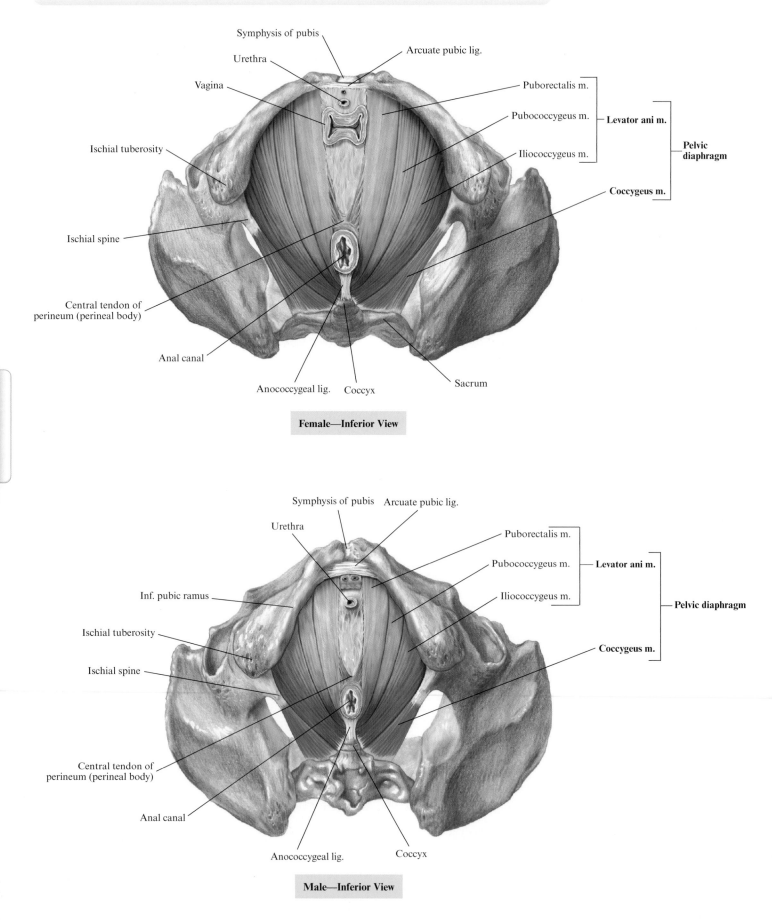

Symphysis of pubis

Urethra

Arcuate pubic lig.

Vagina

Puborectalis m.

Pubococcygeus m.

Iliococcygeus m.

Levator ani m.

Pelvic diaphragm

Ischial tuberosity

Coccygeus m.

Ischial spine

Central tendon of perineum (perineal body)

Anal canal

Anococcygeal lig.   Coccyx

Sacrum

Female—Inferior View

Symphysis of pubis   Arcuate pubic lig.

Urethra

Puborectalis m.

Pubococcygeus m.

Iliococcygeus m.

Levator ani m.

Inf. pubic ramus

Pelvic diaphragm

Ischial tuberosity

Coccygeus m.

Ischial spine

Central tendon of perineum (perineal body)

Anal canal

Anococcygeal lig.   Coccyx

Male—Inferior View

Muscle	Superior or Lateral Attachment	Inferior or Medial Attachment	Innervation	Action(s)
Ischiocavernosus	Int. surface of ischial ramus & tuberosity laterally	Sides & ventrum of crus of penis in ♂ or clitoris medially in ♀	Perineal brr. of pudendal n. (S2–4)	Maintains erection of penis or clitoris
Bulbospongiosus	Dorsum of clitoris in ♀; inf. fascia of urogenital diaphragm, sides & dorsum of penile bulb in ♂	Perineal body, inf. fascia of urogenital diaphragm & median raphe of penile bulb in ♂		Compresses vaginal orifice & erection of clitoris in ♀; compresses urethra, assist in erection & ejaculation in ♂
Superficial transverse perineal	Int. surface of ischial tuberosity laterally	Perineal body (central perineal tendon) medially		Supports pelvic viscera
Ext. anal sphincter	Anococcygeal lig. to coccyx & int. anal sphincter m. superiorly	Perineal body anteriorly & skin superficially	Inf. rectal n. (S2–3) and perineal br. of S4 spinal n.	Compresses anus
Sphincter urethrae	Inf. pubic ramus laterally	Perineal body posteriorly & fibers from opposite side medially	Perineal brr. of pudendal n. (S2–4)	Compresses urethra in ♂ & ♀ & vagina in ♀
Deep transverse perineal	Ischial ramus laterally	Perineal body medially		Supports pelvic viscera

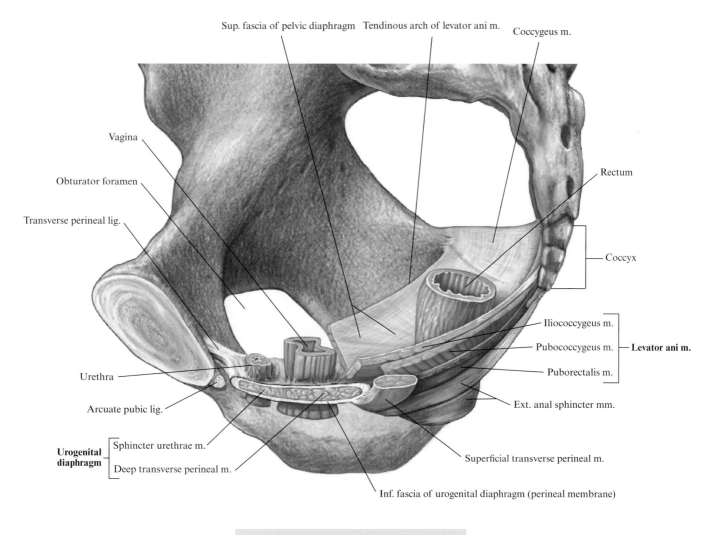

Female Perineum & Muscles—Left Lateral View

PLATE 4.10   PELVIC MUSCLES—MALE

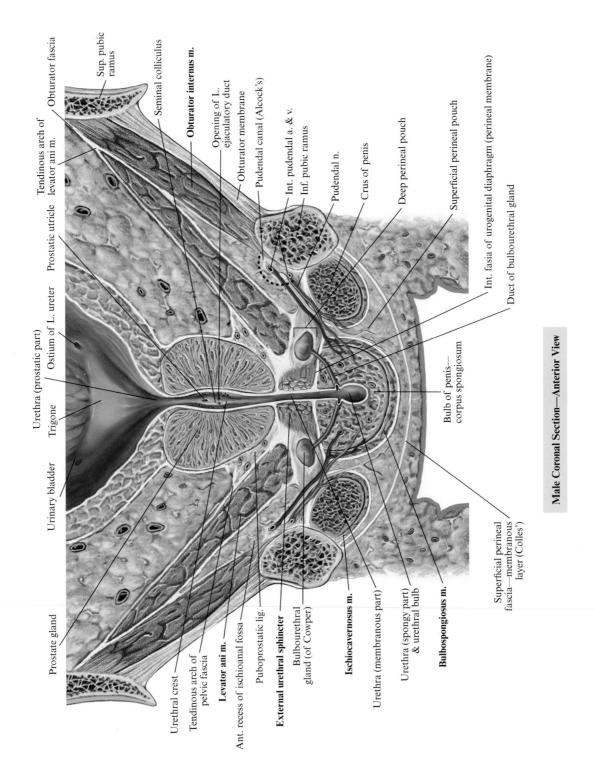

Obturator fascia

Sup. pubic ramus

Tendinous arch of levator ani m.

Seminal colliculus

Obturator internus m.

Opening of L. ejaculatory duct

Obturator membrane

Pudendal canal (Alcock's)

Int. pudendal a. & v.

Inf. pubic ramus

Pudendal n.

Crus of penis

Deep perineal pouch

Superficial perineal pouch

Int. fasia of urogenital diaphragm (perineal membrane)

Duct of bulbourethral gland

Prostatic utricle

Urethra (prostatic part)

Ostium of L. ureter

Trigone

Urinary bladder

Bulb of penis— corpus spongiosum

Superficial perineal fascia—membranous layer (Colles')

Prostate gland

Urethral crest

Tendinous arch of pelvic fascia

Levator ani m.

Ant. recess of ischioanal fossa

Puboprostatic lig.

External urethral sphincter

Bulbourethral gland (of Cowper)

Ischiocavernosus m.

Urethra (membranous part)

Urethra (spongy part) & urethral bulb

Bulbospongiosus m.

Male Coronal Section—Anterior View

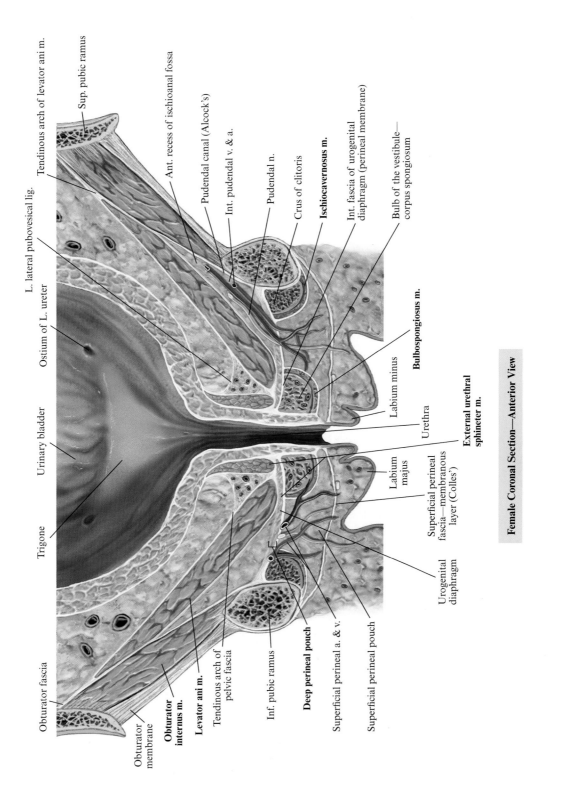

Sup. pubic ramus

Tendinous arch of levator ani m.

Ant. recess of ischioanal fossa

Pudendal canal (Alcock's)

Int. pudendal v. & a.

Pudendal n.

Crus of clitoris

Ischiocavernosus m.

Int. fascia of urogenital diaphragm (perineal membrane)

Bulb of the vestibule— corpus spongiosum

L. lateral pubovesical lig.

Ostium of L. ureter

Bulbospongiosus m.

Urinary bladder

Labium minus

Urethra

Trigone

External urethral sphineter m.

Labium majus

Superficial perineal fascia—membranous layer (Colles')

Obturator fascia

Urogenital diaphragm

Obturator membrane

Obturator internus m.

Levator ani m.

Tendinous arch of pelvic fascia

Inf. pubic ramus

Deep perineal pouch

Superficial perineal a. & v.

Superficial perineal pouch

Female Coronal Section—Anterior View

PLATE 4.12   FEMOROPELVIC MUSCLES

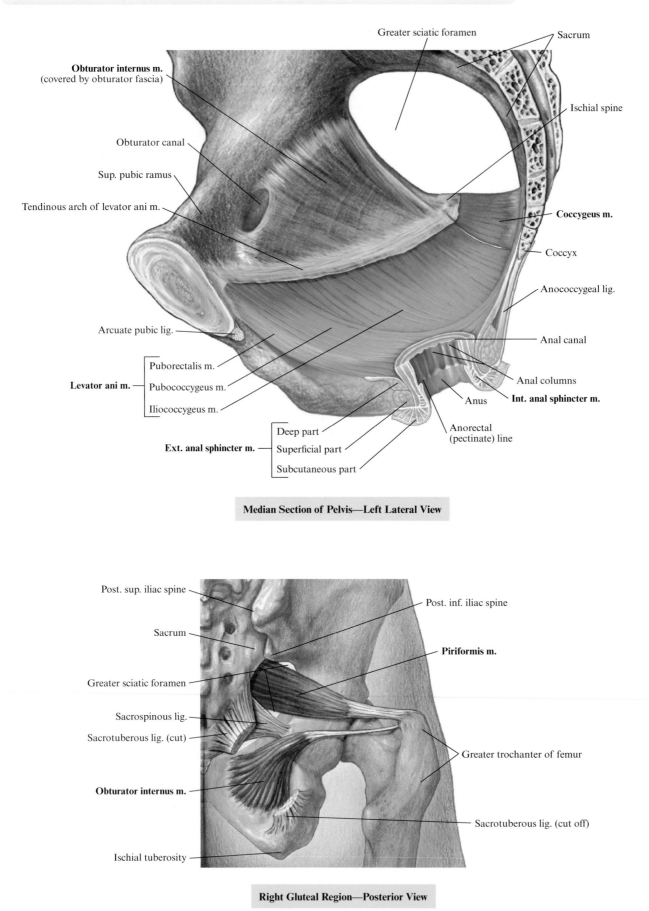

Greater sciatic foramen

Sacrum

Obturator internus m.
(covered by obturator fascia)

Ischial spine

Obturator canal

Sup. pubic ramus

Coccygeus m.

Tendinous arch of levator ani m.

Coccyx

Anococcygeal lig.

Arcuate pubic lig.

Anal canal

Puborectalis m.

Anal columns

Levator ani m.   Pubococcygeus m.

Int. anal sphincter m.

Iliococcygeus m.

Anus

Deep part

Anorectal
(pectinate) line

Ext. anal sphincter m.   Superficial part

Subcutaneous part

Median Section of Pelvis—Left Lateral View

Post. sup. iliac spine

Post. inf. iliac spine

Sacrum

Piriformis m.

Greater sciatic foramen

Sacrospinous lig.

Sacrotuberous lig. (cut)

Greater trochanter of femur

Obturator internus m.

Sacrotuberous lig. (cut off)

Ischial tuberosity

Right Gluteal Region—Posterior View

Muscles of the Pelvic Diaphragm

Muscle	Superior or Lateral Attachment	Inferior or Medial Attachment	Innervation	Action(s)
Puborectalis	Body of pubis anteriorly	Fibers of opposite side post. to rectum	Inf. rectal n. (S2, 3) & perineal brr. of S3, 4 spinal n.	Maintains anorectal flexure by drawing anal canal anteriorly
Pubococcygeus	Body of pubis and obturator fascia anteriorly	Coccyx & anococcygeal lig. posteriorly		Supports pelvic viscera
Iliococcygeus	Ischial spine & tendinous arch of pelvic fascia laterally	Coccyx & anococcygeal lig. posteriorly		Supports pelvic viscera
Coccygeus	Ischial spine & sacrospinous lig. laterally	Coccyx & S5 vertebra medially	Brr. of S3–5 spinal nn.	Supports pelvic viscera

Muscles of the Pelvic Walls

Muscle	Superior or Medial Attachment	Inferior or Lateral Attachment	Innervation	Action(s)
Obturator internus	Pelvic surfaces of ilium & ischium; obturator membrane	Greater trochanter of femur	N. to obturator internus (L5–S2)	Rotates thigh laterally
Piriformis	Pelvic surface of 2nd–4th sacral segments; sup. margin of greater sciatic notch, & sacrotuberous lig.		Ventral rami of S1 & S2	Rotates thigh laterally

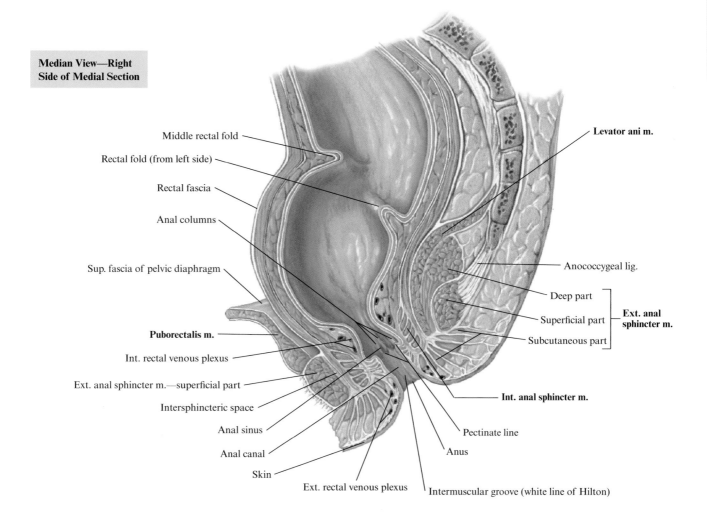

Median View—Right Side of Medial Section

Middle rectal fold

Rectal fold (from left side)

Rectal fascia

Anal columns

Sup. fascia of pelvic diaphragm

Puborectalis m.

Int. rectal venous plexus

Ext. anal sphincter m.—superficial part

Intersphincteric space

Anal sinus

Anal canal

Skin

Ext. rectal venous plexus

Levator ani m.

Anococcygeal lig.

Deep part
Superficial part } **Ext. anal sphincter m.**
Subcutaneous part

Int. anal sphincter m.

Pectinate line

Anus

Intermuscular groove (white line of Hilton)

PLATE 4.13   ARTERIES OF THE PELVIS—MALE

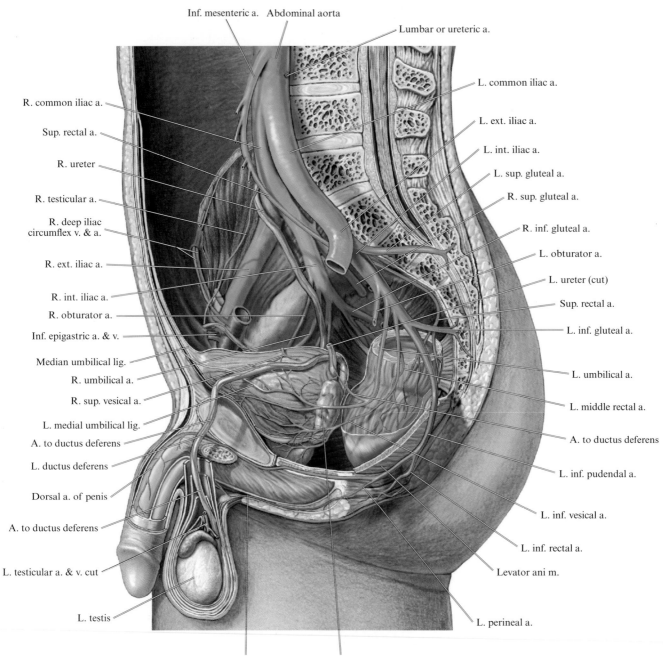

Inf. mesenteric a.   Abdominal aorta

Lumbar or ureteric a.

R. common iliac a.

Sup. rectal a.

R. ureter

R. testicular a.

R. deep iliac
circumflex v. & a.

R. ext. iliac a.

R. int. iliac a.

R. obturator a.

Inf. epigastric a. & v.

Median umbilical lig.

R. umbilical a.

R. sup. vesical a.

L. medial umbilical lig.

A. to ductus deferens

L. ductus deferens

Dorsal a. of penis

A. to ductus deferens

L. testicular a. & v. cut

L. testis

L. common iliac a.

L. ext. iliac a.

L. int. iliac a.

L. sup. gluteal a.

R. sup. gluteal a.

R. inf. gluteal a.

L. obturator a.

L. ureter (cut)

Sup. rectal a.

L. inf. gluteal a.

L. umbilical a.

L. middle rectal a.

A. to ductus deferens

L. inf. pudendal a.

L. inf. vesical a.

L. inf. rectal a.

Levator ani m.

L. perineal a.

L. post. scrotal a. & v.   L. sup. vesical a.

Medial View with Peritoneum Removed

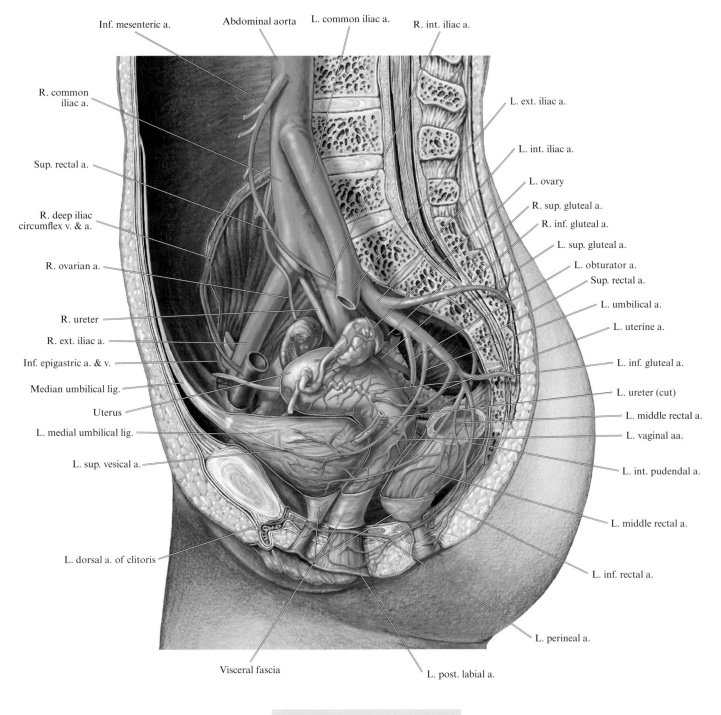

Inf. mesenteric a.

Abdominal aorta

L. common iliac a.

R. int. iliac a.

R. common iliac a.

L. ext. iliac a.

Sup. rectal a.

L. int. iliac a.

L. ovary

R. deep iliac circumflex v. & a.

R. sup. gluteal a.

R. inf. gluteal a.

L. sup. gluteal a.

R. ovarian a.

L. obturator a.

Sup. rectal a.

L. umbilical a.

R. ureter

L. uterine a.

R. ext. iliac a.

Inf. epigastric a. & v.

L. inf. gluteal a.

L. ureter (cut)

Median umbilical lig.

L. middle rectal a.

Uterus

L. vaginal aa.

L. medial umbilical lig.

L. int. pudendal a.

L. sup. vesical a.

L. middle rectal a.

L. dorsal a. of clitoris

L. inf. rectal a.

L. perineal a.

Visceral fascia

L. post. labial a.

Medial View with Peritoneum Removed

PLATE 4.15   VEINS OF THE PELVIS—MALE

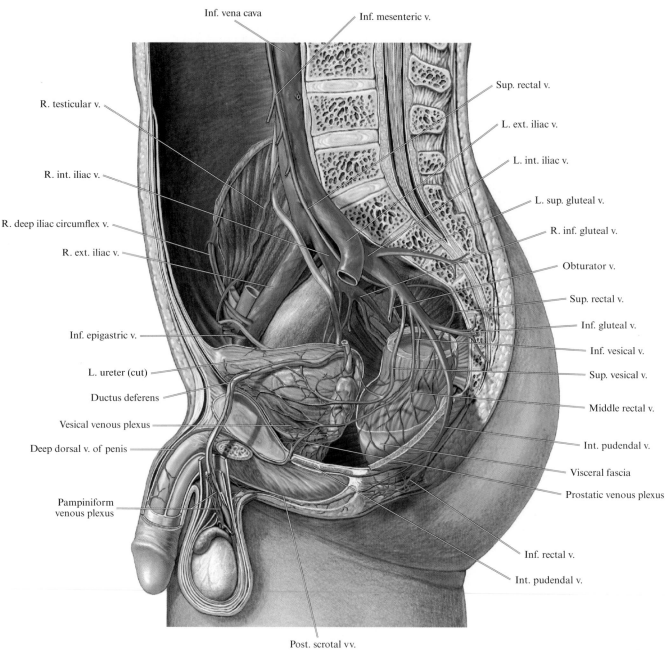

Inf. vena cava

Inf. mesenteric v.

R. testicular v.

R. int. iliac v.

R. deep iliac circumflex v.

R. ext. iliac v.

Inf. epigastric v.

L. ureter (cut)

Ductus deferens

Vesical venous plexus

Deep dorsal v. of penis

Pampiniform
venous plexus

Sup. rectal v.

L. ext. iliac v.

L. int. iliac v.

L. sup. gluteal v.

R. inf. gluteal v.

Obturator v.

Sup. rectal v.

Inf. gluteal v.

Inf. vesical v.

Sup. vesical v.

Middle rectal v.

Int. pudendal v.

Visceral fascia

Prostatic venous plexus

Inf. rectal v.

Int. pudendal v.

Post. scrotal vv.

Medial View with Peritoneum Removed

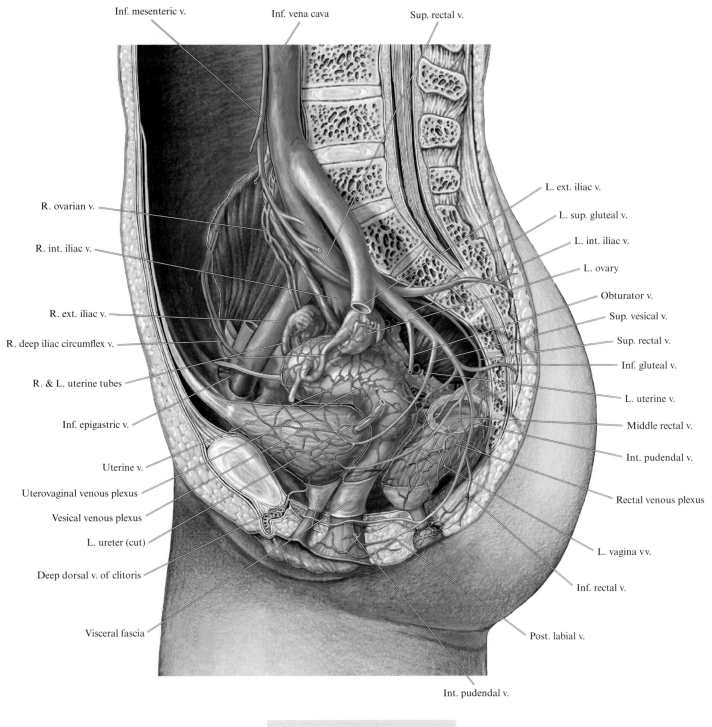

Inf. mesenteric v.

Inf. vena cava

Sup. rectal v.

R. ovarian v.

R. int. iliac v.

R. ext. iliac v.

R. deep iliac circumflex v.

R. & L. uterine tubes

Inf. epigastric v.

Uterine v.

Uterovaginal venous plexus

Vesical venous plexus

L. ureter (cut)

Deep dorsal v. of clitoris

Visceral fascia

L. ext. iliac v.

L. sup. gluteal v.

L. int. iliac v.

L. ovary

Obturator v.

Sup. vesical v.

Sup. rectal v.

Inf. gluteal v.

L. uterine v.

Middle rectal v.

Int. pudendal v.

Rectal venous plexus

L. vagina vv.

Inf. rectal v.

Post. labial v.

Int. pudendal v.

Medial View with Peritoneum Removed

PLATE 4.17   DERMATOMES & CUTANEOUS NERVES—MALE

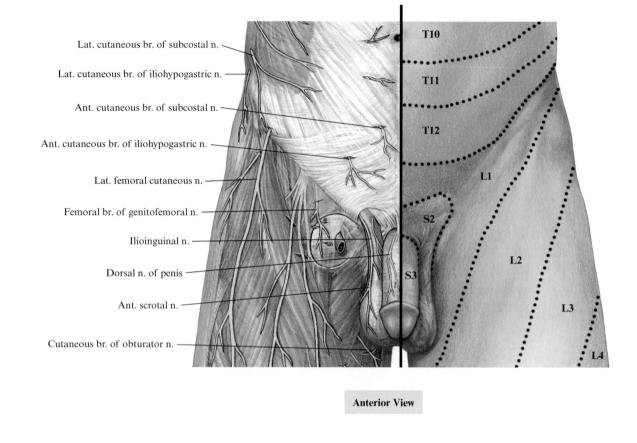

Lat. cutaneous br. of subcostal n.

Lat. cutaneous br. of iliohypogastric n.

Ant. cutaneous br. of subcostal n.

Ant. cutaneous br. of iliohypogastric n.

Lat. femoral cutaneous n.

Femoral br. of genitofemoral n.

Ilioinguinal n.

Dorsal n. of penis

Ant. scrotal n.

Cutaneous br. of obturator n.

T10

T11

T12

L1

S2

L2

S3

L3

L4

Anterior View

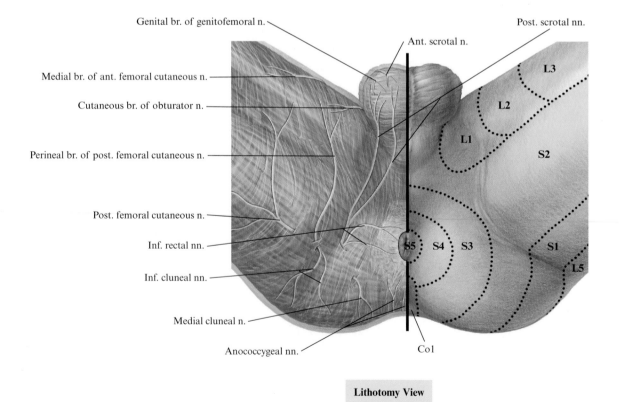

Genital br. of genitofemoral n.

Ant. scrotal n.

Post. scrotal nn.

Medial br. of ant. femoral cutaneous n.

Cutaneous br. of obturator n.

Perineal br. of post. femoral cutaneous n.

Post. femoral cutaneous n.

Inf. rectal nn.

Inf. cluneal nn.

Medial cluneal n.

Anococcygeal nn.

L3

L2

L1

S2

S5

S4

S3

S1

L5

Co1

Lithotomy View

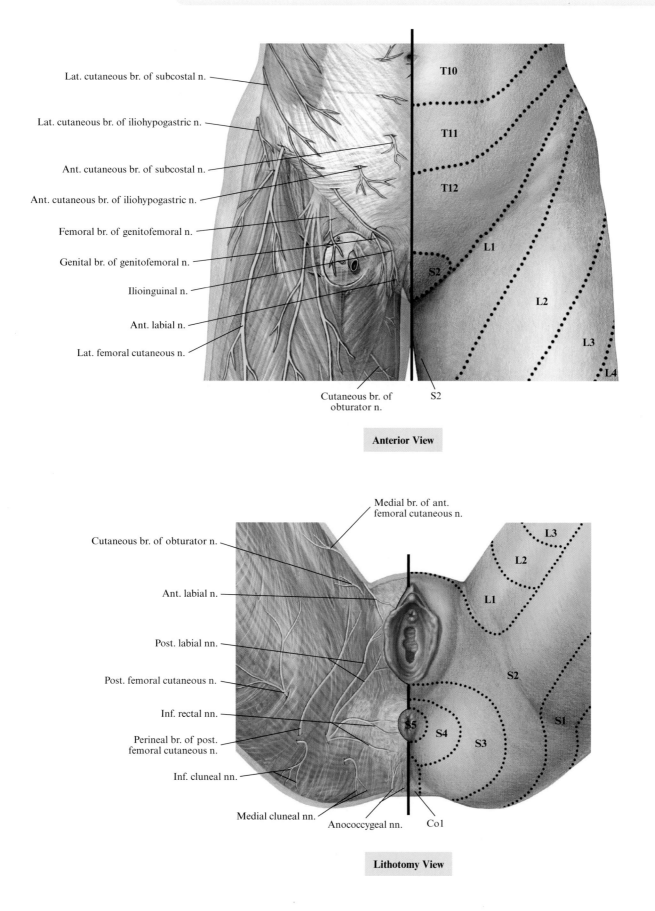

Lat. cutaneous br. of subcostal n.

Lat. cutaneous br. of iliohypogastric n.

Ant. cutaneous br. of subcostal n.

Ant. cutaneous br. of iliohypogastric n.

Femoral br. of genitofemoral n.

Genital br. of genitofemoral n.

Ilioinguinal n.

Ant. labial n.

Lat. femoral cutaneous n.

T10

T11

T12

L1

S2

L2

L3

L4

Cutaneous br. of
obturator n.

S2

Anterior View

Medial br. of ant.
femoral cutaneous n.

Cutaneous br. of obturator n.

Ant. labial n.

Post. labial nn.

Post. femoral cutaneous n.

Inf. rectal nn.

Perineal br. of post.
femoral cutaneous n.

Inf. cluneal nn.

Medial cluneal nn.

Anococcygeal nn.

Co1

L3

L2

L1

S2

S1

S5

S4

S3

Lithotomy View

PLATE 4.19   PELVIC NERVES—MALE

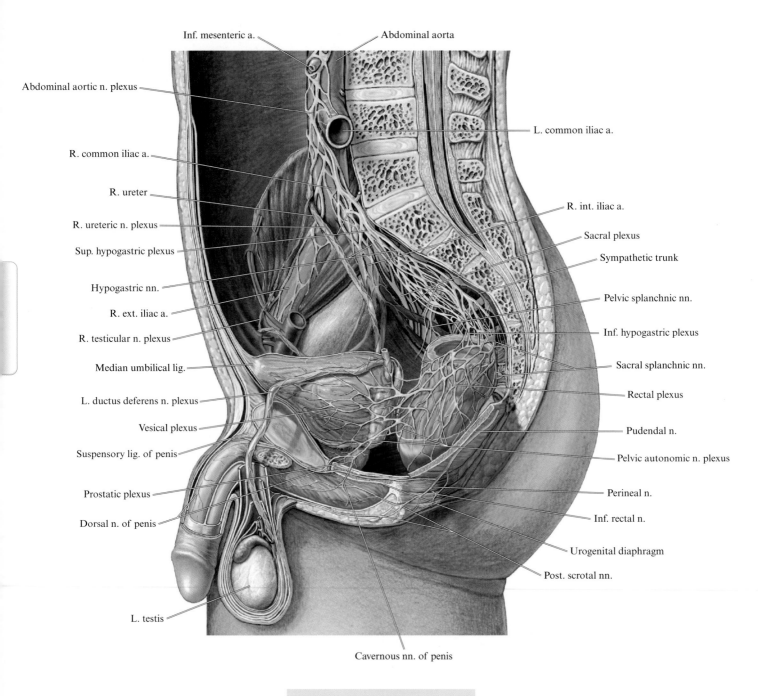

Inf. mesenteric a.

Abdominal aorta

Abdominal aortic n. plexus

L. common iliac a.

R. common iliac a.

R. ureter

R. int. iliac a.

R. ureteric n. plexus

Sacral plexus

Sup. hypogastric plexus

Sympathetic trunk

Hypogastric nn.

Pelvic splanchnic nn.

R. ext. iliac a.

Inf. hypogastric plexus

R. testicular n. plexus

Sacral splanchnic nn.

Median umbilical lig.

Rectal plexus

L. ductus deferens n. plexus

Vesical plexus

Pudendal n.

Suspensory lig. of penis

Pelvic autonomic n. plexus

Prostatic plexus

Perineal n.

Dorsal n. of penis

Inf. rectal n.

Urogenital diaphragm

Post. scrotal nn.

L. testis

Cavernous nn. of penis

Medial View with Peritoneum Removed

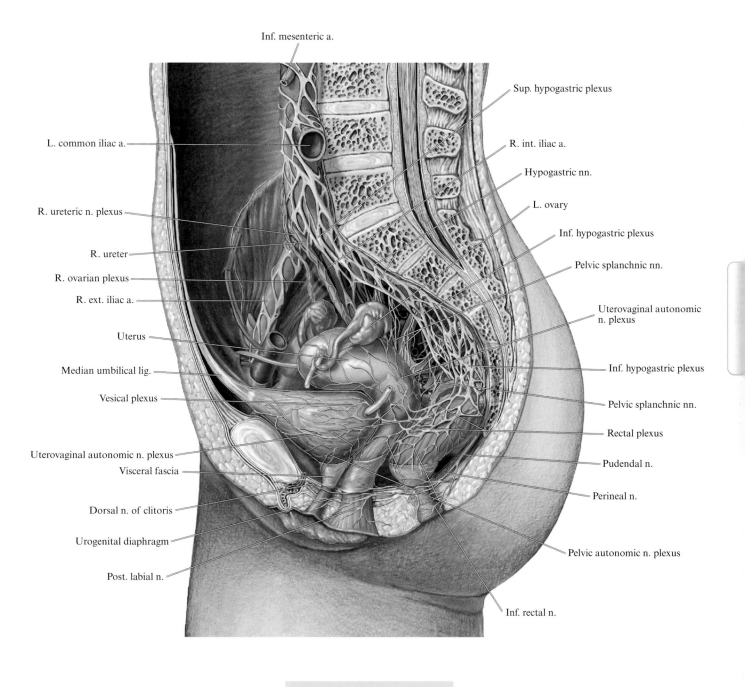

Inf. mesenteric a.

Sup. hypogastric plexus

L. common iliac a.

R. int. iliac a.

Hypogastric nn.

R. ureteric n. plexus

L. ovary

R. ureter

Inf. hypogastric plexus

R. ovarian plexus

Pelvic splanchnic nn.

R. ext. iliac a.

Uterovaginal autonomic
n. plexus

Uterus

Median umbilical lig.

Inf. hypogastric plexus

Vesical plexus

Pelvic splanchnic nn.

Rectal plexus

Uterovaginal autonomic n. plexus

Pudendal n.

Visceral fascia

Perineal n.

Dorsal n. of clitoris

Urogenital diaphragm

Pelvic autonomic n. plexus

Post. labial n.

Inf. rectal n.

Medial View Peritoneum Removed

PLATE **4.21** PELVIC AUTONOMIC NERVES—MALE

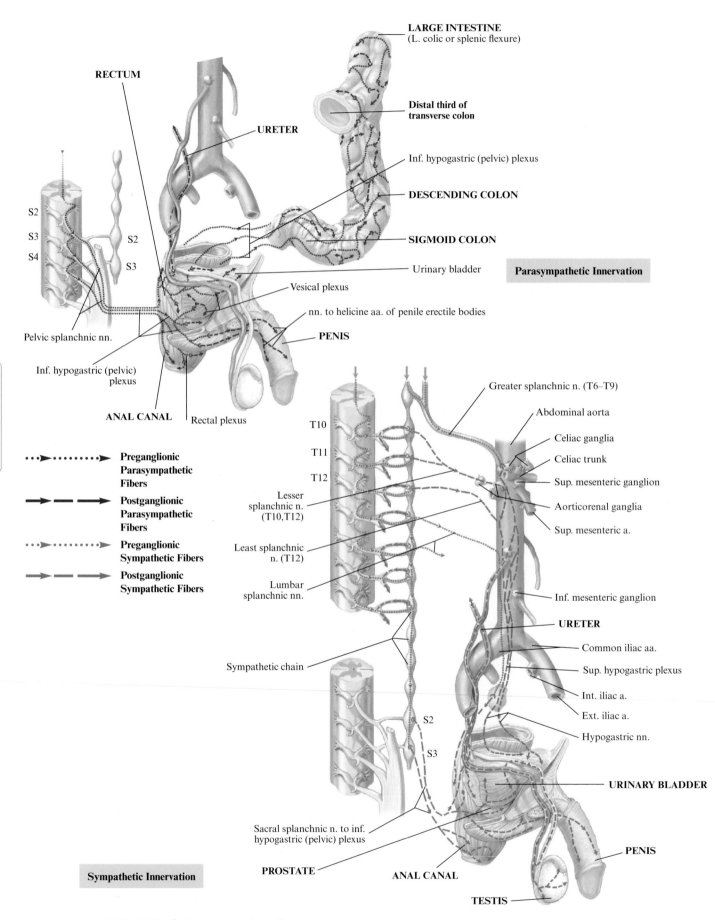

LARGE INTESTINE
(L. colic or splenic flexure)

RECTUM

URETER

Distal third of
transverse colon

Inf. hypogastric (pelvic) plexus

DESCENDING COLON

S2
S3
S4

S2
S3

SIGMOID COLON

Urinary bladder

Parasympathetic Innervation

Vesical plexus

nn. to helicine aa. of penile erectile bodies

Pelvic splanchnic nn.

PENIS

Inf. hypogastric (pelvic)
plexus

ANAL CANAL | Rectal plexus

•••▶•••••••▶ **Preganglionic
Parasympathetic
Fibers**

—————▶ **Postganglionic
Parasympathetic
Fibers**

•••▶•••••••▶ **Preganglionic
Sympathetic Fibers**

———▶ **Postganglionic
Sympathetic Fibers**

Greater splanchnic n. (T6–T9)

Abdominal aorta

Celiac ganglia

Celiac trunk

Sup. mesenteric ganglion

Aorticorenal ganglia

Sup. mesenteric a.

T10
T11
T12

Lesser
splanchnic n.
(T10,T12)

Least splanchnic
n. (T12)

Lumbar
splanchnic nn.

Inf. mesenteric ganglion

URETER

Common iliac aa.

Sup. hypogastric plexus

Int. iliac a.

Ext. iliac a.

Hypogastric nn.

Sympathetic chain

S2

S3

URINARY BLADDER

Sacral splanchnic n. to inf.
hypogastric (pelvic) plexus

PROSTATE

ANAL CANAL

PENIS

TESTIS

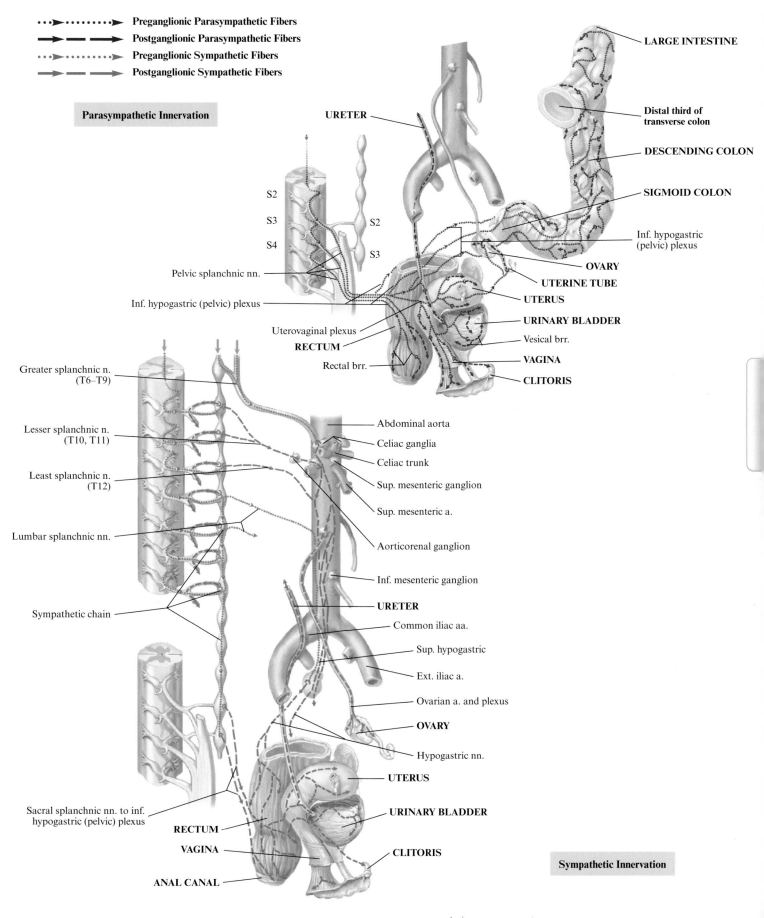

Preganglionic Parasympathetic Fibers
Postganglionic Parasympathetic Fibers
Preganglionic Sympathetic Fibers
Postganglionic Sympathetic Fibers

Parasympathetic Innervation

URETER

LARGE INTESTINE

Distal third of
transverse colon

DESCENDING COLON

SIGMOID COLON

S2
S3
S4

S2

S3

Inf. hypogastric
(pelvic) plexus

OVARY

UTERINE TUBE

Pelvic splanchnic nn.

UTERUS

Inf. hypogastric (pelvic) plexus

URINARY BLADDER

Uterovaginal plexus

Vesical brr.

RECTUM

VAGINA

Rectal brr.

CLITORIS

Greater splanchnic n.
(T6–T9)

Abdominal aorta

Celiac ganglia

Celiac trunk

Lesser splanchnic n.
(T10, T11)

Sup. mesenteric ganglion

Sup. mesenteric a.

Least splanchnic n.
(T12)

Aorticorenal ganglion

Lumbar splanchnic nn.

Inf. mesenteric ganglion

URETER

Common iliac aa.

Sympathetic chain

Sup. hypogastric

Ext. iliac a.

Ovarian a. and plexus

OVARY

Hypogastric nn.

UTERUS

URINARY BLADDER

Sacral splanchnic nn. to inf.
hypogastric (pelvic) plexus

RECTUM

VAGINA

CLITORIS

ANAL CANAL

Sympathetic Innervation

PLATE 4.23   SUPERFICIAL LYMPHATICS

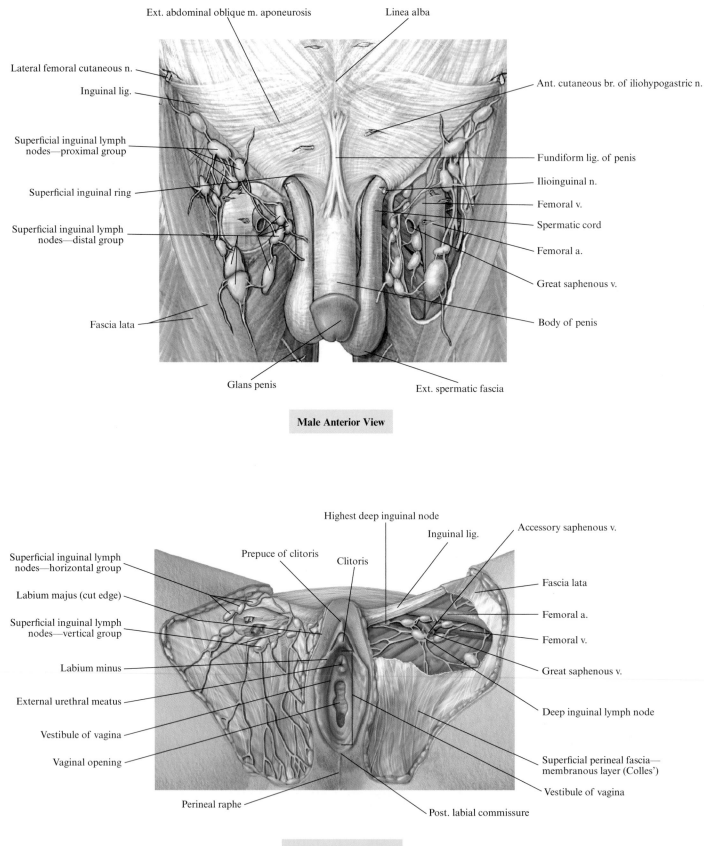

Ext. abdominal oblique m. aponeurosis

Linea alba

Lateral femoral cutaneous n.

Inguinal lig.

Superficial inguinal lymph nodes—proximal group

Superficial inguinal ring

Superficial inguinal lymph nodes—distal group

Fascia lata

Glans penis

Ant. cutaneous br. of iliohypogastric n.

Fundiform lig. of penis

Ilioinguinal n.

Femoral v.

Spermatic cord

Femoral a.

Great saphenous v.

Body of penis

Ext. spermatic fascia

Male Anterior View

Highest deep inguinal node

Inguinal lig.

Accessory saphenous v.

Superficial inguinal lymph nodes—horizontal group

Prepuce of clitoris

Clitoris

Labium majus (cut edge)

Superficial inguinal lymph nodes—vertical group

Labium minus

External urethral meatus

Vestibule of vagina

Vaginal opening

Perineal raphe

Fascia lata

Femoral a.

Femoral v.

Great saphenous v.

Deep inguinal lymph node

Superficial perineal fascia—membranous layer (Colles')

Vestibule of vagina

Post. labial commissure

Female Lithotomy View

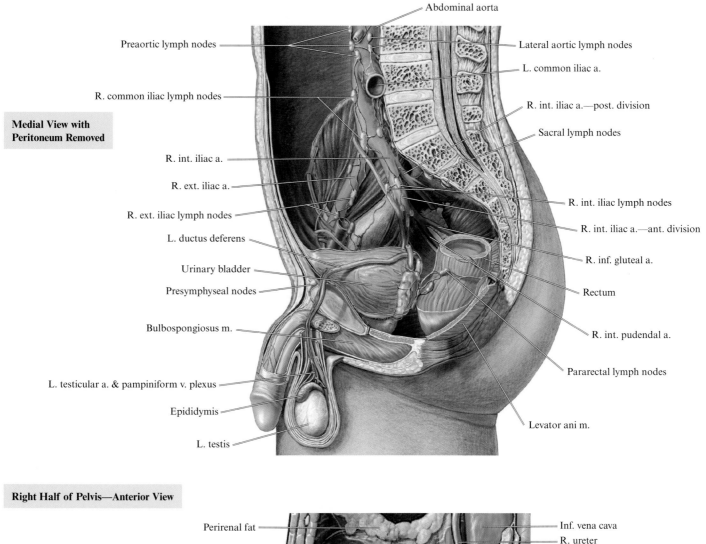

Medial View with Peritoneum Removed

Abdominal aorta

Preaortic lymph nodes

Lateral aortic lymph nodes

L. common iliac a.

R. common iliac lymph nodes

R. int. iliac a.—post. division

Sacral lymph nodes

R. int. iliac a.

R. ext. iliac a.

R. int. iliac lymph nodes

R. ext. iliac lymph nodes

R. int. iliac a.—ant. division

L. ductus deferens

R. inf. gluteal a.

Urinary bladder

Presymphyseal nodes

Rectum

Bulbospongiosus m.

R. int. pudendal a.

Pararectal lymph nodes

L. testicular a. & pampiniform v. plexus

Epididymis

Levator ani m.

L. testis

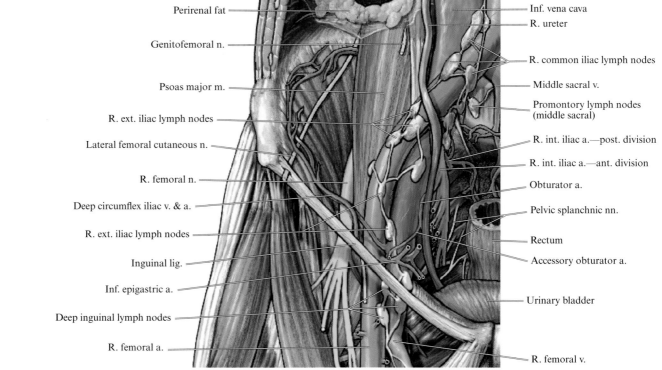

Right Half of Pelvis—Anterior View

Perirenal fat

Inf. vena cava

R. ureter

Genitofemoral n.

R. common iliac lymph nodes

Psoas major m.

Middle sacral v.

Promontory lymph nodes (middle sacral)

R. ext. iliac lymph nodes

R. int. iliac a.—post. division

Lateral femoral cutaneous n.

R. int. iliac a.—ant. division

R. femoral n.

Obturator a.

Deep circumflex iliac v. & a.

Pelvic splanchnic nn.

R. ext. iliac lymph nodes

Rectum

Inguinal lig.

Accessory obturator a.

Inf. epigastric a.

Urinary bladder

Deep inguinal lymph nodes

R. femoral a.

R. femoral v.

CHAPTER 4 | **PELVIS AND PERINEUM**   175

PLATE 4.25   UROGENITAL TRACT—FEMALE

♀ = **Characteristic Female Structures**

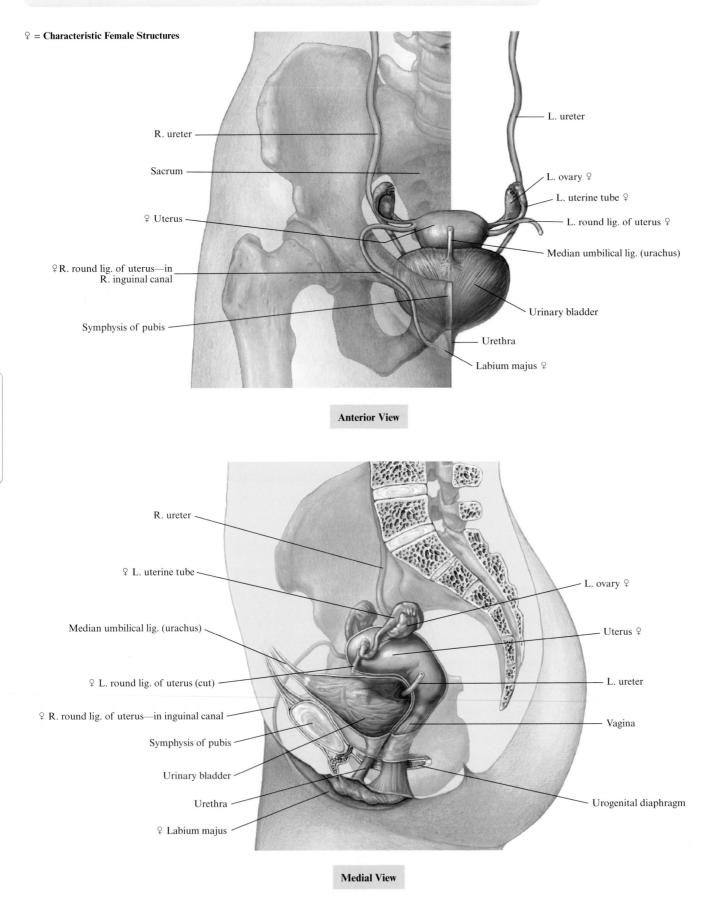

R. ureter

Sacrum

♀ Uterus

♀R. round lig. of uterus—in
R. inguinal canal

Symphysis of pubis

L. ureter

L. ovary ♀

L. uterine tube ♀

L. round lig. of uterus ♀

Median umbilical lig. (urachus)

Urinary bladder

Urethra

Labium majus ♀

Anterior View

R. ureter

♀ L. uterine tube

Median umbilical lig. (urachus)

♀ L. round lig. of uterus (cut)

♀ R. round lig. of uterus—in inguinal canal

Symphysis of pubis

Urinary bladder

Urethra

♀ Labium majus

L. ovary ♀

Uterus ♀

L. ureter

Vagina

Urogenital diaphragm

Medial View

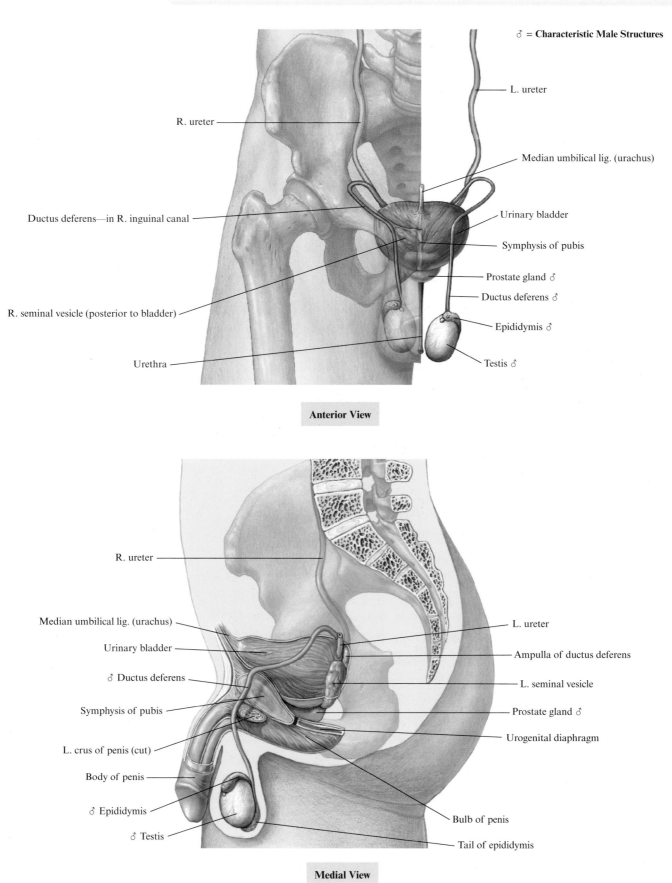

♂ = **Characteristic Male Structures**

L. ureter

R. ureter

Median umbilical lig. (urachus)

Ductus deferens—in R. inguinal canal

Urinary bladder

Symphysis of pubis

Prostate gland ♂

Ductus deferens ♂

Epididymis ♂

R. seminal vesicle (posterior to bladder)

Testis ♂

Urethra

Anterior View

R. ureter

Median umbilical lig. (urachus)

L. ureter

Urinary bladder

Ampulla of ductus deferens

♂ Ductus deferens

L. seminal vesicle

Symphysis of pubis

Prostate gland ♂

Urogenital diaphragm

L. crus of penis (cut)

Body of penis

♂ Epididymis

Bulb of penis

♂ Testis

Tail of epididymis

Medial View

PLATE 4.27   PELVIC CONTENTS—FEMALE

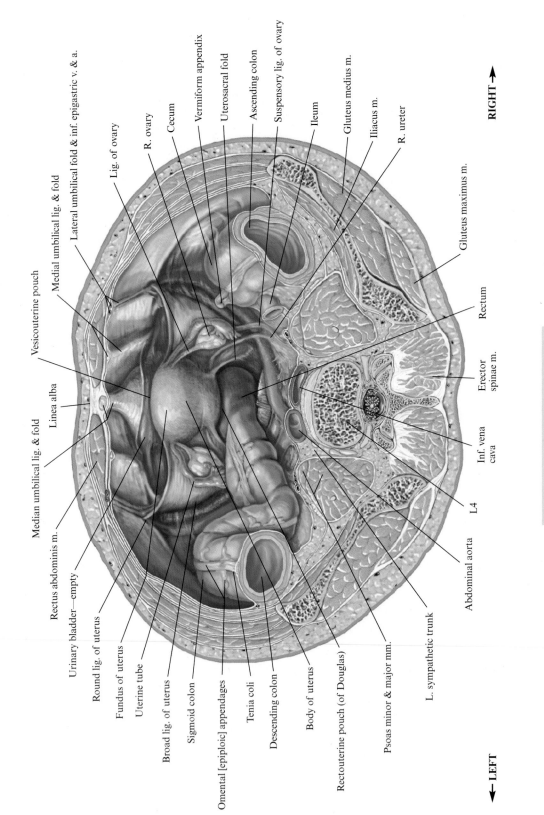

Medial umbilical lig. & fold
Lateral umbilical fold & inf. epigastric v. & a.
Lig. of ovary
R. ovary
Cecum
Vermiform appendix
Uterosacral fold
Ascending colon
Suspensory lig. of ovary
Ileum
Gluteus medius m.
Iliacus m.
R. ureter

RIGHT →

Vesicouterine pouch

Gluteus maximus m.

Median umbilical lig. & fold
Linea alba
Rectus abdominis m.
Urinary bladder—empty
Round lig. of uterus
Fundus of uterus
Uterine tube
Broad lig. of uterus
Sigmoid colon
Omental [epiploic] appendages
Tenia coli
Descending colon
Body of uterus
Rectouterine pouch (of Douglas)
Psoas minor & major mm.
L. sympathetic trunk

Rectum
Erector spinae m.
L4
Inf. vena cava
Abdominal aorta

Transverse Section at L4—Superior View

← LEFT

Medial umbilical lig. & fold

Broad lig. of uterus

R. ovary

Pelvic diaphragm (covered by peritoneum)

Fundus of uterus

Sigmoid colon

Urinary bladder—empty

Rectum

Vesicouterine pouch

Omental [epiploic] appendages

Medial umbilical lig. & fold

Lateral umbilical fold & inf. epigastric v. & a.

Round lig. of uterus

Broad lig. of uterus

Uterine tube

Sigmoid colon

Uterosacral fold

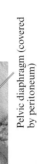

Pelvic Cavity—Superior View

PLATE 4.29   PELVIC CONTENTS—FEMALE

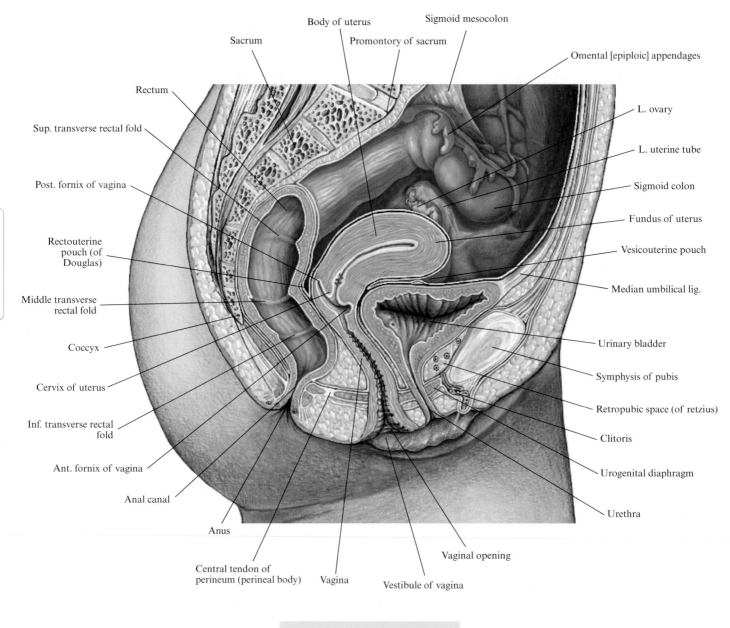

Body of uterus

Sigmoid mesocolon

Sacrum

Promontory of sacrum

Omental [epiploic] appendages

Rectum

L. ovary

Sup. transverse rectal fold

L. uterine tube

Post. fornix of vagina

Sigmoid colon

Fundus of uterus

Rectouterine
pouch (of
Douglas)

Vesicouterine pouch

Median umbilical lig.

Middle transverse
rectal fold

Coccyx

Urinary bladder

Cervix of uterus

Symphysis of pubis

Inf. transverse rectal
fold

Retropubic space (of retzius)

Ant. fornix of vagina

Clitoris

Anal canal

Urogenital diaphragm

Anus

Urethra

Central tendon of
perineum (perineal body)

Vagina

Vaginal opening

Vestibule of vagina

Median Section—Right Lateral View

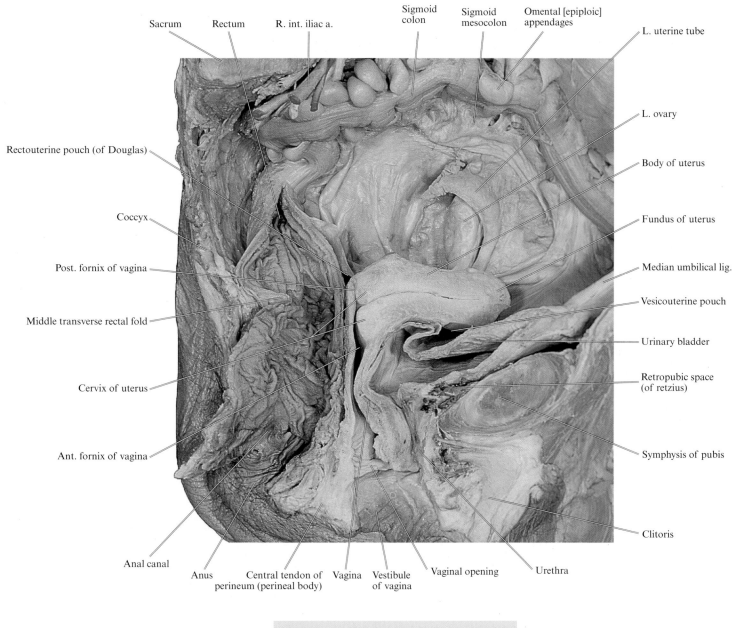

Sacrum   Rectum   R. int. iliac a.

Sigmoid colon

Sigmoid mesocolon

Omental [epiploic] appendages

L. uterine tube

Rectouterine pouch (of Douglas)

L. ovary

Body of uterus

Coccyx

Fundus of uterus

Post. fornix of vagina

Median umbilical lig.

Middle transverse rectal fold

Vesicouterine pouch

Urinary bladder

Cervix of uterus

Retropubic space (of retzius)

Ant. fornix of vagina

Symphysis of pubis

Anal canal

Clitoris

Anus   Central tendon of perineum (perineal body)   Vagina   Vestibule of vagina   Vaginal opening   Urethra

Median Section—Right Lateral View of Left Pelvis

PLATE 4.31   PELVIC CONTENTS—FEMALE

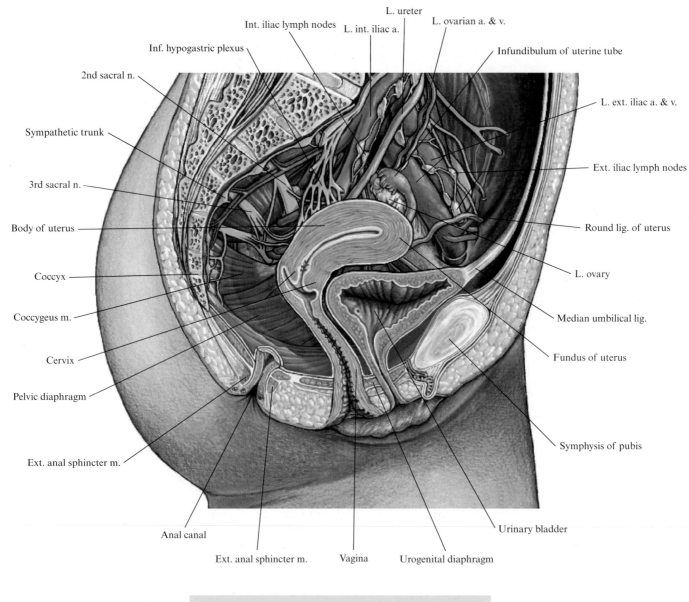

L. ureter

Int. iliac lymph nodes

L. int. iliac a.

L. ovarian a. & v.

Inf. hypogastric plexus

Infundibulum of uterine tube

2nd sacral n.

L. ext. iliac a. & v.

Sympathetic trunk

Ext. iliac lymph nodes

3rd sacral n.

Round lig. of uterus

Body of uterus

L. ovary

Coccyx

Median umbilical lig.

Coccygeus m.

Fundus of uterus

Cervix

Pelvic diaphragm

Symphysis of pubis

Ext. anal sphincter m.

Urinary bladder

Anal canal

Ext. anal sphincter m.

Vagina

Urogenital diaphragm

Median Section—Right Lateral View with Peritoneum Removed

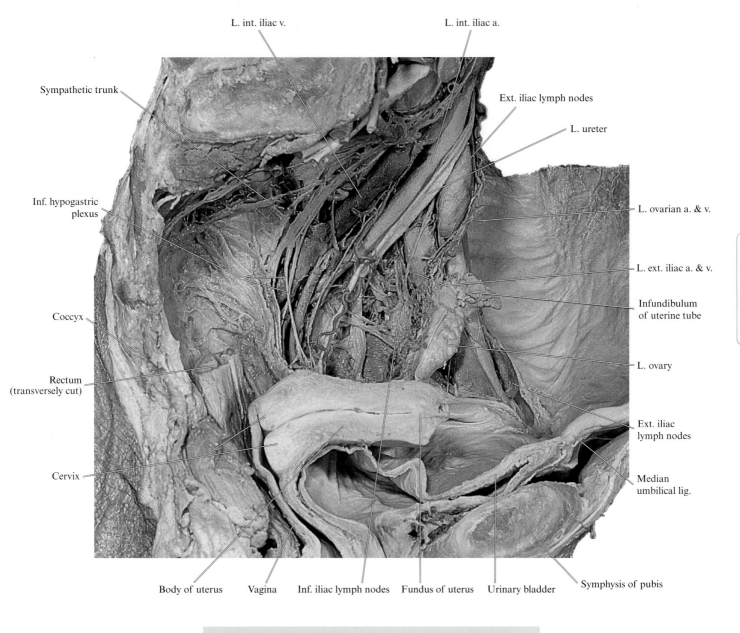

L. int. iliac v.

L. int. iliac a.

Sympathetic trunk

Ext. iliac lymph nodes

L. ureter

Inf. hypogastric
plexus

L. ovarian a. & v.

L. ext. iliac a. & v.

Infundibulum
of uterine tube

Coccyx

L. ovary

Rectum
(transversely cut)

Ext. iliac
lymph nodes

Cervix

Median
umbilical lig.

Body of uterus   Vagina   Inf. iliac lymph nodes   Fundus of uterus   Urinary bladder   Symphysis of pubis

Left Half of Hemisected Pelvis—Medial View with Peritoneum Removed

PLATE 4.33   PELVIC CONTENTS—FEMALE

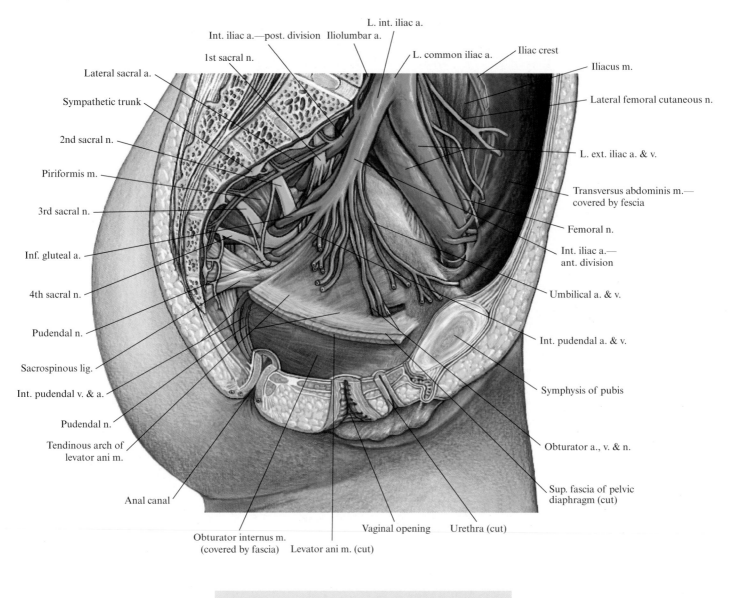

Lateral sacral a.

Sympathetic trunk

2nd sacral n.

Piriformis m.

3rd sacral n.

Inf. gluteal a.

4th sacral n.

Pudendal n.

Sacrospinous lig.

Int. pudendal v. & a.

Pudendal n.

Tendinous arch of
levator ani m.

Anal canal

Int. iliac a.—post. division   Iliolumbar a.

1st sacral n.

L. int. iliac a.

L. common iliac a.   Iliac crest

Iliacus m.

Lateral femoral cutaneous n.

L. ext. iliac a. & v.

Transversus abdominis m.—
covered by fescia

Femoral n.

Int. iliac a.—
ant. division

Umbilical a. & v.

Int. pudendal a. & v.

Symphysis of pubis

Obturator a., v. & n.

Sup. fascia of pelvic
diaphragm (cut)

Obturator internus m.
(covered by fascia)   Levator ani m. (cut)

Vaginal opening   Urethra (cut)

Median Section—Right Lateral View with Peritoneum Removed

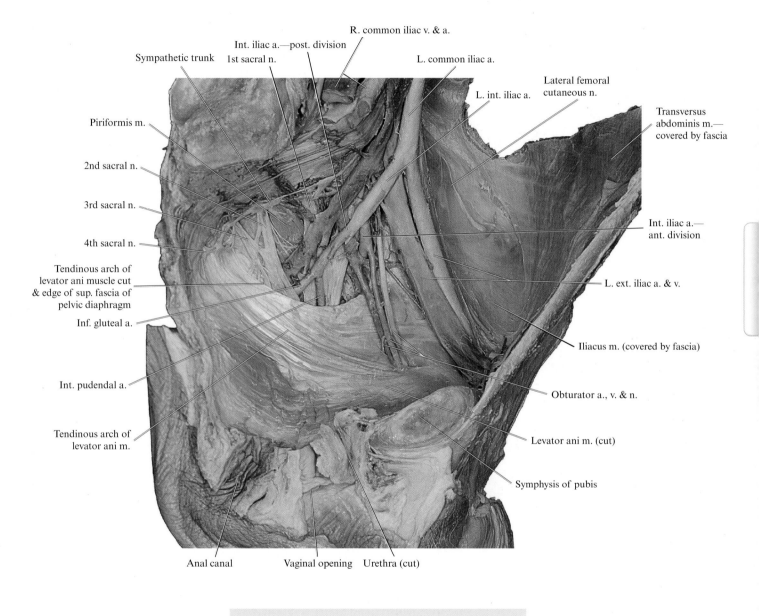

Sympathetic trunk

Int. iliac a.—post. division

1st sacral n.

R. common iliac v. & a.

L. common iliac a.

L. int. iliac a.

Lateral femoral cutaneous n.

Transversus abdominis m.—covered by fascia

Piriformis m.

2nd sacral n.

3rd sacral n.

4th sacral n.

Int. iliac a.—ant. division

Tendinous arch of levator ani muscle cut & edge of sup. fascia of pelvic diaphragm

Inf. gluteal a.

L. ext. iliac a. & v.

Iliacus m. (covered by fascia)

Int. pudendal a.

Obturator a., v. & n.

Tendinous arch of levator ani m.

Levator ani m. (cut)

Symphysis of pubis

Anal canal   Vaginal opening   Urethra (cut)

Median Section—Right Lateral View with Peritoneum Removed

PLATE 4.35   LATERAL PELVIC WALL—FEMALE

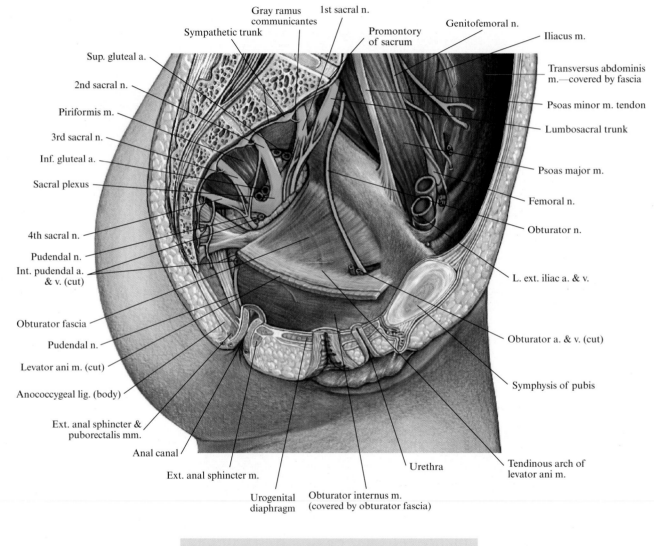

Gray ramus
communicantes

1st sacral n.

Sympathetic trunk

Promontory
of sacrum

Genitofemoral n.

Iliacus m.

Sup. gluteal a.

Transversus abdominis
m.—covered by fascia

2nd sacral n.

Psoas minor m. tendon

Piriformis m.

Lumbosacral trunk

3rd sacral n.

Inf. gluteal a.

Psoas major m.

Sacral plexus

Femoral n.

Obturator n.

4th sacral n.

Pudendal n.

Int. pudendal a.
& v. (cut)

L. ext. iliac a. & v.

Obturator fascia

Pudendal n.

Obturator a. & v. (cut)

Levator ani m. (cut)

Anococcygeal lig. (body)

Symphysis of pubis

Ext. anal sphincter &
puborectalis mm.

Anal canal

Urethra

Tendinous arch of
levator ani m.

Ext. anal sphincter m.

Urogenital
diaphragm

Obturator internus m.
(covered by obturator fascia)

Median Section—Right Lateral View with Peritoneum Removed

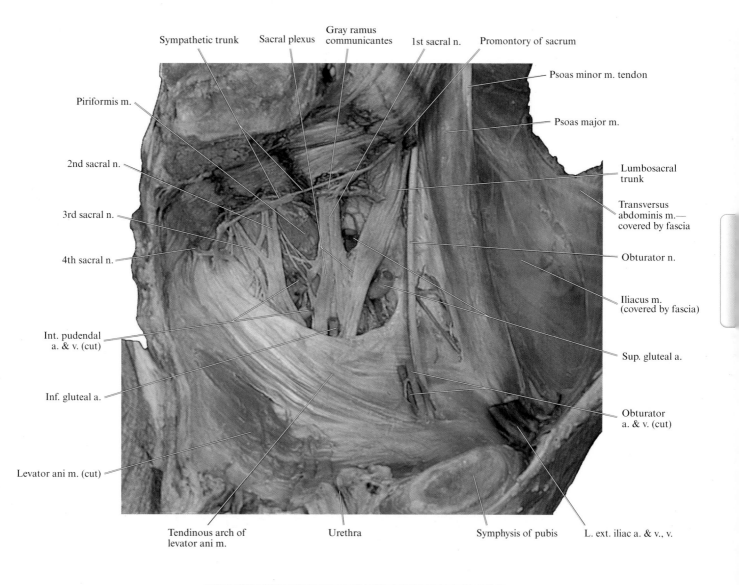

Sympathetic trunk

Sacral plexus

Gray ramus
communicantes

1st sacral n.

Promontory of sacrum

Piriformis m.

Psoas minor m. tendon

Psoas major m.

2nd sacral n.

Lumbosacral
trunk

Transversus
abdominis m.—
covered by fascia

3rd sacral n.

Obturator n.

4th sacral n.

Iliacus m.
(covered by fascia)

Int. pudendal
a. & v. (cut)

Sup. gluteal a.

Inf. gluteal a.

Obturator
a. & v. (cut)

Levator ani m. (cut)

Tendinous arch of
levator ani m.

Urethra

Symphysis of pubis

L. ext. iliac a. & v., v.

Median Section—Right Lateral View with Peritoneum Removed

PLATE 4.37 PELVIC CONTENTS—MALE

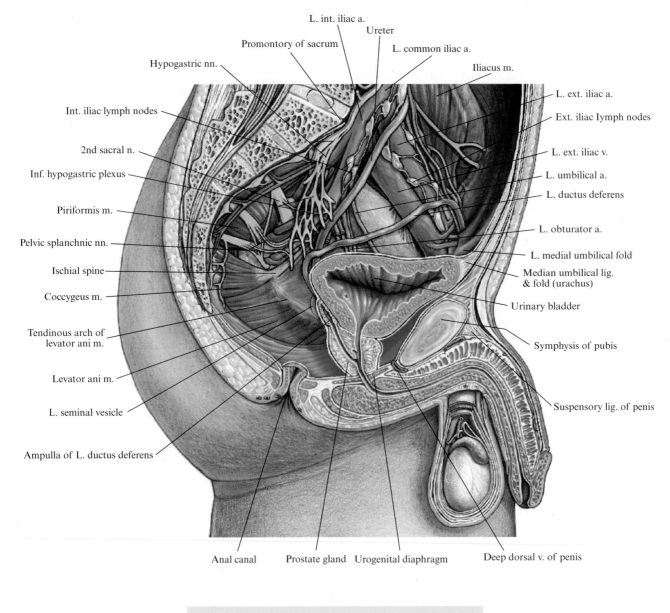

L. int. iliac a.

Ureter

Promontory of sacrum

L. common iliac a.

Hypogastric nn.

Iliacus m.

L. ext. iliac a.

Int. iliac lymph nodes

Ext. iliac lymph nodes

2nd sacral n.

L. ext. iliac v.

Inf. hypogastric plexus

L. umbilical a.

L. ductus deferens

Piriformis m.

L. obturator a.

Pelvic splanchnic nn.

L. medial umbilical fold

Ischial spine

Median umbilical lig.
& fold (urachus)

Coccygeus m.

Urinary bladder

Tendinous arch of
levator ani m.

Symphysis of pubis

Levator ani m.

L. seminal vesicle

Suspensory lig. of penis

Ampulla of L. ductus deferens

Anal canal   Prostate gland   Urogenital diaphragm   Deep dorsal v. of penis

Median Section—Right Lateral View with Peritoneum Removed

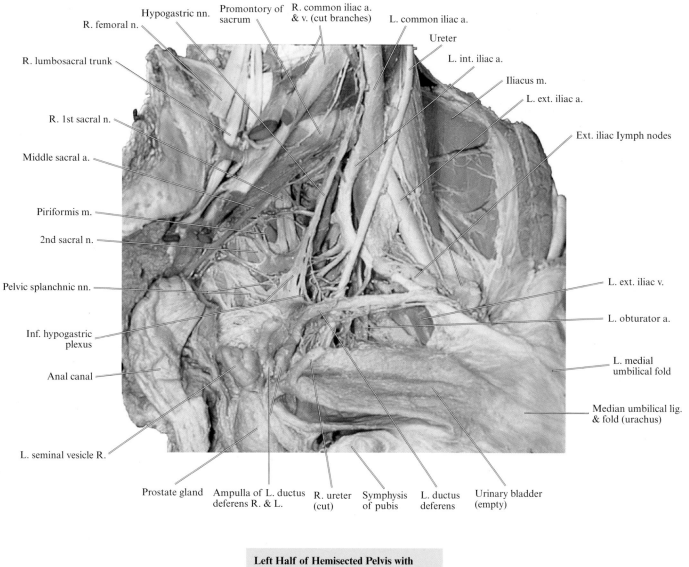

R. femoral n.

Hypogastric nn.

Promontory of sacrum

R. common iliac a. & v. (cut branches)

L. common iliac a.

R. lumbosacral trunk

Ureter

L. int. iliac a.

Iliacus m.

L. ext. iliac a.

R. 1st sacral n.

Ext. iliac lymph nodes

Middle sacral a.

Piriformis m.

2nd sacral n.

Pelvic splanchnic nn.

L. ext. iliac v.

L. obturator a.

Inf. hypogastric plexus

L. medial umbilical fold

Anal canal

Median umbilical lig. & fold (urachus)

L. seminal vesicle R.

Prostate gland

Ampulla of L. ductus deferens R. & L.

R. ureter (cut)

Symphysis of pubis

L. ductus deferens

Urinary bladder (empty)

Left Half of Hemisected Pelvis with Bladder Pulled Anteriorly—Medial View

PLATE 4.39   PERITONEAL FASCIAE & SPACES—FEMALE

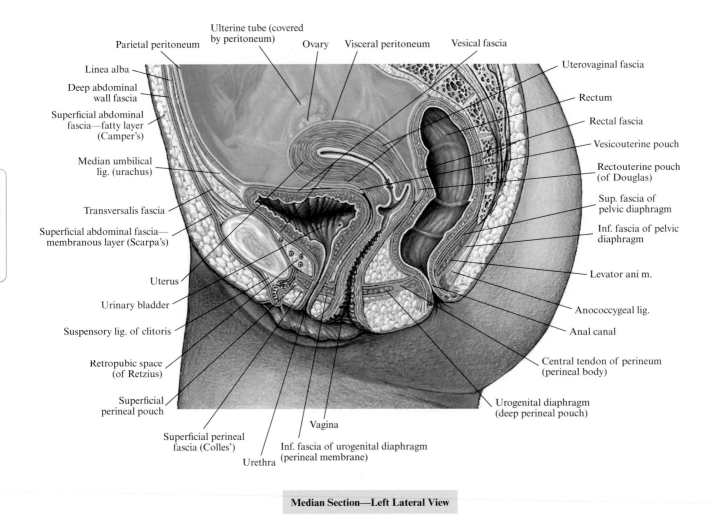

Ulterine tube (covered by peritoneum)

Parietal peritoneum

Ovary

Visceral peritoneum

Vesical fascia

Uterovaginal fascia

Linea alba

Deep abdominal wall fascia

Superficial abdominal fascia—fatty layer (Camper's)

Median umbilical lig. (urachus)

Transversalis fascia

Superficial abdominal fascia— membranous layer (Scarpa's)

Uterus

Urinary bladder

Suspensory lig. of clitoris

Retropubic space (of Retzius)

Superficial perineal pouch

Rectum

Rectal fascia

Vesicouterine pouch

Rectouterine pouch (of Douglas)

Sup. fascia of pelvic diaphragm

Inf. fascia of pelvic diaphragm

Levator ani m.

Anococcygeal lig.

Anal canal

Central tendon of perineum (perineal body)

Urogenital diaphragm (deep perineal pouch)

Superficial perineal fascia (Colles')

Urethra

Vagina

Inf. fascia of urogenital diaphragm (perineal membrane)

Median Section—Left Lateral View

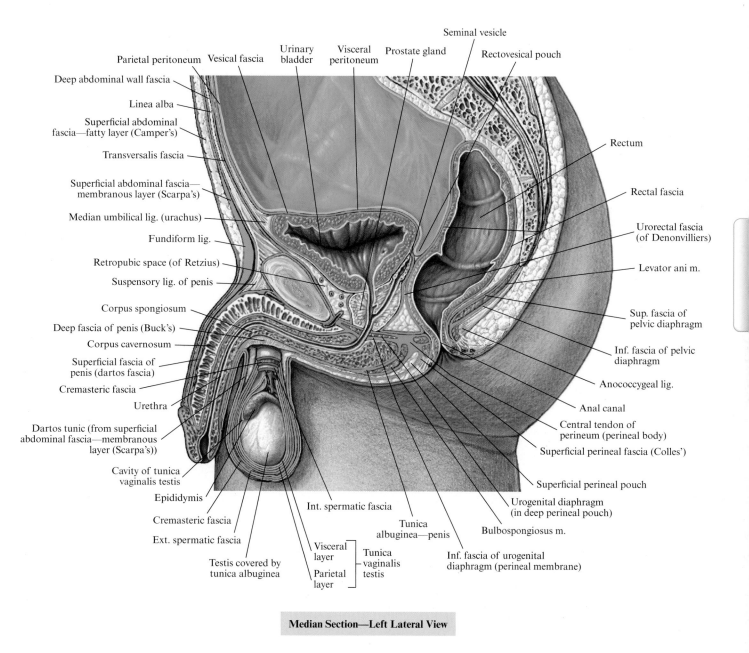

Parietal peritoneum

Vesical fascia

Urinary bladder

Visceral peritoneum

Prostate gland

Seminal vesicle

Rectovesical pouch

Deep abdominal wall fascia

Linea alba

Superficial abdominal fascia—fatty layer (Camper's)

Transversalis fascia

Superficial abdominal fascia—membranous layer (Scarpa's)

Median umbilical lig. (urachus)

Fundiform lig.

Retropubic space (of Retzius)

Suspensory lig. of penis

Corpus spongiosum

Deep fascia of penis (Buck's)

Corpus cavernosum

Superficial fascia of penis (dartos fascia)

Cremasteric fascia

Urethra

Dartos tunic (from superficial abdominal fascia—membranous layer (Scarpa's))

Cavity of tunica vaginalis testis

Epididymis

Cremasteric fascia

Ext. spermatic fascia

Testis covered by tunica albuginea

Int. spermatic fascia

Visceral layer
Parietal layer
Tunica vaginalis testis

Tunica albuginea—penis

Inf. fascia of urogenital diaphragm (perineal membrane)

Bulbospongiosus m.

Urogenital diaphragm (in deep perineal pouch)

Superficial perineal pouch

Superficial perineal fascia (Colles')

Central tendon of perineum (perineal body)

Anal canal

Anococcygeal lig.

Inf. fascia of pelvic diaphragm

Sup. fascia of pelvic diaphragm

Levator ani m.

Urorectal fascia (of Denonvilliers)

Rectal fascia

Rectum

Median Section—Left Lateral View

PLATE 4.41   PERINEUM—FEMALE I

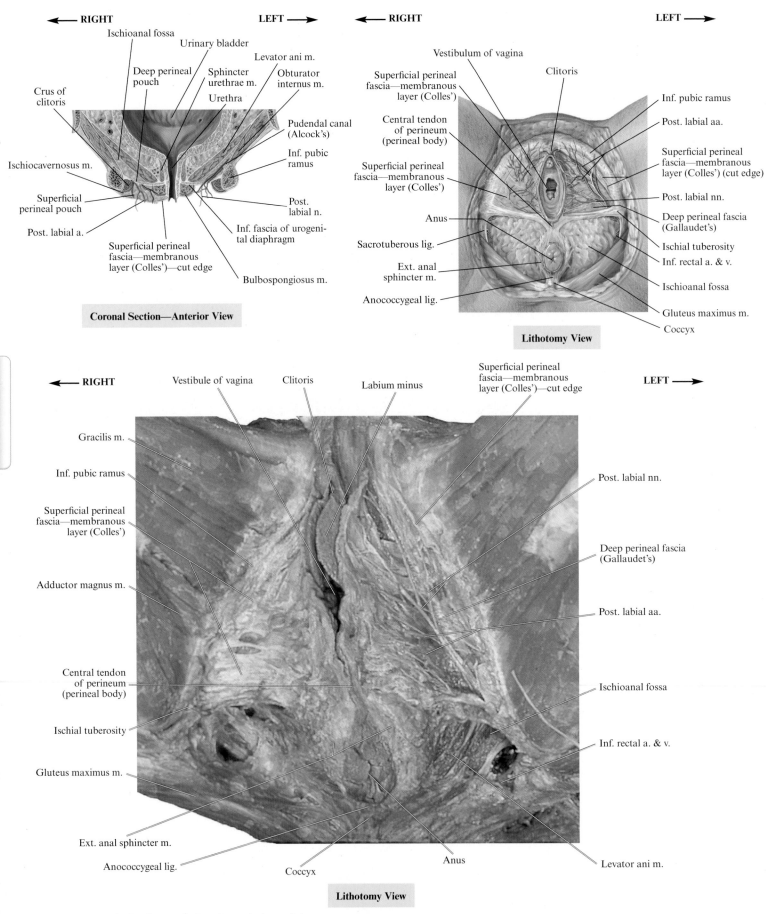

← RIGHT   LEFT →   ← RIGHT   LEFT →

Ischioanal fossa

Urinary bladder

Deep perineal
pouch   Sphincter
urethrae m.   Levator ani m.

Crus of   Urethra   Obturator
clitoris   internus m.

Pudendal canal
(Alcock's)

Ischiocavernosus m.   Inf. pubic
ramus

Superficial
perineal pouch   Post.
labial n.

Post. labial a.   Inf. fascia of urogenital diaphragm

Superficial perineal
fascia—membranous
layer (Colles')—cut edge   Bulbospongiosus m.

Coronal Section—Anterior View

Vestibulum of vagina   Clitoris

Superficial perineal
fascia—membranous
layer (Colles')   Inf. pubic ramus

Central tendon
of perineum   Post. labial aa.
(perineal body)   Superficial perineal
fascia—membranous
Superficial perineal   layer (Colles') (cut edge)
fascia—membranous
layer (Colles')   Post. labial nn.

Anus   Deep perineal fascia
(Gallaudet's)

Sacrotuberous lig.   Ischial tuberosity

Ext. anal   Inf. rectal a. & v.
sphincter m.

Anococcygeal lig.   Ischioanal fossa

Gluteus maximus m.

Coccyx

Lithotomy View

← RIGHT   Vestibule of vagina   Clitoris   Labium minus   Superficial perineal
fascia—membranous   LEFT →
layer (Colles')—cut edge

Gracilis m.

Inf. pubic ramus   Post. labial nn.

Superficial perineal
fascia—membranous
layer (Colles')   Deep perineal fascia
(Gallaudet's)

Adductor magnus m.   Post. labial aa.

Central tendon
of perineum
(perineal body)   Ischioanal fossa

Ischial tuberosity   Inf. rectal a. & v.

Gluteus maximus m.

Ext. anal sphincter m.   Anus   Levator ani m.

Anococcygeal lig.   Coccyx

Lithotomy View

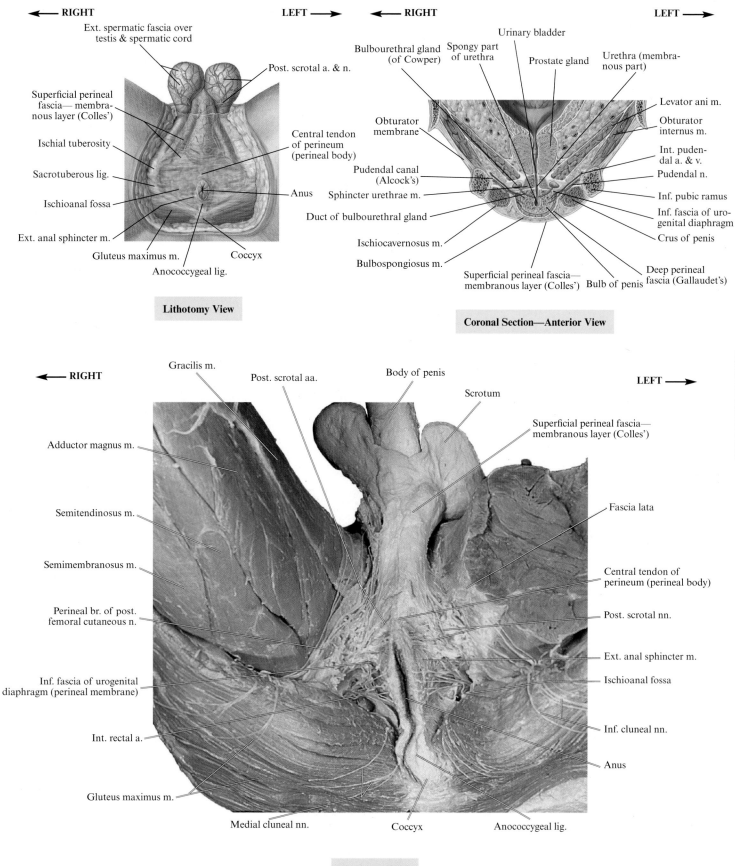

← RIGHT   LEFT →   ← RIGHT   LEFT →

Ext. spermatic fascia over
testis & spermatic cord

Post. scrotal a. & n.

Bulbourethral gland
(of Cowper)   Spongy part
of urethra   Urinary bladder   Urethra (membra-
Prostate gland   nous part)

Superficial perineal
fascia— membra-
nous layer (Colles')

Levator ani m.

Obturator
membrane   Obturator
internus m.

Ischial tuberosity

Central tendon
of perineum
(perineal body)

Int. puden-
dal a. & v.
Pudendal n.

Sacrotuberous lig.

Pudendal canal
(Alcock's)

Ischioanal fossa

Anus   Sphincter urethrae m.   Inf. pubic ramus

Ext. anal sphincter m.   Duct of bulbourethral gland   Inf. fascia of urogenital diaphragm

Gluteus maximus m.   Coccyx   Ischiocavernosus m.   Crus of penis

Anococcygeal lig.   Bulbospongiosus m.

Superficial perineal fascia—   Deep perineal
membranous layer (Colles')   Bulb of penis   fascia (Gallaudet's)

Lithotomy View

Coronal Section—Anterior View

Gracilis m.   Body of penis

← RIGHT   Post. scrotal aa.   Scrotum   LEFT →

Adductor magnus m.   Superficial perineal fascia—
membranous layer (Colles')

Semitendinosus m.

Fascia lata

Semimembranosus m.

Central tendon of
perineum (perineal body)

Perineal br. of post.
femoral cutaneous n.   Post. scrotal nn.

Ext. anal sphincter m.

Inf. fascia of urogenital
diaphragm (perineal membrane)   Ischioanal fossa

Int. rectal a.   Inf. cluneal nn.

Anus

Gluteus maximus m.

Medial cluneal nn.   Coccyx   Anococcygeal lig.

Lithotomy View

PLATE 4.43   **PERINEUM—FEMALE II**

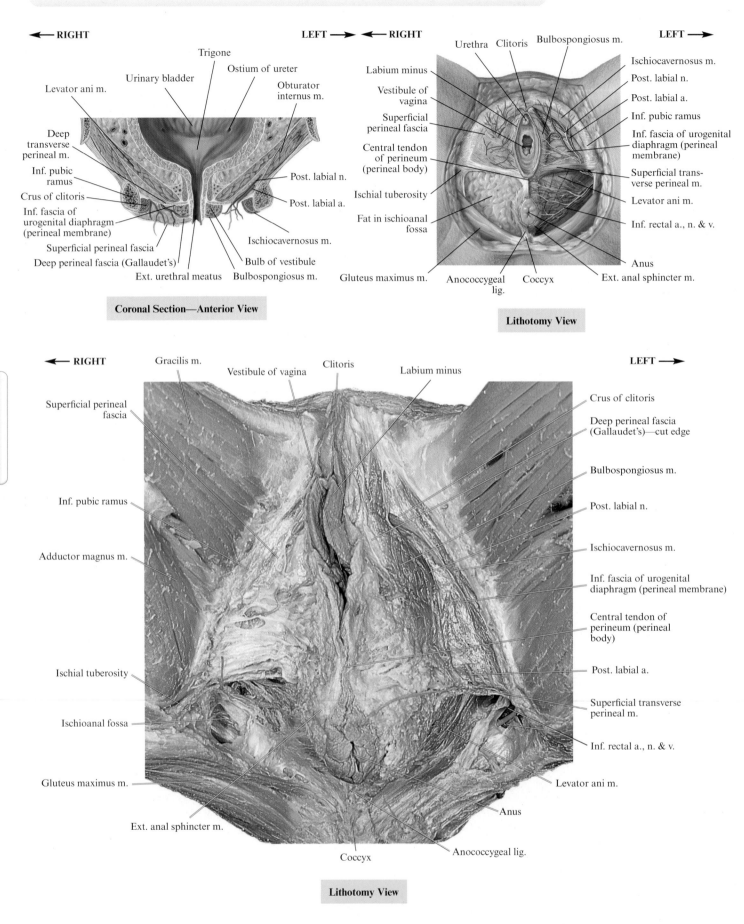

← **RIGHT**   **LEFT** →

Trigone
Urinary bladder
Ostium of ureter
Obturator internus m.
Levator ani m.
Deep transverse perineal m.
Inf. pubic ramus
Crus of clitoris
Inf. fascia of urogenital diaphragm (perineal membrane)
Superficial perineal fascia
Deep perineal fascia (Gallaudet's)
Ext. urethral meatus
Post. labial n.
Post. labial a.
Ischiocavernosus m.
Bulb of vestibule
Bulbospongiosus m.

Coronal Section—Anterior View

← **RIGHT**   **LEFT** →

Urethra   Clitoris   Bulbospongiosus m.
Labium minus
Vestibule of vagina
Superficial perineal fascia
Central tendon of perineum (perineal body)
Ischial tuberosity
Fat in ischioanal fossa
Gluteus maximus m.
Anococcygeal lig.
Coccyx
Ischiocavernosus m.
Post. labial n.
Post. labial a.
Inf. pubic ramus
Inf. fascia of urogenital diaphragm (perineal membrane)
Superficial transverse perineal m.
Levator ani m.
Inf. rectal a., n. & v.
Anus
Ext. anal sphincter m.

Lithotomy View

← **RIGHT**   **LEFT** →

Gracilis m.
Vestibule of vagina
Clitoris
Labium minus
Superficial perineal fascia
Inf. pubic ramus
Adductor magnus m.
Ischial tuberosity
Ischioanal fossa
Gluteus maximus m.
Ext. anal sphincter m.
Coccyx
Anococcygeal lig.
Crus of clitoris
Deep perineal fascia (Gallaudet's)—cut edge
Bulbospongiosus m.
Post. labial n.
Ischiocavernosus m.
Inf. fascia of urogenital diaphragm (perineal membrane)
Central tendon of perineum (perineal body)
Post. labial a.
Superficial transverse perineal m.
Inf. rectal a., n. & v.
Levator ani m.
Anus

Lithotomy View

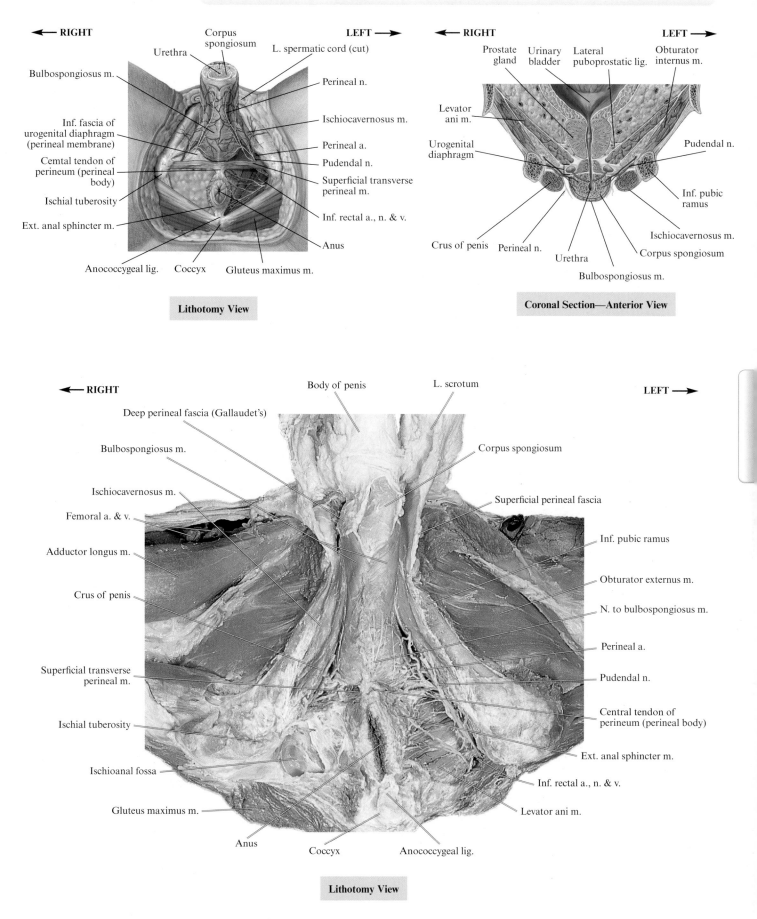

← RIGHT   LEFT →

Bulbospongiosus m.

Urethra

Corpus spongiosum

L. spermatic cord (cut)

Perineal n.

Ischiocavernosus m.

Inf. fascia of urogenital diaphragm (perineal membrane)

Perineal a.

Pudendal n.

Cemtal tendon of perineum (perineal body)

Superficial transverse perineal m.

Ischial tuberosity

Inf. rectal a., n. & v.

Ext. anal sphincter m.

Anus

Anococcygeal lig.   Coccyx   Gluteus maximus m.

Lithotomy View

← RIGHT   LEFT →

Prostate gland   Urinary bladder   Lateral puboprostatic lig.   Obturator internus m.

Levator ani m.

Urogenital diaphragm

Pudendal n.

Inf. pubic ramus

Ischiocavernosus m.

Crus of penis   Perineal n.   Corpus spongiosum

Urethra

Bulbospongiosus m.

Coronal Section—Anterior View

← RIGHT   Body of penis   L. scrotum   LEFT →

Deep perineal fascia (Gallaudet's)

Bulbospongiosus m.

Corpus spongiosum

Ischiocavernosus m.

Superficial perineal fascia

Femoral a. & v.

Inf. pubic ramus

Adductor longus m.

Obturator externus m.

Crus of penis

N. to bulbospongiosus m.

Perineal a.

Pudendal n.

Superficial transverse perineal m.

Central tendon of perineum (perineal body)

Ischial tuberosity

Ext. anal sphincter m.

Ischioanal fossa

Inf. rectal a., n. & v.

Gluteus maximus m.

Levator ani m.

Anus   Coccyx   Anococcygeal lig.

Lithotomy View

PLATE 4.45   PERINEUM—FEMALE III

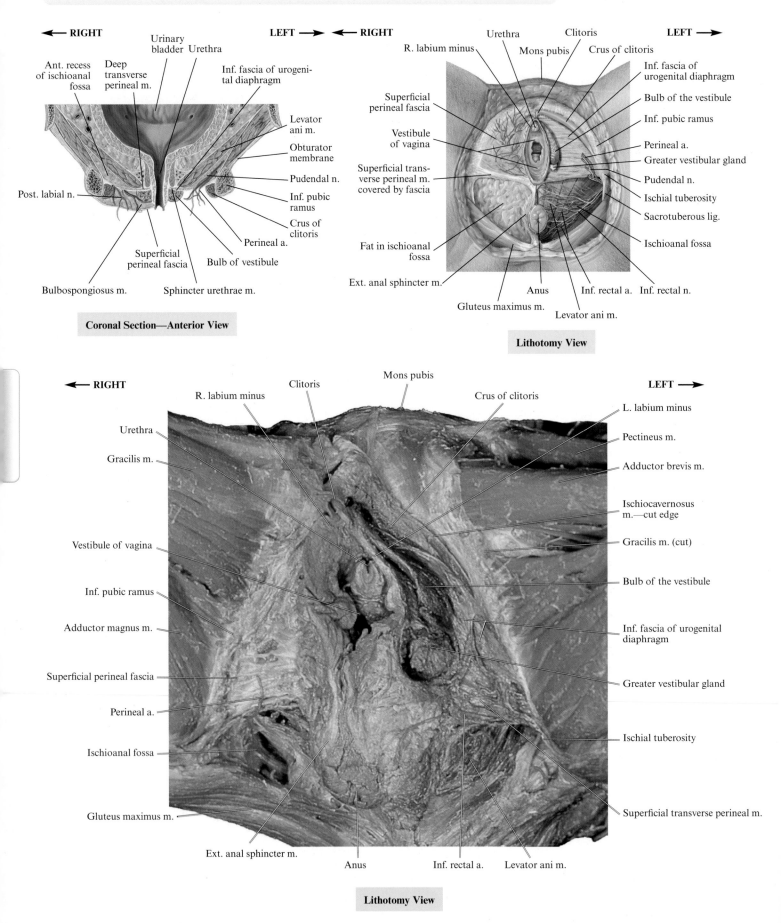

← RIGHT   LEFT → ← RIGHT   LEFT →

Urinary
bladder Urethra

Ant. recess   Deep
of ischioanal transverse   Inf. fascia of urogeni-
fossa   perineal m.   tal diaphragm

Levator
ani m.

Obturator
membrane

Pudendal n.

Post. labial n.   Inf. pubic
ramus

Crus of
clitoris

Perineal a.

Superficial
perineal fascia   Bulb of vestibule

Bulbospongiosus m.   Sphincter urethrae m.

Coronal Section—Anterior View

Urethra   Clitoris

R. labium minus   Mons pubis   Crus of clitoris

Inf. fascia of
urogenital diaphragm

Superficial
perineal fascia

Bulb of the vestibule

Vestibule
of vagina

Inf. pubic ramus

Superficial trans-
verse perineal m.
covered by fascia

Perineal a.

Greater vestibular gland

Pudendal n.

Ischial tuberosity

Sacrotuberous lig.

Fat in ischioanal
fossa

Ischioanal fossa

Ext. anal sphincter m.

Anus   Inf. rectal a.   Inf. rectal n.

Gluteus maximus m.   Levator ani m.

Lithotomy View

← RIGHT   LEFT →

Clitoris   Mons pubis

R. labium minus   Crus of clitoris

L. labium minus

Urethra

Pectineus m.

Gracilis m.

Adductor brevis m.

Ischiocavernosus
m.—cut edge

Gracilis m. (cut)

Vestibule of vagina

Bulb of the vestibule

Inf. pubic ramus

Adductor magnus m.

Inf. fascia of urogenital
diaphragm

Superficial perineal fascia

Greater vestibular gland

Perineal a.

Ischial tuberosity

Ischioanal fossa

Superficial transverse perineal m.

Gluteus maximus m.

Ext. anal sphincter m.

Anus   Inf. rectal a.   Levator ani m.

Lithotomy View

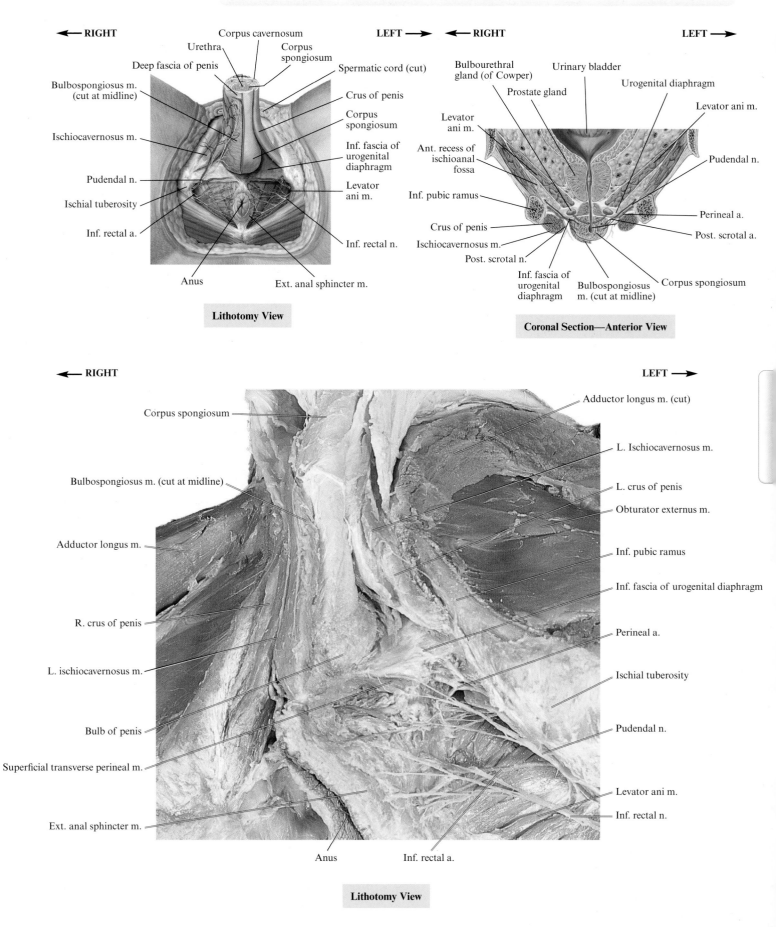

← **RIGHT**   Corpus cavernosum   **LEFT** →   ← **RIGHT**   **LEFT** →

Urethra

Corpus
spongiosum

Deep fascia of penis

Spermatic cord (cut)

Bulbospongiosus m.
(cut at midline)

Crus of penis

Corpus
spongiosum

Ischiocavernosus m.

Inf. fascia of
urogenital
diaphragm

Pudendal n.

Levator
ani m.

Ischial tuberosity

Inf. rectal a.

Inf. rectal n.

Anus   Ext. anal sphincter m.

Lithotomy View

Bulbourethral
gland (of Cowper)   Urinary bladder

Prostate gland   Urogenital diaphragm

Levator
ani m.   Levator ani m.

Ant. recess of
ischioanal
fossa   Pudendal n.

Inf. pubic ramus

Perineal a.

Crus of penis   Post. scrotal a.

Ischiocavernosus m.

Post. scrotal n.

Inf. fascia of
urogenital
diaphragm   Bulbospongiosus
m. (cut at midline)   Corpus spongiosum

Coronal Section—Anterior View

← **RIGHT**   **LEFT** →

Corpus spongiosum

Adductor longus m. (cut)

L. Ischiocavernosus m.

Bulbospongiosus m. (cut at midline)

L. crus of penis

Obturator externus m.

Adductor longus m.

Inf. pubic ramus

Inf. fascia of urogenital diaphragm

R. crus of penis

Perineal a.

L. ischiocavernosus m.

Ischial tuberosity

Bulb of penis

Pudendal n.

Superficial transverse perineal m.

Levator ani m.

Inf. rectal n.

Ext. anal sphincter m.

Anus   Inf. rectal a.

Lithotomy View

PLATE 4.47   PERINEUM—FEMALE IV

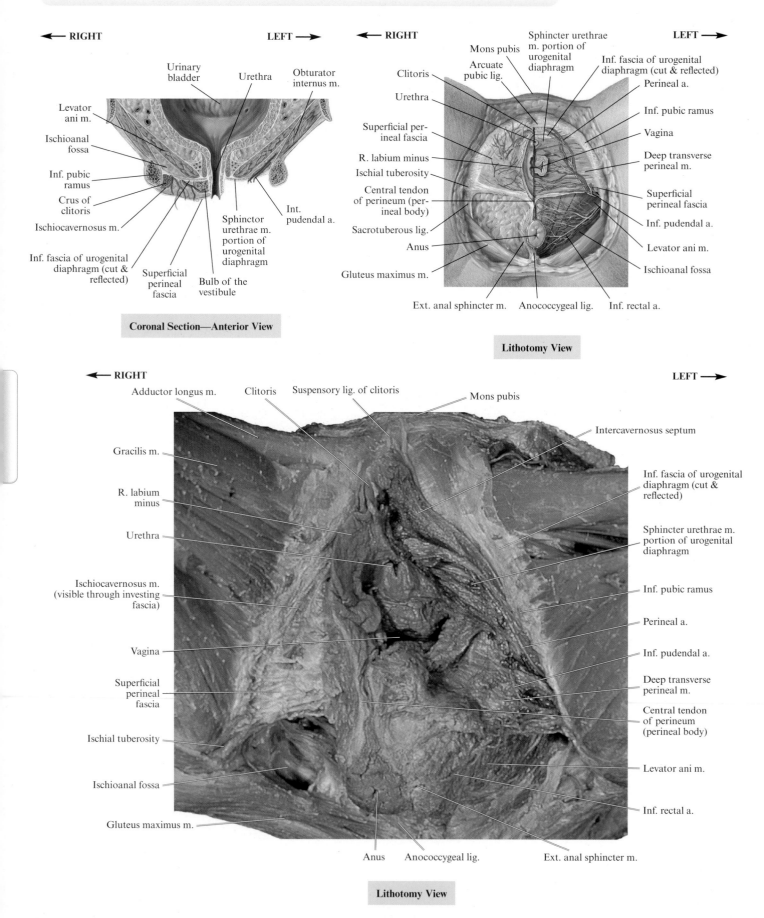

← RIGHT   LEFT →

Urinary bladder
Urethra
Obturator internus m.

Levator ani m.
Ischioanal fossa
Inf. pubic ramus
Crus of clitoris
Ischiocavernosus m.
Inf. fascia of urogenital diaphragm (cut & reflected)
Superficial perineal fascia
Bulb of the vestibule
Sphinctor urethrae m. portion of urogenital diaphragm
Int. pudendal a.

Coronal Section—Anterior View

← RIGHT   LEFT →

Mons pubis
Arcuate pubic lig.
Clitoris
Urethra
Superficial perineal fascia
R. labium minus
Ischial tuberosity
Central tendon of perineum (perineal body)
Sacrotuberous lig.
Anus
Gluteus maximus m.
Ext. anal sphincter m.
Anococcygeal lig.
Inf. rectal a.
Sphincter urethrae m. portion of urogenital diaphragm
Inf. fascia of urogenital diaphragm (cut & reflected)
Perineal a.
Inf. pubic ramus
Vagina
Deep transverse perineal m.
Superficial perineal fascia
Inf. pudendal a.
Levator ani m.
Ischioanal fossa

Lithotomy View

← RIGHT   LEFT →

Adductor longus m.
Clitoris
Suspensory lig. of clitoris
Mons pubis
Gracilis m.
R. labium minus
Urethra
Ischiocavernosus m. (visible through investing fascia)
Vagina
Superficial perineal fascia
Ischial tuberosity
Ischioanal fossa
Gluteus maximus m.
Anus
Anococcygeal lig.
Ext. anal sphincter m.
Intercavernosus septum
Inf. fascia of urogenital diaphragm (cut & reflected)
Sphincter urethrae m. portion of urogenital diaphragm
Inf. pubic ramus
Perineal a.
Inf. pudendal a.
Deep transverse perineal m.
Central tendon of perineum (perineal body)
Levator ani m.
Inf. rectal a.

Lithotomy View

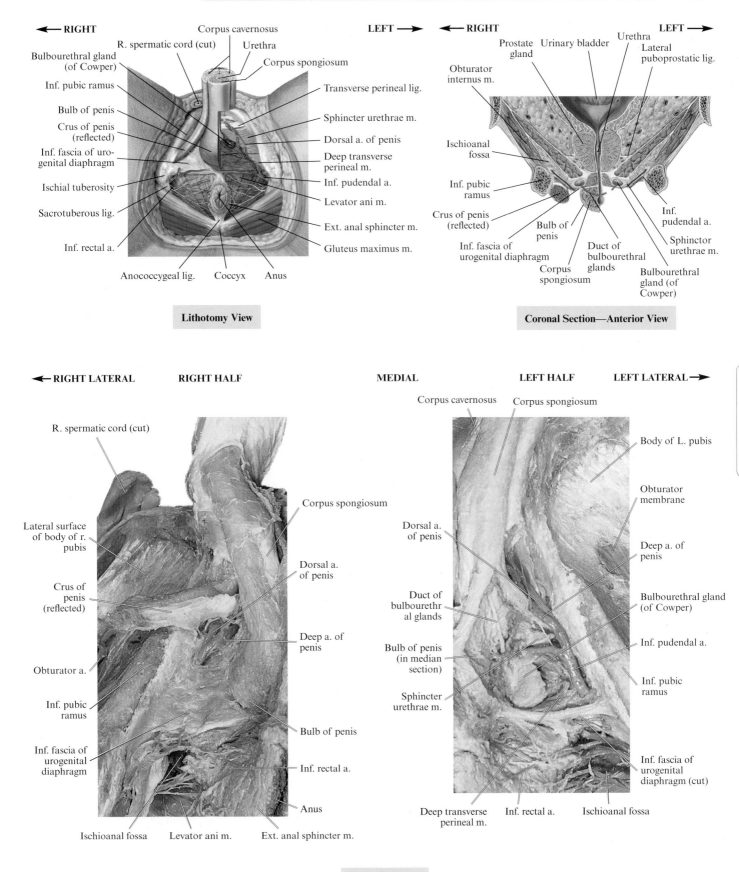

◄— RIGHT   LEFT —►   ◄— RIGHT   LEFT —►

R. spermatic cord (cut)
Corpus cavernosus
Urethra
Corpus spongiosum

Bulbourethral gland (of Cowper)
Inf. pubic ramus
Bulb of penis
Crus of penis (reflected)
Inf. fascia of uro-genital diaphragm
Ischial tuberosity
Sacrotuberous lig.
Inf. rectal a.

Transverse perineal lig.
Sphincter urethrae m.
Dorsal a. of penis
Deep transverse perineal m.
Inf. pudendal a.
Levator ani m.
Ext. anal sphincter m.
Gluteus maximus m.

Anococcygeal lig.   Coccyx   Anus

Lithotomy View

Prostate gland   Urinary bladder   Urethra   Lateral puboprostatic lig.
Obturator internus m.
Ischioanal fossa
Inf. pubic ramus
Crus of penis (reflected)
Bulb of penis
Inf. fascia of urogenital diaphragm
Corpus spongiosum
Duct of bulbourethral glands
Inf. pudendal a.
Sphinctor urethrae m.
Bulbourethral gland (of Cowper)

Coronal Section—Anterior View

◄— RIGHT LATERAL   RIGHT HALF   MEDIAL   LEFT HALF   LEFT LATERAL —►

R. spermatic cord (cut)

Lateral surface of body of r. pubis
Crus of penis (reflected)
Obturator a.
Inf. pubic ramus
Inf. fascia of urogenital diaphragm

Corpus spongiosum
Dorsal a. of penis
Deep a. of penis
Bulb of penis
Inf. rectal a.
Anus

Ischioanal fossa   Levator ani m.   Ext. anal sphincter m.

Corpus cavernosus   Corpus spongiosum

Dorsal a. of penis
Duct of bulbourethral glands
Bulb of penis (in median section)
Sphincter urethrae m.
Deep transverse perineal m.   Inf. rectal a.   Ischioanal fossa

Body of L. pubis
Obturator membrane
Deep a. of penis
Bulbourethral gland (of Cowper)
Inf. pudendal a.
Inf. pubic ramus
Inf. fascia of urogenital diaphragm (cut)

Lithotomy View

PLATE 4.49   PERINEUM—FEMALE V

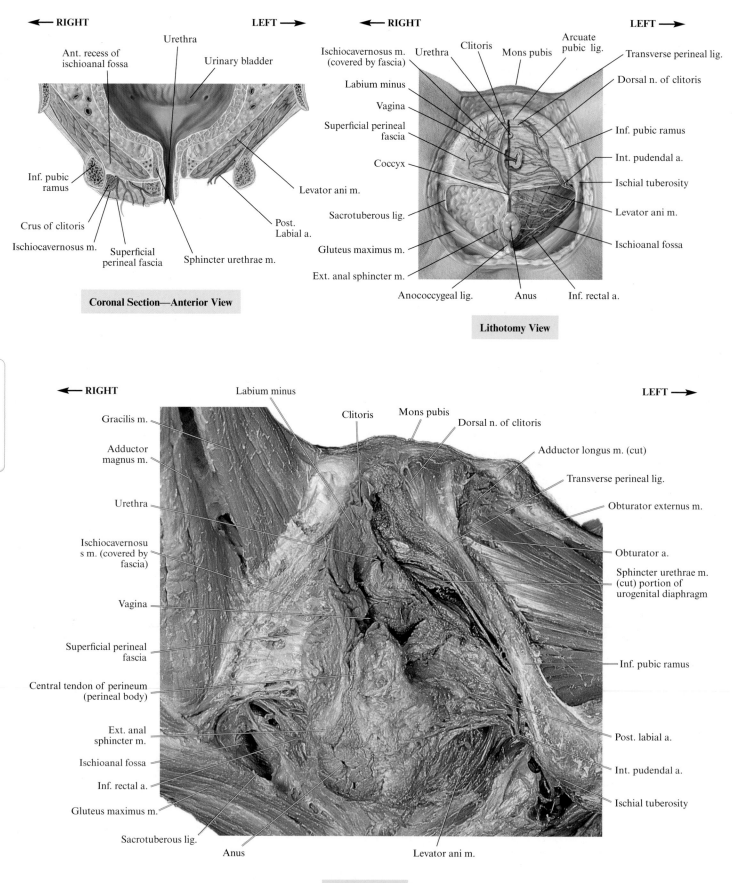

← RIGHT   LEFT →

Ant. recess of
ischioanal fossa

Urethra

Urinary bladder

Inf. pubic
ramus

Crus of clitoris

Ischiocavernosus m.

Superficial
perineal fascia

Levator ani m.

Post.
Labial a.

Sphincter urethrae m.

Coronal Section—Anterior View

← RIGHT   LEFT →

Ischiocavernosus m.
(covered by fascia)

Urethra

Clitoris

Mons pubis

Arcuate
pubic lig.

Transverse perineal lig.

Labium minus

Vagina

Superficial perineal
fascia

Coccyx

Sacrotuberous lig.

Gluteus maximus m.

Ext. anal sphincter m.

Anococcygeal lig.

Anus

Inf. rectal a.

Dorsal n. of clitoris

Inf. pubic ramus

Int. pudendal a.

Ischial tuberosity

Levator ani m.

Ischioanal fossa

Lithotomy View

← RIGHT   LEFT →

Labium minus

Clitoris

Mons pubis

Dorsal n. of clitoris

Gracilis m.

Adductor
magnus m.

Urethra

Ischiocavernosu
s m. (covered by
fascia)

Vagina

Superficial perineal
fascia

Central tendon of perineum
(perineal body)

Ext. anal
sphincter m.

Ischioanal fossa

Inf. rectal a.

Gluteus maximus m.

Sacrotuberous lig.

Anus

Levator ani m.

Adductor longus m. (cut)

Transverse perineal lig.

Obturator externus m.

Obturator a.

Sphincter urethrae m.
(cut) portion of
urogenital diaphragm

Inf. pubic ramus

Post. labial a.

Int. pudendal a.

Ischial tuberosity

Lithotomy View

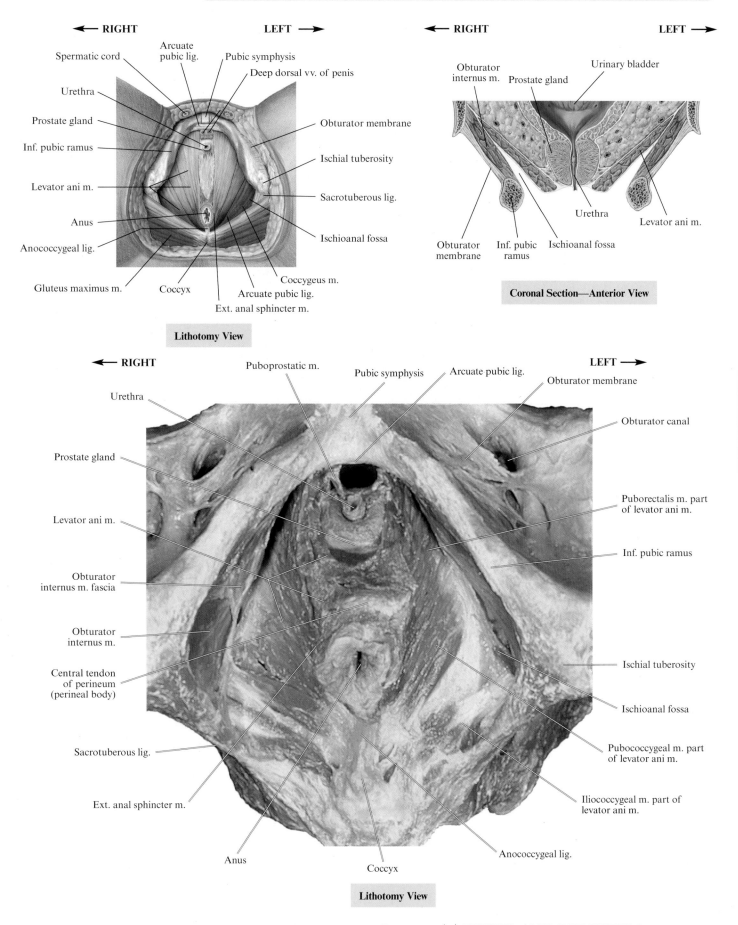

← RIGHT   LEFT →

Spermatic cord
Arcuate pubic lig.
Pubic symphysis
Deep dorsal vv. of penis

Urethra

Prostate gland

Inf. pubic ramus

Levator ani m.

Anus

Anococcygeal lig.

Obturator membrane

Ischial tuberosity

Sacrotuberous lig.

Ischioanal fossa

Gluteus maximus m.   Coccyx   Coccygeus m.
Arcuate pubic lig.
Ext. anal sphincter m.

Lithotomy View

← RIGHT   LEFT →

Obturator internus m.
Prostate gland
Urinary bladder

Obturator membrane   Inf. pubic ramus   Ischioanal fossa
Urethra
Levator ani m.

Coronal Section—Anterior View

← RIGHT   LEFT →

Puboprostatic m.
Pubic symphysis
Arcuate pubic lig.
Obturator membrane

Urethra

Obturator canal

Prostate gland

Puborectalis m. part of levator ani m.

Levator ani m.

Inf. pubic ramus

Obturator internus m. fascia

Obturator internus m.

Central tendon of perineum (perineal body)

Ischial tuberosity

Ischioanal fossa

Sacrotuberous lig.

Pubococcygeal m. part of levator ani m.

Ext. anal sphincter m.

Iliococcygeal m. part of levator ani m.

Anus   Coccyx   Anococcygeal lig.

Lithotomy View

PLATE 4.53 PUDENDAL STRUCTURES

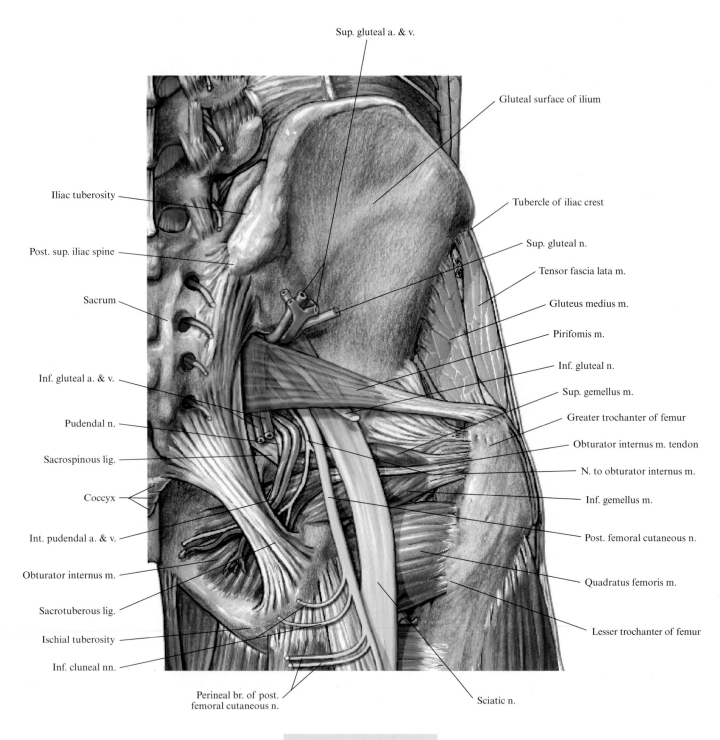

Sup. gluteal a. & v.

Gluteal surface of ilium

Iliac tuberosity

Tubercle of iliac crest

Post. sup. iliac spine

Sup. gluteal n.

Sacrum

Tensor fascia lata m.

Gluteus medius m.

Pirifomis m.

Inf. gluteal a. & v.

Inf. gluteal n.

Pudendal n.

Sup. gemellus m.

Sacrospinous lig.

Greater trochanter of femur

Coccyx

Obturator internus m. tendon

N. to obturator internus m.

Int. pudendal a. & v.

Inf. gemellus m.

Obturator internus m.

Post. femoral cutaneous n.

Sacrotuberous lig.

Quadratus femoris m.

Ischial tuberosity

Inf. cluneal nn.

Lesser trochanter of femur

Perineal br. of post.
femoral cutaneous n.

Sciatic n.

Gluteal Region—Posterior View

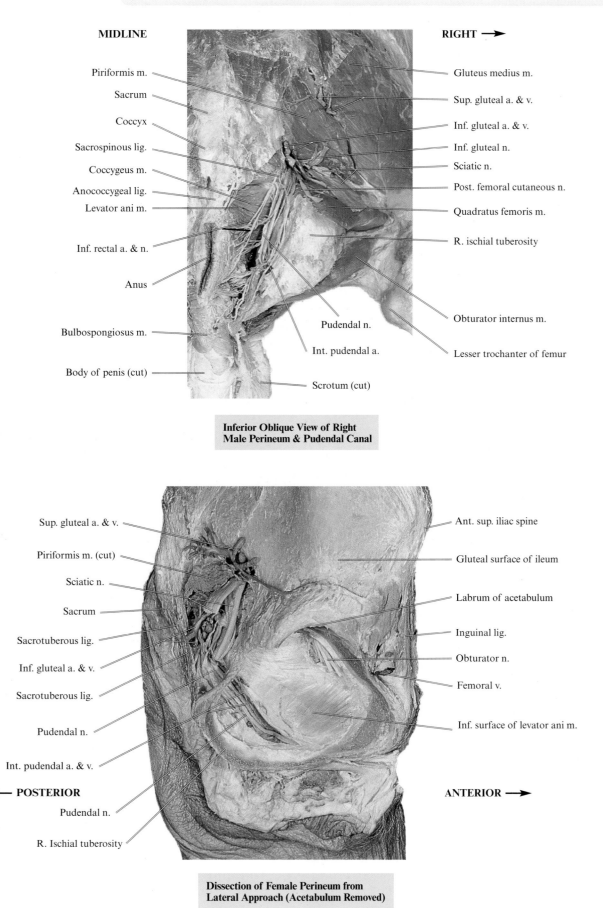

MIDLINE

RIGHT →

Piriformis m.

Sacrum

Coccyx

Sacrospinous lig.

Coccygeus m.

Anococcygeal lig.

Levator ani m.

Inf. rectal a. & n.

Anus

Bulbospongiosus m.

Body of penis (cut)

Gluteus medius m.

Sup. gluteal a. & v.

Inf. gluteal a. & v.

Inf. gluteal n.

Sciatic n.

Post. femoral cutaneous n.

Quadratus femoris m.

R. ischial tuberosity

Obturator internus m.

Lesser trochanter of femur

Pudendal n.

Int. pudendal a.

Scrotum (cut)

**Inferior Oblique View of Right
Male Perineum & Pudendal Canal**

Sup. gluteal a. & v.

Piriformis m. (cut)

Sciatic n.

Sacrum

Sacrotuberous lig.

Inf. gluteal a. & v.

Sacrotuberous lig.

Pudendal n.

Int. pudendal a. & v.

Ant. sup. iliac spine

Gluteal surface of ileum

Labrum of acetabulum

Inguinal lig.

Obturator n.

Femoral v.

Inf. surface of levator ani m.

← POSTERIOR

ANTERIOR →

Pudendal n.

R. Ischial tuberosity

**Dissection of Female Perineum from
Lateral Approach (Acetabulum Removed)**

CHAPTER 4 | **PELVIS AND PERINEUM**

205

PLATE 4.55 RECTUM & ANAL CANAL—ARTERIES

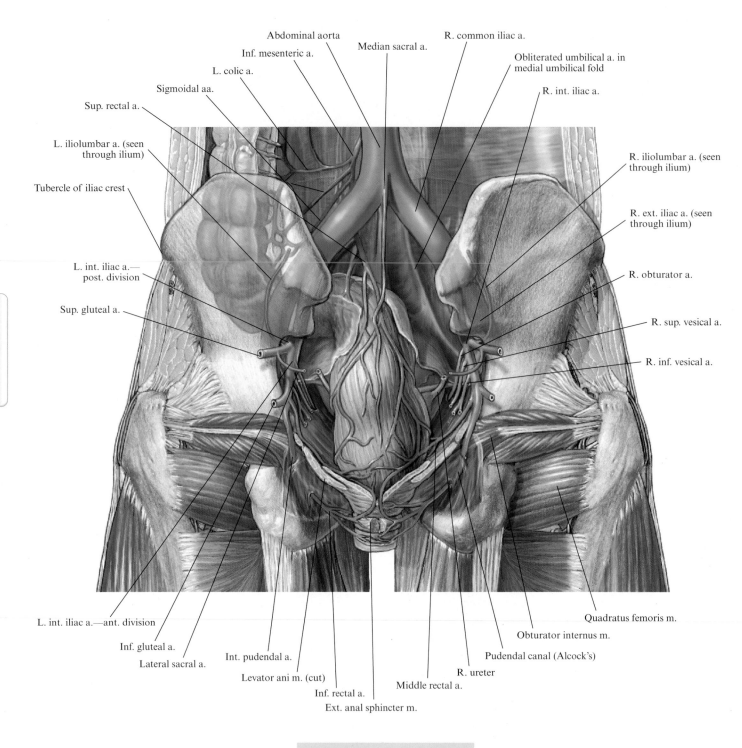

Abdominal aorta

Inf. mesenteric a.

Median sacral a.

R. common iliac a.

Obliterated umbilical a. in medial umbilical fold

L. colic a.

Sigmoidal aa.

R. int. iliac a.

Sup. rectal a.

L. iliolumbar a. (seen through ilium)

R. iliolumbar a. (seen through ilium)

Tubercle of iliac crest

R. ext. iliac a. (seen through ilium)

L. int. iliac a.— post. division

R. obturator a.

Sup. gluteal a.

R. sup. vesical a.

R. inf. vesical a.

L. int. iliac a.—ant. division

Quadratus femoris m.

Inf. gluteal a.

Obturator internus m.

Lateral sacral a.

Int. pudendal a.

Pudendal canal (Alcock's)

Levator ani m. (cut)

R. ureter

Inf. rectal a.

Middle rectal a.

Ext. anal sphincter m.

Posterior View with Sacrum Removed

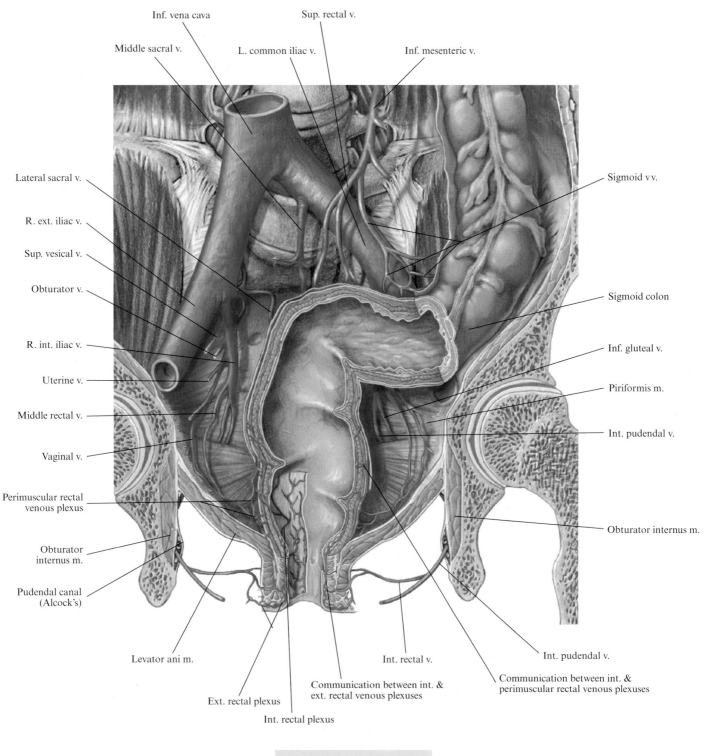

Inf. vena cava

Middle sacral v.

Sup. rectal v.

L. common iliac v.

Inf. mesenteric v.

Lateral sacral v.

R. ext. iliac v.

Sup. vesical v.

Obturator v.

R. int. iliac v.

Uterine v.

Middle rectal v.

Vaginal v.

Perimuscular rectal
venous plexus

Obturator
internus m.

Pudendal canal
(Alcock's)

Sigmoid vv.

Sigmoid colon

Inf. gluteal v.

Piriformis m.

Int. pudendal v.

Obturator internus m.

Int. pudendal v.

Communication between int. &
perimuscular rectal venous plexuses

Levator ani m.

Ext. rectal plexus

Int. rectal plexus

Int. rectal v.

Communication between int. &
ext. rectal venous plexuses

Coronal Section—Anterior View

PLATE 4.57   RECTUM & ANAL CANAL

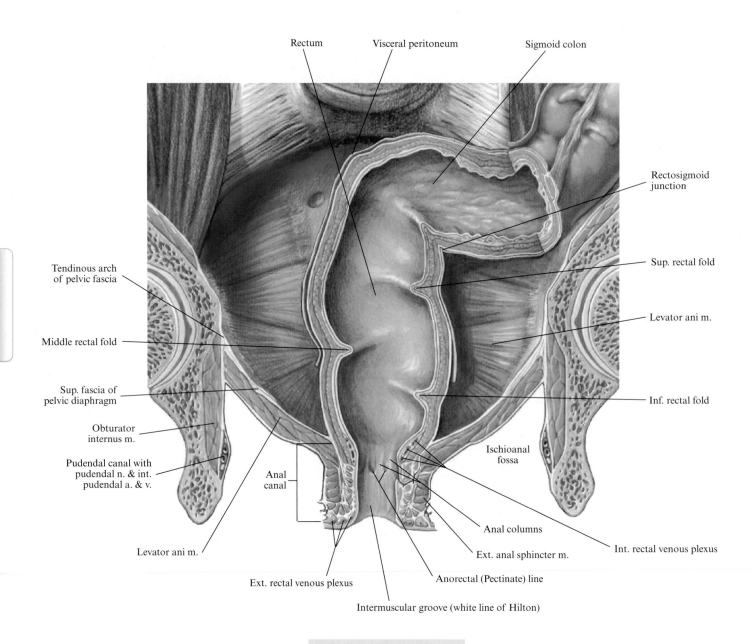

Rectum   Visceral peritoneum   Sigmoid colon

Rectosigmoid
junction

Sup. rectal fold

Tendinous arch
of pelvic fascia

Levator ani m.

Middle rectal fold

Inf. rectal fold

Sup. fascia of
pelvic diaphragm

Obturator
internus m.

Ischioanal
fossa

Pudendal canal with
pudendal n. & int.
pudendal a. & v.

Anal
canal

Int. rectal venous plexus

Levator ani m.

Anal columns

Ext. anal sphincter m.

Ext. rectal venous plexus

Anorectal (Pectinate) line

Intermuscular groove (white line of Hilton)

Coronal Section—Anterior View

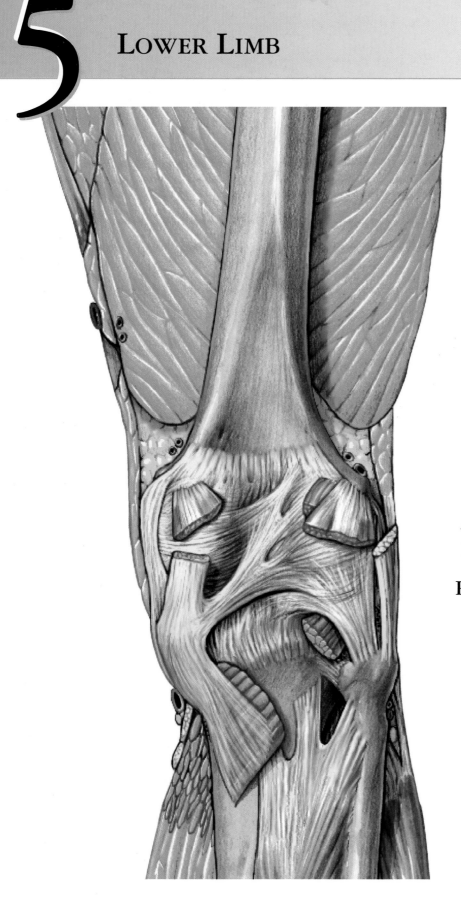

5 LOWER LIMB

SURFACE ANATOMY

SKELETON

MUSCLES

ARTERIES

VEINS

NERVES

LYMPHATICS

ANTERIOR THIGH &
FEMORAL TRIANGLE

POSTERIOR THIGH &
GLUTEAL REGION

MEDIAL &
LATERAL THIGH

ANTERIOR LEG

LATERAL LEG

POSTERIOR LEG

MEDIAL LEG

KNEE REGION

DORSAL SURFACE
OF THE FOOT

PLATE 5.1   SURFACE ANATOMY

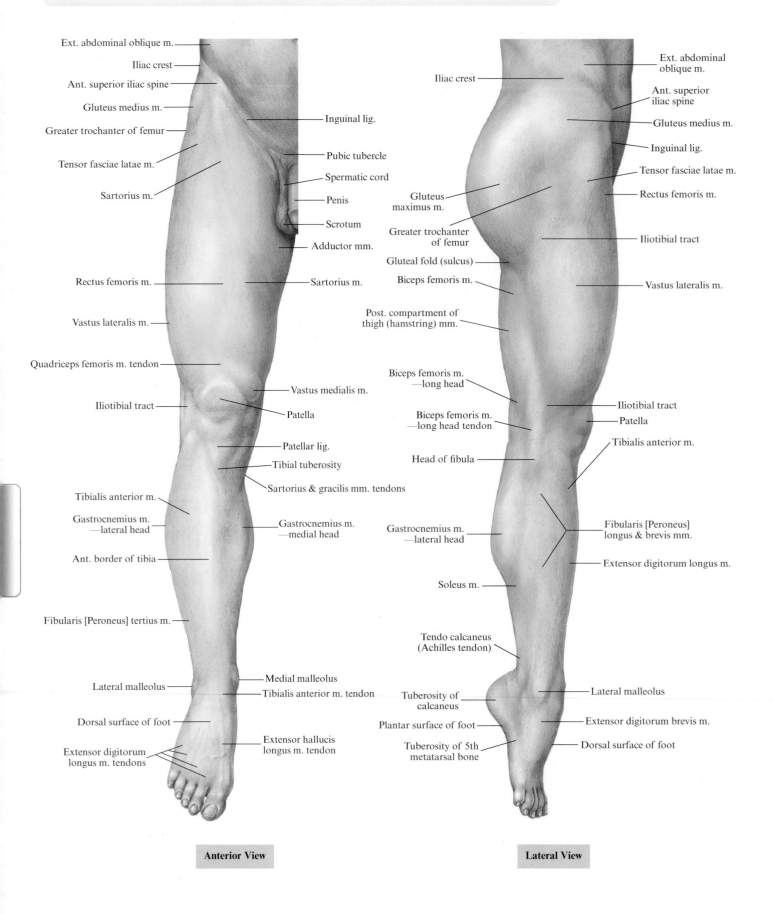

Ext. abdominal oblique m.
Iliac crest
Ant. superior iliac spine
Gluteus medius m.
Greater trochanter of femur
Tensor fasciae latae m.
Sartorius m.

Inguinal lig.

Pubic tubercle
Spermatic cord
Penis
Scrotum
Adductor mm.

Rectus femoris m.
Vastus lateralis m.
Quadriceps femoris m. tendon
Iliotibial tract

Sartorius m.

Vastus medialis m.
Patella

Patellar lig.
Tibial tuberosity
Sartorius & gracilis mm. tendons

Tibialis anterior m.
Gastrocnemius m. —lateral head
Ant. border of tibia

Gastrocnemius m. —medial head

Fibularis [Peroneus] tertius m.

Lateral malleolus
Dorsal surface of foot

Medial malleolus
Tibialis anterior m. tendon

Extensor digitorum longus m. tendons

Extensor hallucis longus m. tendon

Anterior View

Iliac crest

Ext. abdominal oblique m.
Ant. superior iliac spine
Gluteus medius m.
Inguinal lig.

Gluteus maximus m.

Tensor fasciae latae m.
Rectus femoris m.

Greater trochanter of femur

Gluteal fold (sulcus)
Biceps femoris m.

Iliotibial tract

Post. compartment of thigh (hamstring) mm.

Vastus lateralis m.

Biceps femoris m. —long head

Biceps femoris m. —long head tendon

Iliotibial tract
Patella

Head of fibula

Tibialis anterior m.

Gastrocnemius m. —lateral head

Fibularis [Peroneus] longus & brevis mm.

Extensor digitorum longus m.

Soleus m.

Tendo calcaneus (Achilles tendon)

Tuberosity of calcaneus
Plantar surface of foot
Tuberosity of 5th metatarsal bone

Lateral malleolus

Extensor digitorum brevis m.

Dorsal surface of foot

Lateral View

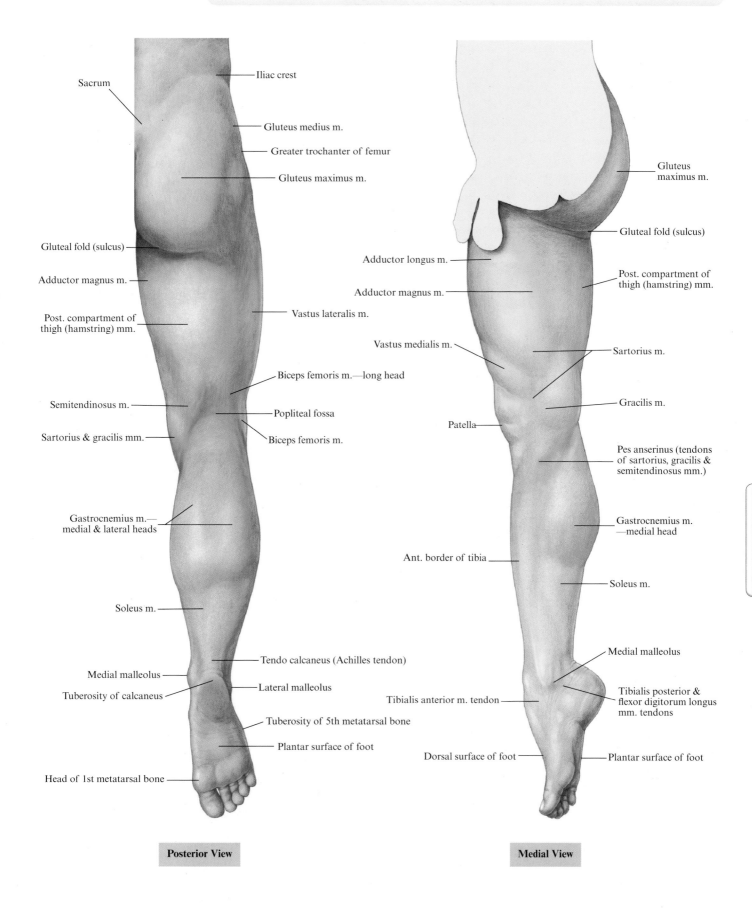

Sacrum

Iliac crest

Gluteus medius m.

Greater trochanter of femur

Gluteus maximus m.

Gluteal fold (sulcus)

Adductor magnus m.

Post. compartment of
thigh (hamstring) mm.

Vastus lateralis m.

Biceps femoris m.—long head

Semitendinosus m.

Popliteal fossa

Sartorius & gracilis mm.

Biceps femoris m.

Gastrocnemius m.—
medial & lateral heads

Soleus m.

Tendo calcaneus (Achilles tendon)

Medial malleolus

Lateral malleolus

Tuberosity of calcaneus

Tuberosity of 5th metatarsal bone

Plantar surface of foot

Head of 1st metatarsal bone

Posterior View

Gluteus
maximus m.

Gluteal fold (sulcus)

Adductor longus m.

Post. compartment of
thigh (hamstring) mm.

Adductor magnus m.

Vastus medialis m.

Sartorius m.

Gracilis m.

Patella

Pes anserinus (tendons
of sartorius, gracilis &
semitendinosus mm.)

Gastrocnemius m.
—medial head

Ant. border of tibia

Soleus m.

Medial malleolus

Tibialis anterior m. tendon

Tibialis posterior &
flexor digitorum longus
mm. tendons

Dorsal surface of foot

Plantar surface of foot

Medial View

PLATE 5.3 SKELETON & MUSCLE ATTACHMENTS

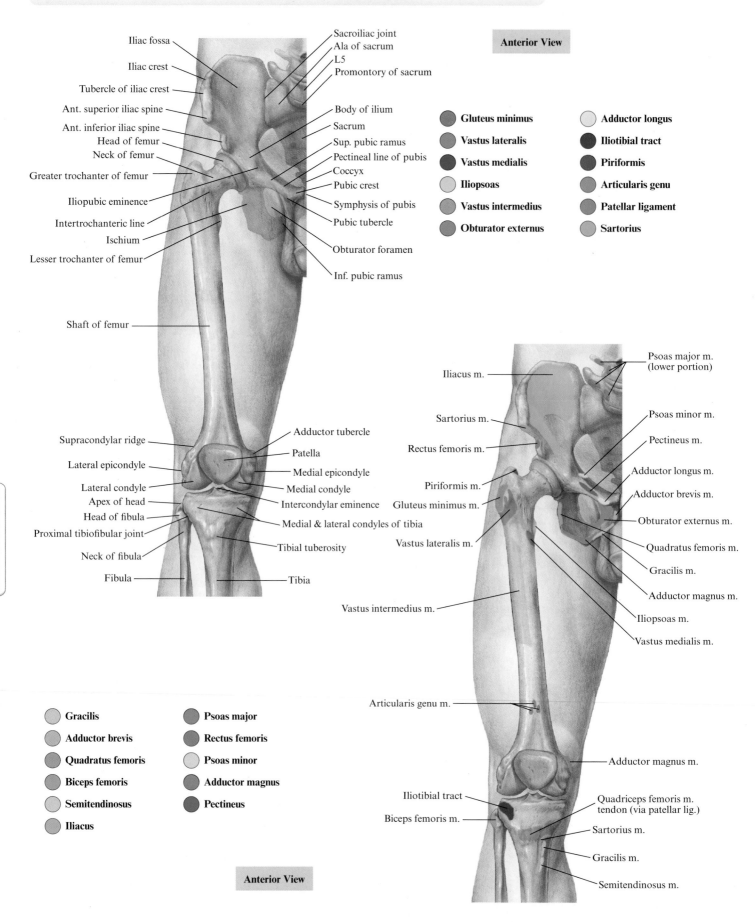

Anterior View

Iliac fossa
Iliac crest
Tubercle of iliac crest
Ant. superior iliac spine
Ant. inferior iliac spine
Head of femur
Neck of femur
Greater trochanter of femur
Iliopubic eminence
Intertrochanteric line
Ischium
Lesser trochanter of femur

Sacroiliac joint
Ala of sacrum
L5
Promontory of sacrum
Body of ilium
Sacrum
Sup. pubic ramus
Pectineal line of pubis
Coccyx
Pubic crest
Symphysis of pubis
Pubic tubercle
Obturator foramen
Inf. pubic ramus

Gluteus minimus
Vastus lateralis
Vastus medialis
Iliopsoas
Vastus intermedius
Obturator externus

Adductor longus
Iliotibial tract
Piriformis
Articularis genu
Patellar ligament
Sartorius

Shaft of femur

Supracondylar ridge
Lateral epicondyle
Lateral condyle
Apex of head
Head of fibula
Proximal tibiofibular joint
Neck of fibula
Fibula

Adductor tubercle
Patella
Medial epicondyle
Medial condyle
Intercondylar eminence
Medial & lateral condyles of tibia
Tibial tuberosity
Tibia

Iliacus m.
Sartorius m.
Rectus femoris m.
Piriformis m.
Gluteus minimus m.
Vastus lateralis m.

Psoas major m. (lower portion)
Psoas minor m.
Pectineus m.
Adductor longus m.
Adductor brevis m.
Obturator externus m.
Quadratus femoris m.
Gracilis m.
Adductor magnus m.
Iliopsoas m.
Vastus medialis m.

Vastus intermedius m.

Articularis genu m.

Iliotibial tract
Biceps femoris m.

Adductor magnus m.
Quadriceps femoris m. tendon (via patellar lig.)
Sartorius m.
Gracilis m.
Semitendinosus m.

Gracilis
Adductor brevis
Quadratus femoris
Biceps femoris
Semitendinosus
Iliacus

Psoas major
Rectus femoris
Psoas minor
Adductor magnus
Pectineus

Anterior View

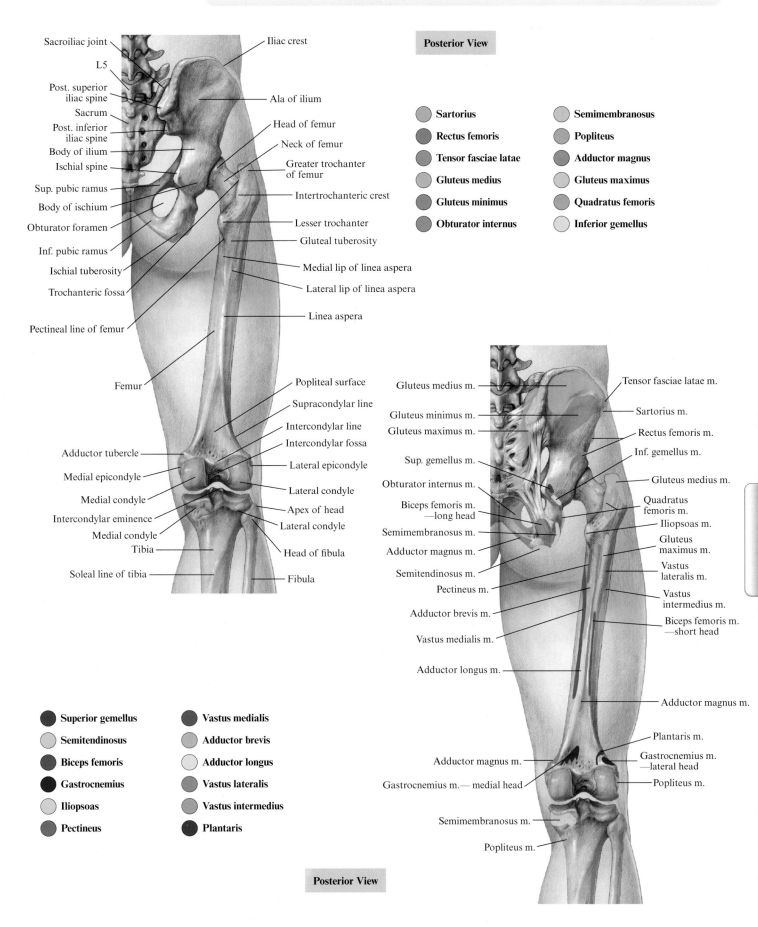

Sacroiliac joint

Iliac crest

L5

Post. superior iliac spine

Ala of ilium

Sacrum

Post. inferior iliac spine

Head of femur

Body of ilium

Neck of femur

Ischial spine

Greater trochanter of femur

Sup. pubic ramus

Intertrochanteric crest

Body of ischium

Lesser trochanter

Obturator foramen

Gluteal tuberosity

Inf. pubic ramus

Medial lip of linea aspera

Ischial tuberosity

Lateral lip of linea aspera

Trochanteric fossa

Linea aspera

Pectineal line of femur

Femur

Popliteal surface

Supracondylar line

Intercondylar line

Intercondylar fossa

Adductor tubercle

Lateral epicondyle

Medial epicondyle

Lateral condyle

Medial condyle

Apex of head

Intercondylar eminence

Lateral condyle

Medial condyle

Tibia

Head of fibula

Soleal line of tibia

Fibula

Sartorius

Semimembranosus

Rectus femoris

Popliteus

Tensor fasciae latae

Adductor magnus

Gluteus medius

Gluteus maximus

Gluteus minimus

Quadratus femoris

Obturator internus

Inferior gemellus

Gluteus medius m.

Tensor fasciae latae m.

Gluteus minimus m.

Sartorius m.

Gluteus maximus m.

Rectus femoris m.

Sup. gemellus m.

Inf. gemellus m.

Obturator internus m.

Gluteus medius m.

Biceps femoris m. —long head

Quadratus femoris m.

Semimembranosus m.

Iliopsoas m.

Adductor magnus m.

Gluteus maximus m.

Semitendinosus m.

Vastus lateralis m.

Pectineus m.

Vastus intermedius m.

Adductor brevis m.

Biceps femoris m. —short head

Vastus medialis m.

Adductor longus m.

Adductor magnus m.

Plantaris m.

Adductor magnus m.

Gastrocnemius m. —lateral head

Gastrocnemius m.— medial head

Popliteus m.

Semimembranosus m.

Popliteus m.

Superior gemellus

Vastus medialis

Semitendinosus

Adductor brevis

Biceps femoris

Adductor longus

Gastrocnemius

Vastus lateralis

Iliopsoas

Vastus intermedius

Pectineus

Plantaris

PLATE 5.5   SKELETON & MUSCLE ATTACHMENTS

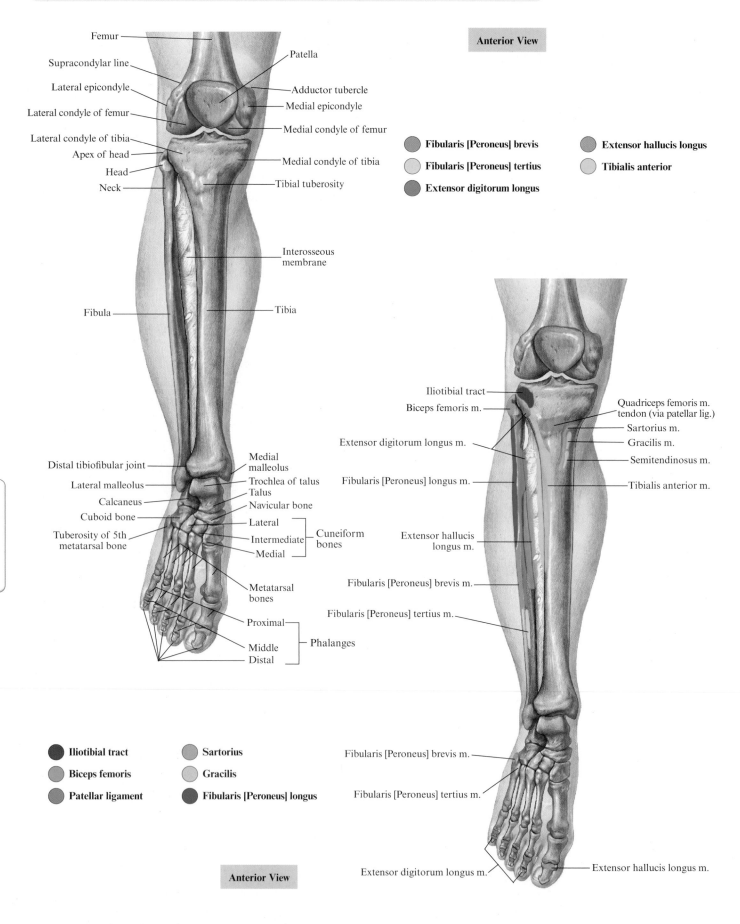

Anterior View

Femur

Supracondylar line

Lateral epicondyle

Lateral condyle of femur

Lateral condyle of tibia

Apex of head

Head

Neck

Patella

Adductor tubercle

Medial epicondyle

Medial condyle of femur

Medial condyle of tibia

Tibial tuberosity

Interosseous membrane

Fibula

Tibia

Distal tibiofibular joint

Lateral malleolus

Calcaneus

Cuboid bone

Tuberosity of 5th metatarsal bone

Medial malleolus

Trochlea of talus

Talus

Navicular bone

Lateral

Intermediate

Medial

Metatarsal bones

Proximal

Middle

Distal

Cuneiform bones

Phalanges

○ Fibularis [Peroneus] brevis

○ Fibularis [Peroneus] tertius

● Extensor digitorum longus

● Extensor hallucis longus

○ Tibialis anterior

Iliotibial tract

Biceps femoris m.

Extensor digitorum longus m.

Fibularis [Peroneus] longus m.

Extensor hallucis longus m.

Fibularis [Peroneus] brevis m.

Fibularis [Peroneus] tertius m.

Quadriceps femoris m. tendon (via patellar lig.)

Sartorius m.

Gracilis m.

Semitendinosus m.

Tibialis anterior m.

Fibularis [Peroneus] brevis m.

Fibularis [Peroneus] tertius m.

Extensor digitorum longus m.

Extensor hallucis longus m.

● Iliotibial tract

● Biceps femoris

● Patellar ligament

● Sartorius

○ Gracilis

● Fibularis [Peroneus] longus

Anterior View

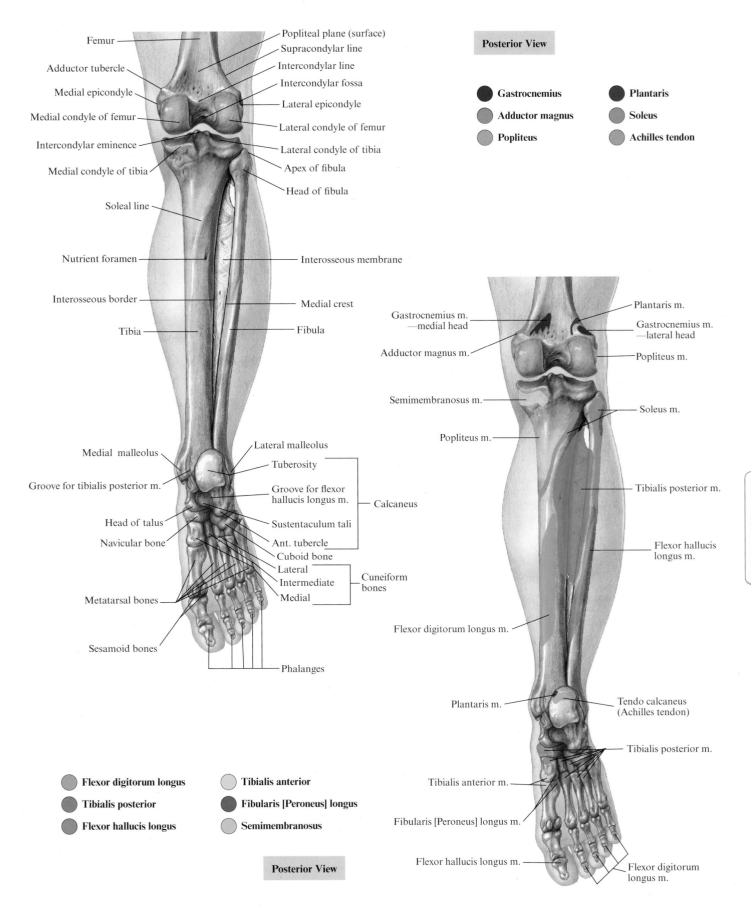

Posterior View

● **Gastrocnemius**   ● **Plantaris**
● **Adductor magnus**   ● **Soleus**
● **Popliteus**   ● **Achilles tendon**

Femur
Adductor tubercle
Medial epicondyle
Medial condyle of femur
Intercondylar eminence
Medial condyle of tibia
Soleal line
Nutrient foramen
Interosseous border
Tibia

Popliteal plane (surface)
Supracondylar line
Intercondylar line
Intercondylar fossa
Lateral epicondyle
Lateral condyle of femur
Lateral condyle of tibia
Apex of fibula
Head of fibula
Interosseous membrane
Medial crest
Fibula

Medial malleolus
Groove for tibialis posterior m.
Head of talus
Navicular bone
Metatarsal bones
Sesamoid bones

Lateral malleolus
Tuberosity
Groove for flexor hallucis longus m.
Sustentaculum tali
Ant. tubercle
Cuboid bone
Lateral
Intermediate
Medial
Phalanges

Calcaneus

Cuneiform bones

Gastrocnemius m. —medial head
Adductor magnus m.
Semimembranosus m.
Popliteus m.

Plantaris m.
Gastrocnemius m. —lateral head
Popliteus m.
Soleus m.
Tibialis posterior m.
Flexor hallucis longus m.

Flexor digitorum longus m.

Plantaris m.
Tibialis anterior m.
Fibularis [Peroneus] longus m.
Flexor hallucis longus m.

Tendo calcaneus (Achilles tendon)
Tibialis posterior m.
Flexor digitorum longus m.

● **Flexor digitorum longus**   ○ **Tibialis anterior**
● **Tibialis posterior**   ● **Fibularis [Peroneus] longus**
● **Flexor hallucis longus**   ● **Semimembranosus**

Posterior View

TABLE 5.1   ANTERIOR THIGH MUSCLES

Muscle	Proximal Attachment	Distal Attachment	Innervation	Main Actions
ILIOPSOAS				
Psoas major	Sides of T12 to L5 vertebral bodies, intervertebral discs between them & transverse processes of L1–L5	Lesser trochanter of femur	Ventral rami of lumbar nn. (**L1, L2** & L3)[a]	Flex pelvis & vertebral column on pelvis when leg & hip are extended and fixed: Act conjointly in flexing thigh at hip joint and in stabilizing this joint
Psoas minor	Sides of T12 & L1 vertebrae & intervertebral disc	Pectineal line, iliopectineal eminence via iliopubic arch lig.	Ventral rami of lumbar nn. (L1 & L2)	
Iliacus	Iliac crest, iliac fossa, ala of sacrum, ant. sacroiliac ligg. & capsule of hip joint	Tendon of psoas major & body of femur, inf. to lesser trochanter	Femoral n. (**L2** & L3)	
Tensor fasciae latae	Ant. sup. iliac spine & ant. part of ext. lip of iliac crest	Anterolateral aspect of lateral tibial condyle via iliotibial tract	Sup. gluteal n. (L4 & L5)	Abducts, flexes hip and helps to keep knee extended; medially rotates hip when it is flexed.
Sartorius	Ant. sup. iliac spine & sup. part of notch inf. to it	Sup. part of medial surface of tibia	Femoral n. (L2 & L3)	Flexes, abducts & laterally rotates thigh at hip joint & flexes leg at knee joint
QUADRICEPS FEMORIS				
Rectus femoris	Ant. inf. iliac spine & groove sup. to acetabulum	Base of patella & via patellar lig. to tibial tuberosity	Femoral n. (L2, **L3** & **L4**)	Extend leg at knee joint; rectus femoris also helps iliopsoas to flex thigh
Vastus lateralis	Greater trochanter & lateral lip of linea aspera of femur			
Vastus medialis	Intertrochanteric line & medial lip of linea aspera of femur			
Vastus intermedius	Ant. & lateral surfaces of shaft of femur			

[a]In this and subsequent tables, the numbers indicate the spinal cord segmental innervation of the nerves. For example, **L1, L2** and L3 indicate that the nerves supplying the psoas major muscle are derived from the first three lumbar segments of the spinal cord; the boldface (**L1, L2**) indicates the main segmental innervation. Damage to one or more of these spinal cord segments or to the motor nerve roots arising from them results in paralysis of the muscles involved.

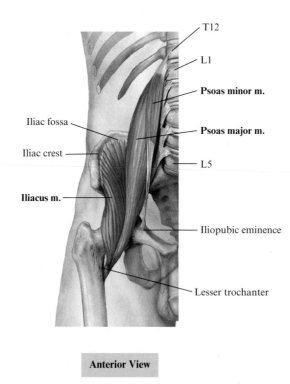

T12

L1

Psoas minor m.

Iliac fossa

Psoas major m.

Iliac crest

L5

Iliacus m.

Iliopubic eminence

Lesser trochanter

Anterior View

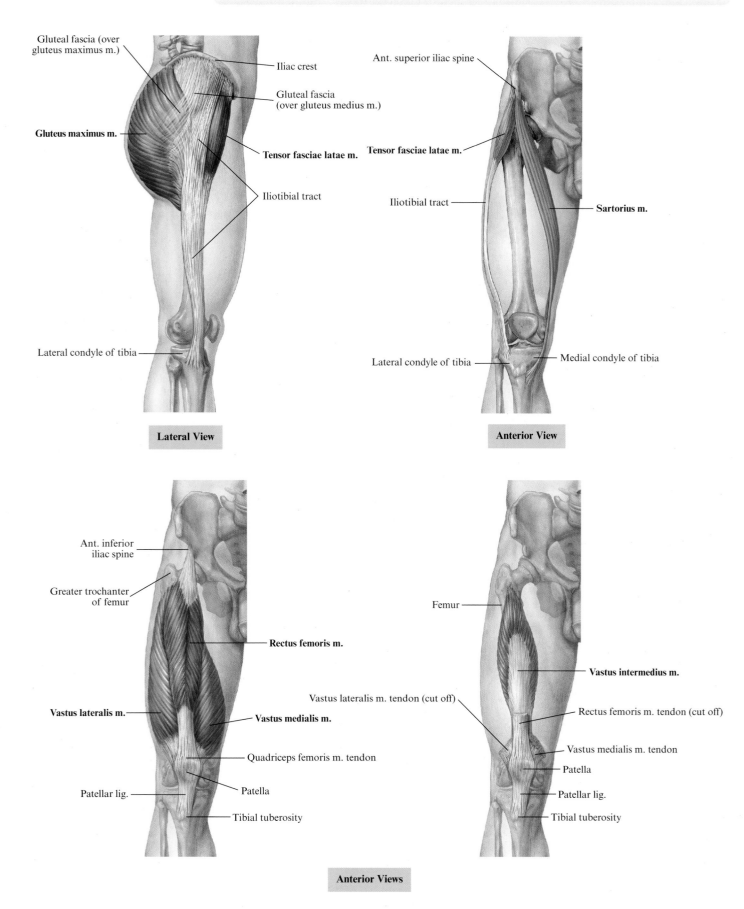

Gluteal fascia (over
gluteus maximus m.)

Iliac crest

Gluteal fascia
(over gluteus medius m.)

Gluteus maximus m.

Tensor fasciae latae m.

Iliotibial tract

Lateral condyle of tibia

Lateral View

Ant. superior iliac spine

Tensor fasciae latae m.

Iliotibial tract

Sartorius m.

Lateral condyle of tibia

Medial condyle of tibia

Anterior View

Ant. inferior
iliac spine

Greater trochanter
of femur

Rectus femoris m.

Vastus lateralis m.

Vastus medialis m.

Quadriceps femoris m. tendon

Patellar lig.

Patella

Tibial tuberosity

Femur

Vastus intermedius m.

Vastus lateralis m. tendon (cut off)

Rectus femoris m. tendon (cut off)

Vastus medialis m. tendon

Patella

Patellar lig.

Tibial tuberosity

Anterior Views

TABLE 5.2   GLUTEAL & POSTERIOR THIGH MUSCLES

Gluteal Muscle	Proximal Attachment	Distal Attachment	Innervation	Main Actions
Gluteus maximus	Ext. surface of ala of ilium, including iliac crest, dorsal surface of sacrum & coccyx and sacrotuberous lig.	Most fibers end in iliotibial tract which inserts into lateral condyle of tibia; some fibers insert on gluteal tuberosity of femur	Inf. gluteal n. (L5, **S1** & **S2**)	Extends thigh & assists in its lat. rotation; also assists in raising trunk from flexed position
Gluteus medius	Ext. surface of ilium between ant. & post. gluteal lines	Lateral surface of greater trochanter of femur	Sup. gluteal n. (**L5** & S1)	Abduct & medially rotate thigh; steady pelvis
Gluteus minimus	Ext. surface of ilium between ant. & inf. gluteal lines	Ant. surface of greater trochanter of femur		
Piriformis	Ant. surface of sacrum between S2 & S4	Superior border of greater trochanter of femur	Brr. from ventral rami of **S1** & S2	Laterally rotate extended thigh & abduct flexed thigh
Obturator internus	Pelvic surface of obturator membrane & surrounding bones	Trochanteric fossa[a]	N. to obturator internus (L5 & **S1**)	
Superior gemellus	Ischial spine		Same nerve supply as obturator internus	
Inferior gemellus	Ischial tuberosity		Same nerve supply as quadratus femoris	
Quadratus femoris	Lateral border of ischial tuberosity	Quadrate tubercle and intertrochanteric crest of femur	N. to quadratus femoris (L5 & S1)	Laterally rotates thigh[b]

[a]The gemelli muscles join the tendon of the obturator internus muscle as it attaches to the trochanteric fossa.
[b]There are six lateral rotators of the thigh: piriformis, obturator internus, gemelli (superior and inferior), quadratus femoris and obturator externus. These muscles also help to stabilize the hip joint.

Post. Thigh Muscle	Proximal Attachment	Distal Attachment	Innervation	Main Actions
Semitendinosus	Ischial tuberosity	Medial surface of sup. part of tibia	Tibial division of sciatic n. (**L5**, **S1** & S2)	Extend thigh; flex leg and rotate it medially; when thigh & leg are flexed, they can extend pelvis (and trunk)
Semimembranous		Post. part of medial condyle of tibia		
Biceps femoris *Long head* *Short head*	Ischial tuberosity Lateral lip of distal half of linea aspera & lateral supracondylar line	Lateral side of head of fibula	Tibial division of sciatic n. (L5, **S1** & S2) Common fibular (peroneal) division of sciatic n. (L5, **S1** & S2)	Flexes leg & rotates it laterally; extends thigh (*e.g.,* when starting to walk)

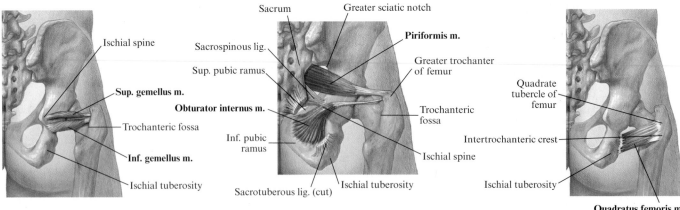

Posterior Views

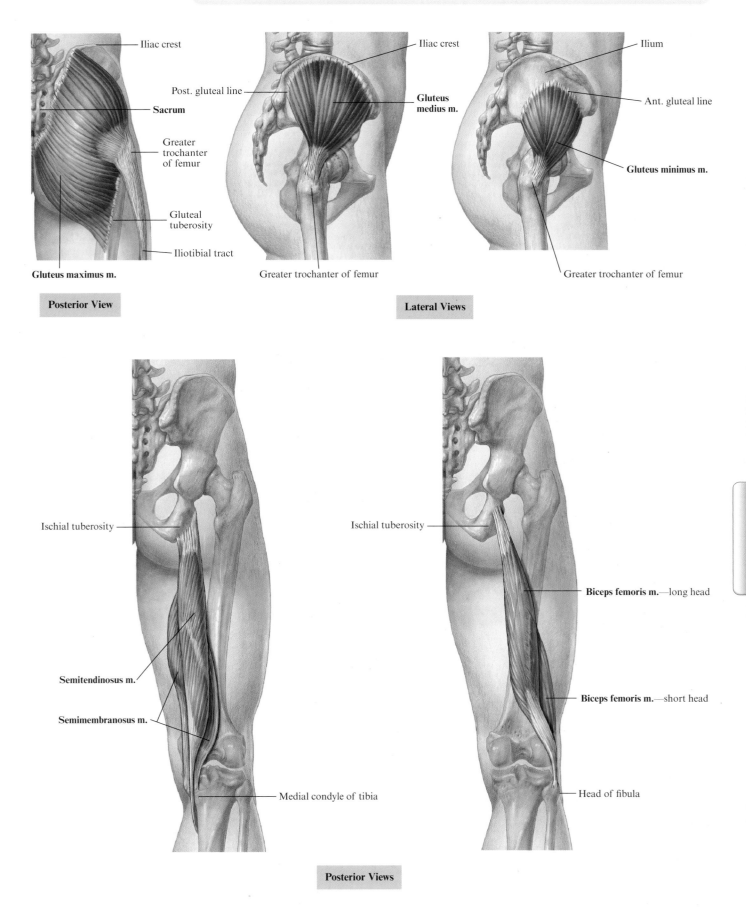

Iliac crest

Post. gluteal line

Sacrum

Greater trochanter of femur

Gluteal tuberosity

Iliotibial tract

Gluteus maximus m.

Posterior View

Iliac crest

Gluteus medius m.

Greater trochanter of femur

Lateral Views

Ilium

Ant. gluteal line

Gluteus minimus m.

Greater trochanter of femur

Ischial tuberosity

Semitendinosus m.

Semimembranosus m.

Medial condyle of tibia

Ischial tuberosity

Biceps femoris m.—long head

Biceps femoris m.—short head

Head of fibula

Posterior Views

TABLE 5.3   MEDIAL THIGH MUSCLES

Muscle[a]	Proximal Attachment	Distal Attachment	Innervation	Main Actions
Pectineus	Pecten pubis	Pectineal line of femur	Femoral nerve (**L2** & L3) & br. from obturator n. (L2, L3)	Adducts; flexes & laterally rotates thigh
Adductor longus	Body of pubis, inf. to pubic crest	Middle third of linea aspera of femur	Obturator n. ant. br. (L2, **L3** & L4)	Adducts thigh
Adductor brevis	Body & inf. ramus of pubis	Pectineal line & proximal part of linea aspera of femur	Obturator n. (L2, **L3** & L4)	Adducts thigh & may act to flex hip
Adductor magnus	Inf. ramus of pubis, ramus of ischium (adductor part) & ischial tuberosity	Gluteal tuberosity, linea aspera med. supracondylar line (adductor part) & adductor tubercle of femur (hamstring part)	*Adductor part*, obturator n. (L2, **L3** & L4) *Hamstring part*, tibial portion of sciatic n. (**L4**)	Adducts thigh; its adductor part also flexes thigh & its hamstring part extends it
Gracilis	Body & inf. ramus of pubis	Sup. part of med. surface of tibia	Obturator n. (**L2**, L3 & L4)	Adducts thigh, flexes leg & helps to rotate it medially
Obturator externus	Margins of obturator foramen & ext. surface of obturator membrane	Trochanteric fossa of femur	Obturator n. (L3 & **L4**)	Laterally rotates thigh

[a]The last five muscles are called the *adductors of the thigh.*

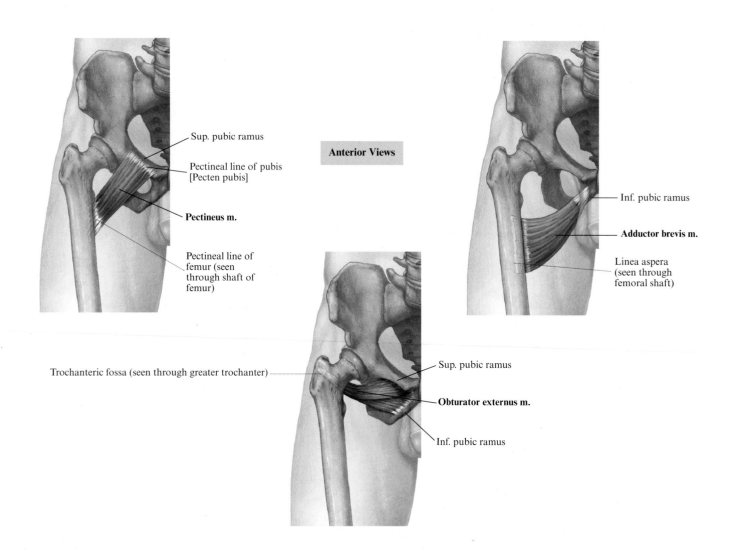

Anterior Views

Sup. pubic ramus

Pectineal line of pubis [Pecten pubis]

Pectineus m.

Pectineal line of femur (seen through shaft of femur)

Inf. pubic ramus

Adductor brevis m.

Linea aspera (seen through femoral shaft)

Trochanteric fossa (seen through greater trochanter)

Sup. pubic ramus

Obturator externus m.

Inf. pubic ramus

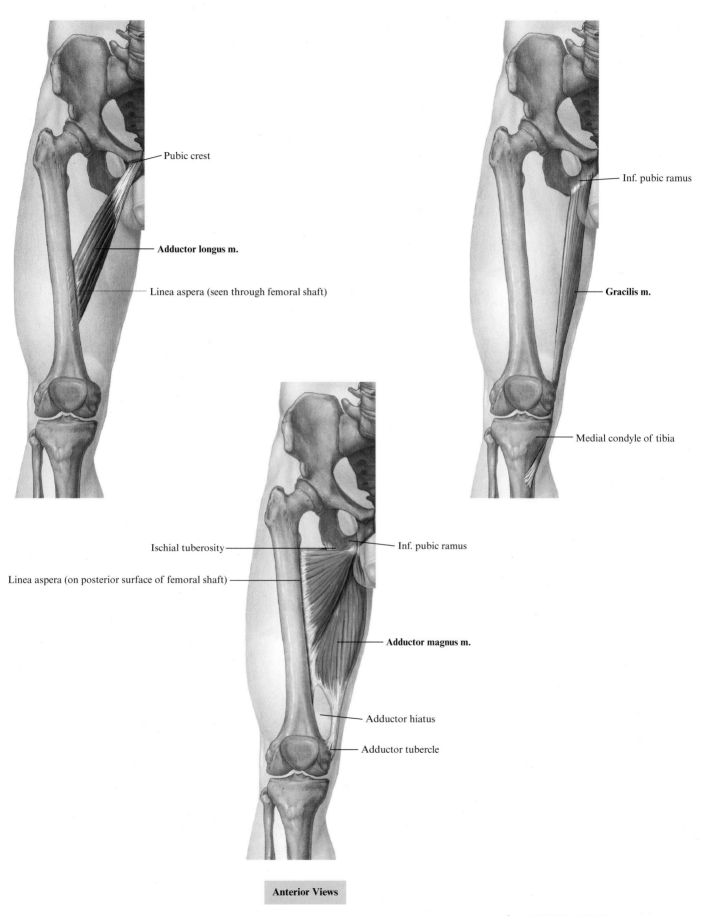

Pubic crest

Adductor longus m.

Linea aspera (seen through femoral shaft)

Inf. pubic ramus

Gracilis m.

Medial condyle of tibia

Ischial tuberosity

Inf. pubic ramus

Linea aspera (on posterior surface of femoral shaft)

Adductor magnus m.

Adductor hiatus

Adductor tubercle

Anterior Views

TABLE 5.4 ANTERIOR & LATERAL LEG MUSCLES

Anterior Muscle	Proximal Attachment	Distal Attachment	Innervation	Main Actions
Tibialis anterior	Lateral condyle & sup. half of lateral surface of tibia	Medial & inf. surfaces of medial cuneiform bone & base of 1st metatarsal bone	Deep fibular [peroneal] n. (L4 & L5)	Dorsiflexes & inverts foot
Extensor hallucis longus	Middle part of ant. surface of fibula & interosseous membrane	Dorsal aspect of base of distal phalanx of 1st digit (hallux)	Deep fibular [peroneal] n. (L5 & S1)	Extends 1st digit & dorsiflexes foot
Extensor digitorum longus	Lateral condyle of tibia, sup. 3/4 of ant. surface of fibula & interosseous membrane	Middle & distal phalanges of lateral 4 digits via extensor expansions		Extends lateral 4 digits & dorsiflexes foot
Fibularis [Peroneus] tertius	Inferior third of ant. surface of fibula & interosseous membrane	Dorsum of base of 5th metatarsal bone		Dorsiflexes foot & aids in eversion of it

Lateral Muscle[a]	Proximal Attachment	Distal Attachment	Innervation	Main Actions
Fibularis [Peroneus] longus	Head & sup. 2/3 of lateral surface of fibula	Base of 1st metatarsal bone & medial cuneiform bone	Superficial fibular (peroneal) n. (L5, S1 & S2)	Everts & plantarflexes foot
Fibularis [Peroneus] brevis	Inf. 2/3 of lateral surface of fibula	Dorsal surface of tuberosity of 5th metatarsal bone		Everts foot & weakly plantarflexes foot

[a]The fibularis [peroneus] longus and brevis were named because their proximal attachment is to the fibula. *Peroneus* is the Greek word for the Latin term *fibula* and has also been used to identify these muscles.

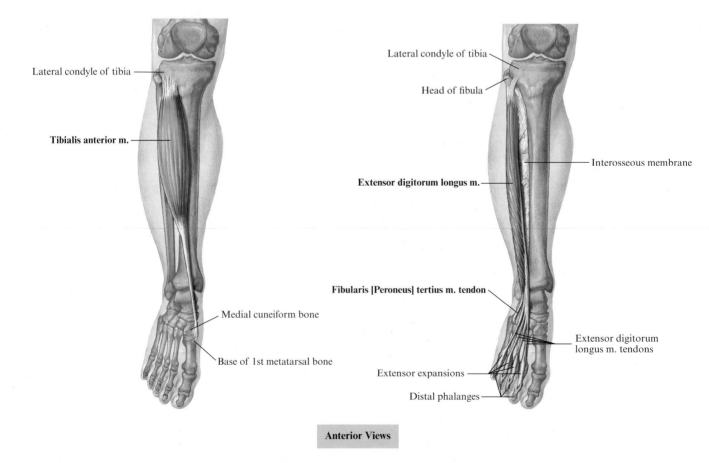

Anterior Views

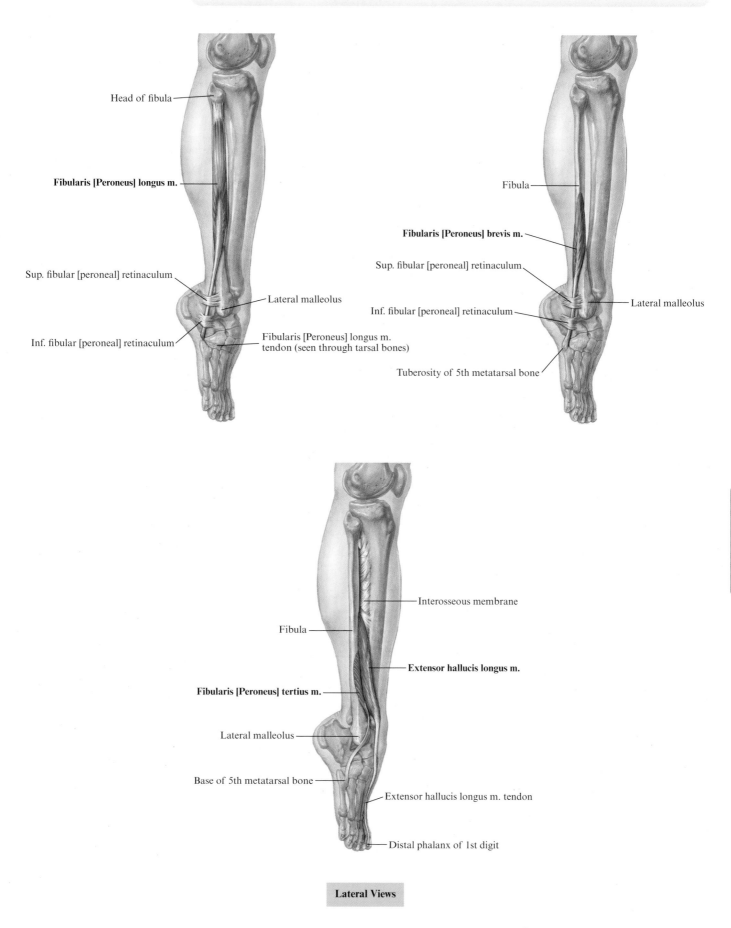

Head of fibula

Fibularis [Peroneus] longus m.

Sup. fibular [peroneal] retinaculum

Lateral malleolus

Inf. fibular [peroneal] retinaculum

Fibularis [Peroneus] longus m.
tendon (seen through tarsal bones)

Fibula

Fibularis [Peroneus] brevis m.

Sup. fibular [peroneal] retinaculum

Inf. fibular [peroneal] retinaculum

Lateral malleolus

Tuberosity of 5th metatarsal bone

Interosseous membrane

Fibula

Extensor hallucis longus m.

Fibularis [Peroneus] tertius m.

Lateral malleolus

Base of 5th metatarsal bone

Extensor hallucis longus m. tendon

Distal phalanx of 1st digit

Lateral Views

TABLE 5.5   POSTERIOR LEG MUSCLES

Muscles	Proximal Attachment	Distal Attachment	Innervation	Main Actions
SUPERFICIAL GROUP				
Gastrocnemius	*Lateral head:* Lateral aspect of lateral condyle of femur *Medial head:* Popliteal surface of femur, sup. to medial condyle	Post. surface of tuberosity of calcaneus via tendo calcaneus	Tibial n. (L5, S1 & **S2**)	Plantarflexes foot, raises heel during walking & flexes knee joint
Soleus	Post. aspect of head of fibula, sup. 1/4th of post. surface of fibula, soleal line & medial border of tibia			Plantarflexes foot
Plantaris	Inf. end of lat. supracondylar line of femur & oblique popliteal lig.	Medial side of tendo calcaneus		Weakly assists gastronemius in plantarflexing foot & flexing knee joint

Muscles	Proximal Attachment	Distal Attachment	Innervation	Main Actions
DEEP GROUP				
Popliteus	Lateral epicondyle of femur & lateral meniscus	Post. surface of tibia, sup. to soleal line	Tibial n. (**L4, L5** & S1)	Weakly flexes knee & unlocks it
Flexor hallucis longus	Inf. 2/3 of post. surface of fibula & inf. part of interosseous membrane	Base of distal phalanx of 1st digit (hallux)	Tibial n. (**S2**–S3)	Flexes 1st digit at all joints and plantarflexes foot
Flexor digitorum longus	Medial part of post. surface of tibia, inf. to soleal line & by a broad aponeurosis to fibula	Bases of distal phalanges of lateral 4 digits		Flexes 4 digits & plantarflexes foot
Tibialis posterior	Interosseus membrane, post. surface of tibia inf. to soleal line & post. surface of fibula	Tuberosity of navicular, cuneiform & cuboid bones, & bases of 2nd, 3rd & 4th metatarsal bones	Tibial n. (L4–L5)	Plantarflexes & inverts foot

Posterior Views of Superficial Muscles

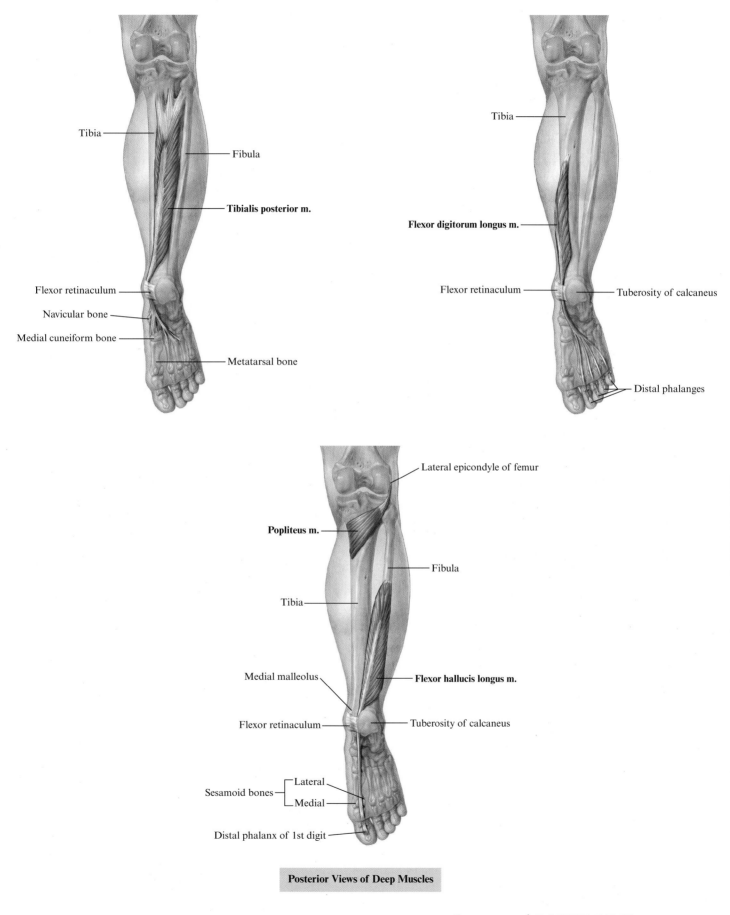

Tibia

Fibula

Tibialis posterior m.

Flexor retinaculum

Navicular bone

Medial cuneiform bone

Metatarsal bone

Tibia

Flexor digitorum longus m.

Flexor retinaculum

Tuberosity of calcaneus

Distal phalanges

Lateral epicondyle of femur

Popliteus m.

Fibula

Tibia

Medial malleolus

Flexor hallucis longus m.

Flexor retinaculum

Tuberosity of calcaneus

Sesamoid bones — Lateral

Medial

Distal phalanx of 1st digit

Posterior Views of Deep Muscles

TABLE 5.6 INTRINSIC FOOT MUSCLES

Muscle	Proximal Attachment	Distal Attachment	Innervation	Main Actions
FIRST LAYER[a]				
Abductor hallucis	Medial process of calcaneal tuberosity, flexor retinaculum & plantar aponeurosis	Medial side of base of proximal phalanx & medial sesamoid bone of 1st digit (hallux)	Medial plantar n. (S2 & **S3**)	Abducts & flexes 1st digit
Flexor digitorum brevis	Medial process of tuber calcanei, plantar aponeurosis & intermuscular septa	Both sides of middle phalanges of lateral 4 digits		Flexes lateral 4 digits (toes)
Abductor digiti minimi	Medial & lateral processes of calcaneal tuberosity, plantar aponeurosis & intermuscular septa	Lateral side of base of proximal phalanx of 5th digit (little toe)	Lateral plantar n. (S2 & **S3**)	Abducts & flexes 5th digit
SECOND LAYER				
Quadratus plantae	Medial surface & lateral margin of plantar surface of calcaneus	Posterolateral margin of tendon of flexor digitorum longus	Lateral plantar n. (S2 & **S3**)	Assists flexor digitorum longus in flexing lateral 4 digits
Lumbricalis	Tendons of flexor digitorum longus	Medial sides of bases of proximal phalanges of lateral 4 digits & extensor expansions of extensor digitorum longus m. tendons	*Medial one:* medial plantar n. (S2 & **S3**) *Lateral three:* lateral plantar n. (S2 & **S3**)	Flex proximal phalanges & extend middle & distal phalanges of lateral 4 digits
THIRD LAYER				
Flexor hallucis brevis	Plantar surfaces of cuboid & lateral cuneiform bones	Both sides of base of proximal phalanx of 1st digit	Medial plantar n. (S2 & **S3**)	Flexes proximal phalanx of 1st digit (hallux)
Adductor hallucis	*Oblique head:* Bases of metatarsal bones 2–4 *Transverse head:* Plantar ligg. of metatarsophalangeal joints 2–5	Tendons of both heads attached to lateral side of base of proximal phalanx & lat. sesamoid bone of 1st digit (hallux)	Deep br. of lateral plantar n. (S2 & **S3**)	Adducts 1st digit; assists in maintaining transverse arch of foot
Flexor digiti minimi brevis	Base of 5th metatarsal bone	Base of proximal phalanx of 5th digit	Superficial br. of lateral plantar n. (S2 & **S3**)	Flexes proximal phalanx of 5th digit
FOURTH LAYER				
Plantar interossei (3 muscles)	Bases & medial sides of metatarsal bones 3–5	Medial sides of bases of proximal phalanges of digits 3–5	Lateral plantar n. (S2 & **S3**)	Adduct digits (2–4) & flex metatarsophalangeal joints
Dorsal interossei (4 muscles)	Adjacent side of metatarsal bones 1–5	*1st:* medial side of proximal phalanx of 2nd digit *2nd–4th:* lateral sides of digits 2–4		Abduct digits (2–4) & flex metatarsorphalangeal joints

[a]Independent of the individual actions associated with them, the primary function of the first layer of intrinsic muscles of the foot is to sustain the longitudinal arch of the foot (i.e., resisting forces tending to spread or flatten it).

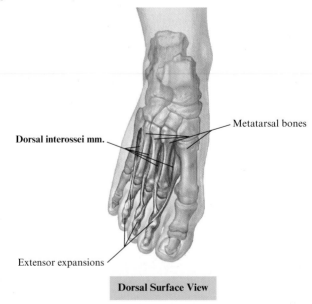

Metatarsal bones

Dorsal interossei mm.

Extensor expansions

Dorsal Surface View

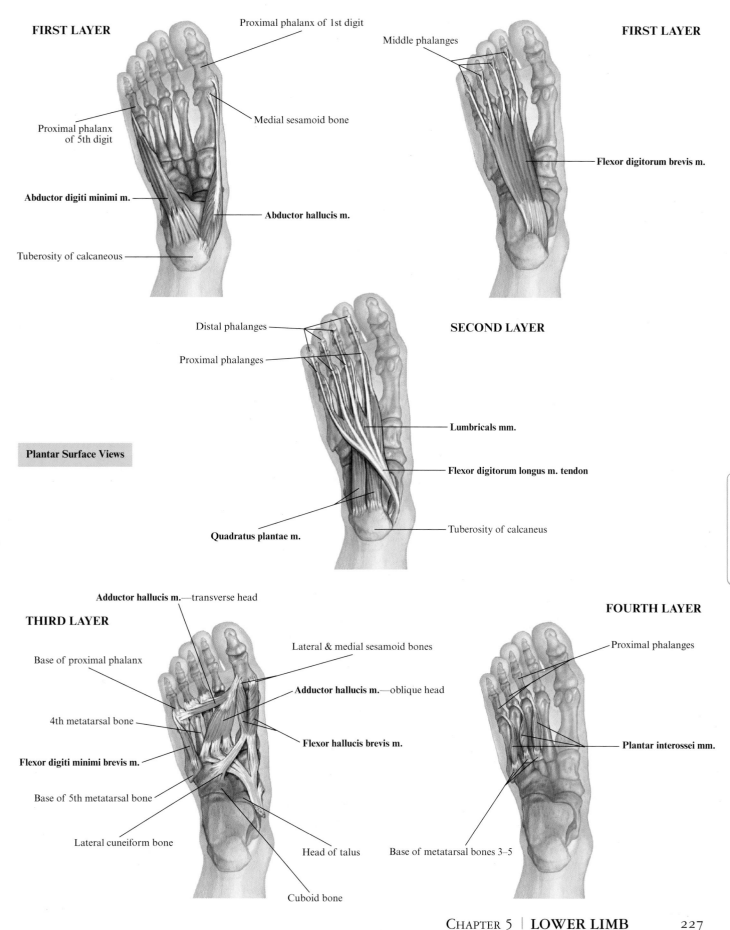

FIRST LAYER

Proximal phalanx of 1st digit

Middle phalanges

FIRST LAYER

Medial sesamoid bone

Flexor digitorum brevis m.

Proximal phalanx of 5th digit

Abductor digiti minimi m.

Abductor hallucis m.

Tuberosity of calcaneous

Distal phalanges

SECOND LAYER

Proximal phalanges

Lumbricals mm.

Plantar Surface Views

Flexor digitorum longus m. tendon

Tuberosity of calcaneus

Quadratus plantae m.

Adductor hallucis m.—transverse head

FOURTH LAYER

THIRD LAYER

Lateral & medial sesamoid bones

Proximal phalanges

Base of proximal phalanx

Adductor hallucis m.—oblique head

4th metatarsal bone

Flexor hallucis brevis m.

Flexor digiti minimi brevis m.

Plantar interossei mm.

Base of 5th metatarsal bone

Lateral cuneiform bone

Head of talus

Base of metatarsal bones 3–5

Cuboid bone

PLATE 5.13   GAIT CYCLE—STANCE PHASE

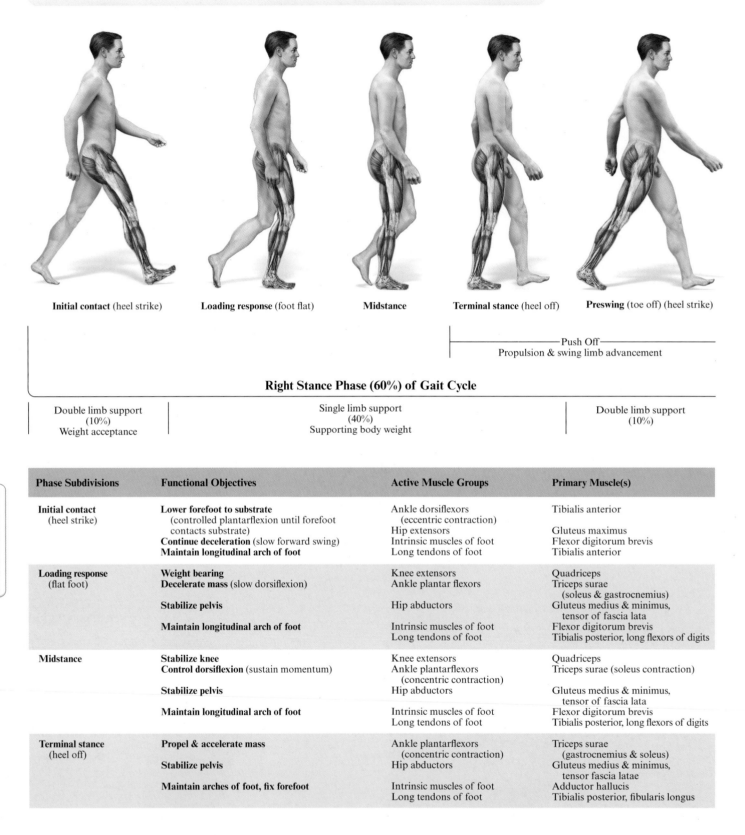

Initial contact (heel strike)   **Loading response** (foot flat)   **Midstance**   **Terminal stance** (heel off)   **Preswing** (toe off) (heel strike)

Push Off
Propulsion & swing limb advancement

Right Stance Phase (60%) of Gait Cycle

| Double limb support (10%) Weight acceptance | Single limb support (40%) Supporting body weight | Double limb support (10%) |

Phase Subdivisions	Functional Objectives	Active Muscle Groups	Primary Muscle(s)
Initial contact (heel strike)	**Lower forefoot to substrate** (controlled plantarflexion until forefoot contacts substrate) **Continue deceleration** (slow forward swing) **Maintain longitudinal arch of foot**	Ankle dorsiflexors (eccentric contraction) Hip extensors Intrinsic muscles of foot Long tendons of foot	Tibialis anterior Gluteus maximus Flexor digitorum brevis Tibialis anterior
Loading response (flat foot)	**Weight bearing** **Decelerate mass** (slow dorsiflexion) **Stabilize pelvis** **Maintain longitudinal arch of foot**	Knee extensors Ankle plantar flexors Hip abductors Intrinsic muscles of foot Long tendons of foot	Quadriceps Triceps surae (soleus & gastrocnemius) Gluteus medius & minimus, tensor of fascia lata Flexor digitorum brevis Tibialis posterior, long flexors of digits
Midstance	**Stabilize knee** **Control dorsiflexion** (sustain momentum) **Stabilize pelvis** **Maintain longitudinal arch of foot**	Knee extensors Ankle plantarflexors (concentric contraction) Hip abductors Intrinsic muscles of foot Long tendons of foot	Quadriceps Triceps surae (soleus contraction) Gluteus medius & minimus, tensor of fascia lata Flexor digitorum brevis Tibialis posterior, long flexors of digits
Terminal stance (heel off)	**Propel & accelerate mass** **Stabilize pelvis** **Maintain arches of foot, fix forefoot**	Ankle plantarflexors (concentric contraction) Hip abductors Intrinsic muscles of foot Long tendons of foot	Triceps surae (gastrocnemius & soleus) Gluteus medius & minimus, tensor fascia latae Adductor hallucis Tibialis posterior, fibularis longus

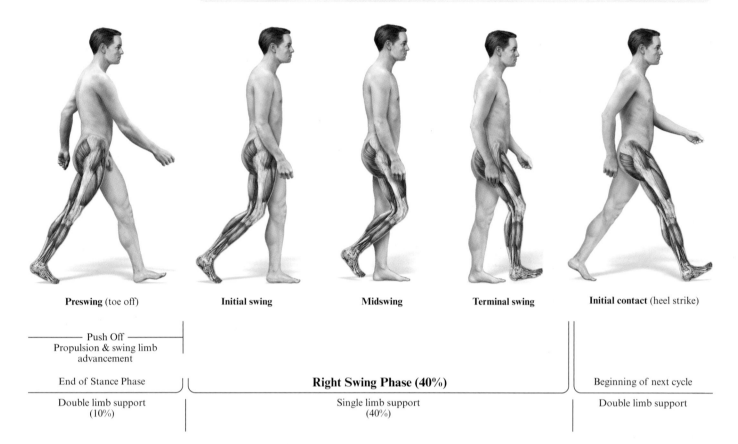

Preswing (toe off)   **Initial swing**   **Midswing**   **Terminal swing**   **Initial contact** (heel strike)

Push Off
Propulsion & swing limb
advancement

End of Stance Phase   **Right Swing Phase (40%)**   Beginning of next cycle

Double limb support   Single limb support   Double limb support
(10%)   (40%)

Phase Subdivisions	Functional Objectives	Active Muscle Groups	Primary Muscle(s)
Preswing (toe off)	Propel & accelerate mass	Long flexors of digits	Flexor hallucis longus, flexor digitorum longus
	Maintain arches of foot, fix forefoot	Intrinsic muscles of foot	Adductor hallucis
		Long tendons of foot	Tibialis posterior, fibularis longus
	Accelerate thigh; swing	Flexors of hip (eccentric contraction)	Iliopsoas, rectus femoris
Initial swing	Accelerate thigh	Flexors of hip (concentric contraction)	Illiopsoas, rectus femoris, sartorius
	Clear foot	Ankle dorsiflexors	Tibialis anterior
Midswing	Maintain flexed knee	Knee flexors (concentric contraction)	Hamstrings, sartorius
	Clear foot	Ankle dorsiflexors	Tibialis anterior
Terminal swing (heel strike)	Decelerate thigh & leg	Hip extensors (eccentric contraction)	Gluteus maximus, hamstrings
	Extend knee for heel strike (control stride length), prepare for contact with substrate	Knee extensors (concentric contraction)	Quadriceps
	Position foot	Ankle dorsiflexors	Tibialis anterior
	Absorb shock at impact	Knee extensors (eccentric contraction)	Quadriceps

During normal walking on a level surface in a straight line at a constant speed, a single gait cycle begins with heel strike (initial contact) of one foot and ends with the heel strike (initial contact) of the same foot. Each cycle is divided into stance and swing phases and each phase is further subdivided into component parts.

The **stance phase** for each limb is that interval of the cycle that begins with heel strike (initial contact) and ends with toe off. During stance phase, the foot is stationary relative to the substrate and is weight bearing.

Swing phase occurs between toe off and heel strike (initial contact). The limb in swing phase is non-weight bearing and moves in the desired direction of travel.

Tables under each set of figures indicate the functional objectives of the major muscle groups and primary muscles that are active during each subdivision of stance and swing phases.

PLATE 5.15   ARTERIES OF LOWER LIMB

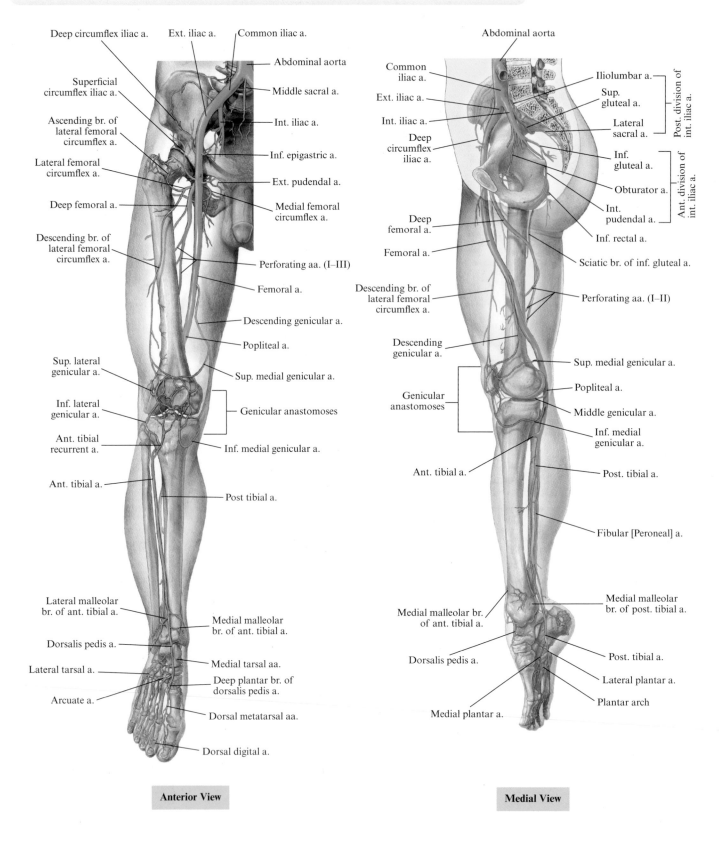

Deep circumflex iliac a.

Ext. iliac a.

Common iliac a.

Abdominal aorta

Middle sacral a.

Int. iliac a.

Inf. epigastric a.

Ext. pudendal a.

Medial femoral circumflex a.

Superficial circumflex iliac a.

Ascending br. of lateral femoral circumflex a.

Lateral femoral circumflex a.

Deep femoral a.

Descending br. of lateral femoral circumflex a.

Perforating aa. (I–III)

Femoral a.

Descending genicular a.

Popliteal a.

Sup. medial genicular a.

Sup. lateral genicular a.

Inf. lateral genicular a.

Ant. tibial recurrent a.

Ant. tibial a.

Genicular anastomoses

Inf. medial genicular a.

Post tibial a.

Lateral malleolar br. of ant. tibial a.

Dorsalis pedis a.

Lateral tarsal a.

Arcuate a.

Medial malleolar br. of ant. tibial a.

Medial tarsal aa.

Deep plantar br. of dorsalis pedis a.

Dorsal metatarsal aa.

Dorsal digital a.

Anterior View

Abdominal aorta

Common iliac a.

Ext. iliac a.

Int. iliac a.

Deep circumflex iliac a.

Deep femoral a.

Femoral a.

Iliolumbar a.

Sup. gluteal a.

Lateral sacral a.

Post. division of int. iliac a.

Inf. gluteal a.

Obturator a.

Int. pudendal a.

Ant. division of int. iliac a.

Inf. rectal a.

Sciatic br. of inf. gluteal a.

Descending br. of lateral femoral circumflex a.

Perforating aa. (I–II)

Descending genicular a.

Sup. medial genicular a.

Popliteal a.

Middle genicular a.

Genicular anastomoses

Inf. medial genicular a.

Ant. tibial a.

Post. tibial a.

Fibular [Peroneal] a.

Medial malleolar br. of ant. tibial a.

Medial malleolar br. of post. tibial a.

Dorsalis pedis a.

Post. tibial a.

Lateral plantar a.

Medial plantar a.

Plantar arch

Medial View

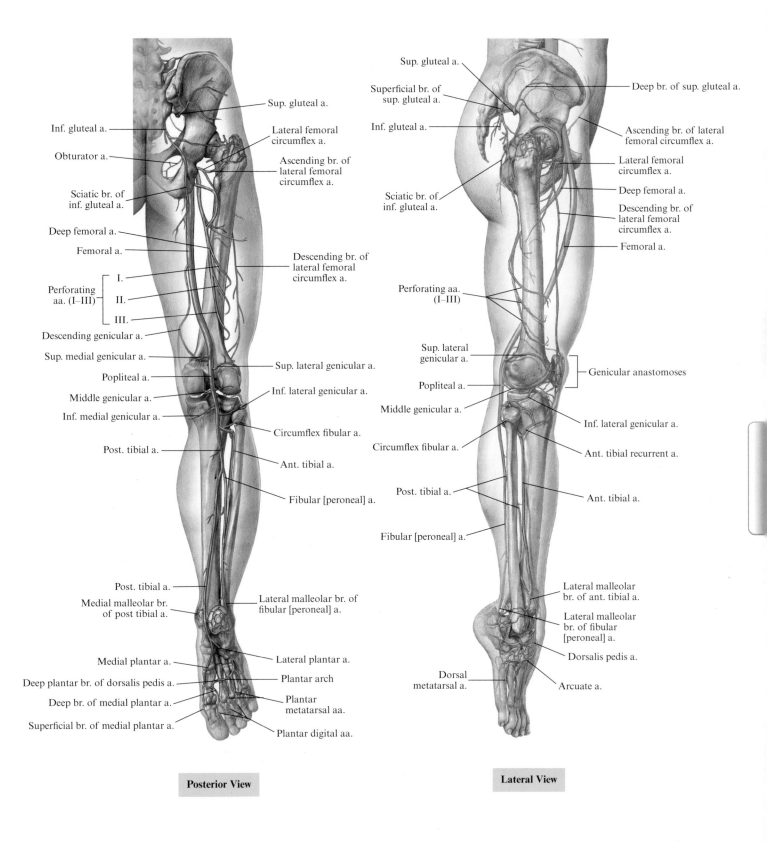

Sup. gluteal a.

Inf. gluteal a.

Obturator a.

Sciatic br. of
inf. gluteal a.

Deep femoral a.

Femoral a.

Perforating
aa. (I–III)
I.
II.
III.

Descending genicular a.

Sup. medial genicular a.

Popliteal a.

Middle genicular a.

Inf. medial genicular a.

Post. tibial a.

Post. tibial a.

Medial malleolar br.
of post tibial a.

Medial plantar a.

Deep plantar br. of dorsalis pedis a.

Deep br. of medial plantar a.

Superficial br. of medial plantar a.

Sup. gluteal a.

Lateral femoral
circumflex a.

Ascending br. of
lateral femoral
circumflex a.

Descending br. of
lateral femoral
circumflex a.

Sup. lateral genicular a.

Inf. lateral genicular a.

Circumflex fibular a.

Ant. tibial a.

Fibular [peroneal] a.

Lateral malleolar br. of
fibular [peroneal] a.

Lateral plantar a.

Plantar arch

Plantar
metatarsal aa.

Plantar digital aa.

Posterior View

Sup. gluteal a.

Superficial br. of
sup. gluteal a.

Inf. gluteal a.

Sciatic br. of
inf. gluteal a.

Perforating aa.
(I–III)

Sup. lateral
genicular a.

Popliteal a.

Middle genicular a.

Circumflex fibular a.

Post. tibial a.

Fibular [peroneal] a.

Deep br. of sup. gluteal a.

Ascending br. of lateral
femoral circumflex a.

Lateral femoral
circumflex a.

Deep femoral a.

Descending br. of
lateral femoral
circumflex a.

Femoral a.

Genicular anastomoses

Inf. lateral genicular a.

Ant. tibial recurrent a.

Ant. tibial a.

Lateral malleolar
br. of ant. tibial a.

Lateral malleolar
br. of fibular
[peroneal] a.

Dorsalis pedis a.

Dorsal
metatarsal a.

Arcuate a.

Lateral View

PLATE 5.17   SUPERFICIAL VEINS OF LOWER LIMB

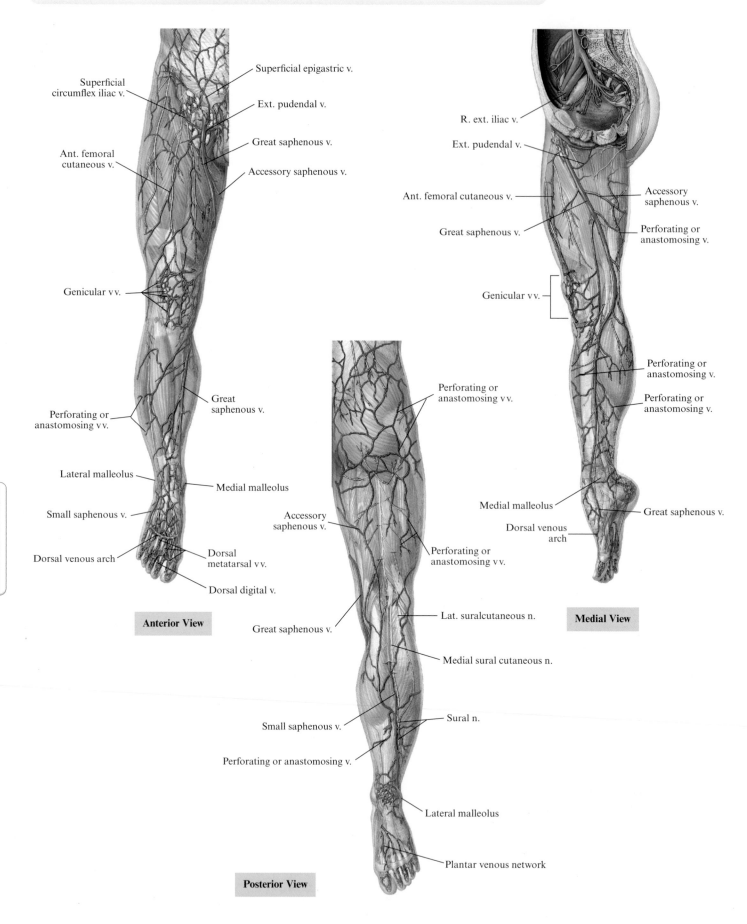

Superficial epigastric v.

Superficial circumflex iliac v.

Ext. pudendal v.

Great saphenous v.

Ant. femoral cutaneous v.

Accessory saphenous v.

R. ext. iliac v.

Ext. pudendal v.

Ant. femoral cutaneous v.

Accessory saphenous v.

Great saphenous v.

Perforating or anastomosing v.

Genicular v v.

Genicular v v.

Perforating or anastomosing v.

Perforating or anastomosing v.

Great saphenous v.

Perforating or anastomosing v v.

Perforating or anastomosing v v.

Lateral malleolus

Medial malleolus

Small saphenous v.

Accessory saphenous v.

Medial malleolus

Great saphenous v.

Dorsal venous arch

Dorsal metatarsal v v.

Perforating or anastomosing v v.

Dorsal venous arch

Dorsal digital v.

Lat. suralcutaneous n.

Great saphenous v.

Medial sural cutaneous n.

Anterior View

Medial View

Sural n.

Small saphenous v.

Perforating or anastomosing v.

Lateral malleolus

Plantar venous network

Posterior View

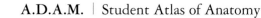

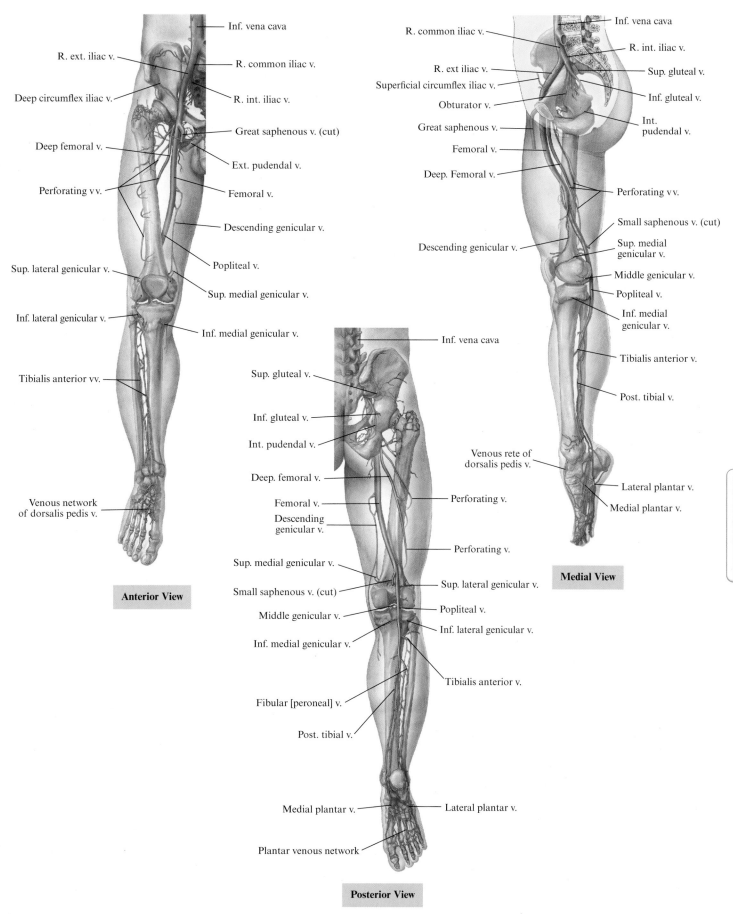

Anterior View

Inf. vena cava

R. ext. iliac v.

Deep circumflex iliac v.

Deep femoral v.

Perforating v v.

Sup. lateral genicular v.

Inf. lateral genicular v.

Tibialis anterior vv.

Venous network
of dorsalis pedis v.

R. common iliac v.

R. int. iliac v.

Great saphenous v. (cut)

Ext. pudendal v.

Femoral v.

Descending genicular v.

Popliteal v.

Sup. medial genicular v.

Inf. medial genicular v.

Medial View

R. common iliac v.

R. ext iliac v.

Superficial circumflex iliac v.

Obturator v.

Great saphenous v.

Femoral v.

Deep. Femoral v.

Descending genicular v.

Inf. vena cava

R. int. iliac v.

Sup. gluteal v.

Inf. gluteal v.

Int. pudendal v.

Perforating v v.

Small saphenous v. (cut)

Sup. medial genicular v.

Middle genicular v.

Popliteal v.

Inf. medial genicular v.

Tibialis anterior v.

Post. tibial v.

Venous rete of dorsalis pedis v.

Lateral plantar v.

Medial plantar v.

Posterior View

Inf. vena cava

Sup. gluteal v.

Inf. gluteal v.

Int. pudendal v.

Deep. femoral v.

Femoral v.

Descending genicular v.

Sup. medial genicular v.

Small saphenous v. (cut)

Middle genicular v.

Inf. medial genicular v.

Fibular [peroneal] v.

Post. tibial v.

Perforating v.

Perforating v.

Sup. lateral genicular v.

Popliteal v.

Inf. lateral genicular v.

Tibialis anterior v.

Medial plantar v.

Lateral plantar v.

Plantar venous network

PLATE 5.19   DERMATOMES & CUTANEOUS NERVES OF LOWER LIMB

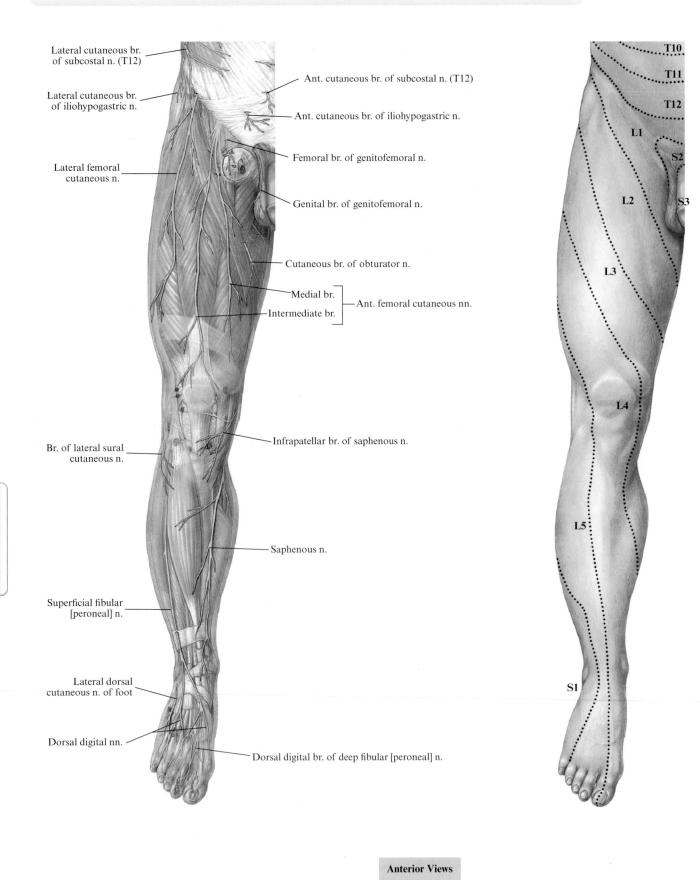

Lateral cutaneous br.
of subcostal n. (T12)

Lateral cutaneous br.
of iliohypogastric n.

Lateral femoral
cutaneous n.

Br. of lateral sural
cutaneous n.

Superficial fibular
[peroneal] n.

Lateral dorsal
cutaneous n. of foot

Dorsal digital nn.

Ant. cutaneous br. of subcostal n. (T12)

Ant. cutaneous br. of iliohypogastric n.

Femoral br. of genitofemoral n.

Genital br. of genitofemoral n.

Cutaneous br. of obturator n.

Medial br.
Intermediate br.   } Ant. femoral cutaneous nn.

Infrapatellar br. of saphenous n.

Saphenous n.

Dorsal digital br. of deep fibular [peroneal] n.

T10
T11
T12
L1
S2
L2
S3
L3
L4
L5
S1

Anterior Views

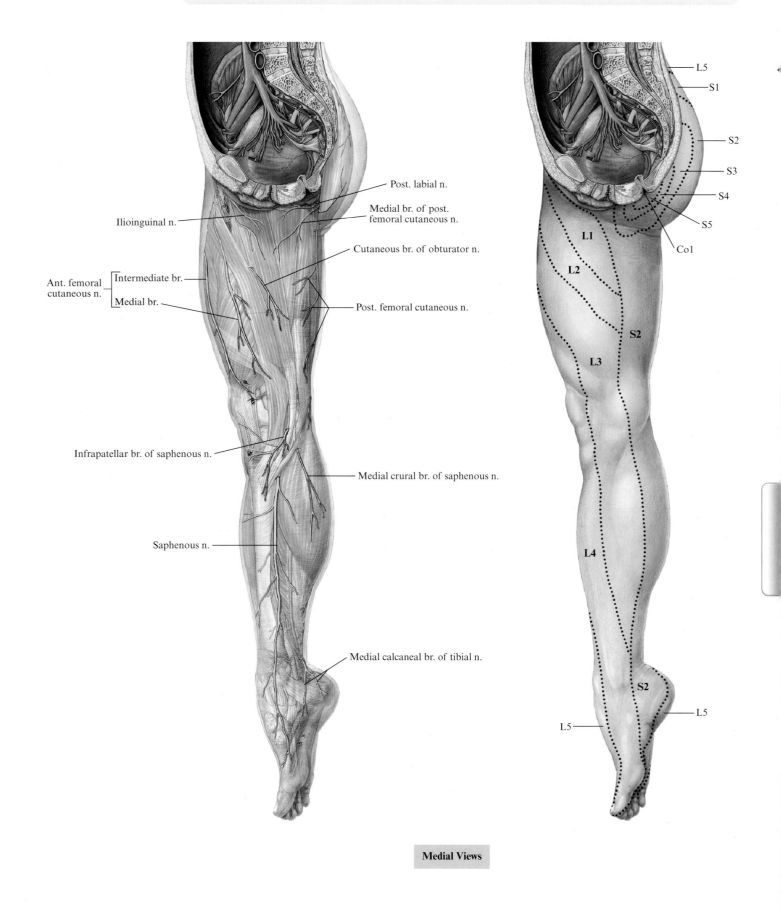

Post. labial n.

Ilioinguinal n.

Medial br. of post. femoral cutaneous n.

Cutaneous br. of obturator n.

Ant. femoral cutaneous n. — Intermediate br. — Medial br.

Post. femoral cutaneous n.

Infrapatellar br. of saphenous n.

Medial crural br. of saphenous n.

Saphenous n.

Medial calcaneal br. of tibial n.

L5
S1
S2
S3
S4
S5
Co1

L1
L2
L3
L4
S2
S2
L5
L5
L5

Medial Views

PLATE 5.21   DERMATOMES & CUTANEOUS NERVES OF LOWER LIMB

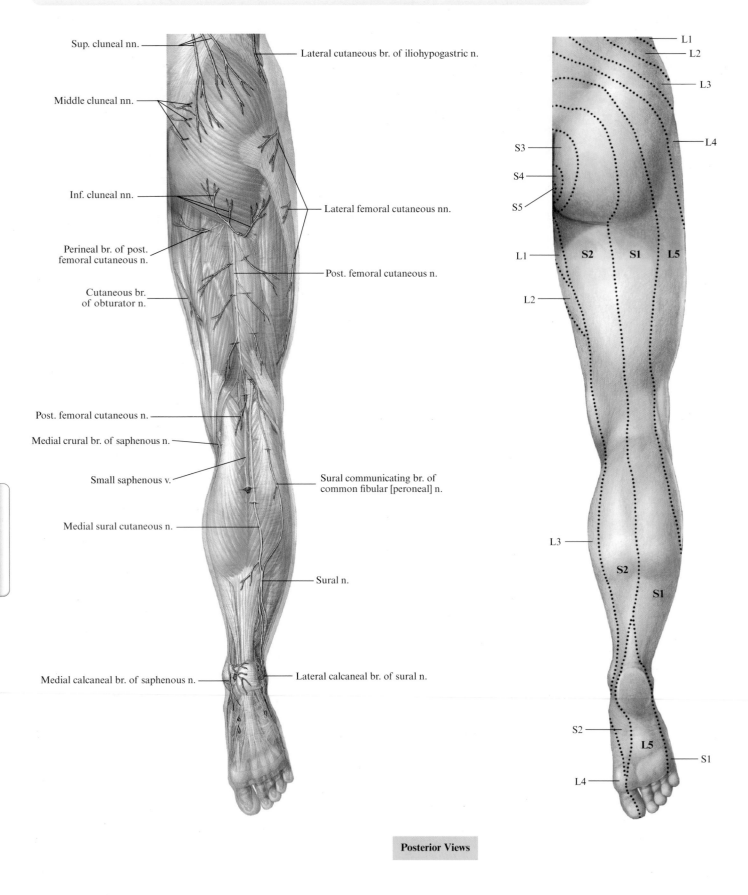

Sup. cluneal nn.

Lateral cutaneous br. of iliohypogastric n.

Middle cluneal nn.

Inf. cluneal nn.

Lateral femoral cutaneous nn.

Perineal br. of post. femoral cutaneous n.

Post. femoral cutaneous n.

Cutaneous br. of obturator n.

Post. femoral cutaneous n.

Medial crural br. of saphenous n.

Small saphenous v.

Sural communicating br. of common fibular [peroneal] n.

Medial sural cutaneous n.

Sural n.

Medial calcaneal br. of saphenous n.

Lateral calcaneal br. of sural n.

L1
L2
L3
L4
S3
S4
S5
L1
L2
S2
S1
L5
L3
S2
S1
S2
L5
L4
S1

Posterior Views

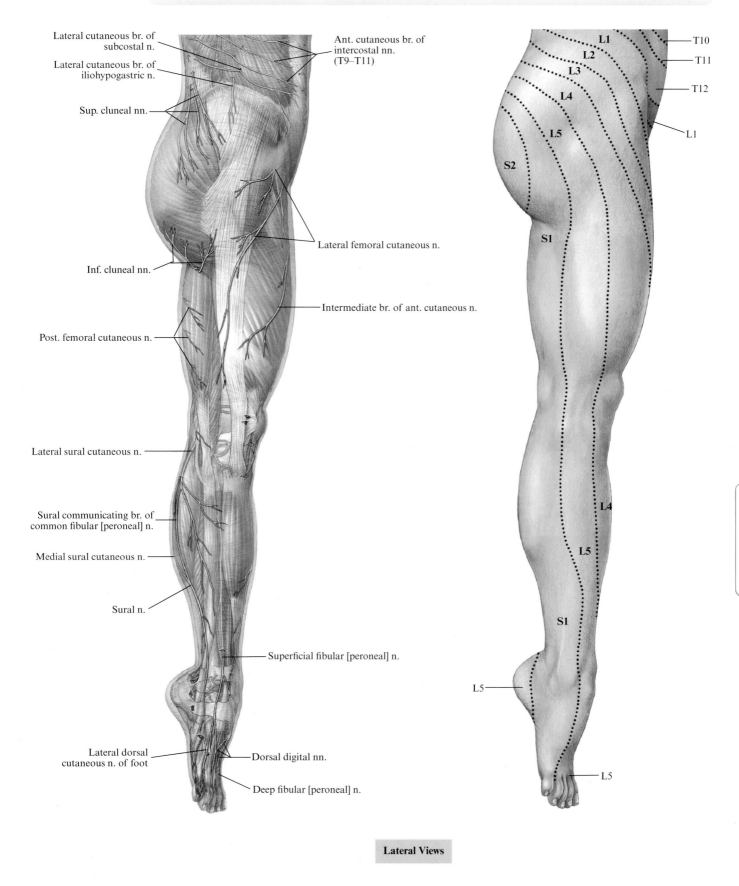

Lateral cutaneous br. of subcostal n.

Ant. cutaneous br. of intercostal nn. (T9–T11)

Lateral cutaneous br. of iliohypogastric n.

Sup. cluneal nn.

Inf. cluneal nn.

Lateral femoral cutaneous n.

Intermediate br. of ant. cutaneous n.

Post. femoral cutaneous n.

Lateral sural cutaneous n.

Sural communicating br. of common fibular [peroneal] n.

Medial sural cutaneous n.

Sural n.

Superficial fibular [peroneal] n.

Lateral dorsal cutaneous n. of foot

Dorsal digital nn.

Deep fibular [peroneal] n.

T10
T11
T12
L1
L1
L2
L3
L4
L5
S2
S1
L4
L5
S1
L5
L5

Lateral Views

PLATE 5.23   SEGMENTAL INNERVATION & JOINT ACTIONS

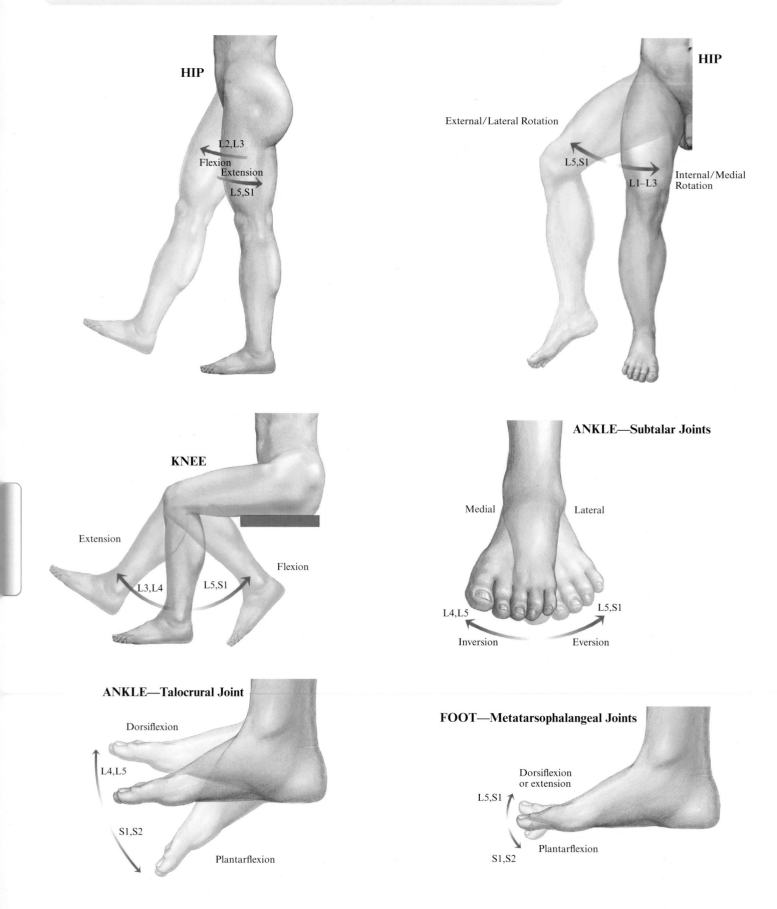

HIP

L2,L3

Flexion

Extension

L5,S1

HIP

External/Lateral Rotation

L5,S1

L1–L3

Internal/Medial Rotation

KNEE

Extension

Flexion

L3,L4   L5,S1

ANKLE—Subtalar Joints

Medial   Lateral

L4,L5   L5,S1

Inversion   Eversion

ANKLE—Talocrural Joint

Dorsiflexion

L4,L5

S1,S2

Plantarflexion

FOOT—Metatarsophalangeal Joints

Dorsiflexion or extension

L5,S1

Plantarflexion

S1,S2

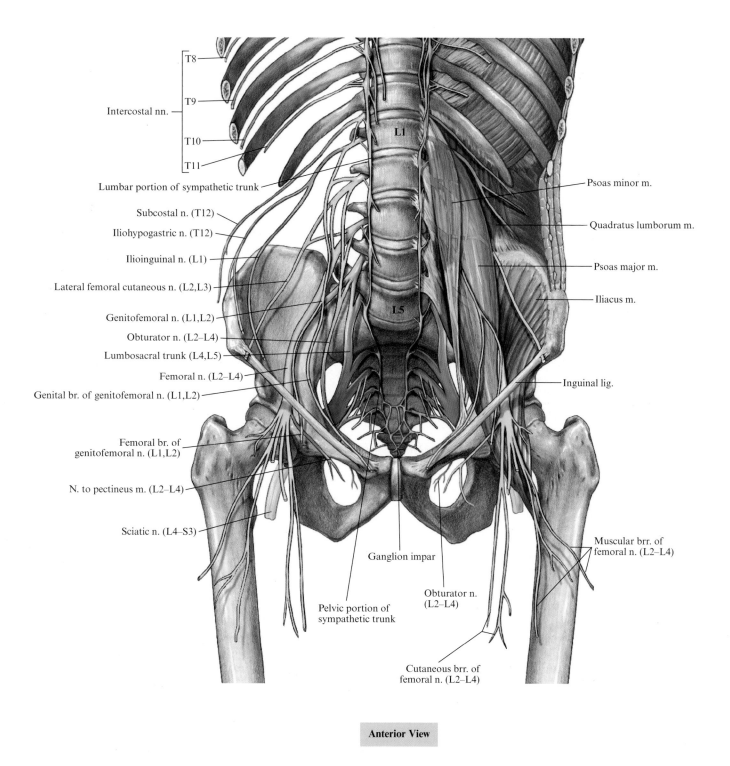

T8

Intercostal nn.

T9

T10

T11

Lumbar portion of sympathetic trunk

Subcostal n. (T12)

Iliohypogastric n. (T12)

Ilioinguinal n. (L1)

Lateral femoral cutaneous n. (L2,L3)

Genitofemoral n. (L1,L2)

Obturator n. (L2–L4)

Lumbosacral trunk (L4,L5)

Femoral n. (L2–L4)

Genital br. of genitofemoral n. (L1,L2)

Femoral br. of
genitofemoral n. (L1,L2)

N. to pectineus m. (L2–L4)

Sciatic n. (L4–S3)

L1

L5

Psoas minor m.

Quadratus lumborum m.

Psoas major m.

Iliacus m.

Inguinal lig.

Muscular brr. of
femoral n. (L2–L4)

Ganglion impar

Pelvic portion of
sympathetic trunk

Obturator n.
(L2–L4)

Cutaneous brr. of
femoral n. (L2–L4)

Anterior View

PLATE 5.25   DEEP NERVES OF LOWER LIMB

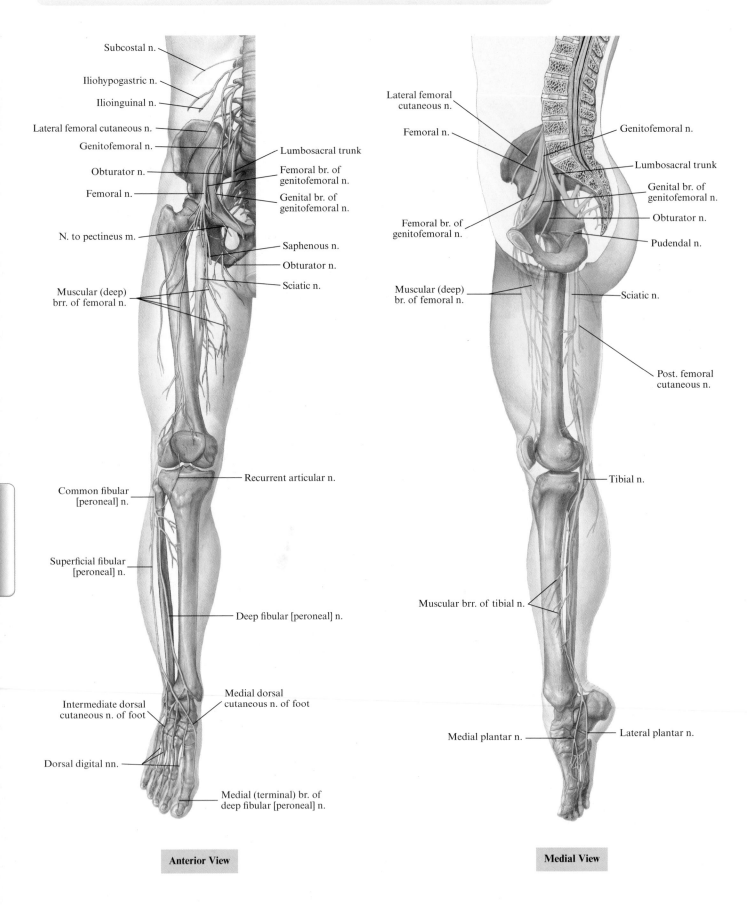

Subcostal n.

Iliohypogastric n.

Ilioinguinal n.

Lateral femoral cutaneous n.

Genitofemoral n.

Obturator n.

Femoral n.

N. to pectineus m.

Muscular (deep) brr. of femoral n.

Common fibular [peroneal] n.

Superficial fibular [peroneal] n.

Intermediate dorsal cutaneous n. of foot

Dorsal digital nn.

Lumbosacral trunk

Femoral br. of genitofemoral n.

Genital br. of genitofemoral n.

Saphenous n.

Obturator n.

Sciatic n.

Recurrent articular n.

Deep fibular [peroneal] n.

Medial dorsal cutaneous n. of foot

Medial (terminal) br. of deep fibular [peroneal] n.

Anterior View

Lateral femoral cutaneous n.

Femoral n.

Femoral br. of genitofemoral n.

Muscular (deep) br. of femoral n.

Muscular brr. of tibial n.

Medial plantar n.

Genitofemoral n.

Lumbosacral trunk

Genital br. of genitofemoral n.

Obturator n.

Pudendal n.

Sciatic n.

Post. femoral cutaneous n.

Tibial n.

Lateral plantar n.

Medial View

A.D.A.M. | Student Atlas of Anatomy

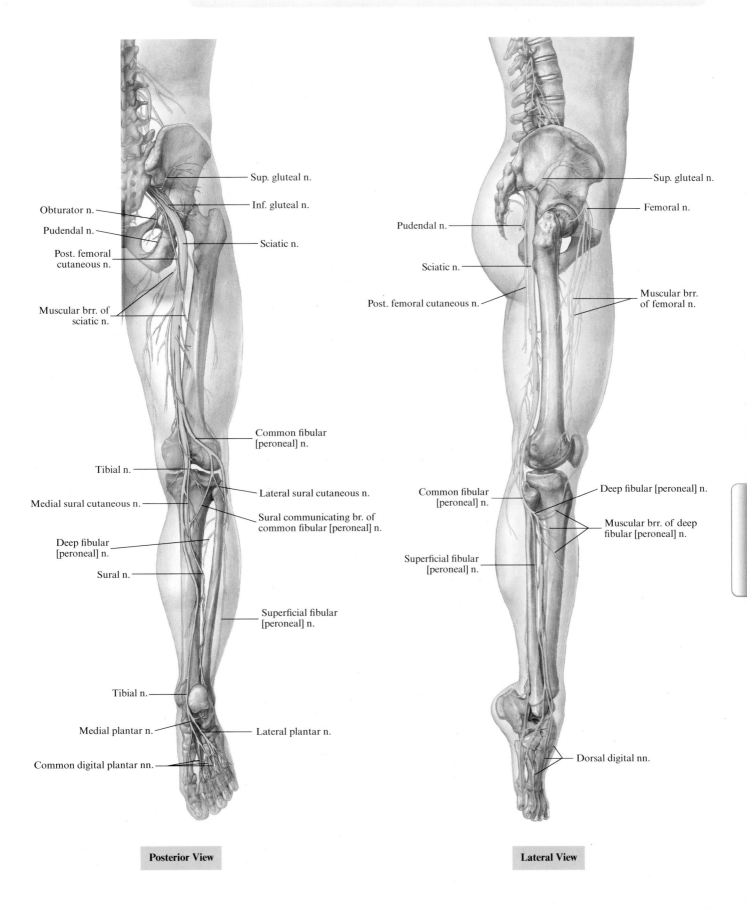

Sup. gluteal n.

Inf. gluteal n.

Obturator n.

Pudendal n.

Sciatic n.

Post. femoral
cutaneous n.

Muscular brr. of
sciatic n.

Common fibular
[peroneal] n.

Tibial n.

Lateral sural cutaneous n.

Medial sural cutaneous n.

Sural communicating br. of
common fibular [peroneal] n.

Deep fibular
[peroneal] n.

Sural n.

Superficial fibular
[peroneal] n.

Tibial n.

Medial plantar n.

Lateral plantar n.

Common digital plantar nn.

Posterior View

Sup. gluteal n.

Femoral n.

Pudendal n.

Sciatic n.

Post. femoral cutaneous n.

Muscular brr.
of femoral n.

Common fibular
[peroneal] n.

Deep fibular [peroneal] n.

Muscular brr. of deep
fibular [peroneal] n.

Superficial fibular
[peroneal] n.

Dorsal digital nn.

Lateral View

PLATE 5.27   LUMBAR PLEXUS

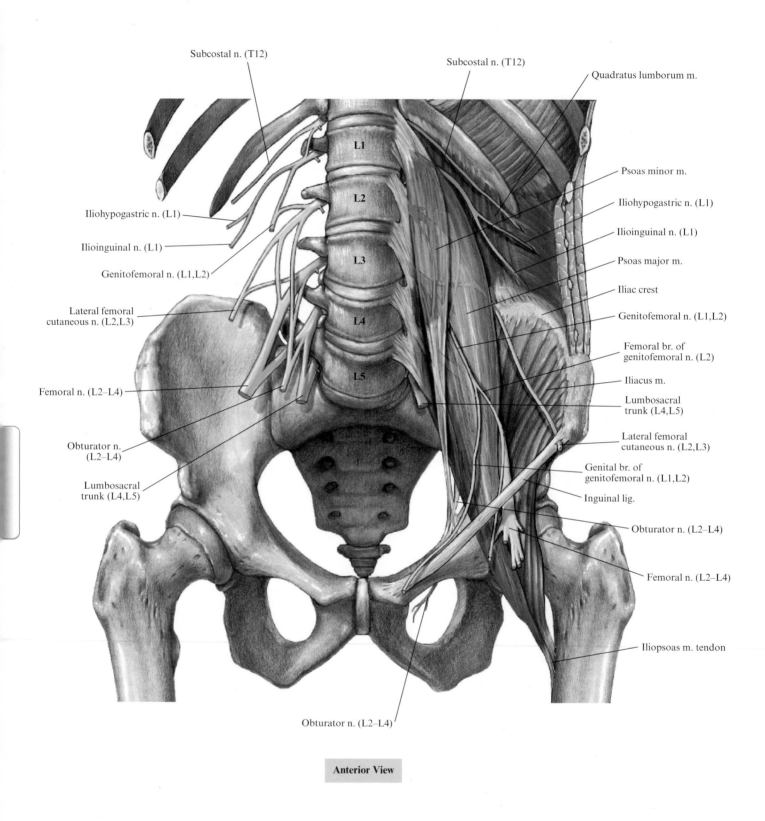

Subcostal n. (T12)

Subcostal n. (T12)

Quadratus lumborum m.

L1

L2

L3

L4

L5

Iliohypogastric n. (L1)

Ilioinguinal n. (L1)

Genitofemoral n. (L1,L2)

Lateral femoral
cutaneous n. (L2,L3)

Femoral n. (L2–L4)

Obturator n.
(L2–L4)

Lumbosacral
trunk (L4,L5)

Psoas minor m.

Iliohypogastric n. (L1)

Ilioinguinal n. (L1)

Psoas major m.

Iliac crest

Genitofemoral n. (L1,L2)

Femoral br. of
genitofemoral n. (L2)

Iliacus m.

Lumbosacral
trunk (L4,L5)

Lateral femoral
cutaneous n. (L2,L3)

Genital br. of
genitofemoral n. (L1,L2)

Inguinal lig.

Obturator n. (L2–L4)

Femoral n. (L2–L4)

Iliopsoas m. tendon

Obturator n. (L2–L4)

Anterior View

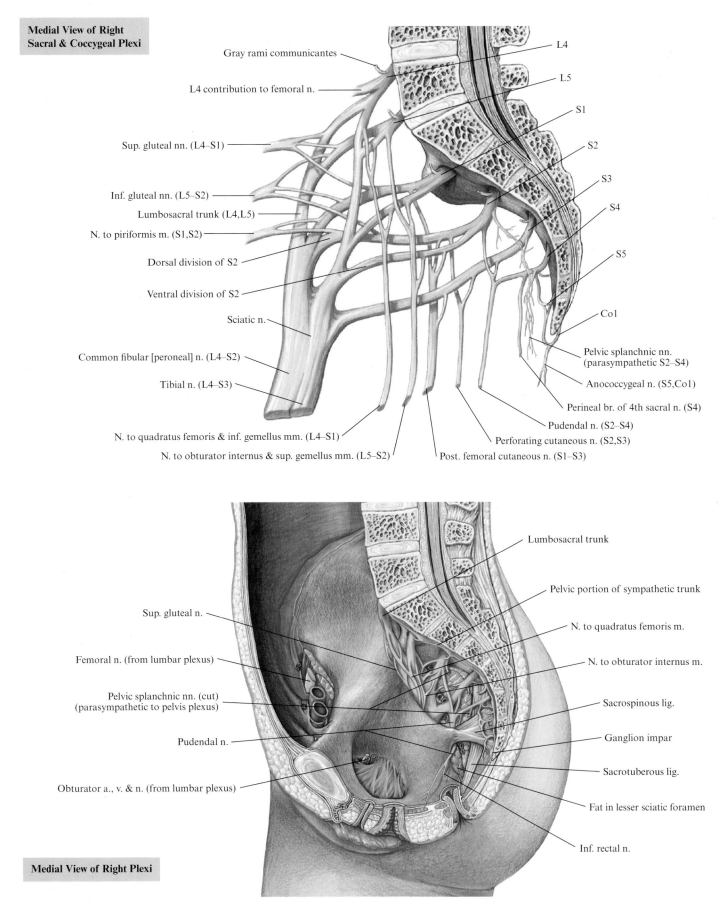

Medial View of Right Sacral & Coccygeal Plexi

Gray rami communicantes

L4 contribution to femoral n.

Sup. gluteal nn. (L4–S1)

Inf. gluteal nn. (L5–S2)

Lumbosacral trunk (L4,L5)

N. to piriformis m. (S1,S2)

Dorsal division of S2

Ventral division of S2

Sciatic n.

Common fibular [peroneal] n. (L4–S2)

Tibial n. (L4–S3)

N. to quadratus femoris & inf. gemellus mm. (L4–S1)

N. to obturator internus & sup. gemellus mm. (L5–S2)

L4

L5

S1

S2

S3

S4

S5

Co1

Pelvic splanchnic nn. (parasympathetic S2–S4)

Anococcygeal n. (S5,Co1)

Perineal br. of 4th sacral n. (S4)

Pudendal n. (S2–S4)

Perforating cutaneous n. (S2,S3)

Post. femoral cutaneous n. (S1–S3)

Sup. gluteal n.

Femoral n. (from lumbar plexus)

Pelvic splanchnic nn. (cut) (parasympathetic to pelvis plexus)

Pudendal n.

Obturator a., v. & n. (from lumbar plexus)

Lumbosacral trunk

Pelvic portion of sympathetic trunk

N. to quadratus femoris m.

N. to obturator internus m.

Sacrospinous lig.

Ganglion impar

Sacrotuberous lig.

Fat in lesser sciatic foramen

Inf. rectal n.

Medial View of Right Plexi

CHAPTER 5 │ **LOWER LIMB**   243

PLATE **5.29** SUPERFICIAL LYMPHATICS

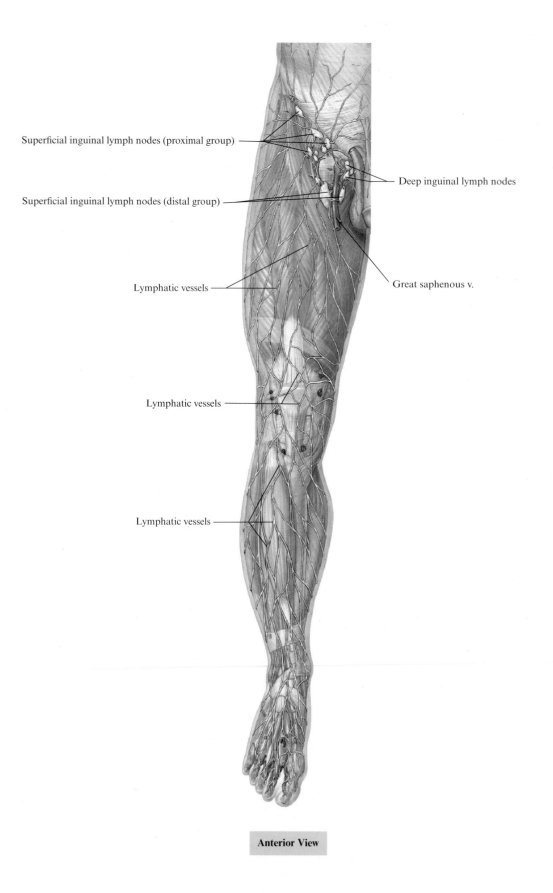

Superficial inguinal lymph nodes (proximal group)

Deep inguinal lymph nodes

Superficial inguinal lymph nodes (distal group)

Lymphatic vessels

Great saphenous v.

Lymphatic vessels

Lymphatic vessels

Anterior View

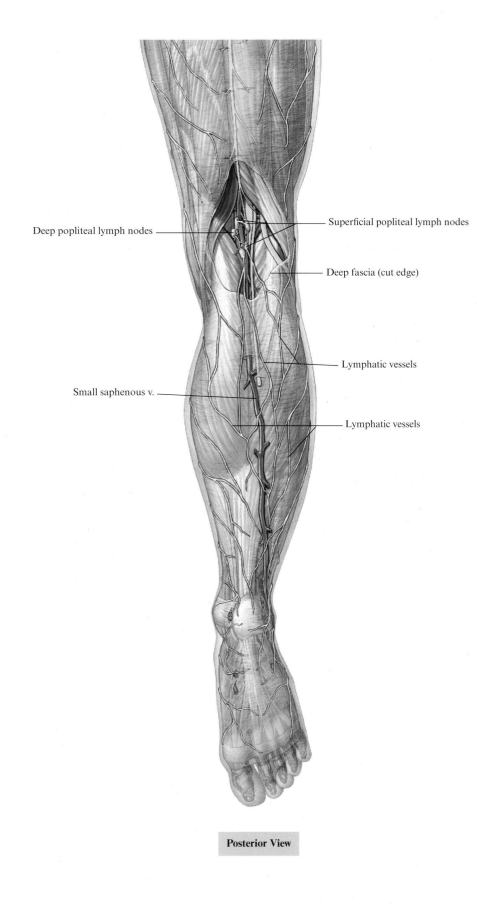

Deep popliteal lymph nodes

Superficial popliteal lymph nodes

Deep fascia (cut edge)

Lymphatic vessels

Small saphenous v.

Lymphatic vessels

Posterior View

PLATE 5.31   ANTERIOR THIGH

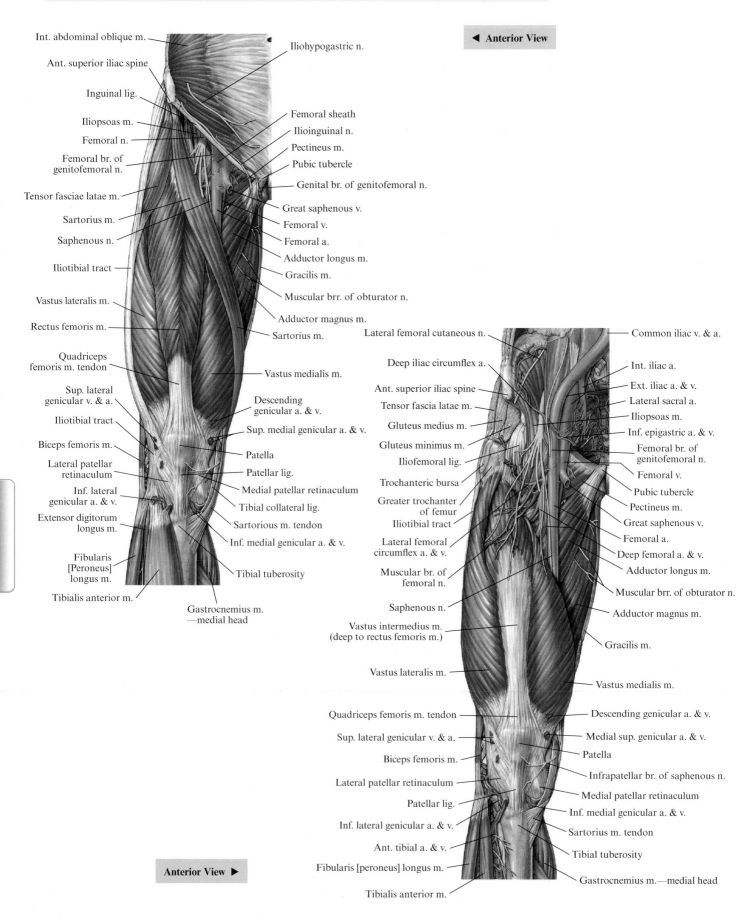

Int. abdominal oblique m.

Ant. superior iliac spine

Inguinal lig.

Iliopsoas m.

Femoral n.

Femoral br. of
genitofemoral n.

Tensor fasciae latae m.

Sartorius m.

Saphenous n.

Iliotibial tract

Vastus lateralis m.

Rectus femoris m.

Quadriceps
femoris m. tendon

Sup. lateral
genicular v. & a.

Iliotibial tract

Biceps femoris m.

Lateral patellar
retinaculum

Inf. lateral
genicular a. & v.

Extensor digitorum
longus m.

Fibularis
[Peroneus]
longus m.

Tibialis anterior m.

Iliohypogastric n.

Femoral sheath

Ilioinguinal n.

Pectineus m.

Pubic tubercle

Genital br. of genitofemoral n.

Great saphenous v.

Femoral v.

Femoral a.

Adductor longus m.

Gracilis m.

Muscular brr. of obturator n.

Adductor magnus m.

Sartorius m.

Vastus medialis m.

Descending
genicular a. & v.

Sup. medial genicular a. & v.

Patella

Patellar lig.

Medial patellar retinaculum

Tibial collateral lig.

Sartorious m. tendon

Inf. medial genicular a. & v.

Tibial tuberosity

Gastrocnemius m.
—medial head

◄ Anterior View

Lateral femoral cutaneous n.

Deep iliac circumflex a.

Ant. superior iliac spine

Tensor fascia latae m.

Gluteus medius m.

Gluteus minimus m.

Iliofemoral lig.

Trochanteric bursa

Greater trochanter
of femur

Iliotibial tract

Lateral femoral
circumflex a. & v.

Muscular br. of
femoral n.

Saphenous n.

Vastus intermedius m.
(deep to rectus femoris m.)

Vastus lateralis m.

Quadriceps femoris m. tendon

Sup. lateral genicular v. & a.

Biceps femoris m.

Lateral patellar retinaculum

Patellar lig.

Inf. lateral genicular a. & v.

Ant. tibial a. & v.

Fibularis [peroneus] longus m.

Tibialis anterior m.

Common iliac v. & a.

Int. iliac a.

Ext. iliac a. & v.

Lateral sacral a.

Iliopsoas m.

Inf. epigastric a. & v.

Femoral br. of
genitofemoral n.

Femoral v.

Pubic tubercle

Pectineus m.

Great saphenous v.

Femoral a.

Deep femoral a. & v.

Adductor longus m.

Muscular brr. of obturator n.

Adductor magnus m.

Gracilis m.

Vastus medialis m.

Descending genicular a. & v.

Medial sup. genicular a. & v.

Patella

Infrapatellar br. of saphenous n.

Medial patellar retinaculum

Inf. medial genicular a. & v.

Sartorius m. tendon

Tibial tuberosity

Gastrocnemius m.—medial head

Anterior View ►

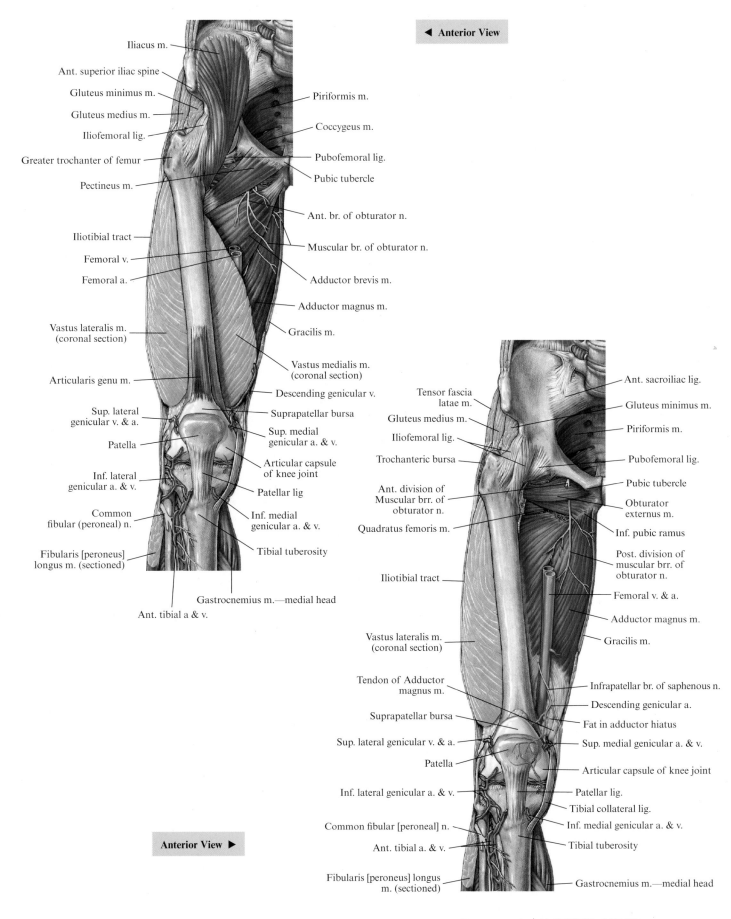

◄ Anterior View

Iliacus m.

Ant. superior iliac spine

Gluteus minimus m.

Gluteus medius m.

Iliofemoral lig.

Greater trochanter of femur

Pectineus m.

Iliotibial tract

Femoral v.

Femoral a.

Vastus lateralis m.
(coronal section)

Articularis genu m.

Sup. lateral
genicular v. & a.

Patella

Inf. lateral
genicular a. & v.

Common
fibular (peroneal) n.

Fibularis [peroneus]
longus m. (sectioned)

Piriformis m.

Coccygeus m.

Pubofemoral lig.

Pubic tubercle

Ant. br. of obturator n.

Muscular br. of obturator n.

Adductor brevis m.

Adductor magnus m.

Gracilis m.

Vastus medialis m.
(coronal section)

Descending genicular v.

Suprapatellar bursa

Sup. medial
genicular a. & v.

Articular capsule
of knee joint

Patellar lig

Inf. medial
genicular a. & v.

Gastrocnemius m.—medial head

Ant. tibial a & v.

Tibial tuberosity

Anterior View ►

Tensor fascia
latae m.

Gluteus medius m.

Iliofemoral lig.

Trochanteric bursa

Ant. division of
Muscular brr. of
obturator n.

Quadratus femoris m.

Iliotibial tract

Vastus lateralis m.
(coronal section)

Tendon of Adductor
magnus m.

Suprapatellar bursa

Sup. lateral genicular v. & a.

Patella

Inf. lateral genicular a. & v.

Common fibular [peroneal] n.

Ant. tibial a. & v.

Fibularis [peroneus] longus
m. (sectioned)

Ant. sacroiliac lig.

Gluteus minimus m.

Piriformis m.

Pubofemoral lig.

Pubic tubercle

Obturator
externus m.

Inf. pubic ramus

Post. division of
muscular brr. of
obturator n.

Femoral v. & a.

Adductor magnus m.

Gracilis m.

Infrapatellar br. of saphenous n.

Descending genicular a.

Fat in adductor hiatus

Sup. medial genicular a. & v.

Articular capsule of knee joint

Patellar lig.

Tibial collateral lig.

Inf. medial genicular a. & v.

Tibial tuberosity

Gastrocnemius m.—medial head

PLATE 5.33   FEMORAL TRIANGLE

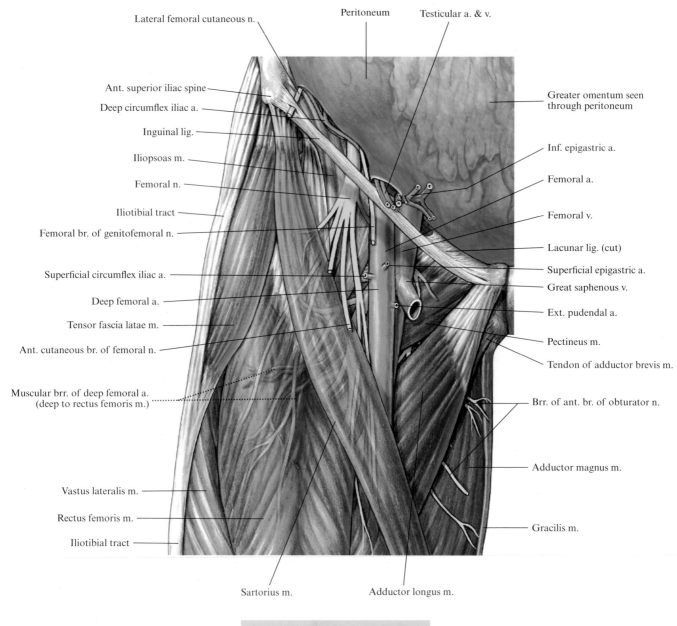

Lateral femoral cutaneous n.

Peritoneum

Testicular a. & v.

Ant. superior iliac spine

Deep circumflex iliac a.

Inguinal lig.

Iliopsoas m.

Femoral n.

Iliotibial tract

Femoral br. of genitofemoral n.

Superficial circumflex iliac a.

Deep femoral a.

Tensor fascia latae m.

Ant. cutaneous br. of femoral n.

Muscular brr. of deep femoral a.
(deep to rectus femoris m.)

Vastus lateralis m.

Rectus femoris m.

Iliotibial tract

Greater omentum seen
through peritoneum

Inf. epigastric a.

Femoral a.

Femoral v.

Lacunar lig. (cut)

Superficial epigastric a.

Great saphenous v.

Ext. pudendal a.

Pectineus m.

Tendon of adductor brevis m.

Brr. of ant. br. of obturator n.

Adductor magnus m.

Gracilis m.

Sartorius m.

Adductor longus m.

Anterior View of Right Proximal Thigh

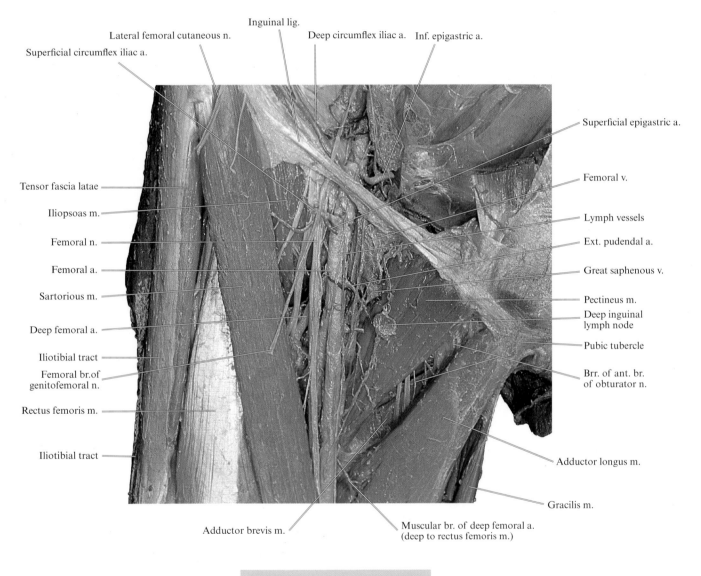

Superficial circumflex iliac a.

Lateral femoral cutaneous n.

Inguinal lig.

Deep circumflex iliac a.   Inf. epigastric a.

Superficial epigastric a.

Tensor fascia latae

Iliopsoas m.

Femoral n.

Femoral a.

Sartorius m.

Deep femoral a.

Iliotibial tract

Femoral br.of
genitofemoral n.

Rectus femoris m.

Iliotibial tract

Femoral v.

Lymph vessels

Ext. pudendal a.

Great saphenous v.

Pectineus m.

Deep inguinal
lymph node

Pubic tubercle

Brr. of ant. br.
of obturator n.

Adductor longus m.

Gracilis m.

Adductor brevis m.

Muscular br. of deep femoral a.
(deep to rectus femoris m.)

Anterior View of Right Proximal Thigh

PLATE 5.35   POSTERIOR THIGH

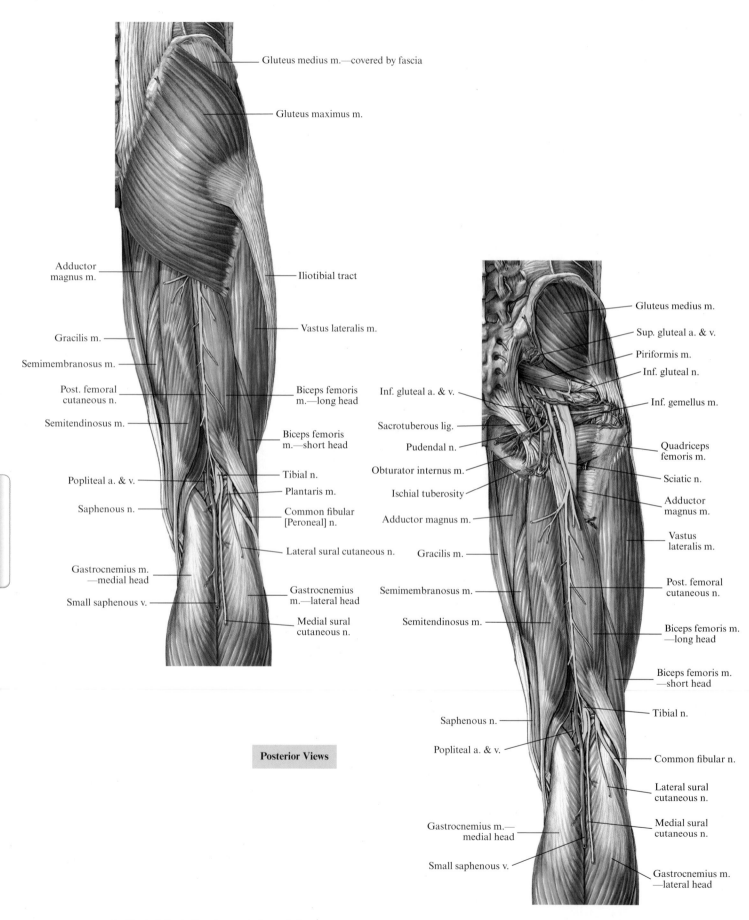

Gluteus medius m.—covered by fascia

Gluteus maximus m.

Adductor magnus m.

Iliotibial tract

Gracilis m.

Vastus lateralis m.

Semimembranosus m.

Post. femoral cutaneous n.

Biceps femoris m.—long head

Semitendinosus m.

Biceps femoris m.—short head

Popliteal a. & v.

Tibial n.

Saphenous n.

Plantaris m.

Common fibular [Peroneal] n.

Lateral sural cutaneous n.

Gastrocnemius m.—medial head

Small saphenous v.

Gastrocnemius m.—lateral head

Medial sural cutaneous n.

Posterior Views

Gluteus medius m.

Sup. gluteal a. & v.

Piriformis m.

Inf. gluteal n.

Inf. gluteal a. & v.

Inf. gemellus m.

Sacrotuberous lig.

Pudendal n.

Quadriceps femoris m.

Obturator internus m.

Sciatic n.

Ischial tuberosity

Adductor magnus m.

Adductor magnus m.

Vastus lateralis m.

Gracilis m.

Post. femoral cutaneous n.

Semimembranosus m.

Semitendinosus m.

Biceps femoris m.—long head

Biceps femoris m.—short head

Saphenous n.

Tibial n.

Popliteal a. & v.

Common fibular n.

Lateral sural cutaneous n.

Gastrocnemius m.—medial head

Medial sural cutaneous n.

Small saphenous v.

Gastrocnemius m.—lateral head

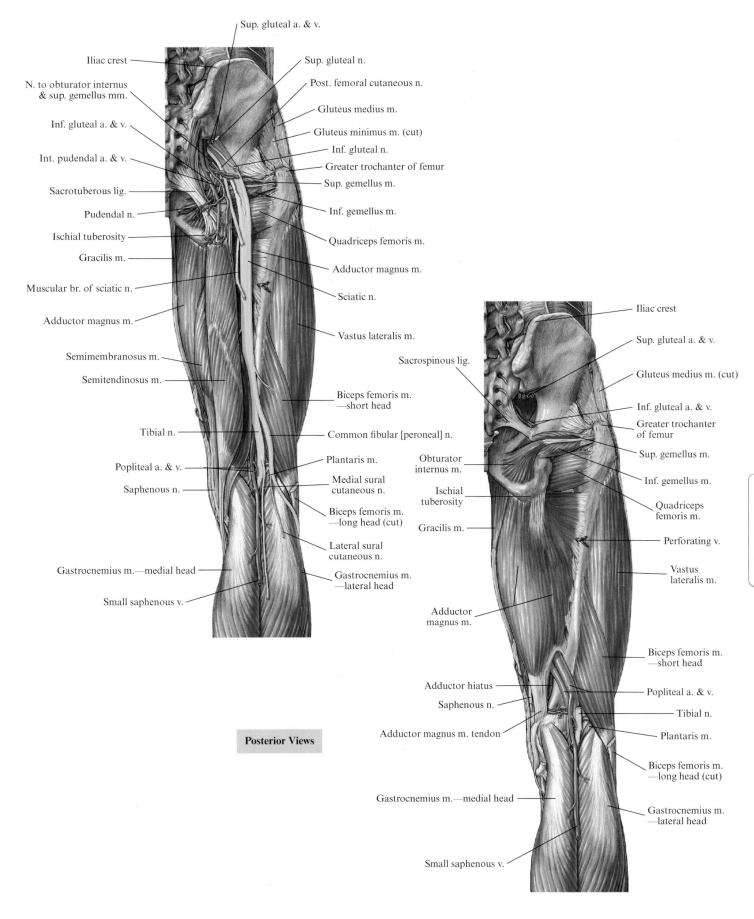

Sup. gluteal a. & v.

Iliac crest

N. to obturator internus & sup. gemellus mm.

Inf. gluteal a. & v.

Int. pudendal a. & v.

Sacrotuberous lig.

Pudendal n.

Ischial tuberosity

Gracilis m.

Muscular br. of sciatic n.

Adductor magnus m.

Semimembranosus m.

Semitendinosus m.

Tibial n.

Popliteal a. & v.

Saphenous n.

Gastrocnemius m.—medial head

Small saphenous v.

Sup. gluteal n.

Post. femoral cutaneous n.

Gluteus medius m.

Gluteus minimus m. (cut)

Inf. gluteal n.

Greater trochanter of femur

Sup. gemellus m.

Inf. gemellus m.

Quadriceps femoris m.

Adductor magnus m.

Sciatic n.

Vastus lateralis m.

Biceps femoris m. —short head

Common fibular [peroneal] n.

Plantaris m.

Medial sural cutaneous n.

Biceps femoris m. —long head (cut)

Lateral sural cutaneous n.

Gastrocnemius m. —lateral head

Sacrospinous lig.

Obturator internus m.

Ischial tuberosity

Gracilis m.

Adductor magnus m.

Adductor hiatus

Saphenous n.

Adductor magnus m. tendon

Gastrocnemius m.—medial head

Small saphenous v.

Iliac crest

Sup. gluteal a. & v.

Gluteus medius m. (cut)

Inf. gluteal a. & v.

Greater trochanter of femur

Sup. gemellus m.

Inf. gemellus m.

Quadriceps femoris m.

Perforating v.

Vastus lateralis m.

Biceps femoris m. —short head

Popliteal a. & v.

Tibial n.

Plantaris m.

Biceps femoris m. —long head (cut)

Gastrocnemius m. —lateral head

Posterior Views

PLATE 5.37   GLUTEAL REGION

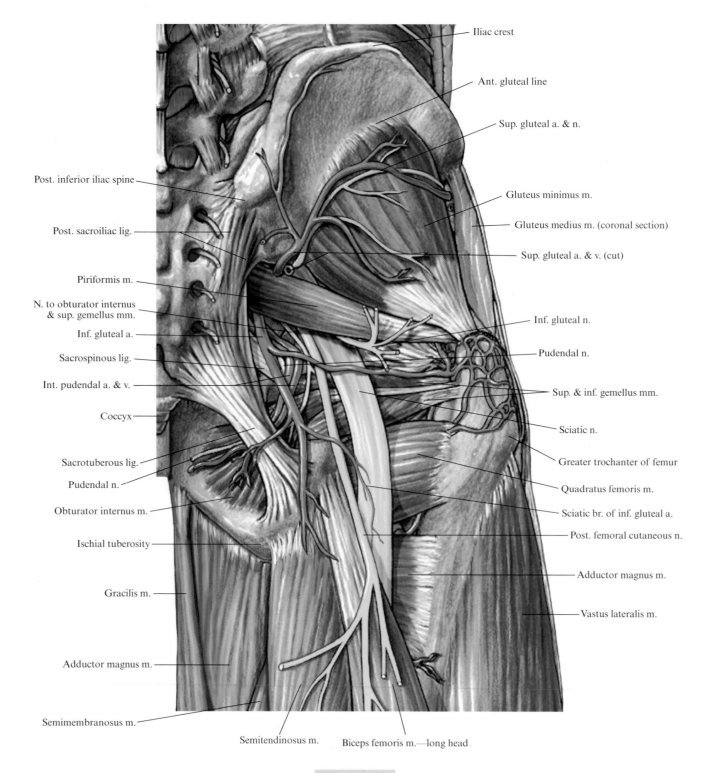

Iliac crest

Ant. gluteal line

Sup. gluteal a. & n.

Post. inferior iliac spine

Gluteus minimus m.

Post. sacroiliac lig.

Gluteus medius m. (coronal section)

Sup. gluteal a. & v. (cut)

Piriformis m.

N. to obturator internus & sup. gemellus mm.

Inf. gluteal n.

Inf. gluteal a.

Pudendal n.

Sacrospinous lig.

Int. pudendal a. & v.

Sup. & inf. gemellus mm.

Coccyx

Sciatic n.

Sacrotuberous lig.

Greater trochanter of femur

Pudendal n.

Quadratus femoris m.

Obturator internus m.

Sciatic br. of inf. gluteal a.

Ischial tuberosity

Post. femoral cutaneous n.

Adductor magnus m.

Gracilis m.

Vastus lateralis m.

Adductor magnus m.

Semimembranosus m.

Semitendinosus m.   Biceps femoris m.—long head

Posterior View

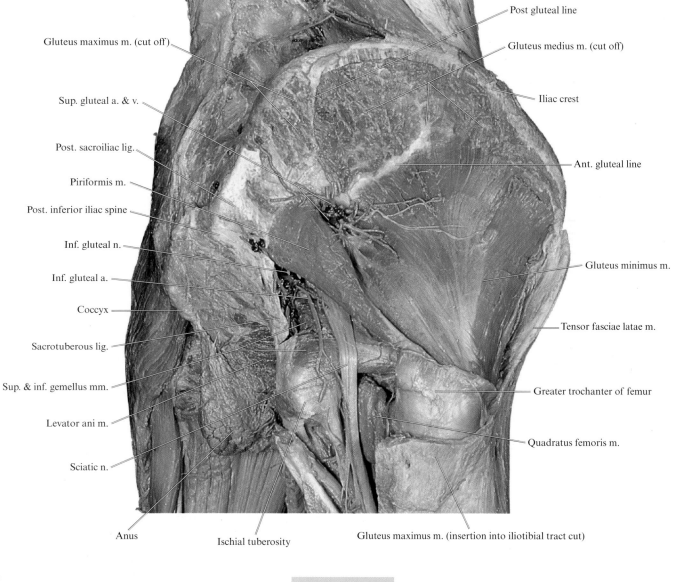

Post gluteal line

Gluteus maximus m. (cut off)

Gluteus medius m. (cut off)

Sup. gluteal a. & v.

Iliac crest

Post. sacroiliac lig.

Piriformis m.

Ant. gluteal line

Post. inferior iliac spine

Inf. gluteal n.

Inf. gluteal a.

Gluteus minimus m.

Coccyx

Sacrotuberous lig.

Tensor fasciae latae m.

Sup. & inf. gemellus mm.

Levator ani m.

Greater trochanter of femur

Sciatic n.

Quadratus femoris m.

Anus

Ischial tuberosity

Gluteus maximus m. (insertion into iliotibial tract cut)

Posterolateral View

PLATE 5.39   MEDIAL & LATERAL THIGH

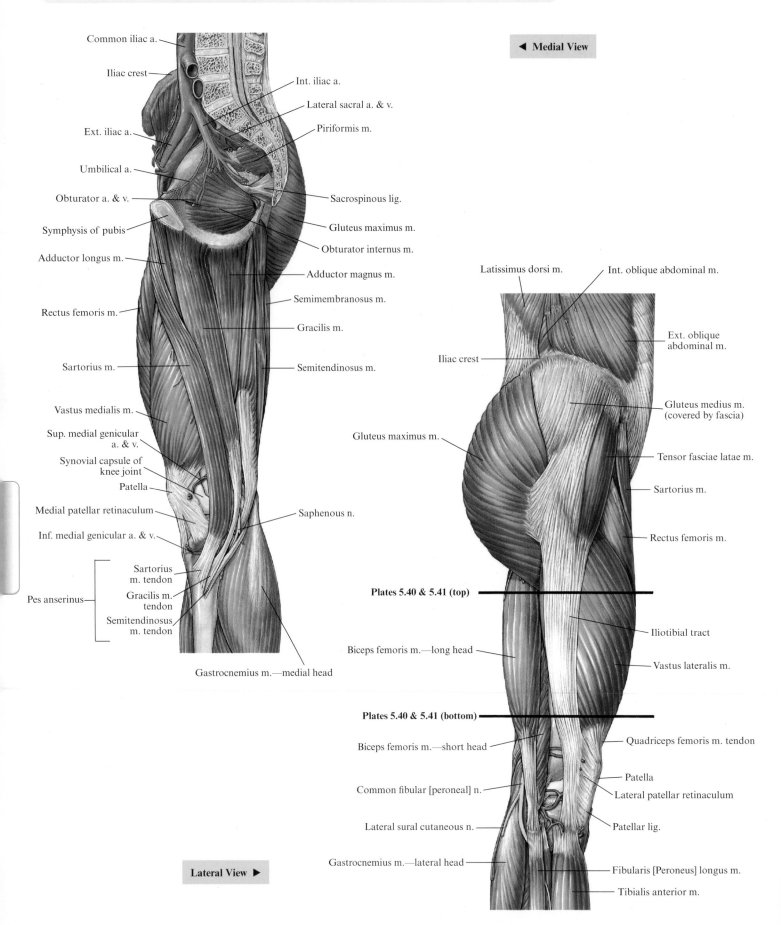

◀ **Medial View**

Common iliac a.

Iliac crest

Int. iliac a.

Lateral sacral a. & v.

Ext. iliac a.

Piriformis m.

Umbilical a.

Obturator a. & v.

Sacrospinous lig.

Symphysis of pubis

Gluteus maximus m.

Obturator internus m.

Adductor longus m.

Adductor magnus m.

Semimembranosus m.

Rectus femoris m.

Gracilis m.

Sartorius m.

Semitendinosus m.

Vastus medialis m.

Sup. medial genicular a. & v.

Synovial capsule of knee joint

Patella

Medial patellar retinaculum

Saphenous n.

Inf. medial genicular a. & v.

Sartorius m. tendon

Gracilis m. tendon

Pes anserinus

Semitendinosus m. tendon

Gastrocnemius m.—medial head

Latissimus dorsi m.

Int. oblique abdominal m.

Iliac crest

Ext. oblique abdominal m.

Gluteus medius m. (covered by fascia)

Gluteus maximus m.

Tensor fasciae latae m.

Sartorius m.

Rectus femoris m.

Plates 5.40 & 5.41 (top)

Iliotibial tract

Biceps femoris m.—long head

Vastus lateralis m.

Plates 5.40 & 5.41 (bottom)

Biceps femoris m.—short head

Quadriceps femoris m. tendon

Common fibular [peroneal] n.

Patella

Lateral patellar retinaculum

Lateral sural cutaneous n.

Patellar lig.

Gastrocnemius m.—lateral head

Fibularis [Peroneus] longus m.

Tibialis anterior m.

Lateral View ▶

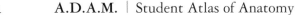

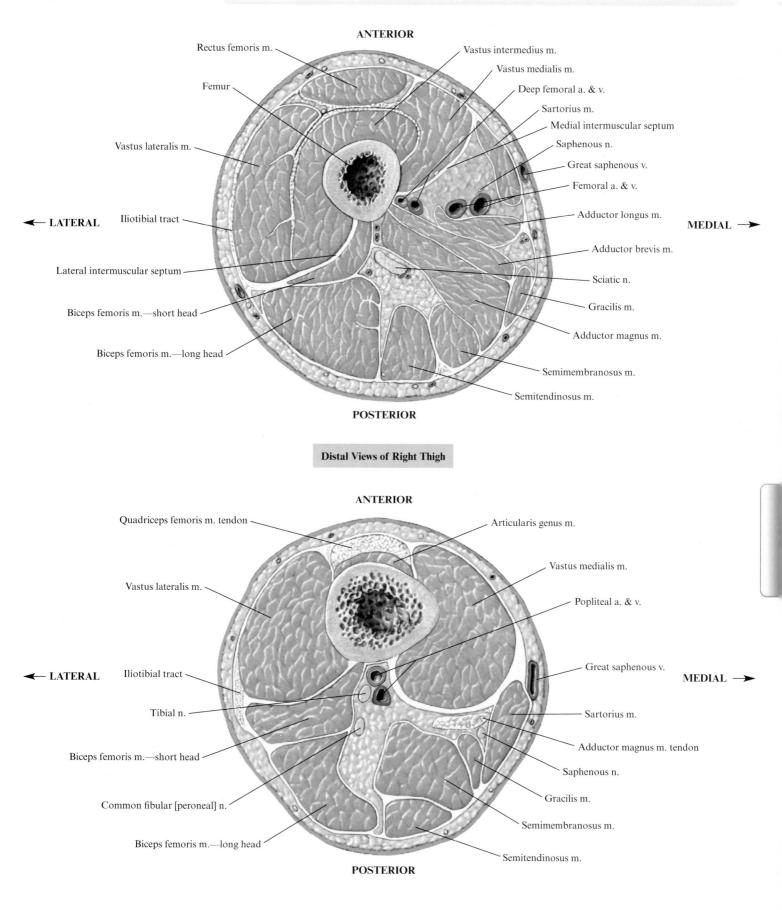

ANTERIOR

Rectus femoris m.

Femur

Vastus lateralis m.

Vastus intermedius m.

Vastus medialis m.

Deep femoral a. & v.

Sartorius m.

Medial intermuscular septum

Saphenous n.

Great saphenous v.

Femoral a. & v.

Adductor longus m.

← LATERAL   Iliotibial tract

MEDIAL →

Lateral intermuscular septum

Adductor brevis m.

Sciatic n.

Biceps femoris m.—short head

Gracilis m.

Biceps femoris m.—long head

Adductor magnus m.

Semimembranosus m.

Semitendinosus m.

POSTERIOR

Distal Views of Right Thigh

ANTERIOR

Quadriceps femoris m. tendon

Articularis genus m.

Vastus lateralis m.

Vastus medialis m.

Popliteal a. & v.

← LATERAL   Iliotibial tract

MEDIAL →

Great saphenous v.

Tibial n.

Sartorius m.

Adductor magnus m. tendon

Biceps femoris m.—short head

Saphenous n.

Common fibular [peroneal] n.

Gracilis m.

Biceps femoris m.—long head

Semimembranosus m.

Semitendinosus m.

POSTERIOR

PLATE 5.41   CROSS SECTIONS OF THIGH

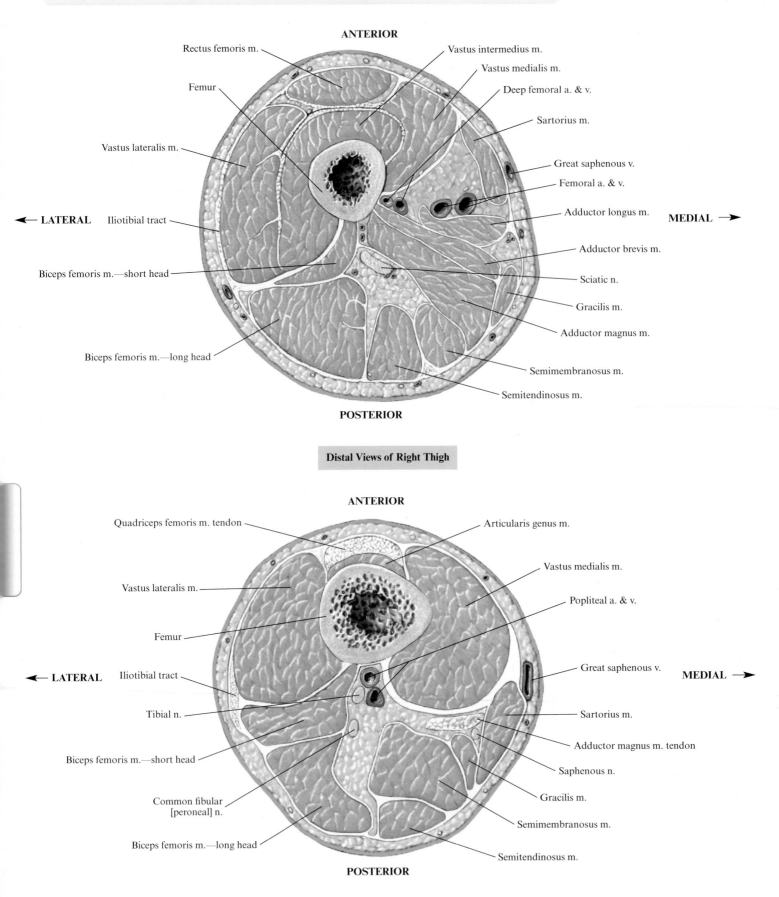

ANTERIOR

Rectus femoris m.

Vastus intermedius m.

Vastus medialis m.

Deep femoral a. & v.

Femur

Sartorius m.

Vastus lateralis m.

Great saphenous v.

Femoral a. & v.

LATERAL   Iliotibial tract

Adductor longus m.   MEDIAL

Adductor brevis m.

Biceps femoris m.—short head

Sciatic n.

Gracilis m.

Adductor magnus m.

Biceps femoris m.—long head

Semimembranosus m.

Semitendinosus m.

POSTERIOR

Distal Views of Right Thigh

ANTERIOR

Quadriceps femoris m. tendon

Articularis genus m.

Vastus medialis m.

Vastus lateralis m.

Popliteal a. & v.

Femur

LATERAL   Iliotibial tract

Great saphenous v.   MEDIAL

Tibial n.

Sartorius m.

Adductor magnus m. tendon

Biceps femoris m.—short head

Saphenous n.

Common fibular
[peroneal] n.

Gracilis m.

Semimembranosus m.

Biceps femoris m.—long head

Semitendinosus m.

POSTERIOR

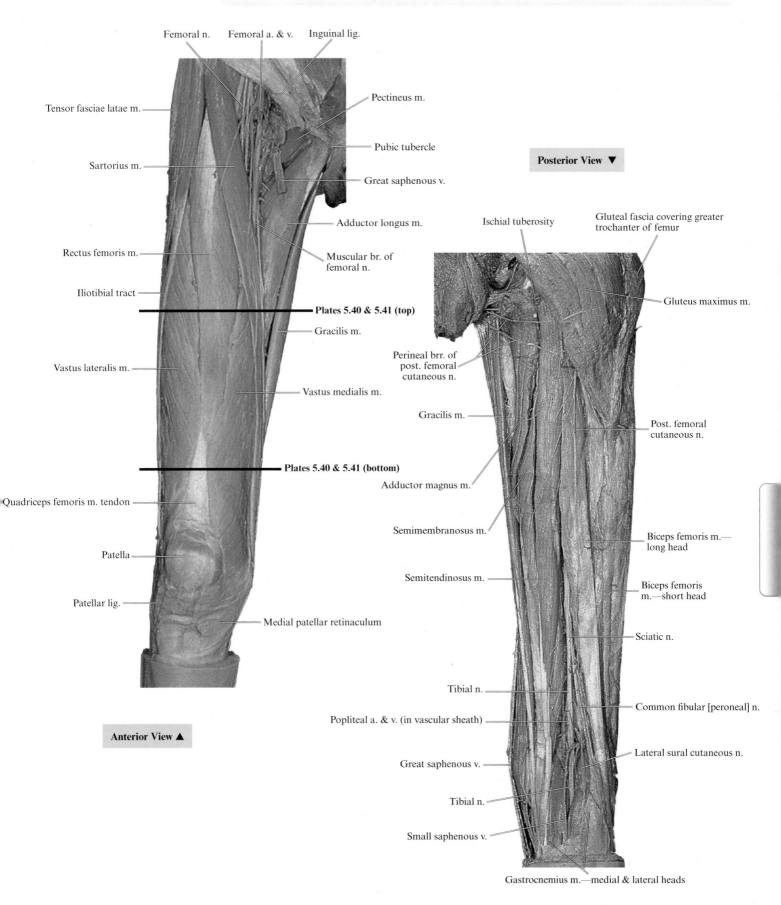

Femoral n.　Femoral a. & v.　Inguinal lig.

Tensor fasciae latae m.

Sartorius m.

Rectus femoris m.

Iliotibial tract

Vastus lateralis m.

Quadriceps femoris m. tendon

Patella

Patellar lig.

Pectineus m.

Pubic tubercle

Great saphenous v.

Adductor longus m.

Muscular br. of femoral n.

Plates 5.40 & 5.41 (top)

Gracilis m.

Vastus medialis m.

Plates 5.40 & 5.41 (bottom)

Medial patellar retinaculum

Anterior View ▲

Posterior View ▼

Ischial tuberosity

Gluteal fascia covering greater trochanter of femur

Gluteus maximus m.

Perineal brr. of post. femoral cutaneous n.

Gracilis m.

Post. femoral cutaneous n.

Adductor magnus m.

Semimembranosus m.

Biceps femoris m.— long head

Semitendinosus m.

Biceps femoris m.—short head

Sciatic n.

Tibial n.

Common fibular [peroneal] n.

Popliteal a. & v. (in vascular sheath)

Lateral sural cutaneous n.

Great saphenous v.

Tibial n.

Small saphenous v.

Gastrocnemius m.—medial & lateral heads

PLATE 5.43 HIP JOINT

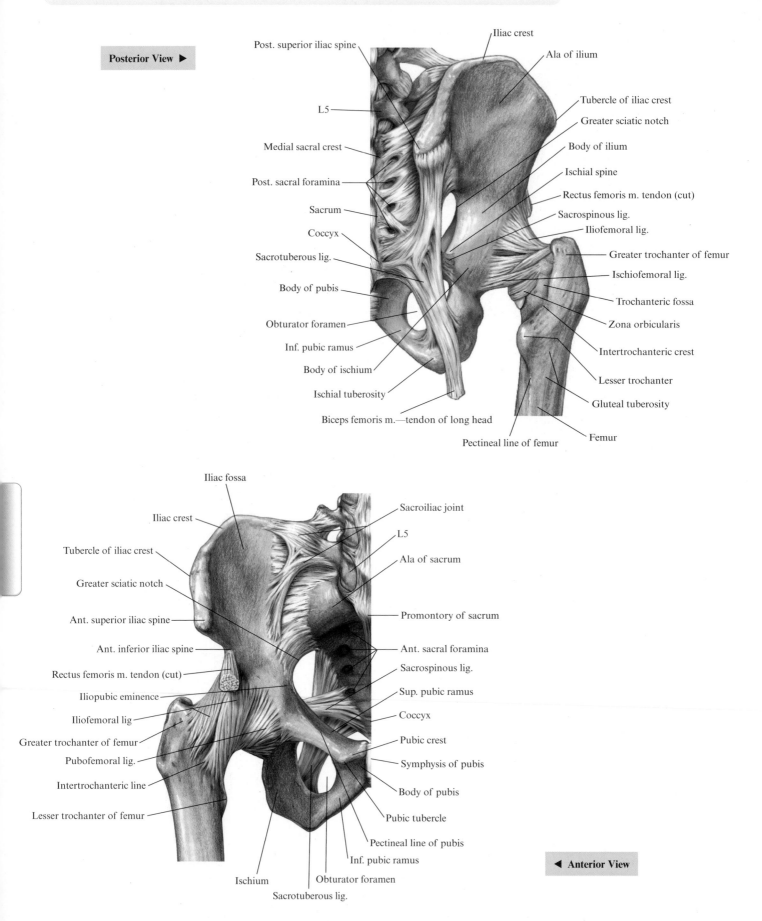

Posterior View ▶

Post. superior iliac spine

Iliac crest

Ala of ilium

L5

Tubercle of iliac crest

Greater sciatic notch

Medial sacral crest

Body of ilium

Post. sacral foramina

Ischial spine

Sacrum

Rectus femoris m. tendon (cut)

Coccyx

Sacrospinous lig.

Sacrotuberous lig.

Iliofemoral lig.

Body of pubis

Greater trochanter of femur

Obturator foramen

Ischiofemoral lig.

Inf. pubic ramus

Trochanteric fossa

Body of ischium

Zona orbicularis

Ischial tuberosity

Intertrochanteric crest

Biceps femoris m.—tendon of long head

Lesser trochanter

Gluteal tuberosity

Pectineal line of femur

Femur

Iliac fossa

Iliac crest

Sacroiliac joint

L5

Tubercle of iliac crest

Ala of sacrum

Greater sciatic notch

Ant. superior iliac spine

Promontory of sacrum

Ant. inferior iliac spine

Ant. sacral foramina

Rectus femoris m. tendon (cut)

Sacrospinous lig.

Iliopubic eminence

Sup. pubic ramus

Iliofemoral lig

Coccyx

Greater trochanter of femur

Pubic crest

Pubofemoral lig.

Symphysis of pubis

Intertrochanteric line

Body of pubis

Lesser trochanter of femur

Pubic tubercle

Pectineal line of pubis

Inf. pubic ramus

Ischium

Obturator foramen

Sacrotuberous lig.

◀ Anterior View

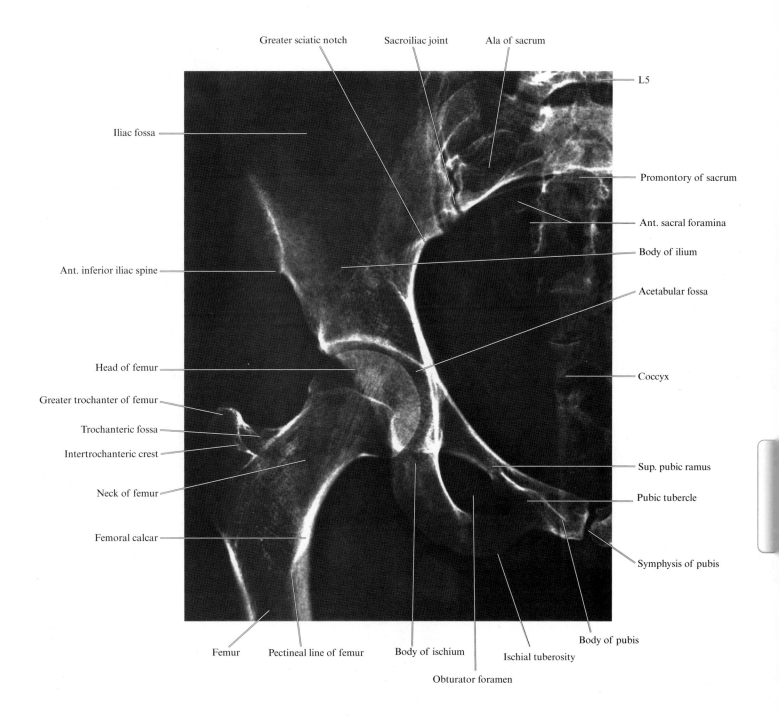

Greater sciatic notch

Sacroiliac joint

Ala of sacrum

L5

Iliac fossa

Promontory of sacrum

Ant. sacral foramina

Body of ilium

Ant. inferior iliac spine

Acetabular fossa

Head of femur

Greater trochanter of femur

Trochanteric fossa

Intertrochanteric crest

Coccyx

Neck of femur

Sup. pubic ramus

Pubic tubercle

Femoral calcar

Symphysis of pubis

Femur

Pectineal line of femur

Body of ischium

Body of pubis

Ischial tuberosity

Obturator foramen

PLATE 5.45   ANTERIOR LEG

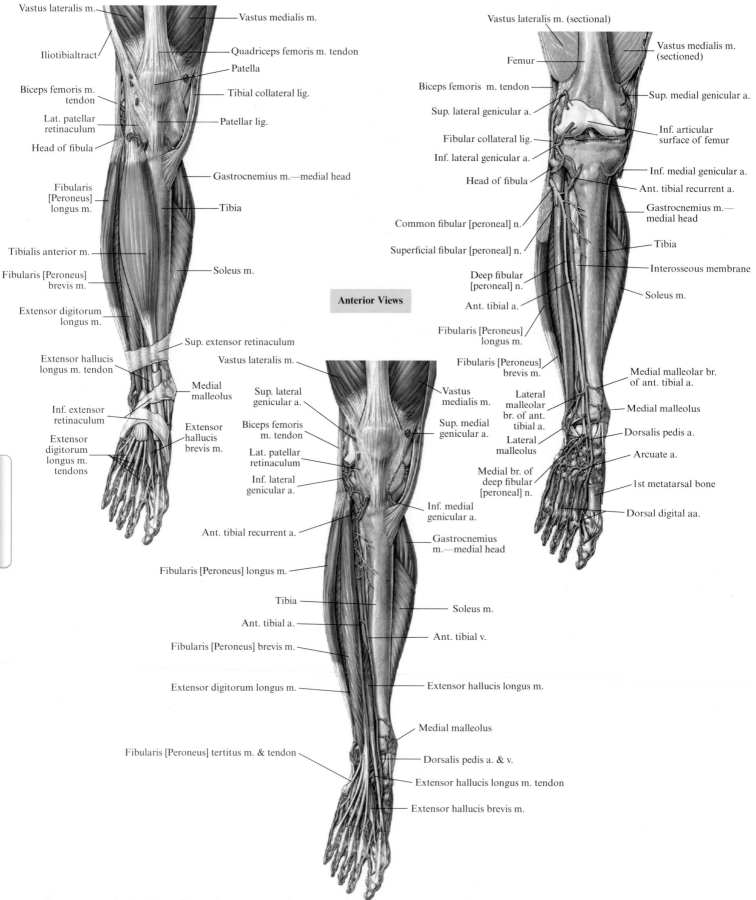

Vastus lateralis m.

Iliotibialtract

Biceps femoris m. tendon

Lat. patellar retinaculum

Head of fibula

Fibularis [Peroneus] longus m.

Tibialis anterior m.

Fibularis [Peroneus] brevis m.

Extensor digitorum longus m.

Extensor hallucis longus m. tendon

Inf. extensor retinaculum

Extensor digitorum longus m. tendons

Vastus medialis m.

Quadriceps femoris m. tendon

Patella

Tibial collateral lig.

Patellar lig.

Gastrocnemius m.—medial head

Tibia

Soleus m.

Sup. extensor retinaculum

Vastus lateralis m.

Medial malleolus

Extensor hallucis brevis m.

Anterior Views

Sup. lateral genicular a.

Biceps femoris m. tendon

Lat. patellar retinaculum

Inf. lateral genicular a.

Ant. tibial recurrent a.

Fibularis [Peroneus] longus m.

Tibia

Ant. tibial a.

Fibularis [Peroneus] brevis m.

Extensor digitorum longus m.

Fibularis [Peroneus] tertitus m. & tendon

Vastus medialis m.

Sup. medial genicular a.

Inf. medial genicular a.

Gastrocnemius m.—medial head

Soleus m.

Ant. tibial v.

Extensor hallucis longus m.

Medial malleolus

Dorsalis pedis a. & v.

Extensor hallucis longus m. tendon

Extensor hallucis brevis m.

Vastus lateralis m. (sectional)

Femur

Biceps femoris m. tendon

Sup. lateral genicular a.

Fibular collateral lig.

Inf. lateral genicular a.

Head of fibula

Common fibular [peroneal] n.

Superficial fibular [peroneal] n.

Deep fibular [peroneal] n.

Ant. tibial a.

Fibularis [Peroneus] longus m.

Fibularis [Peroneus] brevis m.

Lateral malleolar br. of ant. tibial a.

Lateral malleolus

Medial br. of deep fibular [peroneal] n.

Vastus medialis m. (sectioned)

Sup. medial genicular a.

Inf. articular surface of femur

Inf. medial genicular a.

Ant. tibial recurrent a.

Gastrocnemius m.—medial head

Tibia

Interosseous membrane

Soleus m.

Medial malleolar br. of ant. tibial a.

Medial malleolus

Dorsalis pedis a.

Arcuate a.

1st metatarsal bone

Dorsal digital aa.

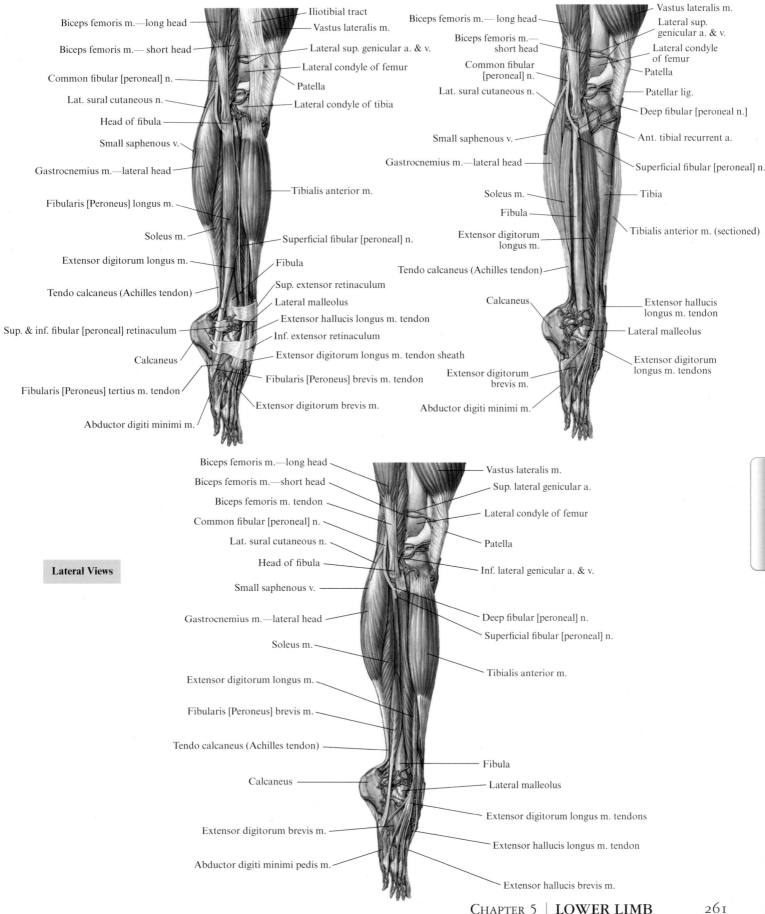

Biceps femoris m.—long head
Biceps femoris m.— short head
Common fibular [peroneal] n.
Lat. sural cutaneous n.
Head of fibula
Small saphenous v.
Gastrocnemius m.—lateral head
Fibularis [Peroneus] longus m.
Soleus m.
Extensor digitorum longus m.
Tendo calcaneus (Achilles tendon)
Sup. & inf. fibular [peroneal] retinaculum
Calcaneus
Fibularis [Peroneus] tertius m. tendon
Abductor digiti minimi m.

Iliotibial tract
Vastus lateralis m.
Lateral sup. genicular a. & v.
Lateral condyle of femur
Patella
Lateral condyle of tibia
Tibialis anterior m.
Superficial fibular [peroneal] n.
Fibula
Sup. extensor retinaculum
Lateral malleolus
Extensor hallucis longus m. tendon
Inf. extensor retinaculum
Extensor digitorum longus m. tendon sheath
Fibularis [Peroneus] brevis m. tendon
Extensor digitorum brevis m.

Biceps femoris m.— long head
Biceps femoris m.— short head
Common fibular [peroneal] n.
Lat. sural cutaneous n.
Small saphenous v.
Gastrocnemius m.—lateral head
Soleus m.
Fibula
Extensor digitorum longus m.
Tendo calcaneus (Achilles tendon)
Calcaneus
Extensor digitorum brevis m.
Abductor digiti minimi m.

Vastus lateralis m.
Lateral sup. genicular a. & v.
Lateral condyle of femur
Patella
Patellar lig.
Deep fibular [peroneal n.]
Ant. tibial recurrent a.
Superficial fibular [peroneal] n.
Tibia
Tibialis anterior m. (sectioned)
Extensor hallucis longus m. tendon
Lateral malleolus
Extensor digitorum longus m. tendons

Lateral Views

Biceps femoris m.—long head
Biceps femoris m.—short head
Biceps femoris m. tendon
Common fibular [peroneal] n.
Lat. sural cutaneous n.
Head of fibula
Small saphenous v.
Gastrocnemius m.—lateral head
Soleus m.
Extensor digitorum longus m.
Fibularis [Peroneus] brevis m.
Tendo calcaneus (Achilles tendon)
Calcaneus
Extensor digitorum brevis m.
Abductor digiti minimi pedis m.

Vastus lateralis m.
Sup. lateral genicular a.
Lateral condyle of femur
Patella
Inf. lateral genicular a. & v.
Deep fibular [peroneal] n.
Superficial fibular [peroneal] n.
Tibialis anterior m.
Fibula
Lateral malleolus
Extensor digitorum longus m. tendons
Extensor hallucis longus m. tendon
Extensor hallucis brevis m.

PLATE 5.47   POSTERIOR LEG & POPLITEAL FOSSA

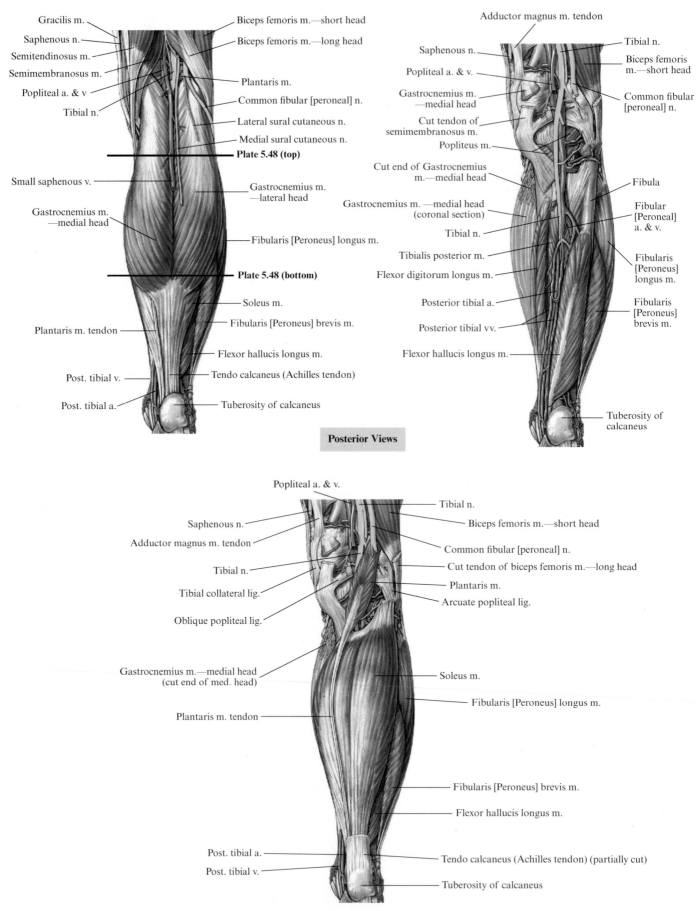

Gracilis m.
Saphenous n.
Semitendinosus m.
Semimembranosus m.
Popliteal a. & v
Tibial n.

Biceps femoris m.—short head
Biceps femoris m.—long head
Plantaris m.
Common fibular [peroneal] n.
Lateral sural cutaneous n.
Medial sural cutaneous n.
Plate 5.48 (top)

Small saphenous v.
Gastrocnemius m. —lateral head

Gastrocnemius m. —medial head

Plate 5.48 (bottom)

Fibularis [Peroneus] longus m.

Soleus m.
Fibularis [Peroneus] brevis m.
Plantaris m. tendon
Flexor hallucis longus m.
Post. tibial v.
Tendo calcaneus (Achilles tendon)
Post. tibial a.
Tuberosity of calcaneus

Adductor magnus m. tendon
Tibial n.
Saphenous n.
Biceps femoris m.—short head
Popliteal a. & v.
Gastrocnemius m. —medial head
Common fibular [peroneal] n.
Cut tendon of semimembranosus m.
Popliteus m.
Cut end of Gastrocnemius m.—medial head
Fibula
Gastrocnemius m.—medial head (coronal section)
Fibular [Peroneal] a. & v.
Tibial n.
Tibialis posterior m.
Fibularis [Peroneus] longus m.
Flexor digitorum longus m.
Posterior tibial a.
Fibularis [Peroneus] brevis m.
Posterior tibial vv.
Flexor hallucis longus m.
Tuberosity of calcaneus

Posterior Views

Popliteal a. & v.
Tibial n.
Saphenous n.
Biceps femoris m.—short head
Adductor magnus m. tendon
Common fibular [peroneal] n.
Tibial n.
Cut tendon of biceps femoris m.—long head
Tibial collateral lig.
Plantaris m.
Oblique popliteal lig.
Arcuate popliteal lig.

Gastrocnemius m.—medial head (cut end of med. head)
Soleus m.
Plantaris m. tendon
Fibularis [Peroneus] longus m.

Fibularis [Peroneus] brevis m.
Flexor hallucis longus m.
Post. tibial a.
Tendo calcaneus (Achilles tendon) (partially cut)
Post. tibial v.
Tuberosity of calcaneus

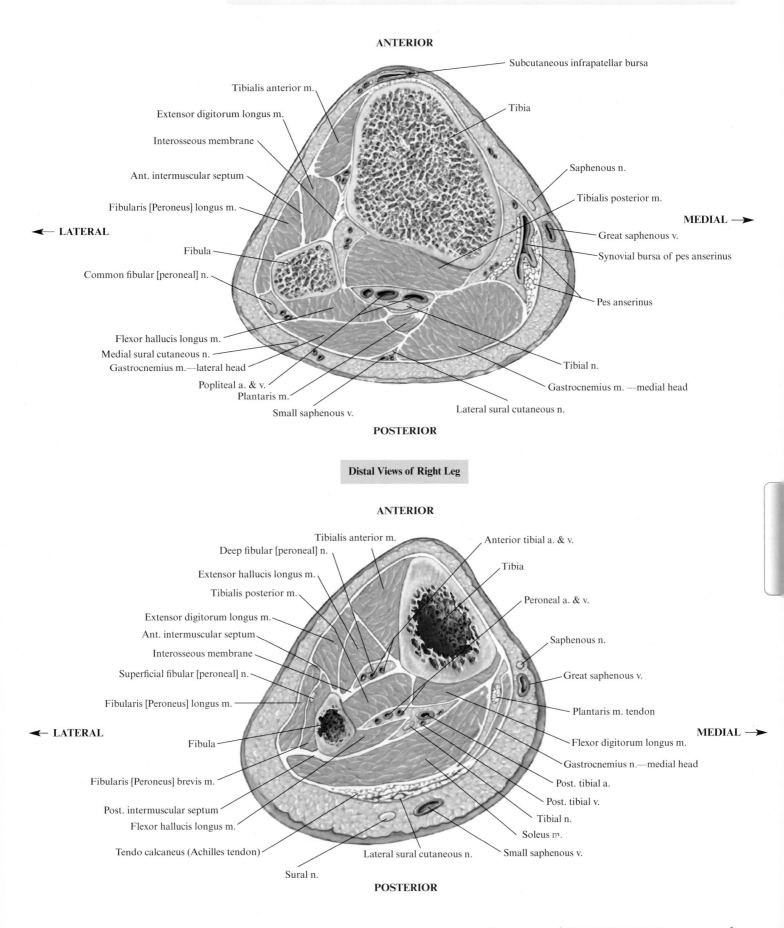

ANTERIOR

Subcutaneous infrapatellar bursa

Tibialis anterior m.

Tibia

Extensor digitorum longus m.

Interosseous membrane

Saphenous n.

Ant. intermuscular septum

Tibialis posterior m.

Fibularis [Peroneus] longus m.

MEDIAL →

← LATERAL

Great saphenous v.

Fibula

Synovial bursa of pes anserinus

Common fibular [peroneal] n.

Pes anserinus

Flexor hallucis longus m.

Medial sural cutaneous n.

Tibial n.

Gastrocnemius m.—lateral head

Gastrocnemius m. —medial head

Popliteal a. & v.

Plantaris m.

Lateral sural cutaneous n.

Small saphenous v.

POSTERIOR

Distal Views of Right Leg

ANTERIOR

Tibialis anterior m.

Anterior tibial a. & v.

Deep fibular [peroneal] n.

Tibia

Extensor hallucis longus m.

Tibialis posterior m.

Peroneal a. & v.

Extensor digitorum longus m.

Ant. intermuscular septum

Saphenous n.

Interosseous membrane

Superficial fibular [peroneal] n.

Great saphenous v.

Fibularis [Peroneus] longus m.

Plantaris m. tendon

← LATERAL

MEDIAL →

Fibula

Flexor digitorum longus m.

Fibularis [Peroneus] brevis m.

Gastrocnemius n.—medial head

Post. intermuscular septum

Post. tibial a.

Flexor hallucis longus m.

Post. tibial v.

Tibial n.

Tendo calcaneus (Achilles tendon)

Soleus m.

Lateral sural cutaneous n.

Small saphenous v.

Sural n.

POSTERIOR

PLATE 5.49   MEDIAL LEG

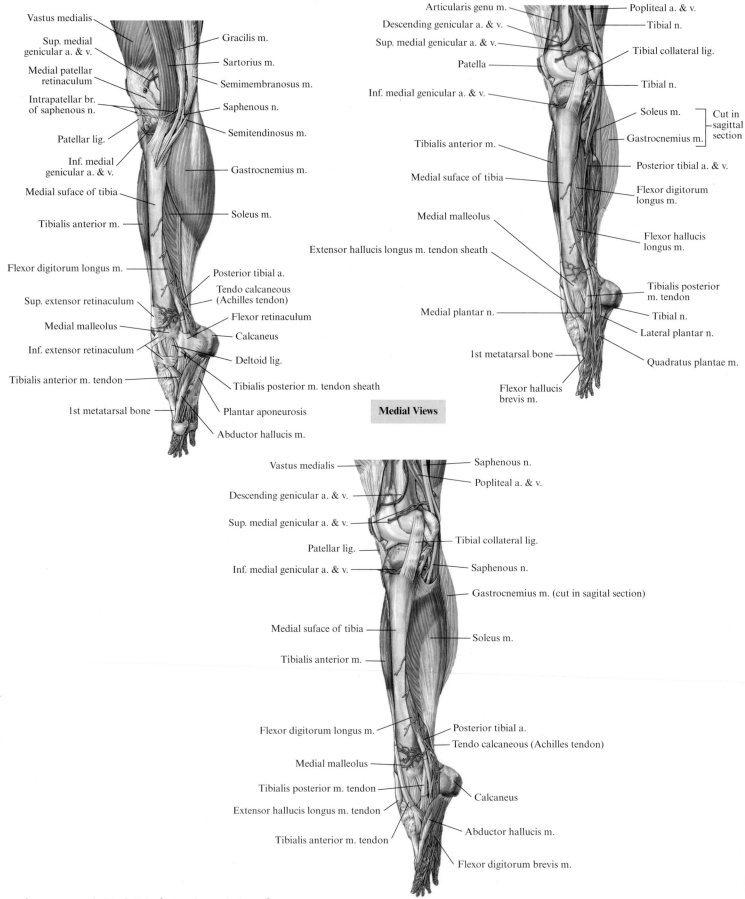

Vastus medialis

Sup. medial
genicular a. & v.

Medial patellar
retinaculum

Intrapatellar br.
of saphenous n.

Patellar lig.

Inf. medial
genicular a. & v.

Medial suface of tibia

Tibialis anterior m.

Flexor digitorum longus m.

Sup. extensor retinaculum

Medial malleolus

Inf. extensor retinaculum

Tibialis anterior m. tendon

1st metatarsal bone

Gracilis m.

Sartorius m.

Semimembranosus m.

Saphenous n.

Semitendinosus m.

Gastrocnemius m.

Soleus m.

Posterior tibial a.

Tendo calcaneous
(Achilles tendon)

Flexor retinaculum

Calcaneus

Deltoid lig.

Tibialis posterior m. tendon sheath

Plantar aponeurosis

Abductor hallucis m.

Articularis genu m.

Descending genicular a. & v.

Sup. medial genicular a. & v.

Patella

Inf. medial genicular a. & v.

Tibialis anterior m.

Medial suface of tibia

Medial malleolus

Extensor hallucis longus m. tendon sheath

Medial plantar n.

1st metatarsal bone

Flexor hallucis
brevis m.

Popliteal a. & v.

Tibial n.

Tibial collateral lig.

Tibial n.

Soleus m.   Cut in
                   sagittal
Gastrocnemius m.   section

Posterior tibial a. & v.

Flexor digitorum
longus m.

Flexor hallucis
longus m.

Tibialis posterior
m. tendon

Tibial n.

Lateral plantar n.

Quadratus plantae m.

Medial Views

Vastus medialis

Descending genicular a. & v.

Sup. medial genicular a. & v.

Patellar lig.

Inf. medial genicular a. & v.

Medial suface of tibia

Tibialis anterior m.

Flexor digitorum longus m.

Medial malleolus

Tibialis posterior m. tendon

Extensor hallucis longus m. tendon

Tibialis anterior m. tendon

Saphenous n.

Popliteal a. & v.

Tibial collateral lig.

Saphenous n.

Gastrocnemius m. (cut in sagital section)

Soleus m.

Posterior tibial a.

Tendo calcaneous (Achilles tendon)

Calcaneus

Abductor hallucis m.

Flexor digitorum brevis m.

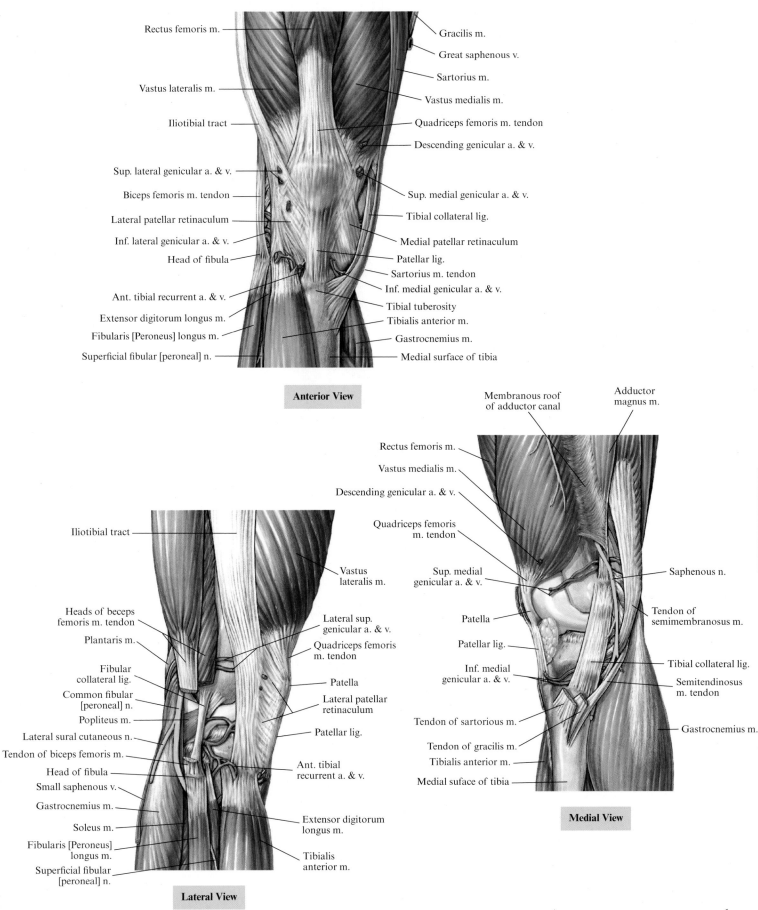

Rectus femoris m.

Vastus lateralis m.

Iliotibial tract

Sup. lateral genicular a. & v.

Biceps femoris m. tendon

Lateral patellar retinaculum

Inf. lateral genicular a. & v.

Head of fibula

Ant. tibial recurrent a. & v.

Extensor digitorum longus m.

Fibularis [Peroneus] longus m.

Superficial fibular [peroneal] n.

Gracilis m.

Great saphenous v.

Sartorius m.

Vastus medialis m.

Quadriceps femoris m. tendon

Descending genicular a. & v.

Sup. medial genicular a. & v.

Tibial collateral lig.

Medial patellar retinaculum

Patellar lig.

Sartorius m. tendon

Inf. medial genicular a. & v.

Tibial tuberosity

Tibialis anterior m.

Gastrocnemius m.

Medial surface of tibia

Anterior View

Iliotibial tract

Heads of beceps femoris m. tendon

Plantaris m.

Fibular collateral lig.

Common fibular [peroneal] n.

Popliteus m.

Lateral sural cutaneous n.

Tendon of biceps femoris m.

Head of fibula

Small saphenous v.

Gastrocnemius m.

Soleus m.

Fibularis [Peroneus] longus m.

Superficial fibular [peroneal] n.

Vastus lateralis m.

Lateral sup. genicular a. & v.

Quadriceps femoris m. tendon

Patella

Lateral patellar retinaculum

Patellar lig.

Ant. tibial recurrent a. & v.

Extensor digitorum longus m.

Tibialis anterior m.

Lateral View

Membranous roof of adductor canal

Adductor magnus m.

Rectus femoris m.

Vastus medialis m.

Descending genicular a. & v.

Quadriceps femoris m. tendon

Sup. medial genicular a. & v.

Patella

Patellar lig.

Inf. medial genicular a. & v.

Tendon of sartorious m.

Tendon of gracilis m.

Tibialis anterior m.

Medial suface of tibia

Saphenous n.

Tendon of semimembranosus m.

Tibial collateral lig.

Semitendinosus m. tendon

Gastrocnemius m.

Medial View

PLATE 5.51   POSTERIOR KNEE

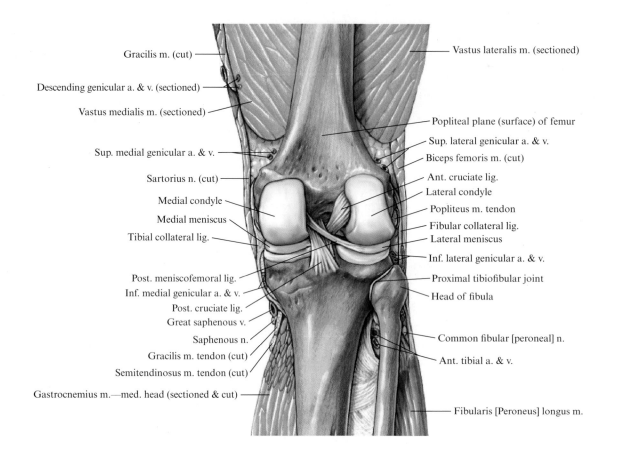

Gracilis m. (cut)

Descending genicular a. & v. (sectioned)

Vastus medialis m. (sectioned)

Sup. medial genicular a. & v.

Sartorius n. (cut)

Medial condyle

Medial meniscus

Tibial collateral lig.

Post. meniscofemoral lig.

Inf. medial genicular a. & v.

Post. cruciate lig.

Great saphenous v.

Saphenous n.

Gracilis m. tendon (cut)

Semitendinosus m. tendon (cut)

Gastrocnemius m.—med. head (sectioned & cut)

Vastus lateralis m. (sectioned)

Popliteal plane (surface) of femur

Sup. lateral genicular a. & v.

Biceps femoris m. (cut)

Ant. cruciate lig.

Lateral condyle

Popliteus m. tendon

Fibular collateral lig.

Lateral meniscus

Inf. lateral genicular a. & v.

Proximal tibiofibular joint

Head of fibula

Common fibular [peroneal] n.

Ant. tibial a. & v.

Fibularis [Peroneus] longus m.

Posterior Views

Gracilis m. (cut)

Descending genicular a. & v.

Vastus medialis m. (sectioned)

Sup. medial genicular a. & v.

Sartorius m. (cut)

Post. surface of articular
capsule of knee joint

Gastrocnemius m.—medial head (cut)

Tibial collateral lig.

Semimembranosus m. tendon

Oblique popliteal lig.

Great saphenous v.

Saphenous n.

Gracilis m. tendon (cut)

Semitendinosus m. tendon (cut)

Gastrocnemius m.—med. head (sectioned & cut)

Vastus lateralis m. (sectioned)

Popliteal plane (surface) of femur

Sup. lateral genicular a. & v.

Plantaris m. (cut)

Biceps femoris m.—short head (coronal section)

Gastrocnemius m.—lateral head (cut)

Fibular collateral lig.

Biceps femoris m.—long head tendon (cut)

Arcuate popliteal lig.

Post. lig. of head of fibula

Head of fibula

Popliteus m. (cut ends)

Common fibular [peroneal] n.

Tibialis posterior m.

Fibularis [Peroneus] longus m.

Distal View of Articular Surface of Right Femur

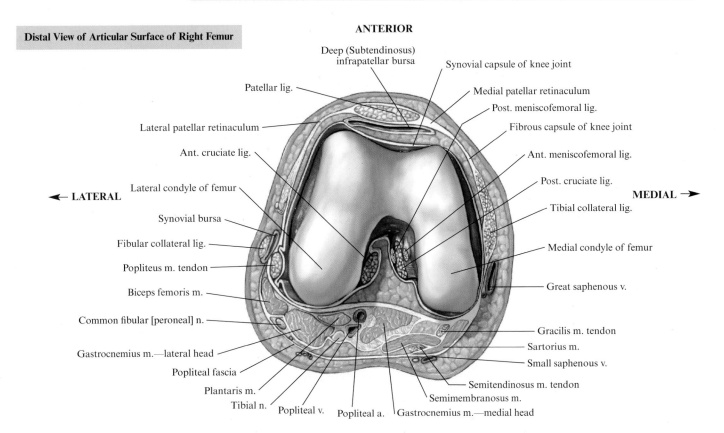

ANTERIOR

Deep (Subtendinosus) infrapatellar bursa

Synovial capsule of knee joint

Patellar lig.

Medial patellar retinaculum

Post. meniscofemoral lig.

Lateral patellar retinaculum

Fibrous capsule of knee joint

Ant. cruciate lig.

Ant. meniscofemoral lig.

Lateral condyle of femur

Post. cruciate lig.

← LATERAL

MEDIAL →

Tibial collateral lig.

Synovial bursa

Medial condyle of femur

Fibular collateral lig.

Popliteus m. tendon

Great saphenous v.

Biceps femoris m.

Common fibular [peroneal] n.

Gracilis m. tendon

Sartorius m.

Gastrocnemius m.—lateral head

Small saphenous v.

Popliteal fascia

Semitendinosus m. tendon

Plantaris m.

Semimembranosus m.

Tibial n.

Popliteal v.

Popliteal a.

Gastrocnemius m.—medial head

POSTERIOR

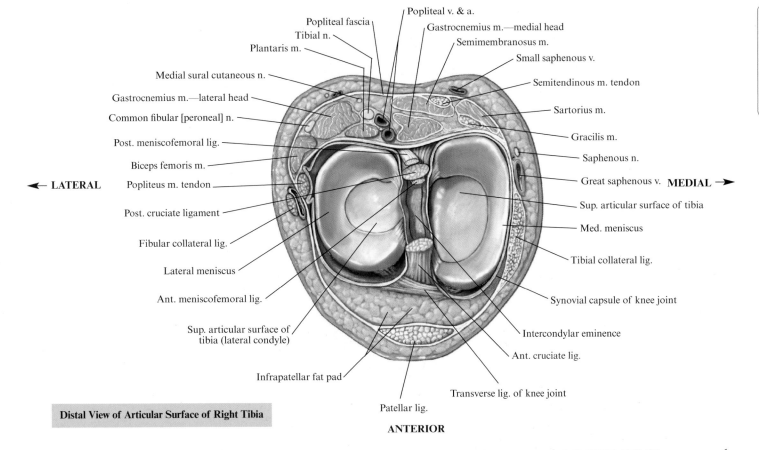

Popliteal v. & a.

Popliteal fascia

Gastrocnemius m.—medial head

Tibial n.

Semimembranosus m.

Plantaris m.

Small saphenous v.

Medial sural cutaneous n.

Semitendinous m. tendon

Gastrocnemius m.—lateral head

Sartorius m.

Common fibular [peroneal] n.

Gracilis m.

Post. meniscofemoral lig.

Saphenous n.

Biceps femoris m.

← LATERAL

Popliteus m. tendon

Great saphenous v. MEDIAL →

Post. cruciate ligament

Sup. articular surface of tibia

Fibular collateral lig.

Med. meniscus

Lateral meniscus

Tibial collateral lig.

Ant. meniscofemoral lig.

Synovial capsule of knee joint

Sup. articular surface of tibia (lateral condyle)

Intercondylar eminence

Ant. cruciate lig.

Infrapatellar fat pad

Transverse lig. of knee joint

Patellar lig.

Distal View of Articular Surface of Right Tibia

ANTERIOR

PLATE 5.53   KNEE JOINT

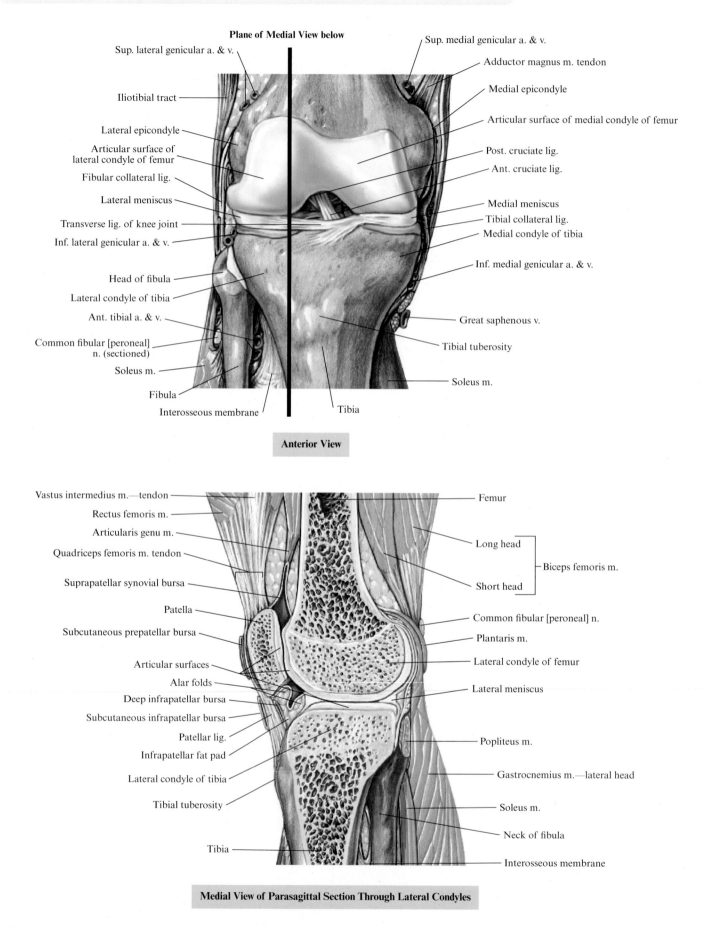

Plane of Medial View below

Anterior View — Labels:

Sup. lateral genicular a. & v.

Iliotibial tract

Lateral epicondyle

Articular surface of lateral condyle of femur

Fibular collateral lig.

Lateral meniscus

Transverse lig. of knee joint

Inf. lateral genicular a. & v.

Head of fibula

Lateral condyle of tibia

Ant. tibial a. & v.

Common fibular [peroneal] n. (sectioned)

Soleus m.

Fibula

Interosseous membrane

Sup. medial genicular a. & v.

Adductor magnus m. tendon

Medial epicondyle

Articular surface of medial condyle of femur

Post. cruciate lig.

Ant. cruciate lig.

Medial meniscus

Tibial collateral lig.

Medial condyle of tibia

Inf. medial genicular a. & v.

Great saphenous v.

Tibial tuberosity

Soleus m.

Tibia

Anterior View

Medial View of Parasagittal Section Through Lateral Condyles — Labels:

Vastus intermedius m.—tendon

Rectus femoris m.

Articularis genu m.

Quadriceps femoris m. tendon

Suprapatellar synovial bursa

Patella

Subcutaneous prepatellar bursa

Articular surfaces

Alar folds

Deep infrapatellar bursa

Subcutaneous infrapatellar bursa

Patellar lig.

Infrapatellar fat pad

Lateral condyle of tibia

Tibial tuberosity

Tibia

Femur

Long head

Biceps femoris m.

Short head

Common fibular [peroneal] n.

Plantaris m.

Lateral condyle of femur

Lateral meniscus

Popliteus m.

Gastrocnemius m.—lateral head

Soleus m.

Neck of fibula

Interosseous membrane

Medial View of Parasagittal Section Through Lateral Condyles

A.D.A.M. | Student Atlas of Anatomy

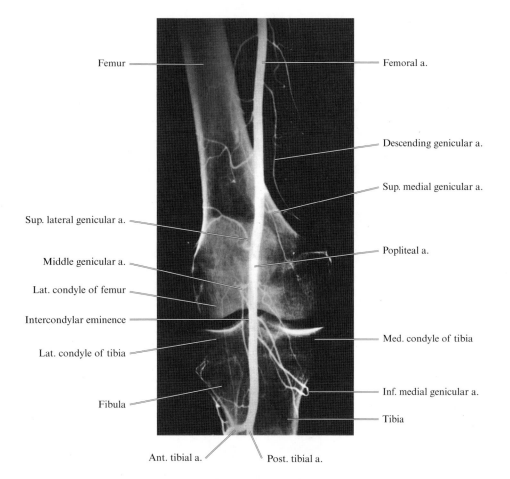

Femur

Femoral a.

Descending genicular a.

Sup. medial genicular a.

Sup. lateral genicular a.

Popliteal a.

Middle genicular a.

Lat. condyle of femur

Intercondylar eminence

Med. condyle of tibia

Lat. condyle of tibia

Inf. medial genicular a.

Fibula

Tibia

Ant. tibial a.

Post. tibial a.

Anteroposterior View of Right Knee Arteriogram

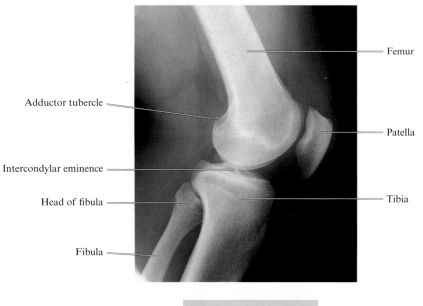

Femur

Adductor tubercle

Patella

Intercondylar eminence

Head of fibula

Tibia

Fibula

Lateral View of Right Knee

PLATE 5.55   SOLE OF FOOT

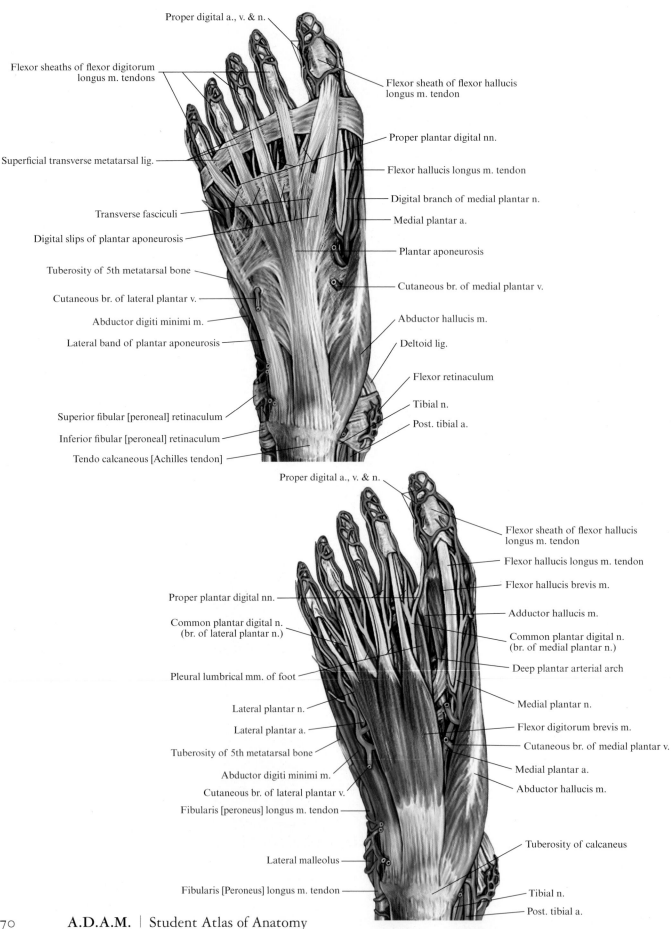

Proper digital a., v. & n.

Flexor sheaths of flexor digitorum
longus m. tendons

Flexor sheath of flexor hallucis
longus m. tendon

Proper plantar digital nn.

Superficial transverse metatarsal lig.

Flexor hallucis longus m. tendon

Digital branch of medial plantar n.

Transverse fasciculi

Medial plantar a.

Digital slips of plantar aponeurosis

Plantar aponeurosis

Tuberosity of 5th metatarsal bone

Cutaneous br. of medial plantar v.

Cutaneous br. of lateral plantar v.

Abductor digiti minimi m.

Abductor hallucis m.

Lateral band of plantar aponeurosis

Deltoid lig.

Flexor retinaculum

Tibial n.

Superior fibular [peroneal] retinaculum

Post. tibial a.

Inferior fibular [peroneal] retinaculum

Tendo calcaneous [Achilles tendon]

Proper digital a., v. & n.

Flexor sheath of flexor hallucis
longus m. tendon

Flexor hallucis longus m. tendon

Flexor hallucis brevis m.

Proper plantar digital nn.

Adductor hallucis m.

Common plantar digital n.
(br. of lateral plantar n.)

Common plantar digital n.
(br. of medial plantar n.)

Deep plantar arterial arch

Pleural lumbrical mm. of foot

Medial plantar n.

Lateral plantar n.

Flexor digitorum brevis m.

Lateral plantar a.

Cutaneous br. of medial plantar v.

Tuberosity of 5th metatarsal bone

Medial plantar a.

Abductor digiti minimi m.

Abductor hallucis m.

Cutaneous br. of lateral plantar v.

Fibularis [peroneus] longus m. tendon

Tuberosity of calcaneus

Lateral malleolus

Fibularis [Peroneus] longus m. tendon

Tibial n.

Post. tibial a.

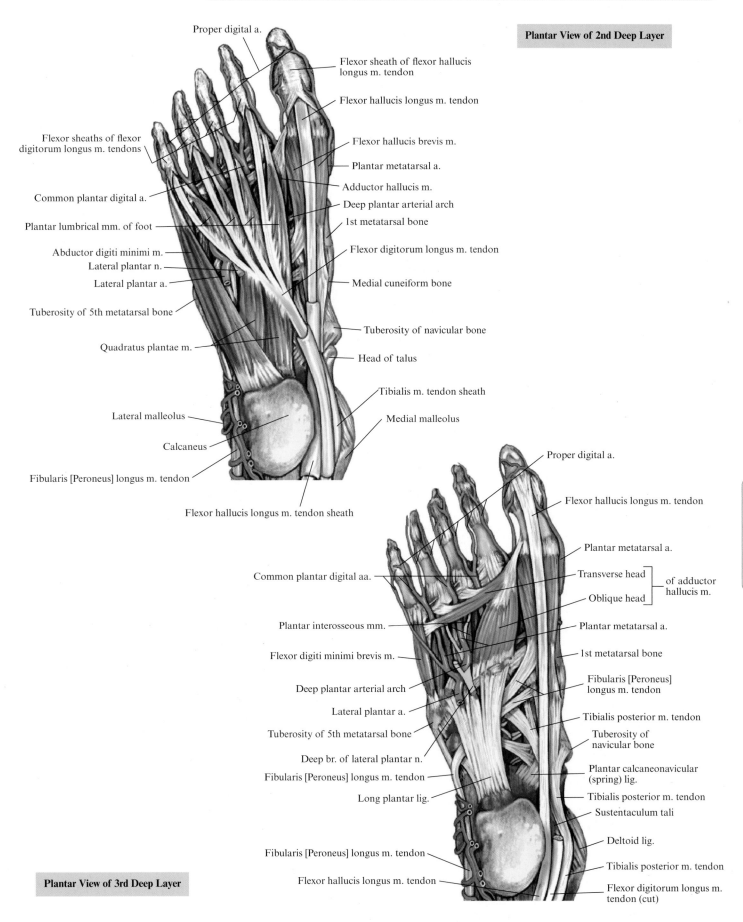

Proper digital a.

Flexor sheath of flexor hallucis longus m. tendon

Flexor hallucis longus m. tendon

Flexor sheaths of flexor digitorum longus m. tendons

Flexor hallucis brevis m.

Plantar metatarsal a.

Common plantar digital a.

Adductor hallucis m.

Plantar lumbrical mm. of foot

Deep plantar arterial arch

1st metatarsal bone

Abductor digiti minimi m.

Flexor digitorum longus m. tendon

Lateral plantar n.

Lateral plantar a.

Medial cuneiform bone

Tuberosity of 5th metatarsal bone

Quadratus plantae m.

Tuberosity of navicular bone

Head of talus

Tibialis m. tendon sheath

Lateral malleolus

Medial malleolus

Calcaneus

Fibularis [Peroneus] longus m. tendon

Flexor hallucis longus m. tendon sheath

Common plantar digital aa.

Proper digital a.

Flexor hallucis longus m. tendon

Plantar metatarsal a.

Transverse head

Plantar interosseous mm.

Oblique head

of adductor hallucis m.

Plantar metatarsal a.

Flexor digiti minimi brevis m.

1st metatarsal bone

Deep plantar arterial arch

Fibularis [Peroneus] longus m. tendon

Lateral plantar a.

Tibialis posterior m. tendon

Tuberosity of 5th metatarsal bone

Tuberosity of navicular bone

Deep br. of lateral plantar n.

Plantar calcaneonavicular (spring) lig.

Fibularis [Peroneus] longus m. tendon

Tibialis posterior m. tendon

Long plantar lig.

Sustentaculum tali

Deltoid lig.

Fibularis [Peroneus] longus m. tendon

Tibialis posterior m. tendon

Flexor hallucis longus m. tendon

Flexor digitorum longus m. tendon (cut)

PLATE 5.57   DORSUM OF FOOT

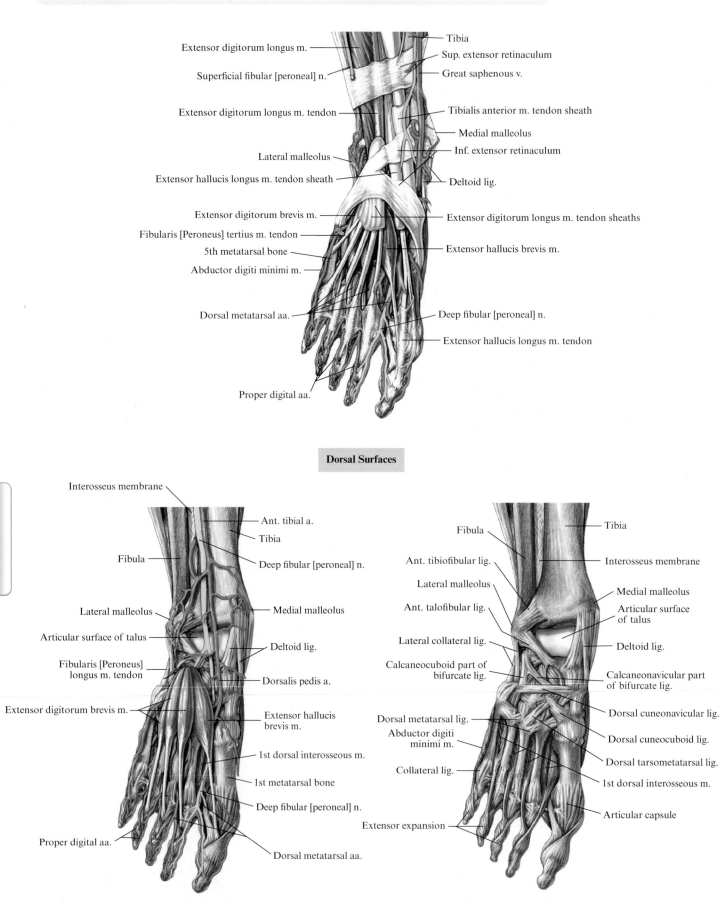

Extensor digitorum longus m.

Superficial fibular [peroneal] n.

Extensor digitorum longus m. tendon

Lateral malleolus

Extensor hallucis longus m. tendon sheath

Extensor digitorum brevis m.

Fibularis [Peroneus] tertius m. tendon

5th metatarsal bone

Abductor digiti minimi m.

Dorsal metatarsal aa.

Proper digital aa.

Tibia

Sup. extensor retinaculum

Great saphenous v.

Tibialis anterior m. tendon sheath

Medial malleolus

Inf. extensor retinaculum

Deltoid lig.

Extensor digitorum longus m. tendon sheaths

Extensor hallucis brevis m.

Deep fibular [peroneal] n.

Extensor hallucis longus m. tendon

Dorsal Surfaces

Interosseus membrane

Fibula

Lateral malleolus

Articular surface of talus

Fibularis [Peroneus] longus m. tendon

Extensor digitorum brevis m.

Proper digital aa.

Ant. tibial a.

Tibia

Deep fibular [peroneal] n.

Medial malleolus

Deltoid lig.

Dorsalis pedis a.

Extensor hallucis brevis m.

1st dorsal interosseous m.

1st metatarsal bone

Deep fibular [peroneal] n.

Dorsal metatarsal aa.

Fibula

Ant. tibiofibular lig.

Lateral malleolus

Ant. talofibular lig.

Lateral collateral lig.

Calcaneocuboid part of bifurcate lig.

Dorsal metatarsal lig.

Abductor digiti minimi m.

Collateral lig.

Extensor expansion

Tibia

Interosseus membrane

Medial malleolus

Articular surface of talus

Deltoid lig.

Calcaneonavicular part of bifurcate lig.

Dorsal cuneonavicular lig.

Dorsal cuneocuboid lig.

Dorsal tarsometatarsal lig.

1st dorsal interosseous m.

Articular capsule

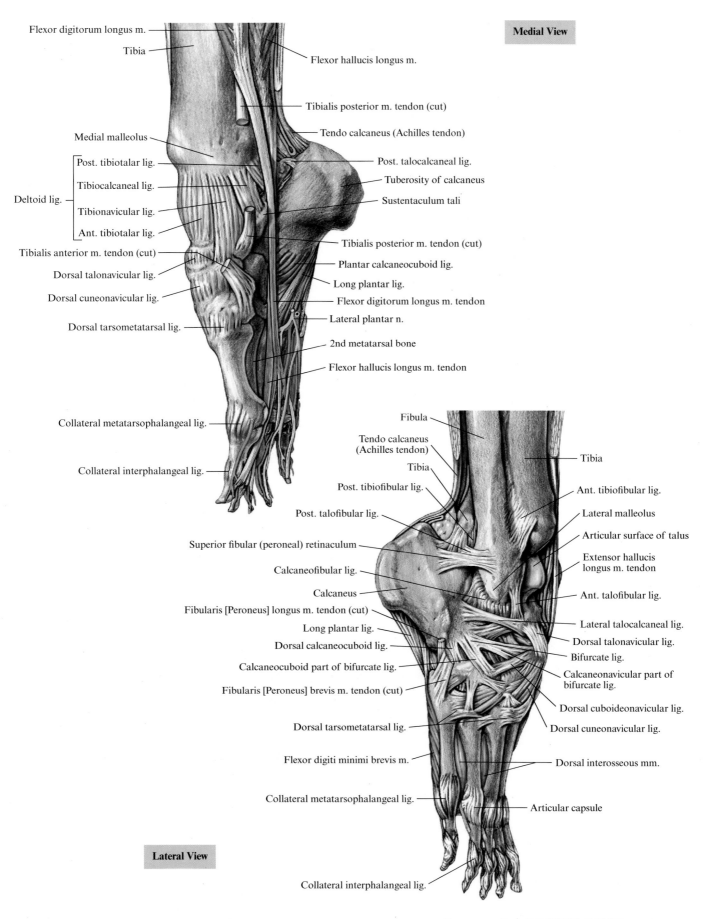

Medial View

Flexor digitorum longus m.

Tibia

Flexor hallucis longus m.

Tibialis posterior m. tendon (cut)

Tendo calcaneus (Achilles tendon)

Medial malleolus

Post. talocalcaneal lig.

Post. tibiotalar lig.

Tuberosity of calcaneus

Tibiocalcaneal lig.

Sustentaculum tali

Deltoid lig.

Tibionavicular lig.

Ant. tibiotalar lig.

Tibialis posterior m. tendon (cut)

Tibialis anterior m. tendon (cut)

Plantar calcaneocuboid lig.

Dorsal talonavicular lig.

Long plantar lig.

Dorsal cuneonavicular lig.

Flexor digitorum longus m. tendon

Lateral plantar n.

Dorsal tarsometatarsal lig.

2nd metatarsal bone

Flexor hallucis longus m. tendon

Collateral metatarsophalangeal lig.

Collateral interphalangeal lig.

Fibula

Tendo calcaneus
(Achilles tendon)

Tibia

Tibia

Ant. tibiofibular lig.

Post. tibiofibular lig.

Lateral malleolus

Post. talofibular lig.

Articular surface of talus

Superior fibular (peroneal) retinaculum

Extensor hallucis
longus m. tendon

Calcaneofibular lig.

Ant. talofibular lig.

Calcaneus

Fibularis [Peroneus] longus m. tendon (cut)

Lateral talocalcaneal lig.

Long plantar lig.

Dorsal talonavicular lig.

Dorsal calcaneocuboid lig.

Bifurcate lig.

Calcaneocuboid part of bifurcate lig.

Calcaneonavicular part of
bifurcate lig.

Fibularis [Peroneus] brevis m. tendon (cut)

Dorsal cuboideonavicular lig.

Dorsal tarsometatarsal lig.

Dorsal cuneonavicular lig.

Flexor digiti minimi brevis m.

Dorsal interosseous mm.

Collateral metatarsophalangeal lig.

Articular capsule

Lateral View

Collateral interphalangeal lig.

PLATE 5.59   FOOT—SKELETON

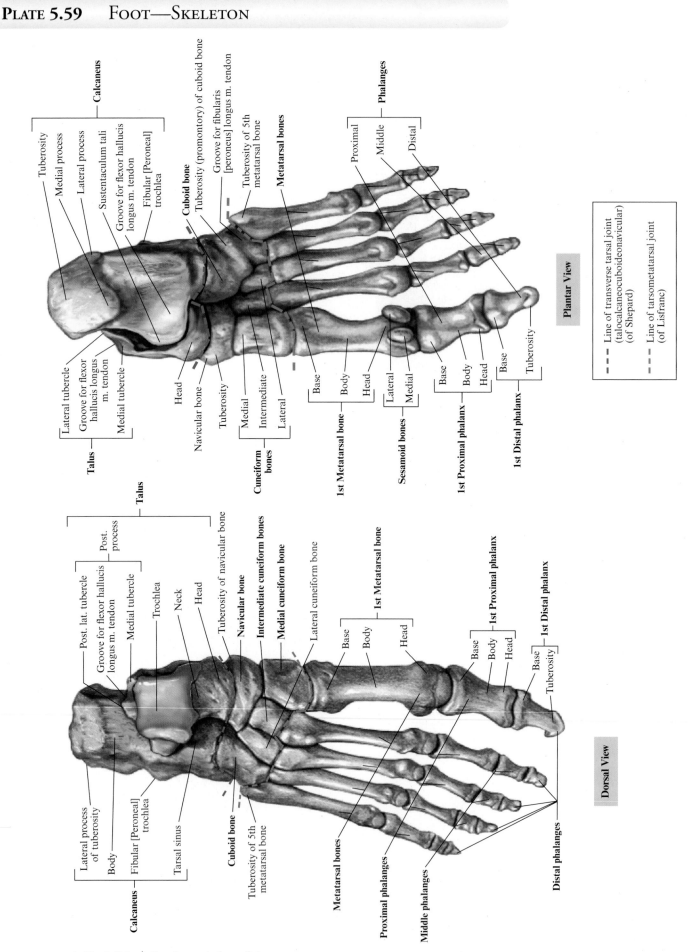

Tuberosity

Medial process

Lateral process

Sustentaculum tali

Groove for flexor hallucis
longus m. tendon

Fibular [Peroneal]
trochlea

Calcaneus

Tuberosity (promontory) of cuboid bone

Groove for fibularis
[peroneus] longus m. tendon

Tuberosity of 5th
metatarsal bone

Cuboid bone

Metatarsal bones

Proximal

Middle

Distal

Phalanges

Lateral tubercle

Groove for flexor
hallucis longus
m. tendon

Medial tubercle

Talus

Head

Navicular bone

Tuberosity

Medial

Intermediate

Lateral

**Cuneiform
bones**

Base

Body

Head

1st Metatarsal bone

Lateral

Medial

Sesamoid bones

Base

Body

Head

1st Proximal phalanx

Base

Tuberosity

1st Distal phalanx

Plantar View

--- Line of transverse tarsal joint
(talocalcaneocuboideonavicular)
(of Shepard)

--- Line of tarsometatarsal joint
(of Lisfranc)

Post. lat. tubercle

Groove for flexor hallucis
longus m. tendon

Medial tubercle

Post.
process

Trochlea

Neck

Head

Tuberosity of navicular bone

Talus

Navicular bone

Intermediate cuneiform bones

Medial cuneiform bone

Lateral cuneiform bone

Base

Body

Head

1st Metatarsal bone

Base

Body

Head

1st Proximal phalanx

Base

Tuberosity

1st Distal phalanx

Lateral process
of tuberosity

Body

Fibular [Peroneal]
trochlea

Tarsal sinus

Calcaneus

Cuboid bone

Tuberosity of 5th
metatarsal bone

Metatarsal bones

Proximal phalanges

Middle phalanges

Distal phalanges

Dorsal View

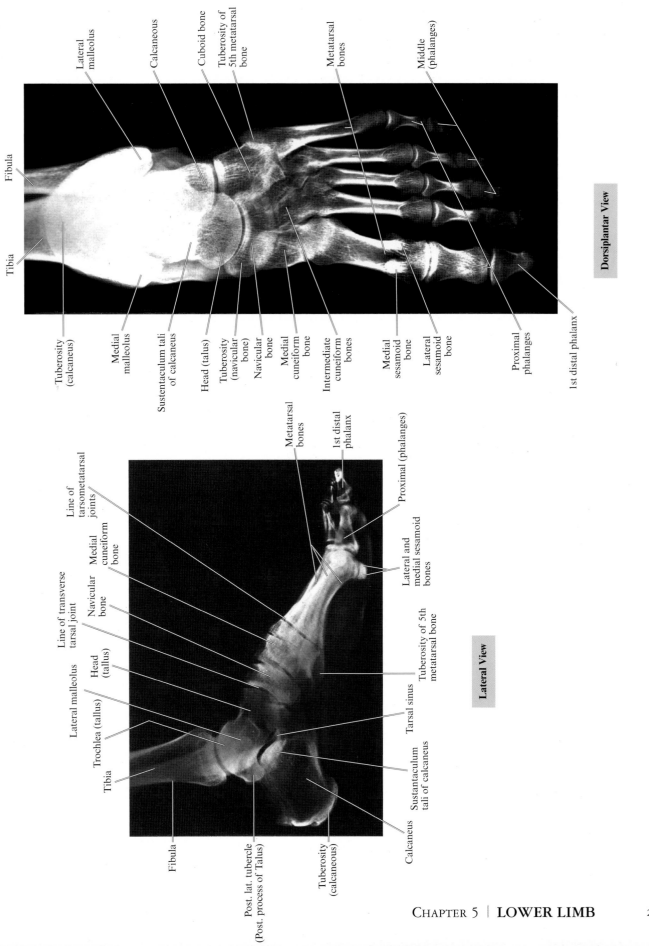

Dorsiplantar View

Lateral malleolus

Calcaneous

Cuboid bone

Tuberosity of 5th metatarsal bone

Metatarsal bones

Middle (phalanges)

Fibula

Tibia

Tuberosity (calcaneus)

Medial malleolus

Sustentaculum tali of calcaneus

Head (talus)

Tuberosity (navicular bone)

Navicular bone

Medial cuneiform bone

Intermediate cuneiform bones

Medial sesamoid bone

Lateral sesamoid bone

Proximal phalanges

1st distal phalanx

Lateral View

Line of tarsometatarsal joints

Medial cuneiform bone

Line of transverse tarsal joint

Navicular bone

Head (tallus)

Lateral malleolus

Trochlea (tallus)

Tibia

Fibula

Post. lat. tubercle (Post. process of Talus)

Tuberosity (calcaneus)

Calcaneus

Sustantaculum tali of calcaneus

Tarsal sinus

Tuberosity of 5th metatarsal bone

Lateral and medial sesamoid bones

Metatarsal bones

1st distal phalanx

Proximal (phalanges)

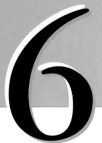

6 UPPER LIMB

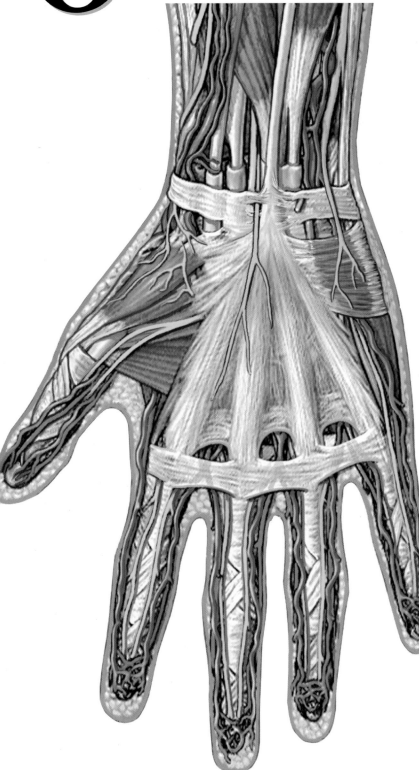

SURFACE ANATOMY

SKELETON

MUSCLES

ARTERIES

VEINS

NERVES

LYMPHATICS

PECTORAL &
SCAPULAR MUSCLES

SHOULDER & AXILLA

POSTERIOR ARM

GLENOHUMERAL JOINT

ANTERIOR &
MEDIAL ARM

ANTERIOR FOREARM

ELBOW &
WRIST JOINTS

LATERAL FOREARM
& HAND

POSTERIOR ARM
& FOREARM

DORSAL SURFACE
OF THE HAND

PALMAR SURFACE
OF THE HAND

WRIST & HAND

PLATE 6.1   SURFACE ANATOMY

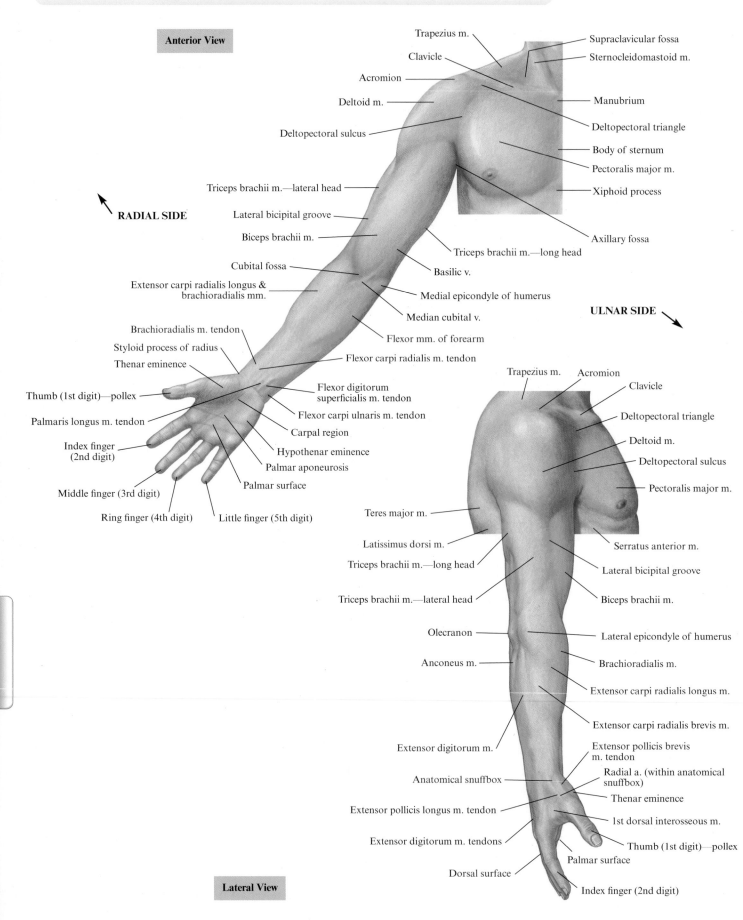

Anterior View

Trapezius m.

Clavicle

Acromion

Deltoid m.

Deltopectoral sulcus

RADIAL SIDE

Triceps brachii m.—lateral head

Lateral bicipital groove

Biceps brachii m.

Cubital fossa

Extensor carpi radialis longus &
brachioradialis mm.

Brachioradialis m. tendon

Styloid process of radius

Thenar eminence

Thumb (1st digit)—pollex

Palmaris longus m. tendon

Index finger
(2nd digit)

Middle finger (3rd digit)

Ring finger (4th digit)

Little finger (5th digit)

Supraclavicular fossa

Sternocleidomastoid m.

Manubrium

Deltopectoral triangle

Body of sternum

Pectoralis major m.

Xiphoid process

Axillary fossa

Triceps brachii m.—long head

Basilic v.

Medial epicondyle of humerus

Median cubital v.

Flexor mm. of forearm

Flexor carpi radialis m. tendon

Flexor digitorum
superficialis m. tendon

Flexor carpi ulnaris m. tendon

Carpal region

Hypothenar eminence

Palmar aponeurosis

Palmar surface

ULNAR SIDE

Trapezius m.   Acromion

Clavicle

Deltopectoral triangle

Deltoid m.

Deltopectoral sulcus

Pectoralis major m.

Teres major m.

Latissimus dorsi m.

Triceps brachii m.—long head

Triceps brachii m.—lateral head

Olecranon

Anconeus m.

Extensor digitorum m.

Anatomical snuffbox

Extensor pollicis longus m. tendon

Extensor digitorum m. tendons

Dorsal surface

Serratus anterior m.

Lateral bicipital groove

Biceps brachii m.

Lateral epicondyle of humerus

Brachioradialis m.

Extensor carpi radialis longus m.

Extensor carpi radialis brevis m.

Extensor pollicis brevis
m. tendon

Radial a. (within anatomical
snuffbox)

Thenar eminence

1st dorsal interosseous m.

Thumb (1st digit)—pollex

Palmar surface

Index finger (2nd digit)

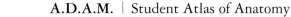

Lateral View

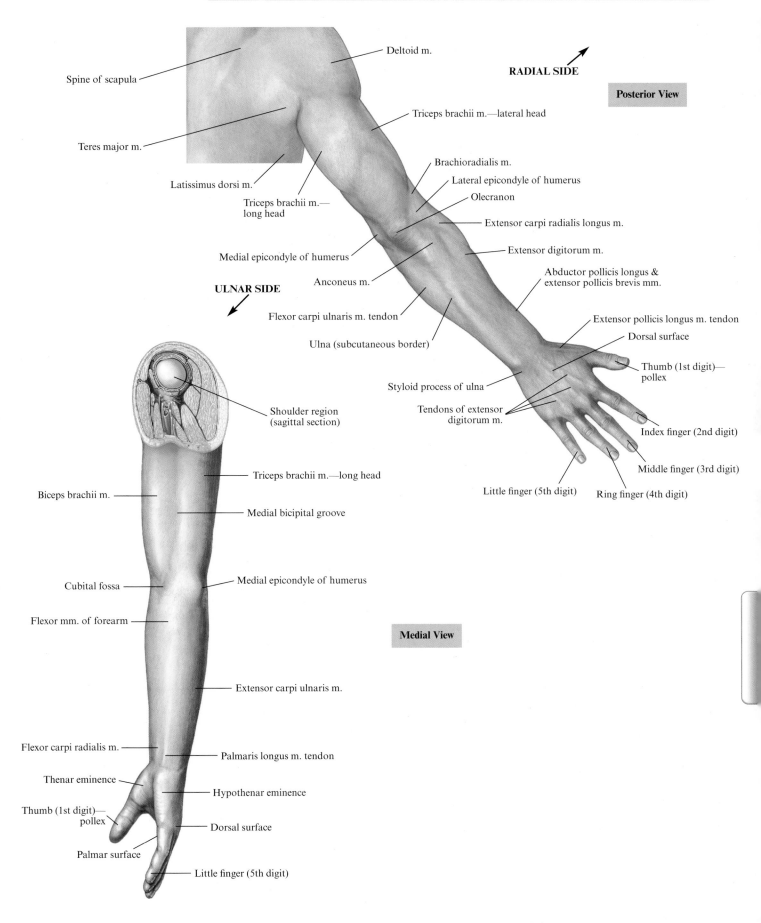

Posterior View

Deltoid m.

RADIAL SIDE

Spine of scapula

Triceps brachii m.—lateral head

Teres major m.

Brachioradialis m.

Lateral epicondyle of humerus

Olecranon

Latissimus dorsi m.

Extensor carpi radialis longus m.

Triceps brachii m.—
long head

Extensor digitorum m.

Abductor pollicis longus &
extensor pollicis brevis mm.

Medial epicondyle of humerus

ULNAR SIDE

Anconeus m.

Extensor pollicis longus m. tendon

Dorsal surface

Flexor carpi ulnaris m. tendon

Ulna (subcutaneous border)

Thumb (1st digit)—
pollex

Styloid process of ulna

Shoulder region
(sagittal section)

Tendons of extensor
digitorum m.

Index finger (2nd digit)

Middle finger (3rd digit)

Triceps brachii m.—long head

Little finger (5th digit)   Ring finger (4th digit)

Biceps brachii m.

Medial bicipital groove

Cubital fossa

Medial epicondyle of humerus

Flexor mm. of forearm

Medial View

Extensor carpi ulnaris m.

Flexor carpi radialis m.

Palmaris longus m. tendon

Thenar eminence

Hypothenar eminence

Thumb (1st digit)—
pollex

Dorsal surface

Palmar surface

Little finger (5th digit)

PLATE 6.3   SKELETON & MUSCLE ATTACHMENTS

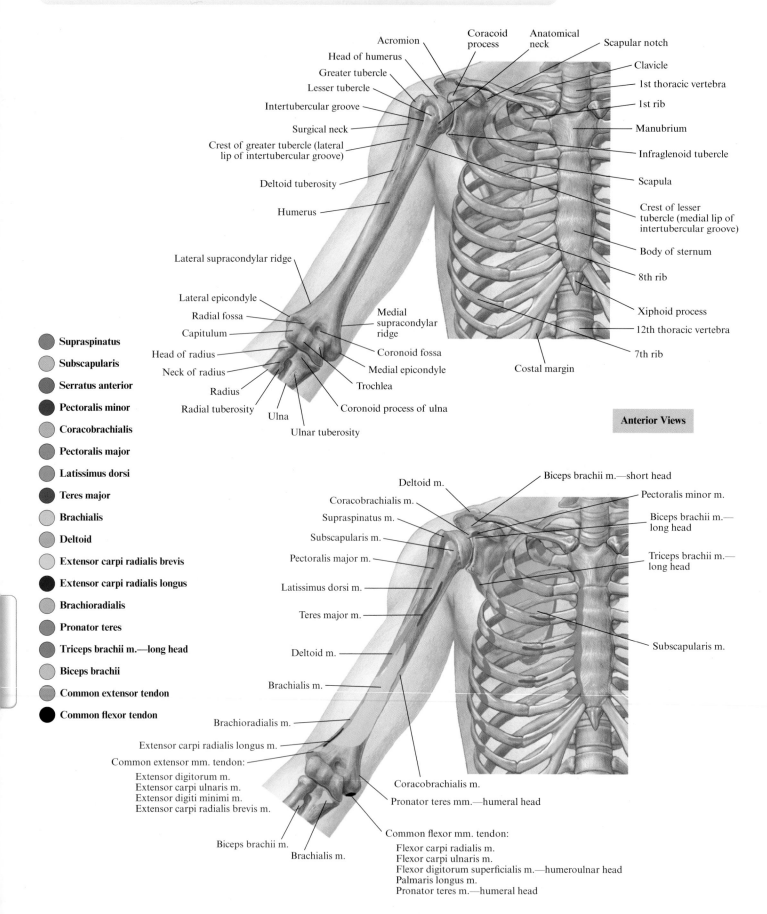

Acromion
Coracoid process
Anatomical neck
Head of humerus
Greater tubercle
Lesser tubercle
Intertubercular groove
Surgical neck
Crest of greater tubercle (lateral lip of intertubercular groove)
Deltoid tuberosity
Humerus
Lateral supracondylar ridge
Lateral epicondyle
Radial fossa
Capitulum
Head of radius
Neck of radius
Radius
Radial tuberosity
Ulna
Ulnar tuberosity

Scapular notch
Clavicle
1st thoracic vertebra
1st rib
Manubrium
Infraglenoid tubercle
Scapula
Crest of lesser tubercle (medial lip of intertubercular groove)
Body of sternum
8th rib
Xiphoid process
12th thoracic vertebra
7th rib
Costal margin

Medial supracondylar ridge
Coronoid fossa
Medial epicondyle
Trochlea
Coronoid process of ulna

Anterior Views

Supraspinatus
Subscapularis
Serratus anterior
Pectoralis minor
Coracobrachialis
Pectoralis major
Latissimus dorsi
Teres major
Brachialis
Deltoid
Extensor carpi radialis brevis
Extensor carpi radialis longus
Brachioradialis
Pronator teres
Triceps brachii m.—long head
Biceps brachii
Common extensor tendon
Common flexor tendon

Deltoid m.
Coracobrachialis m.
Supraspinatus m.
Subscapularis m.
Pectoralis major m.
Latissimus dorsi m.
Teres major m.
Deltoid m.
Brachialis m.
Brachioradialis m.
Extensor carpi radialis longus m.
Common extensor mm. tendon:
    Extensor digitorum m.
    Extensor carpi ulnaris m.
    Extensor digiti minimi m.
    Extensor carpi radialis brevis m.
Biceps brachii m.
Brachialis m.

Biceps brachii m.—short head
Pectoralis minor m.
Biceps brachii m.—long head
Triceps brachii m.—long head
Subscapularis m.

Coracobrachialis m.
Pronator teres mm.—humeral head
Common flexor mm. tendon:
    Flexor carpi radialis m.
    Flexor carpi ulnaris m.
    Flexor digitorum superficialis m.—humeroulnar head
    Palmaris longus m.
    Pronator teres m.—humeral head

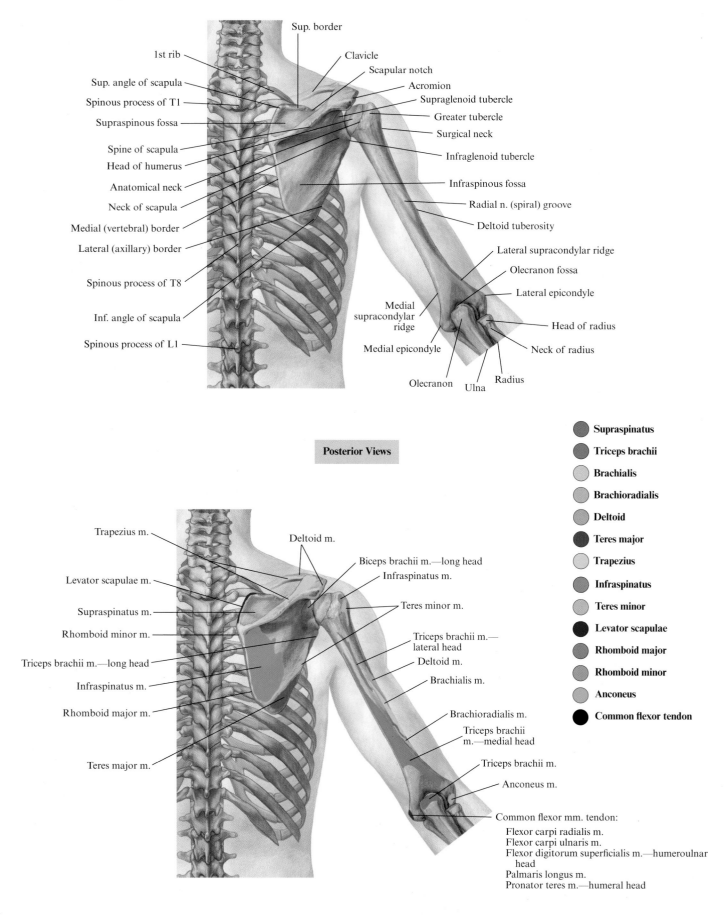

Sup. border

1st rib

Clavicle

Scapular notch

Sup. angle of scapula

Acromion

Spinous process of T1

Supraglenoid tubercle

Supraspinous fossa

Greater tubercle

Surgical neck

Spine of scapula

Head of humerus

Infraglenoid tubercle

Anatomical neck

Infraspinous fossa

Neck of scapula

Radial n. (spiral) groove

Medial (vertebral) border

Deltoid tuberosity

Lateral (axillary) border

Lateral supracondylar ridge

Olecranon fossa

Spinous process of T8

Lateral epicondyle

Medial
supracondylar
ridge

Inf. angle of scapula

Head of radius

Spinous process of L1

Medial epicondyle

Neck of radius

Olecranon   Ulna   Radius

Posterior Views

Supraspinatus

Triceps brachii

Brachialis

Brachioradialis

Deltoid

Teres major

Trapezius

Infraspinatus

Teres minor

Levator scapulae

Rhomboid major

Rhomboid minor

Anconeus

Common flexor tendon

Trapezius m.

Deltoid m.

Biceps brachii m.—long head

Infraspinatus m.

Levator scapulae m.

Teres minor m.

Supraspinatus m.

Triceps brachii m.—
lateral head

Rhomboid minor m.

Deltoid m.

Triceps brachii m.—long head

Brachialis m.

Infraspinatus m.

Brachioradialis m.

Rhomboid major m.

Triceps brachii
m.—medial head

Triceps brachii m.

Teres major m.

Anconeus m.

Common flexor mm. tendon:

Flexor carpi radialis m.
Flexor carpi ulnaris m.
Flexor digitorum superficialis m.—humeroulnar
head
Palmaris longus m.
Pronator teres m.—humeral head

PLATE 6.5   SKELETON & MUSCLE ATTACHMENTS

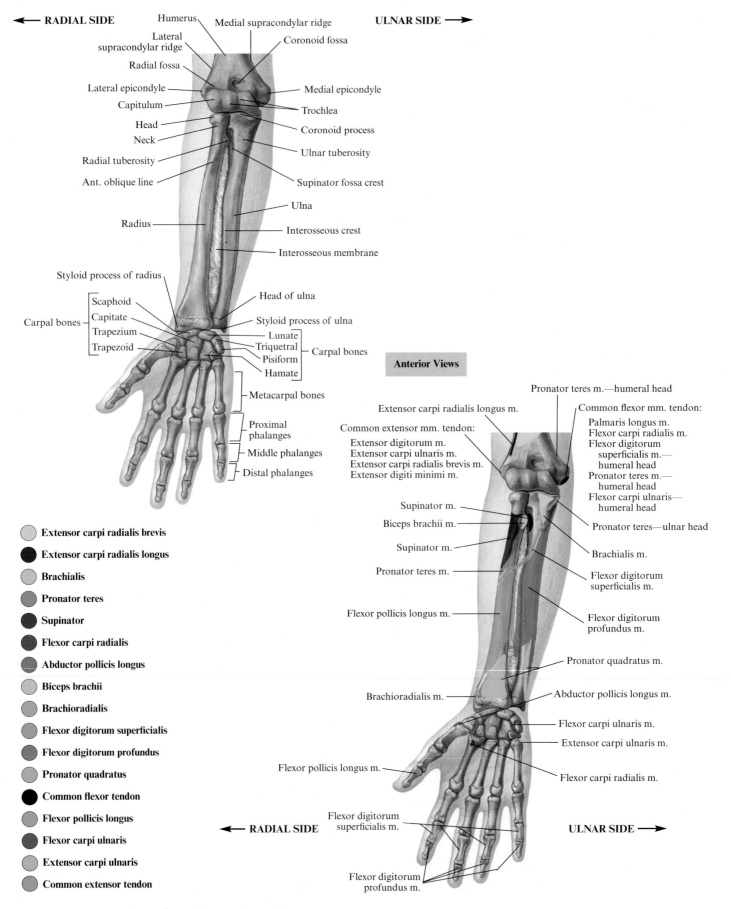

◄── **RADIAL SIDE**

Humerus

Lateral supracondylar ridge

Radial fossa

Lateral epicondyle

Capitulum

Head

Neck

Radial tuberosity

Ant. oblique line

Radius

Styloid process of radius

Carpal bones
- Scaphoid
- Capitate
- Trapezium
- Trapezoid

Medial supracondylar ridge

Coronoid fossa

ULNAR SIDE ──►

Medial epicondyle

Trochlea

Coronoid process

Ulnar tuberosity

Supinator fossa crest

Ulna

Interosseous crest

Interosseous membrane

Head of ulna

Styloid process of ulna

Lunate
Triquetral — Carpal bones
Pisiform
Hamate

Metacarpal bones

Proximal phalanges

Middle phalanges

Distal phalanges

Anterior Views

- Extensor carpi radialis brevis
- Extensor carpi radialis longus
- Brachialis
- Pronator teres
- Supinator
- Flexor carpi radialis
- Abductor pollicis longus
- Biceps brachii
- Brachioradialis
- Flexor digitorum superficialis
- Flexor digitorum profundus
- Pronator quadratus
- Common flexor tendon
- Flexor pollicis longus
- Flexor carpi ulnaris
- Extensor carpi ulnaris
- Common extensor tendon

Extensor carpi radialis longus m.

Common extensor mm. tendon:
Extensor digitorum m.
Extensor carpi ulnaris m.
Extensor carpi radialis brevis m.
Extensor digiti minimi m.

Supinator m.

Biceps brachii m.

Supinator m.

Pronator teres m.

Flexor pollicis longus m.

Pronator teres m.—humeral head

Common flexor mm. tendon:
Palmaris longus m.
Flexor carpi radialis m.
Flexor digitorum superficialis m.—humeral head
Pronator teres m.—humeral head
Flexor carpi ulnaris—humeral head

Pronator teres—ulnar head

Brachialis m.

Flexor digitorum superficialis m.

Flexor digitorum profundus m.

Pronator quadratus m.

Brachioradialis m.

Abductor pollicis longus m.

Flexor carpi ulnaris m.

Extensor carpi ulnaris m.

Flexor pollicis longus m.

Flexor carpi radialis m.

◄── **RADIAL SIDE**

Flexor digitorum superficialis m.

ULNAR SIDE ──►

Flexor digitorum profundus m.

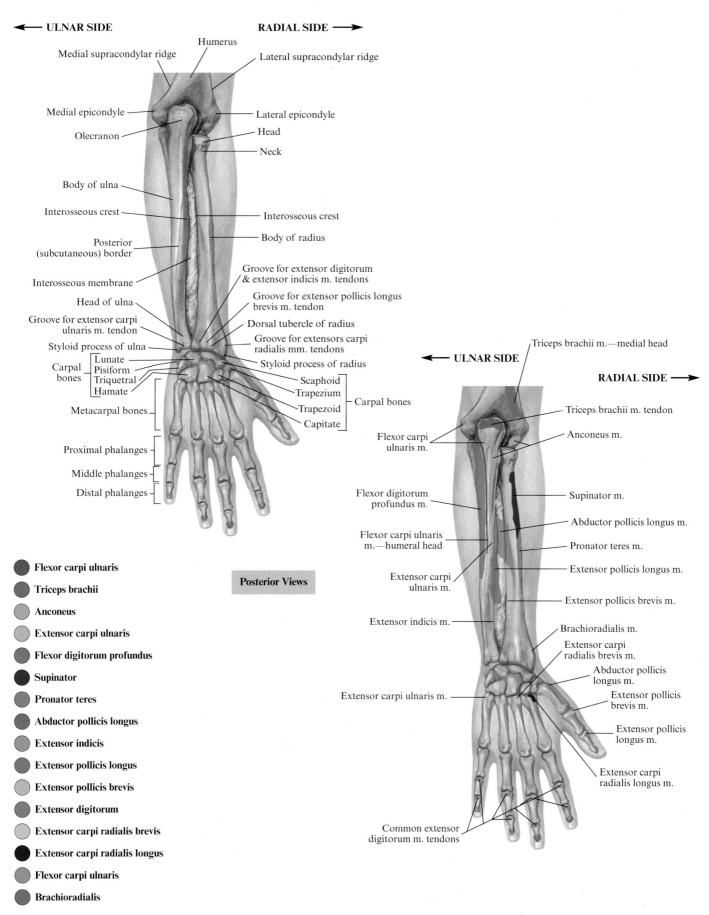

← ULNAR SIDE   RADIAL SIDE →

Humerus

Medial supracondylar ridge

Lateral supracondylar ridge

Medial epicondyle

Lateral epicondyle

Olecranon

Head

Neck

Body of ulna

Interosseous crest

Interosseous crest

Body of radius

Posterior (subcutaneous) border

Groove for extensor digitorum & extensor indicis m. tendons

Interosseous membrane

Groove for extensor pollicis longus brevis m. tendon

Head of ulna

Groove for extensor carpi ulnaris m. tendon

Dorsal tubercle of radius

Styloid process of ulna

Groove for extensors carpi radialis mm. tendons

Styloid process of radius

Carpal bones
- Lunate
- Pisiform
- Triquetral
- Hamate

Scaphoid

Trapezium

Trapezoid

Capitate

Carpal bones

Metacarpal bones

Proximal phalanges

Middle phalanges

Distal phalanges

Posterior Views

Triceps brachii m.—medial head

← ULNAR SIDE

RADIAL SIDE →

Triceps brachii m. tendon

Flexor carpi ulnaris m.

Anconeus m.

Flexor digitorum profundus m.

Supinator m.

Abductor pollicis longus m.

Flexor carpi ulnaris m.—humeral head

Pronator teres m.

Extensor pollicis longus m.

Extensor carpi ulnaris m.

Extensor pollicis brevis m.

Extensor indicis m.

Brachioradialis m.

Extensor carpi radialis brevis m.

Abductor pollicis longus m.

Extensor carpi ulnaris m.

Extensor pollicis brevis m.

Extensor pollicis longus m.

Extensor carpi radialis longus m.

Common extensor digitorum m. tendons

- Flexor carpi ulnaris
- Triceps brachii
- Anconeus
- Extensor carpi ulnaris
- Flexor digitorum profundus
- Supinator
- Pronator teres
- Abductor pollicis longus
- Extensor indicis
- Extensor pollicis longus
- Extensor pollicis brevis
- Extensor digitorum
- Extensor carpi radialis brevis
- Extensor carpi radialis longus
- Flexor carpi ulnaris
- Brachioradialis

TABLE 6.1   PECTORAL & SCAPULAR MUSCLES

Muscles in Pectoral Region

Muscle	Proximal Attachment	Distal Attachment	Innervation[a]	Main Actions
Pectoralis major	*Clavicular head:* ant. surface of the medial half of clavicle *Sternocostal head:* ant. surface of sternum, sup. six costal cartilages & aponeurosis of ext. abdominal oblique muscle	Lateral lip of intertubercular groove of humerus	Lateral & medial pectoral n.: clavicular head (C5 & **C6**) Sternocostal head (**C7, C8,** & T1)	Adducts & medially rotates humerus Draws shoulder joint anteriorly & inferiorly *Acting alone:* Clavicular head flexes humerus & sternoclavicular head extends it
Pectoralis minor	Ribs 3–5 near their costal cartilages	Medial border & sup. surface of coracoid process of scapula	Medial pectoral n. (C8 & T1)	Stabilizes scapula by drawing it inferiorly & anteriorly against thoracic wall
Subclavius	Junction of rib 1 & its costal cartilage	Inf. surface of middle third of clavicle	N. to subclavius (**C5** & C6)	(Draws clavicle medially?)
Serratus anterior	Ext. surfaces of lateral parts of ribs 1–8/9	Ant. surface of medial border of scapula	Long thoracic n. (C5, **C6,** & C7)	Protracts scapula & holds it against thoracic wall; rotates scapula superiorly

Muscles Connecting Upper Limb to Vertebral Column

Muscle	Medial Attachment	Lateral Attachment	Innervation[a]	Main Actions
Trapezius	Medial third of sup. nuchal line; ext. occipital protuberance, ligamentum nuchae & spinous processes of C7–T12 vertebrae	Lateral third of clavicle, acromion & spine of scapula	Accessory n. (CN XI) & cervical nn. (C3 & C4)	Elevates, retracts & rotates scapula; *sup. fibers* elevate, *middle fibers* retract, *inf. fibers* depress scapula; sup. & inf. fibers act together in sup. rotation of scapula
Latissimus dorsi	Spinous processes of the inf. six thoracic vertebrae, thoracolumbar fascia, iliac crest & inf. 3 or 4 ribs	Floor of intertubercular groove & crest of lesser tubercle of humerus	Thoracodorsal n. (**C6, C7,** & C8)	Extends, adducts & medially rotates humerus; raises body toward arms during climbing
Levator scapulae	Post. tubercles of transverse processes of C1–C4 vertebrae	Sup. part of medial border of scapula	Dorsal scapular (C5) & cervical (C3 & C4) nn.	Elevates scapula & tilts its glenoid cavity inferiorly by rotating scapula
Rhomboid minor & major	*Minor:* Ligamentum nuchae & spinous processes of C7 & T1 vertebrae *Major:* Spinous processes of T2–T5 vertebrae	Medial border of scapula from level of spine to inf. angle	Dorsal scapular n. (C4 & **C5**) rotate	Retracts scapula & rotates it to depress glenoid cavity; fixes scapula to thoracic wall

[a]In this and subsequent tables, the numbers indicate the spinal cord segmental innervation of the nerves (*e.g.,* C5 and C6 indicate that the nerves supplying the clavicular head of the pectoralis major muscle are derived from the 5th and 6th cervical segments of the spinal cord). **Boldface** indicates the main segmental innervation. Damage to these segments of the spinal cord, or to the motor nerve roots arising from them, results in paralysis of the muscles concerned.

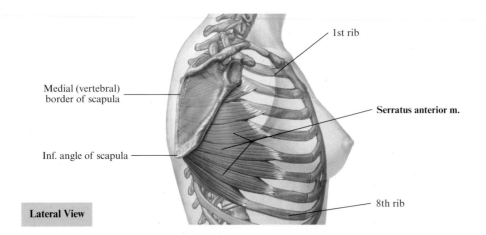

1st rib

Medial (vertebral) border of scapula

Serratus anterior m.

Inf. angle of scapula

8th rib

Lateral View

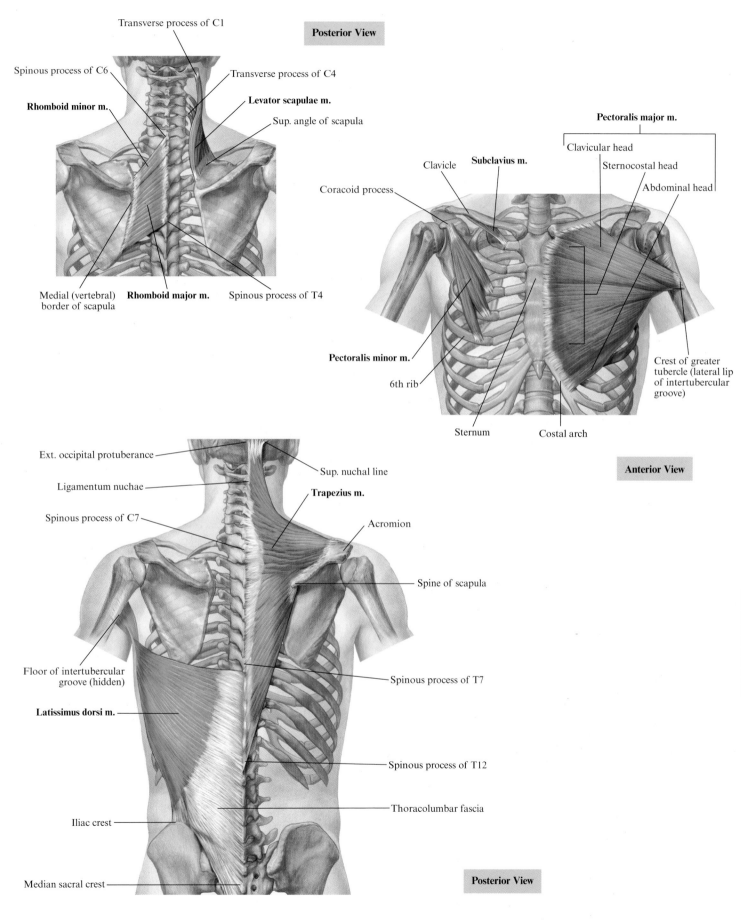

Posterior View

Transverse process of C1

Spinous process of C6

Transverse process of C4

Rhomboid minor m.

Levator scapulae m.

Sup. angle of scapula

Medial (vertebral) border of scapula

Rhomboid major m.

Spinous process of T4

Pectoralis major m.

Clavicular head

Sternocostal head

Abdominal head

Clavicle

Subclavius m.

Coracoid process

Pectoralis minor m.

6th rib

Sternum

Costal arch

Crest of greater tubercle (lateral lip of intertubercular groove)

Anterior View

Ext. occipital protuberance

Ligamentum nuchae

Spinous process of C7

Sup. nuchal line

Trapezius m.

Acromion

Spine of scapula

Floor of intertubercular groove (hidden)

Latissimus dorsi m.

Iliac crest

Median sacral crest

Spinous process of T7

Spinous process of T12

Thoracolumbar fascia

Posterior View

TABLE 6.2   SCAPULAR & POSTERIOR ARM MUSCLES

Scapular Muscles

Muscle	Proximal/Medial Attachment	Distal/Lateral Attachment	Innervation[a]	Main Actions
Deltoid	Lateral third of clavicle, acromion & spine of scapula	Deltoid tuberosity of humerus	Axillary n. (**C5** & **C6**)	*Anterior part:* flexes & medially rolates arm *Middle part:* abducts arm *Posterior part:* extends & laterally rotates arm
Supraspinatus[a]	Supraspinous fossa of scapula	Sup. facet on greater tubercle of humerus	Suprascapular n. (C4, **C5** & C6)	Helps deltoid to abduct arm[a]
Infraspinatus[a]	Infraspinous fossa of scapula	Middle facet on greater tubercle of humerus	Suprascapular n. (C4, **C5** & C6)	Laterally rotates arm; helps to hold humeral head in glenoid cavity of scapula
Teres minor[a]	Sup. part of lateral border of scapula	Inf. facet on greater tubercle of humerus	Axillary n. (**C5** & C6)	
Teres major	Dorsal surface of inf. angle of scapula	Medial lip of intertubular groove of humerus	Lower subscapular n. (**C6** & **C7**)	Adducts & medially rotates arm
Subscapularis[a]	Subscapular fossa	Lesser tubercle of humerus	Upper & lower subscapular nn. (C5, **C6** & C7)	Medially rotates arm & adducts it; helps to hold humeral head in glenoid cavity

[a]Collectively, the supraspinatus, infraspinatus, teres minor, and subscapularis muscles are referred to as the **rotator cuff muscles**. Their prime function during all movements of the shoulder joint is to hold the head of the humerus in the glenoid cavity of the scapula.

Posterior Arm Muscles

Muscle	Proximal Attachment	Distal Attachment	Innervation	Main Actions
Triceps brachii	*Long head:* infraglenoid tubercle of scapula *Lateral head:* post. surface of humerus, sup. to radial n. groove *Medial head:* post. surface of humerus, inf. to radial n. groove	Proximal end of olecranon ulna & fascia of forearm	Radial n. (**C6**, **C7**, & **C8**)	Extends the forearm; it is *chief extensor of forearm,* long head steadies head of abducted humerus
Anconeus	Lateral epicondyle of humerus	Lateral surface of olecranon & sup. part of post. surface of ulna	Radial n. (C7, C8 & T1)	Assists triceps in extending forearm; stabilizes elbow joint; abducts ulna during pronation

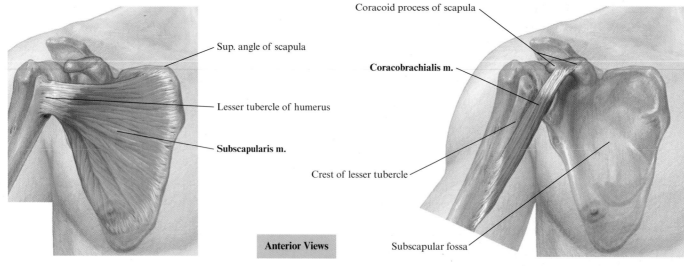

Sup. angle of scapula

Lesser tubercle of humerus

Subscapularis m.

Coracoid process of scapula

Coracobrachialis m.

Crest of lesser tubercle

Anterior Views

Subscapular fossa

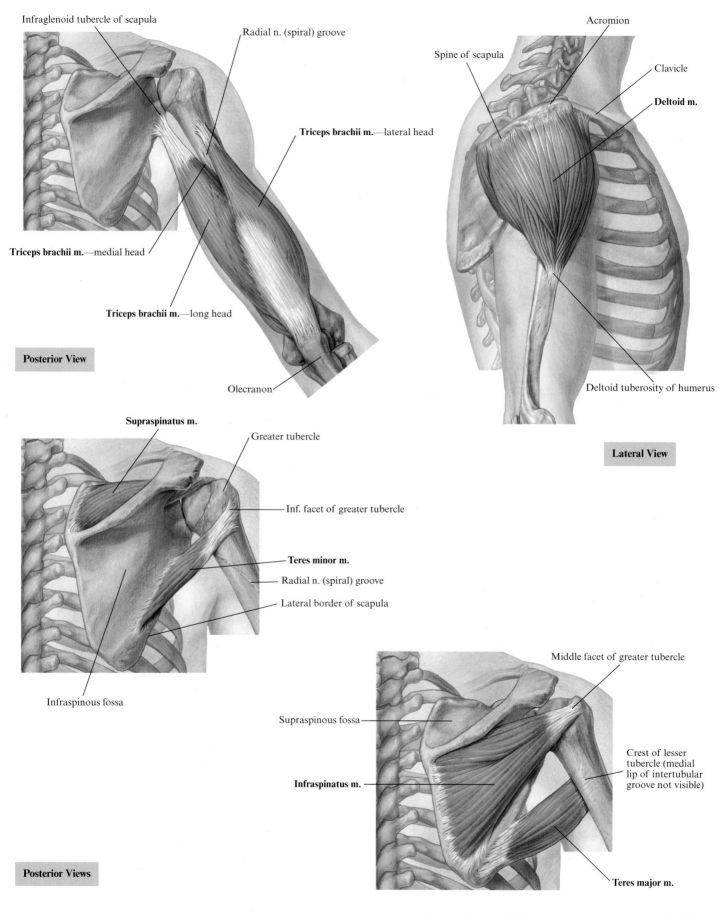

Infraglenoid tubercle of scapula

Radial n. (spiral) groove

Acromion

Spine of scapula

Clavicle

Deltoid m.

Triceps brachii m.—lateral head

Triceps brachii m.—medial head

Triceps brachii m.—long head

Posterior View

Olecranon

Deltoid tuberosity of humerus

Lateral View

Supraspinatus m.

Greater tubercle

Inf. facet of greater tubercle

Teres minor m.

Radial n. (spiral) groove

Lateral border of scapula

Infraspinous fossa

Middle facet of greater tubercle

Supraspinous fossa

Crest of lesser tubercle (medial lip of intertubular groove not visible)

Infraspinatus m.

Posterior Views

Teres major m.

TABLE 6.3   ANTERIOR ARM & FOREARM MUSCLES

Muscles of Anterior Arm

Muscle	Proximal Attachment	Distal Attachment	Innervation[a]	Main Actions
Biceps brachii	*Short head:* Tip of coracoid process of scapula *Long head:* Supraglenoid tubercle of scapula	Tuberosity of radius & fascia of forearm via bicipital aponeurosis	Musculocutaneous n. (C5 & **C6**)	Supinates forearm and, when it is supine, flexes forearm
Brachialis	Distal half of ant. surface of humerus	Coronoid process & tuberosity of ulna		Flexes forearm in all positions
Coracobrachialis	Tip of coracoid process of scapula	Middle third of medial surface of humerus	Musculocutaneous n. (C5, **C6** & C7)	Helps to flex & adduct arm

Superficial and Intermediate Layers of Muscles on Anterior Surface of Forearm[a]

Muscle	Proximal Attachment	Distal Attachment	Innervation[a]	Main Actions
Pronator teres	Medial epicondyle of humerus & coronoid process of ulna	Middle of lateral surface of radius	Median n. (C6 & **C7**)	Pronates forearm & flexes it
Flexor carpi radialis	Medial epicondyle of humerus	Base of 2nd metacarpal bone		Flexes hand & abducts it radially
Palmaris longus	Medial epicondyle of humerus	Distal half of flexor retinaculum & palmar aponeurosis	Median n. (C7 & C8)	Flexes hand & tightens palmar aponeurosis
Flexor carpi ulnaris[b]	*Humeral head:* medial epicondyle of humerus *Ulnar head:* olecranon & post. border of ulna	Pisiform bone (hook of hamate bone & 5th metacarpal bone)	Ulnar n. (C7 & **C8**)	Flexes hand & adducts it ulnarly
Flexor digitorum superficialis[c]	*Humeroulnar head:* medial epicondyle of humerus, ulnar collateral lig. & coronoid process of ulna *Radial head:* sup. half of ant. border of radius	Bodies of the middle phalanges of medial four digits	Median n. (C7, **C8** & T1)	Flexes middle of phalanges of medial four digits; acting more strongly, it flexes proximal phalanges & hand

[a]The superficial muscles of the *flexor-pronator group* are attached, in whole or in part, to the anterior surface of the medial epicondyle by a *common flexor tendon.*
[b]In contrast to the other superficial flexor muscles, the flexor carpi ulnaris is supplied by the ulnar nerve.
[c]This muscle comprises the *intermediate muscle layer* in the anterior part of the forearm. In some clinical texts, this muscle is referred to by its old name, "flexor digitorum sublimis."

Deep Layer of Muscles on Anterior Surface of Forearm

Muscle	Proximal Attachment	Distal Attachment	Innervation	Main Actions
Pronator quadratus	Distal fourth of ant. surface of ulna	Distal fourth of ant. surface of radius	Ant. interosseous n. from median (**C8** & T1)	Pronates forearm; deep fibers bind radius & ulna together

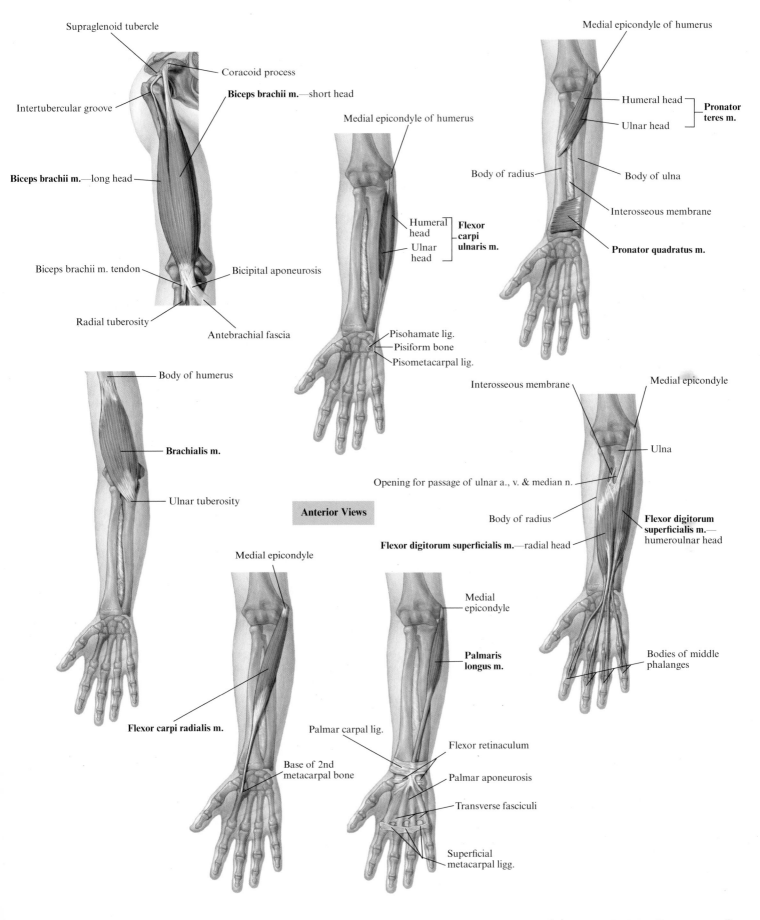

Supraglenoid tubercle

Coracoid process

Biceps brachii m.—short head

Intertubercular groove

Biceps brachii m.—long head

Biceps brachii m. tendon

Radial tuberosity

Bicipital aponeurosis

Antebrachial fascia

Medial epicondyle of humerus

Humeral head

Ulnar head

Flexor carpi ulnaris m.

Pisohamate lig.

Pisiform bone

Pisometacarpal lig.

Medial epicondyle of humerus

Humeral head

Ulnar head

Pronator teres m.

Body of radius

Body of ulna

Interosseous membrane

Pronator quadratus m.

Body of humerus

Brachialis m.

Ulnar tuberosity

Anterior Views

Interosseous membrane

Medial epicondyle

Ulna

Opening for passage of ulnar a., v. & median n.

Body of radius

Flexor digitorum superficialis m.—radial head

Flexor digitorum superficialis m.—humeroulnar head

Bodies of middle phalanges

Medial epicondyle

Flexor carpi radialis m.

Base of 2nd metacarpal bone

Medial epicondyle

Palmaris longus m.

Palmar carpal lig.

Flexor retinaculum

Palmar aponeurosis

Transverse fasciculi

Superficial metacarpal ligg.

TABLE 6.4   FOREARM MUSCLES

Deep Layer of Muscles on Anterior Surface of Forearm

Muscle	Proximal Attachment	Distal Attachment	Innervation	Main Actions
Flexor digitorum profundus	Proximal three-fourths of medial & ant. surfaces of ulna & interosseous membrane	Bases of distal phalanges of medial four digits	*Medial part:* Ulnar n. (**C8** & T1) *Lateral part:* Median n. (**C8** & T1)	Flexes distal phalanges of medial four digits (fingers)
Flexor pollicis longus	Ant. surface of the distal radius & adjacent interosseous membrane	Base of distal phalanx of thumb	Ant. interosseous n. from Median n. (**C8** & T1)	Flexes phalanges of first digit (thumb)

Superficial Muscles on Posterior or Extensor Surface of Forearm

Muscle	Proximal Attachment	Distal Attachment	Innervation	Main Actions
Brachioradialis	Proximal two-thirds of lateral supracondylar ridge of humerus, lat. intermuscular septum	Lateral surface of distal end of radius	Radial n. (C5, **C6** & C7)	Flexes forearm
Extensor carpi radialis longus	Lateral supracondylar ridge of humerus, lat. intermuscular septum	Base of 2nd metacarpal bone	Radial n. (C6 & C7)	Extend & abduct hand at wrist joint
Extensor carpi radialis brevis	Lateral epicondyle of humerus	Base of 3rd metacarpal bone	Deep br. of radial n. (**C7** & C8)	
Extensor digitorum	Lateral epicondyle of humerus	Extensor expansions of medial four digits	Post. interosseous n. (**C7** & C8), a br. of the radial n.	Extends medial four digits at metacarpophalangeal joints; extends hand at wrist joint
Extensor carpi ulnaris	Lateral epicondyle of humerus & post. border of ulna	Base of 5th metacarpal bone		Extends & adducts hand at wrist joint

Body of radius

Flexor pollicis longus m.

Trapezium bone

Base of distal phalanx of thumb

Interosseous membrane

Anterior View

Lateral epicondyle

Extensor carpi ulnaris m.

Base of 5th metacarpal bone

Posterior View

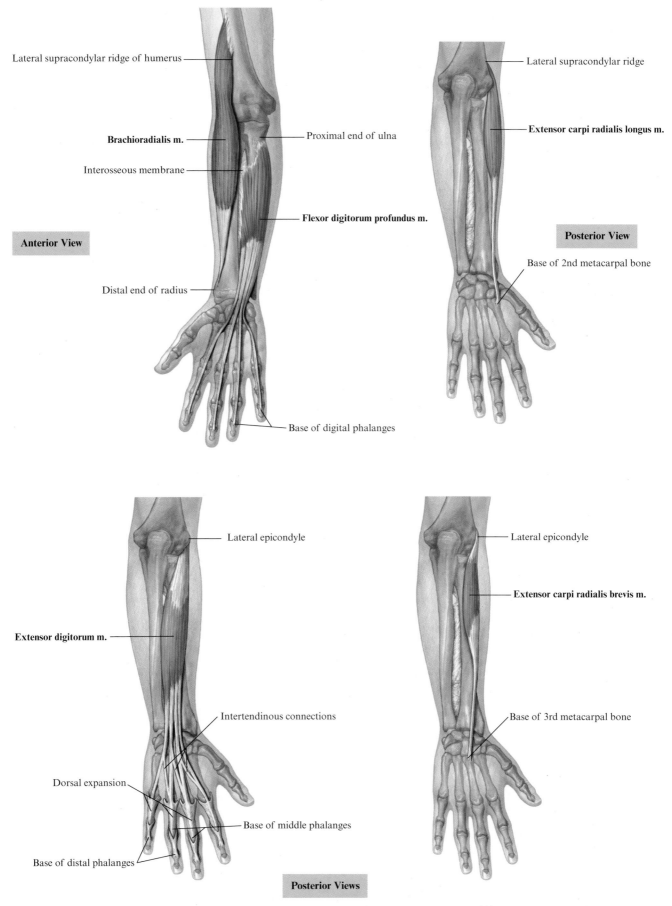

Lateral supracondylar ridge of humerus

Brachioradialis m.

Interosseous membrane

Anterior View

Distal end of radius

Proximal end of ulna

Flexor digitorum profundus m.

Base of digital phalanges

Lateral supracondylar ridge

Extensor carpi radialis longus m.

Posterior View

Base of 2nd metacarpal bone

Extensor digitorum m.

Lateral epicondyle

Intertendinous connections

Dorsal expansion

Base of distal phalanges

Base of middle phalanges

Lateral epicondyle

Extensor carpi radialis brevis m.

Base of 3rd metacarpal bone

Posterior Views

TABLE 6.5   POSTERIOR FOREARM MUSCLES

Deep Muscles on Posterior or Extensor Surface of Forearm

Muscle	Proximal Attachment	Distal Attachment	Innervation	Main Actions
Supinator	Lateral epicondyle of humerus, radial collateral & anular ligaments, supinator fossa & crest of ulna	Lateral, post. & ant. surfaces of proximal third of radius	Deep br. of radial n. (C5 & **C6**)	Supinates forearm, *i.e.,* rotates radius to turn palm anteriorly
Abductor pollicis longus	Post. surfaces of ulna & radius & interosseous membrane	Base of 1st metacarpalbone	Post. interosseous n. (C7 & **C8**)	Abducts thumb & extends it at carpometacarpal joint
Extensor pollicis brevis	Post. surface of radius & interosseous membrane	Base of proximal phalanx of thumb		Extends proximal phalanx of thumb at carpometacarpal joint
Extensor pollicis longus	Post. surface of middle third of ulnar & interosseous membrane	Base of distal phalanx of thumb		Extends distal phalanx of thumb at metacarpophalangeal & interphalangeal joints
Extensor indicis	Post. surface of ulna & interosseous membrane	Extensor expansion of second digit (index finger)		Extends digit 2 & helps to extend wrist
Extensor digit minimi	Lateral epicondyle of humerus	Extensor expansion of 5th digit	Post. interosseous n. (**C7** & C8), a br. of the radial n.	Extends digit 5 at metacarpophalangeal & interphalangeal joints

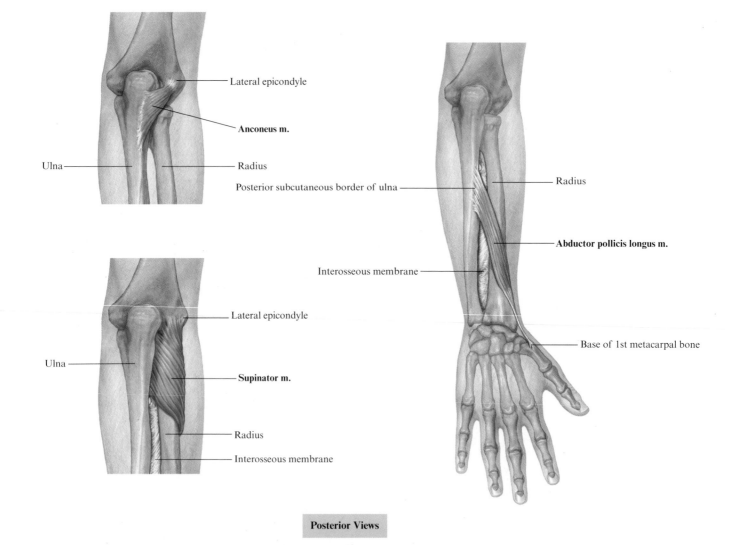

Posterior Views

A.D.A.M. | Student Atlas of Anatomy

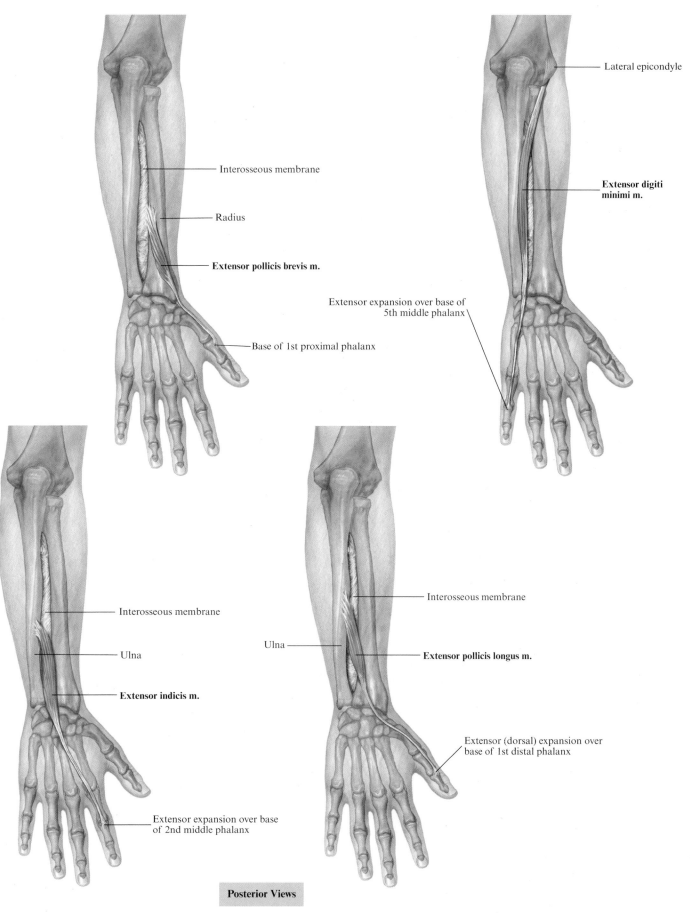

Lateral epicondyle

Extensor digiti minimi m.

Interosseous membrane

Radius

Extensor pollicis brevis m.

Extensor expansion over base of
5th middle phalanx

Base of 1st proximal phalanx

Interosseous membrane

Ulna

Extensor indicis m.

Interosseous membrane

Ulna

Extensor pollicis longus m.

Extensor (dorsal) expansion over
base of 1st distal phalanx

Extensor expansion over base
of 2nd middle phalanx

Posterior Views

TABLE 6.6   INTRINSIC HAND MUSCLES

Short Muscles of Hand

Muscle	Proximal Attachment	Distal Attachment	Innervation	Main Actions
Lumbricalis 1 & 2	Lateral two tendons of flex or digitorum profundus	Lateral sides of extensor expansions of digits 2 to 5	*Lumbricals 1 & 2,* median n. (C8 & **T1**)	Flex digits at metacarpophalangeal joints & extend interphalangeal joints
Lumbricalis 3 & 4	Medial three tendons of flex or digitorum profundus		*Lumbricals 3 & 4,* deep br. of ulnar n. (C8 & **T1**)	
Dorsal interossei 1–4	Adjacent sides of two metacarpal bones	Extensor expansion & bases of proximal phalanges of digits 2–4	Deep br. of ulnar n. (C8 & **T1**)	Abduct digits 2–4
Palmar interossei 1–3	Palmar surfaces of 1st, 2nd, 4th & 5th metacarpal bones	Extensor expansions of digits and bases of proximal phalanges of digits 1, 2, 4 & 5		Adduct digits 2–4
Abductor digiti minimi	Pisiform bone	Medial side of base of proximal phalanx of digit 5 (little finger)	Deep br. of ulnar n. (C8 & **T1**)	Abducts digit 5 (little finger)
Flexor digiti minimi brevis	Hook of hamate bone & flex or retinaculum			Flexes proximal phalanx of digit 5
Opponens digiti minimi		Medial border of 5th metacarpal bone		Draws 5th metacarpal bone anteriorly & rotates it, bringing digit 5 into opposition with thumb
Abductor pollicis brevis	Flexor retinaculum & tubercles of scaphoid & trapezium bones	Lateral side of base of proximal phalanx of thumb	Recurrent br. of median n. (**C8** & T1)	Abducts thumb & helps oppose it
Flexor pollicis brevis	Flexor retinaculum & tubercle of trapezium bone			Flexes thumb
Opponens pollicis		Lateral side of 1st metacarpal bone		Opposes thumb toward center of palm & rotates it medially
Adductor pollicis	*Oblique head:* Bases of 2nd & 3rd metacarpals, captate & adjacent carpal bones *Transverse head:* Ant. surface of body of 3rd metacarpal bone	Medial side of base of proximal phalanx of thumb	Deep br. of ulnar n. (C8 & **T1**)	Adducts thumb toward middle digit

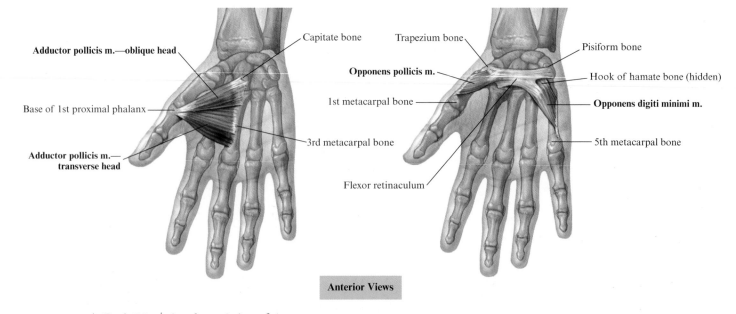

Adductor pollicis m.—oblique head
Capitate bone
Trapezium bone
Pisiform bone
Opponens pollicis m.
Base of 1st proximal phalanx
1st metacarpal bone
Hook of hamate bone (hidden)
Opponens digiti minimi m.
3rd metacarpal bone
5th metacarpal bone
Adductor pollicis m.—transverse head
Flexor retinaculum

Anterior Views

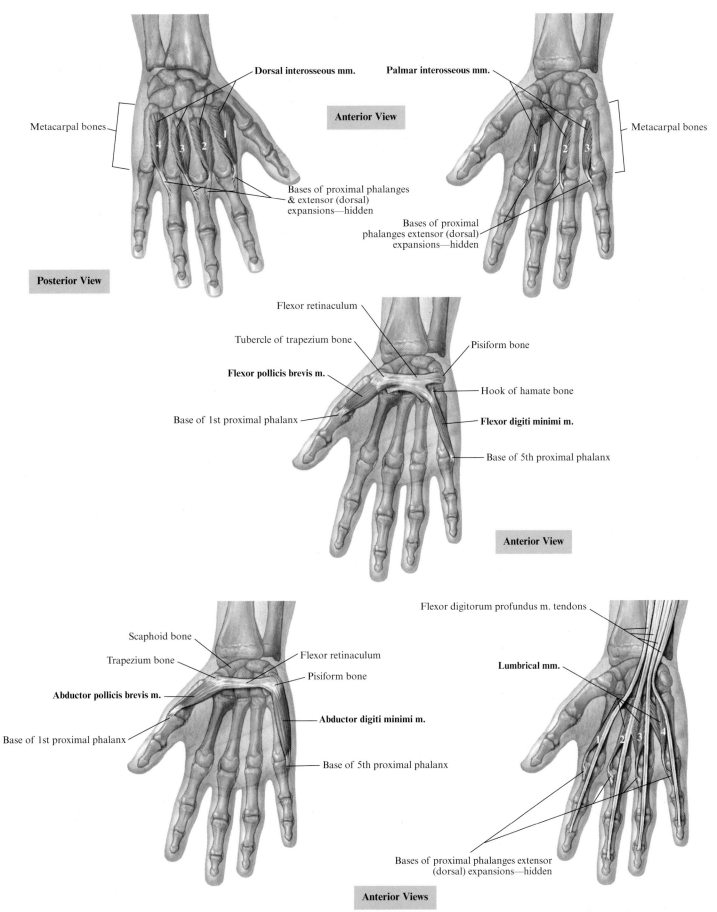

Dorsal interosseous mm.

Palmar interosseous mm.

Anterior View

Metacarpal bones

4 3 2 1

Metacarpal bones

1 2 3

Bases of proximal phalanges
& extensor (dorsal)
expansions—hidden

Bases of proximal
phalanges extensor (dorsal)
expansions—hidden

Posterior View

Flexor retinaculum

Tubercle of trapezium bone

Pisiform bone

Flexor pollicis brevis m.

Hook of hamate bone

Flexor digiti minimi m.

Base of 1st proximal phalanx

Base of 5th proximal phalanx

Anterior View

Flexor digitorum profundus m. tendons

Scaphoid bone

Trapezium bone

Flexor retinaculum

Pisiform bone

Lumbrical mm.

Abductor pollicis brevis m.

Abductor digiti minimi m.

Base of 1st proximal phalanx

Base of 5th proximal phalanx

1 2 3 4

Bases of proximal phalanges extensor
(dorsal) expansions—hidden

Anterior Views

PLATE 6.13   ARTERIES OF UPPER LIMB

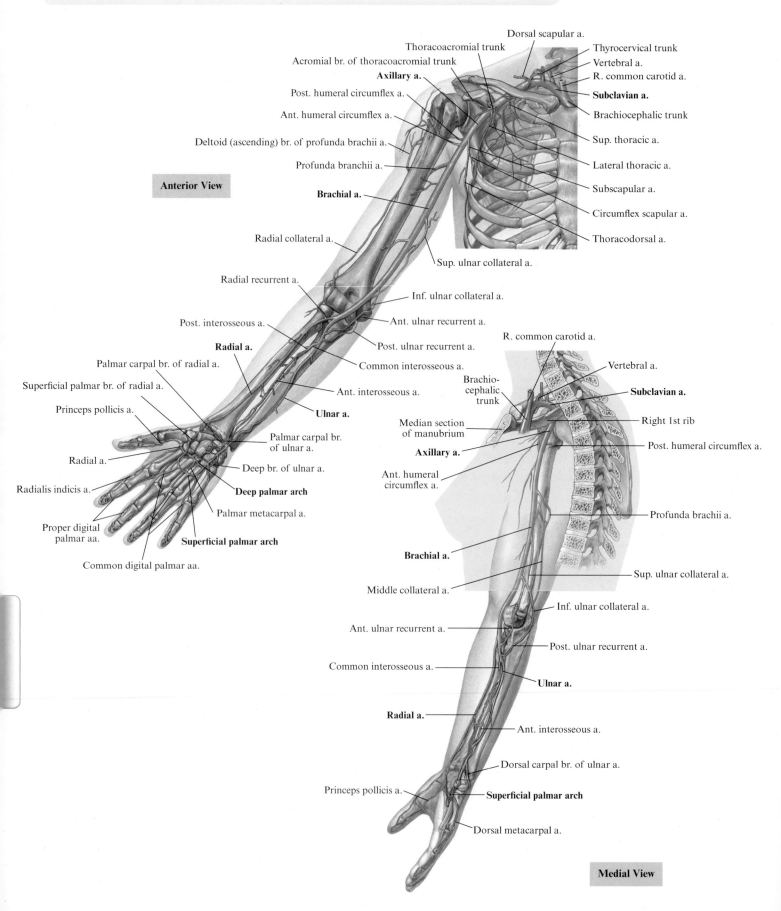

Dorsal scapular a.

Thoracoacromial trunk

Acromial br. of thoracoacromial trunk

Axillary a.

Post. humeral circumflex a.

Ant. humeral circumflex a.

Deltoid (ascending) br. of profunda brachii a.

Profunda branchii a.

Anterior View

Brachial a.

Thyrocervical trunk

Vertebral a.

R. common carotid a.

Subclavian a.

Brachiocephalic trunk

Sup. thoracic a.

Lateral thoracic a.

Subscapular a.

Circumflex scapular a.

Thoracodorsal a.

Radial collateral a.

Radial recurrent a.

Post. interosseous a.

Radial a.

Palmar carpal br. of radial a.

Superficial palmar br. of radial a.

Princeps pollicis a.

Radial a.

Radialis indicis a.

Proper digital palmar aa.

Common digital palmar aa.

Sup. ulnar collateral a.

Inf. ulnar collateral a.

Ant. ulnar recurrent a.

Post. ulnar recurrent a.

Common interosseous a.

Ant. interosseous a.

Ulnar a.

Palmar carpal br. of ulnar a.

Deep br. of ulnar a.

Deep palmar arch

Palmar metacarpal a.

Superficial palmar arch

R. common carotid a.

Vertebral a.

Brachio-cephalic trunk

Subclavian a.

Axillary a.

Median section of manubrium

Ant. humeral circumflex a.

Brachial a.

Middle collateral a.

Ant. ulnar recurrent a.

Common interosseous a.

Radial a.

Princeps pollicis a.

Right 1st rib

Post. humeral circumflex a.

Profunda brachii a.

Sup. ulnar collateral a.

Inf. ulnar collateral a.

Post. ulnar recurrent a.

Ulnar a.

Ant. interosseous a.

Dorsal carpal br. of ulnar a.

Superficial palmar arch

Dorsal metacarpal a.

Medial View

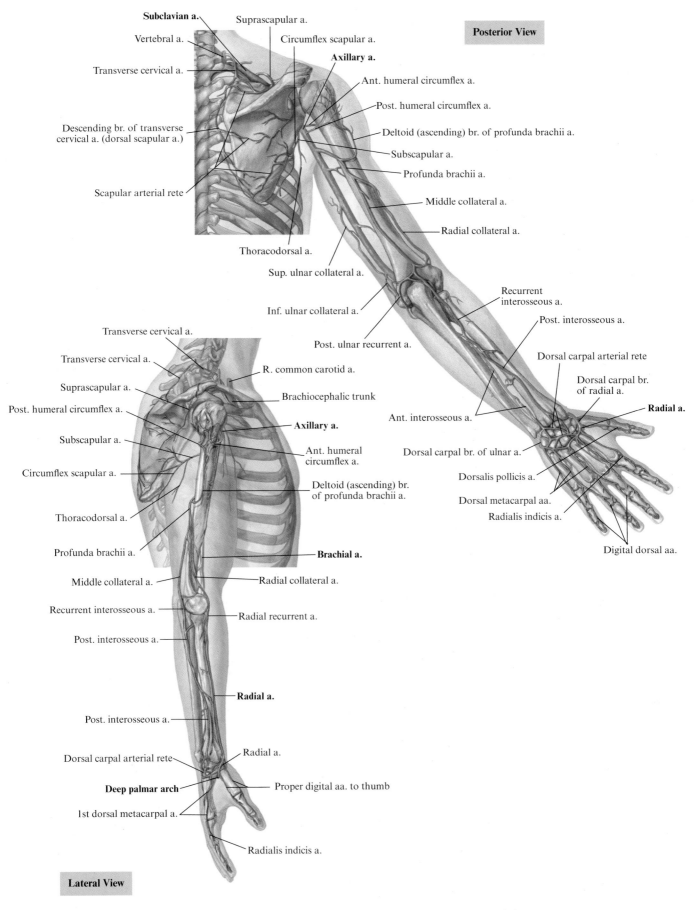

Subclavian a.
Suprascapular a.
Circumflex scapular a.
Vertebral a.
Transverse cervical a.
Axillary a.
Ant. humeral circumflex a.
Post. humeral circumflex a.
Descending br. of transverse cervical a. (dorsal scapular a.)
Deltoid (ascending) br. of profunda brachii a.
Subscapular a.
Profunda brachii a.
Scapular arterial rete
Middle collateral a.
Radial collateral a.
Thoracodorsal a.
Sup. ulnar collateral a.
Recurrent interosseous a.
Inf. ulnar collateral a.
Post. interosseous a.
Post. ulnar recurrent a.
Dorsal carpal arterial rete
Dorsal carpal br. of radial a.
Radial a.
Ant. interosseous a.
Dorsal carpal br. of ulnar a.
Dorsalis pollicis a.
Dorsal metacarpal aa.
Radialis indicis a.
Digital dorsal aa.

Posterior View

Transverse cervical a.
Transverse cervical a.
R. common carotid a.
Suprascapular a.
Brachiocephalic trunk
Post. humeral circumflex a.
Axillary a.
Subscapular a.
Ant. humeral circumflex a.
Circumflex scapular a.
Deltoid (ascending) br. of profunda brachii a.
Thoracodorsal a.
Profunda brachii a.
Brachial a.
Middle collateral a.
Radial collateral a.
Recurrent interosseous a.
Radial recurrent a.
Post. interosseous a.
Radial a.
Post. interosseous a.
Dorsal carpal arterial rete
Radial a.
Deep palmar arch
Proper digital aa. to thumb
1st dorsal metacarpal a.
Radialis indicis a.

Lateral View

PLATE **6.15** VEINS OF UPPER LIMB

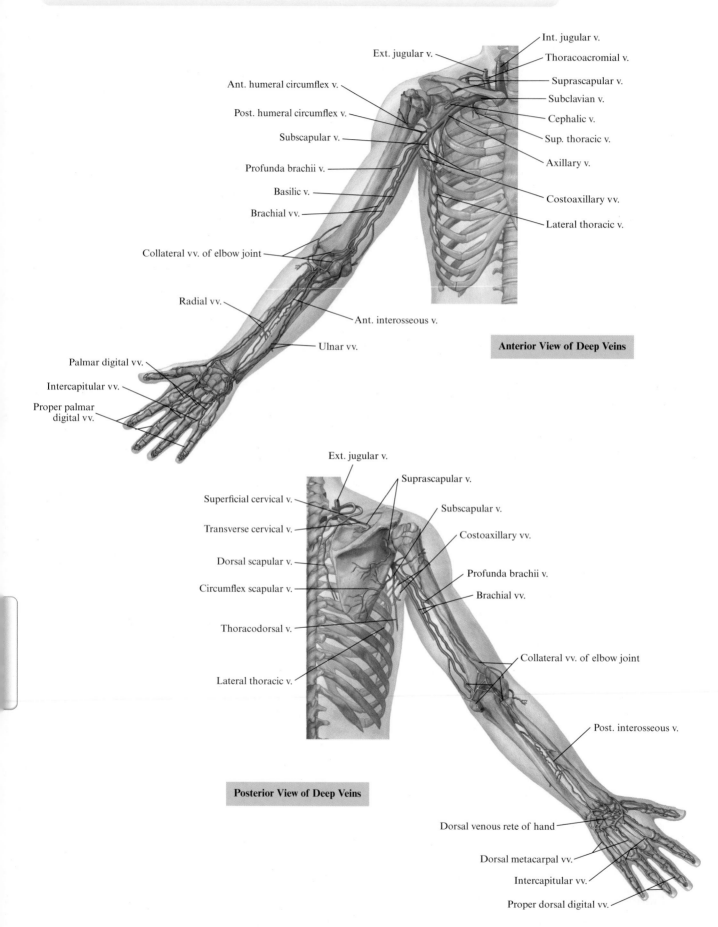

Int. jugular v.

Ext. jugular v.

Thoracoacromial v.

Ant. humeral circumflex v.

Suprascapular v.

Post. humeral circumflex v.

Subclavian v.

Cephalic v.

Subscapular v.

Sup. thoracic v.

Profunda brachii v.

Axillary v.

Basilic v.

Brachial vv.

Costoaxillary vv.

Lateral thoracic v.

Collateral vv. of elbow joint

Radial vv.

Ant. interosseous v.

Ulnar vv.

Palmar digital vv.

Anterior View of Deep Veins

Intercapitular vv.

Proper palmar
digital vv.

Ext. jugular v.

Suprascapular v.

Superficial cervical v.

Subscapular v.

Transverse cervical v.

Costoaxillary vv.

Dorsal scapular v.

Profunda brachii v.

Circumflex scapular v.

Brachial vv.

Thoracodorsal v.

Collateral vv. of elbow joint

Lateral thoracic v.

Post. interosseous v.

Posterior View of Deep Veins

Dorsal venous rete of hand

Dorsal metacarpal vv.

Intercapitular vv.

Proper dorsal digital vv.

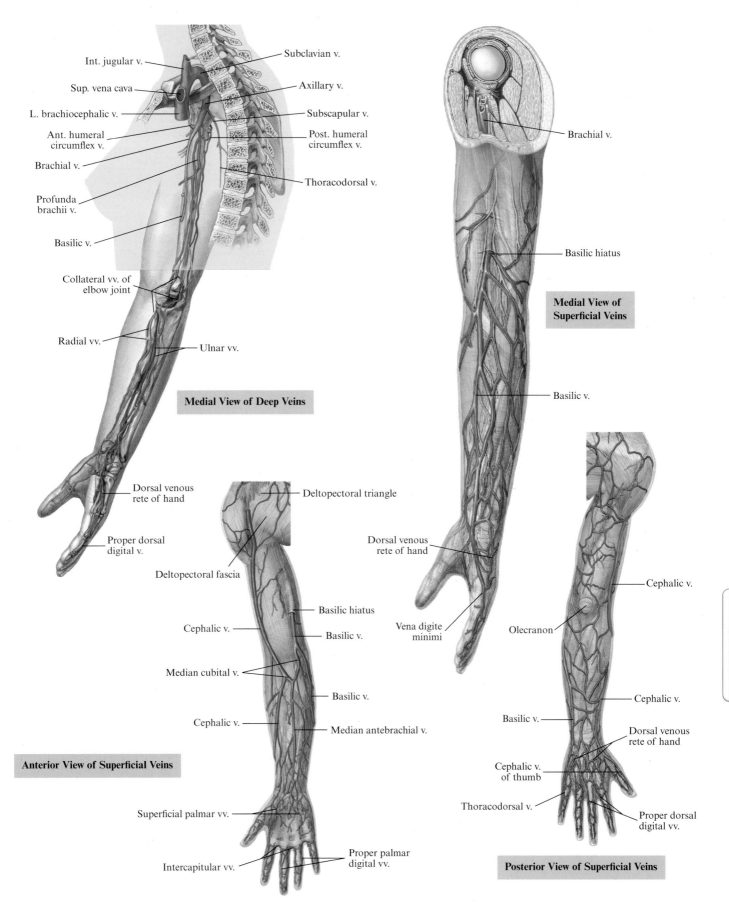

Int. jugular v.

Sup. vena cava

L. brachiocephalic v.

Ant. humeral
circumflex v.

Brachial v.

Profunda
brachii v.

Basilic v.

Collateral vv. of
elbow joint

Radial vv.

Ulnar vv.

Subclavian v.

Axillary v.

Subscapular v.

Post. humeral
circumflex v.

Thoracodorsal v.

Medial View of Deep Veins

Dorsal venous
rete of hand

Proper dorsal
digital v.

Brachial v.

Basilic hiatus

**Medial View of
Superficial Veins**

Basilic v.

Deltopectoral triangle

Deltopectoral fascia

Cephalic v.

Median cubital v.

Cephalic v.

Basilic hiatus

Basilic v.

Basilic v.

Median antebrachial v.

Anterior View of Superficial Veins

Superficial palmar vv.

Intercapitular vv.

Proper palmar
digital vv.

Dorsal venous
rete of hand

Vena digite
minimi

Cephalic v.

Olecranon

Cephalic v.

Basilic v.

Dorsal venous
rete of hand

Cephalic v.
of thumb

Thoracodorsal v.

Proper dorsal
digital vv.

Posterior View of Superficial Veins

PLATE 6.17   DERMATOMES & CUTANEOUS NERVES

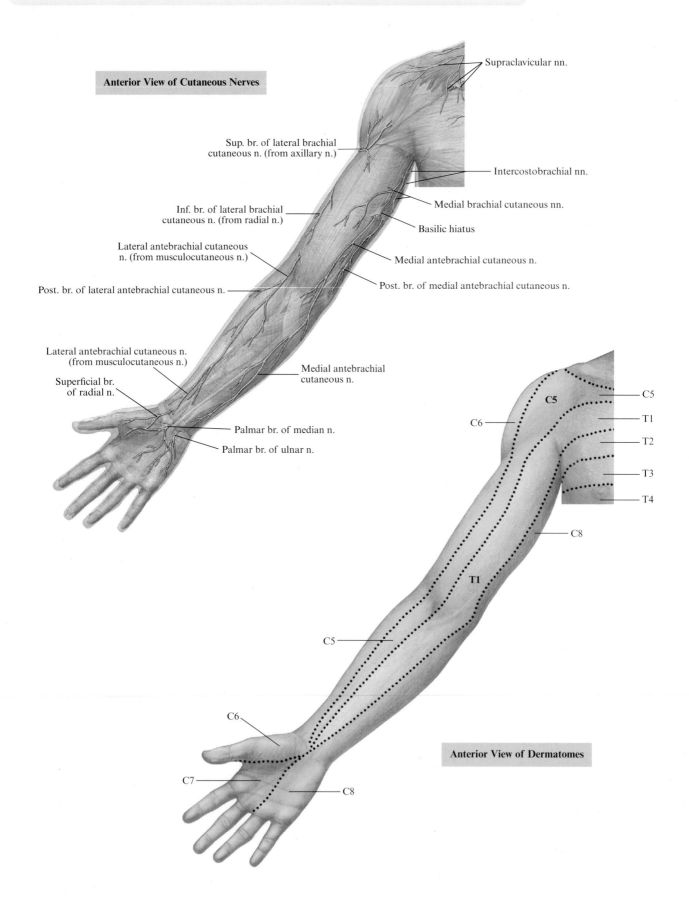

Anterior View of Cutaneous Nerves

Supraclavicular nn.

Sup. br. of lateral brachial cutaneous n. (from axillary n.)

Intercostobrachial nn.

Medial brachial cutaneous nn.

Inf. br. of lateral brachial cutaneous n. (from radial n.)

Basilic hiatus

Lateral antebrachial cutaneous n. (from musculocutaneous n.)

Medial antebrachial cutaneous n.

Post. br. of lateral antebrachial cutaneous n.

Post. br. of medial antebrachial cutaneous n.

Lateral antebrachial cutaneous n. (from musculocutaneous n.)

Medial antebrachial cutaneous n.

Superficial br. of radial n.

Palmar br. of median n.

Palmar br. of ulnar n.

C5

C6

C5

T1

T2

T3

T4

C8

T1

C5

C6

C7

C8

Anterior View of Dermatomes

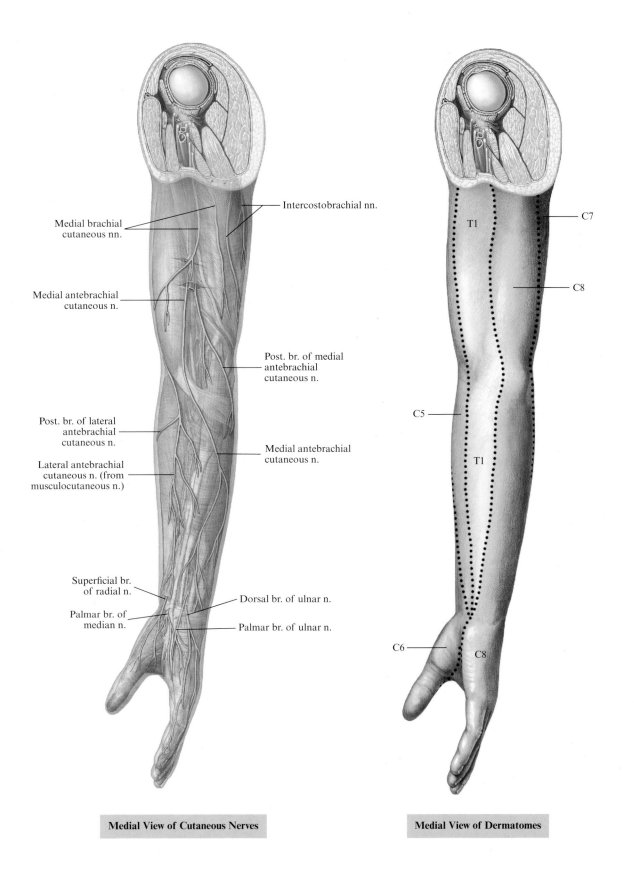

Intercostobrachial nn.

Medial brachial
cutaneous nn.

Medial antebrachial
cutaneous n.

Post. br. of medial
antebrachial
cutaneous n.

Post. br. of lateral
antebrachial
cutaneous n.

Lateral antebrachial
cutaneous n. (from
musculocutaneous n.)

Medial antebrachial
cutaneous n.

Superficial br.
of radial n.

Dorsal br. of ulnar n.

Palmar br. of
median n.

Palmar br. of ulnar n.

Medial View of Cutaneous Nerves

T1

C7

C8

C5

T1

C6

C8

Medial View of Dermatomes

PLATE **6.19**   DERMATOMES & CUTANEOUS NERVES

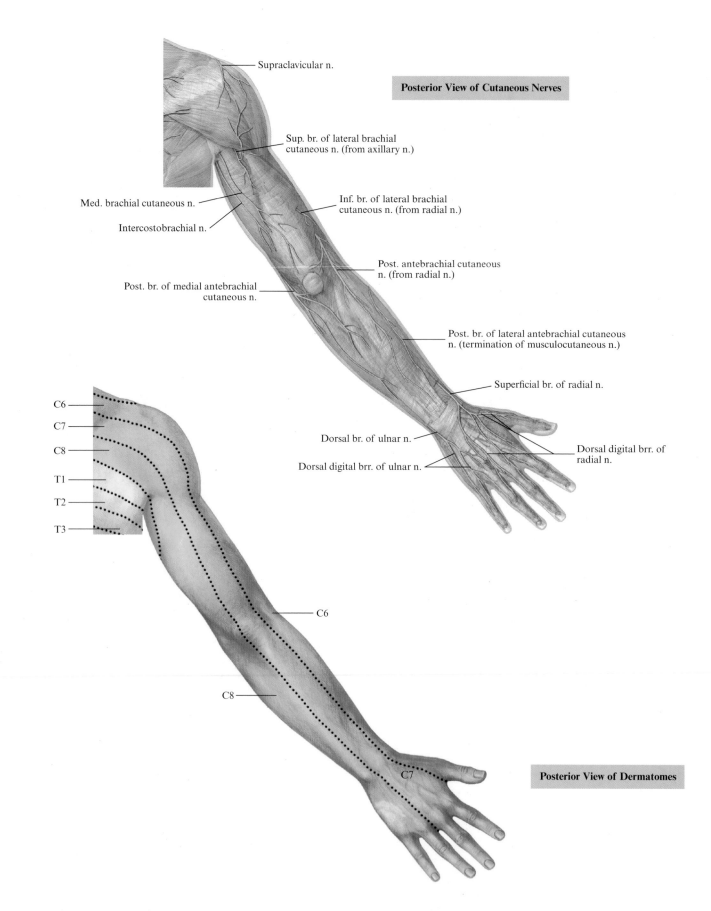

Supraclavicular n.

Posterior View of Cutaneous Nerves

Sup. br. of lateral brachial
cutaneous n. (from axillary n.)

Med. brachial cutaneous n.

Inf. br. of lateral brachial
cutaneous n. (from radial n.)

Intercostobrachial n.

Post. antebrachial cutaneous
n. (from radial n.)

Post. br. of medial antebrachial
cutaneous n.

Post. br. of lateral antebrachial cutaneous
n. (termination of musculocutaneous n.)

Superficial br. of radial n.

Dorsal br. of ulnar n.

Dorsal digital brr. of
radial n.

Dorsal digital brr. of ulnar n.

C6

C7

C8

T1

T2

T3

C6

C8

C7

Posterior View of Dermatomes

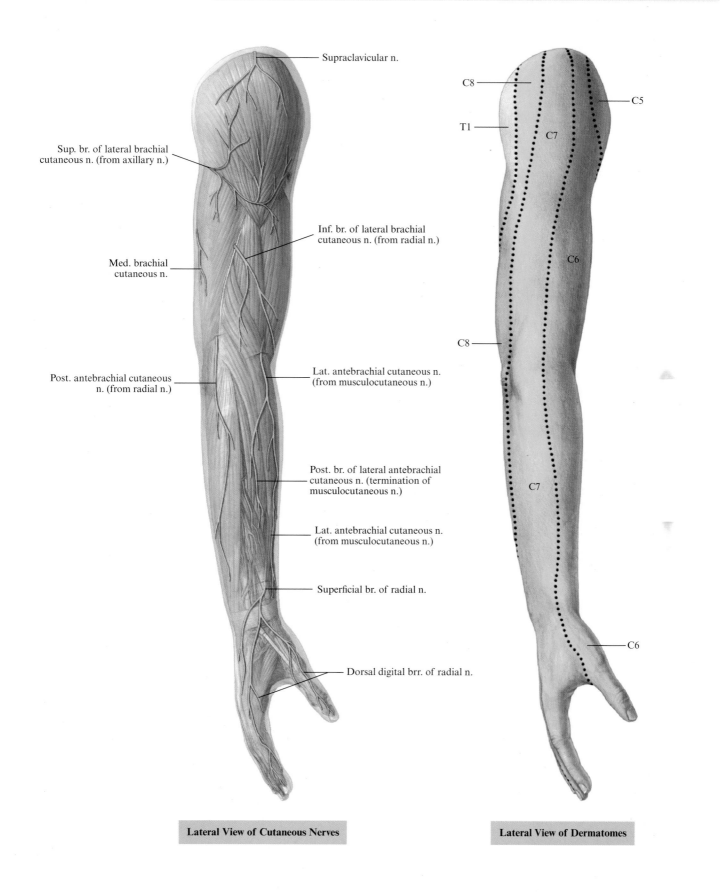

Supraclavicular n.

Sup. br. of lateral brachial
cutaneous n. (from axillary n.)

Inf. br. of lateral brachial
cutaneous n. (from radial n.)

Med. brachial
cutaneous n.

Post. antebrachial cutaneous
n. (from radial n.)

Lat. antebrachial cutaneous n.
(from musculocutaneous n.)

Post. br. of lateral antebrachial
cutaneous n. (termination of
musculocutaneous n.)

Lat. antebrachial cutaneous n.
(from musculocutaneous n.)

Superficial br. of radial n.

Dorsal digital brr. of radial n.

C8

T1

C7

C5

C6

C8

C7

C6

Lateral View of Cutaneous Nerves

Lateral View of Dermatomes

PLATE 6.21   SEGMENTAL INNERVATION OF JOINT ACTIONS

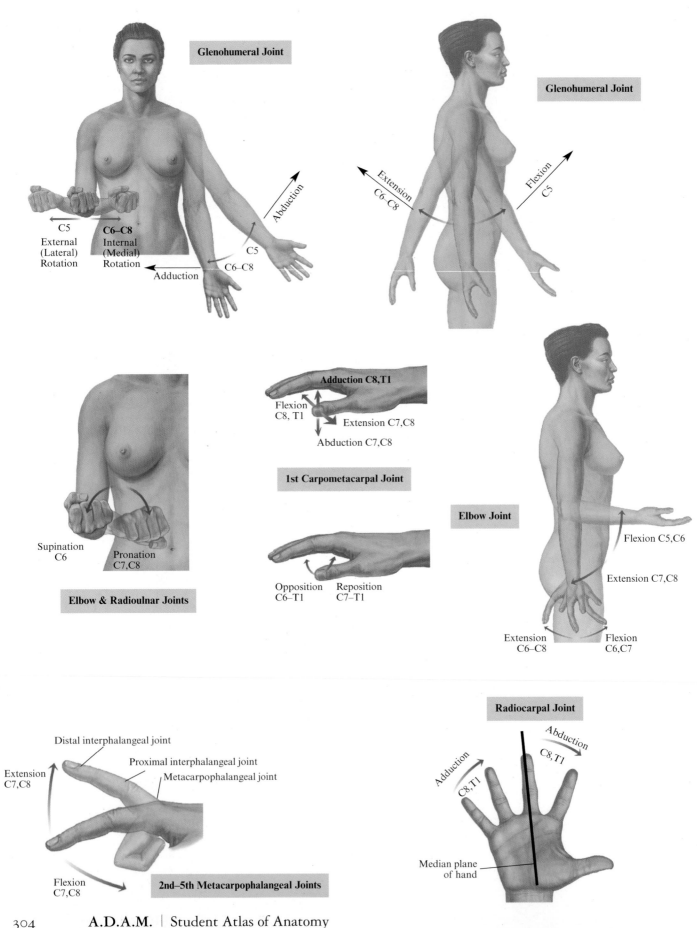

Glenohumeral Joint

Glenohumeral Joint

Abduction

Extension
C6–C8

Flexion
C5

C5
External
(Lateral)
Rotation

C6–C8
Internal
(Medial)
Rotation

C5

C6–C8
Adduction

Adduction C8,T1

Flexion
C8, T1

Extension C7,C8

Abduction C7,C8

1st Carpometacarpal Joint

Elbow Joint

Flexion C5,C6

Extension C7,C8

Supination
C6

Pronation
C7,C8

Opposition
C6–T1

Reposition
C7–T1

Extension
C6–C8

Flexion
C6,C7

Elbow & Radioulnar Joints

Radiocarpal Joint

Distal interphalangeal joint

Proximal interphalangeal joint

Metacarpophalangeal joint

Abduction

Adduction

Extension
C7,C8

C8,T1

C8,T1

Flexion
C7,C8

Median plane
of hand

2nd–5th Metacarpophalangeal Joints

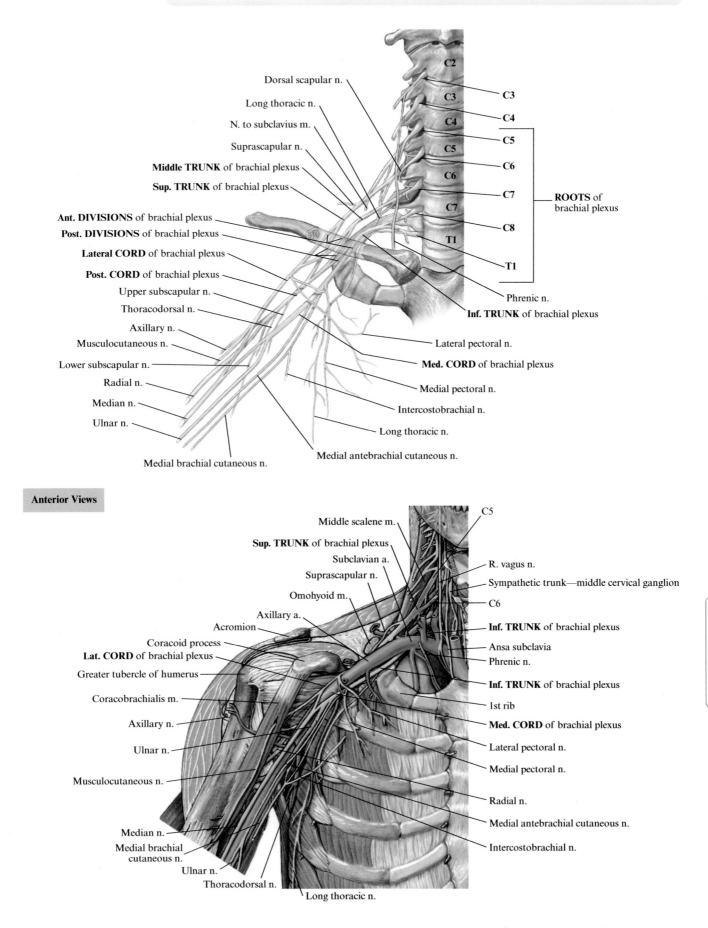

Dorsal scapular n.

Long thoracic n.

N. to subclavius m.

Suprascapular n.

Middle TRUNK of brachial plexus

Sup. TRUNK of brachial plexus

Ant. DIVISIONS of brachial plexus

Post. DIVISIONS of brachial plexus

Lateral CORD of brachial plexus

Post. CORD of brachial plexus

Upper subscapular n.

Thoracodorsal n.

Axillary n.

Musculocutaneous n.

Lower subscapular n.

Radial n.

Median n.

Ulnar n.

Medial brachial cutaneous n.

C2

C3

C4

C5

C6

C7

T1

C3

C4

C5

C6

C7

C8

T1

ROOTS of brachial plexus

Phrenic n.

Inf. TRUNK of brachial plexus

Lateral pectoral n.

Med. CORD of brachial plexus

Medial pectoral n.

Intercostobrachial n.

Long thoracic n.

Medial antebrachial cutaneous n.

Anterior Views

Middle scalene m.

Sup. TRUNK of brachial plexus

Subclavian a.

Suprascapular n.

Omohyoid m.

Axillary a.

Acromion

Lat. CORD of brachial plexus

Greater tubercle of humerus

Coracobrachialis m.

Axillary n.

Ulnar n.

Musculocutaneous n.

Median n.

Medial brachial cutaneous n.

Ulnar n.

Thoracodorsal n.

Long thoracic n.

Coracoid process

C5

R. vagus n.

Sympathetic trunk—middle cervical ganglion

C6

Inf. TRUNK of brachial plexus

Ansa subclavia

Phrenic n.

Inf. TRUNK of brachial plexus

1st rib

Med. CORD of brachial plexus

Lateral pectoral n.

Medial pectoral n.

Radial n.

Medial antebrachial cutaneous n.

Intercostobrachial n.

PLATE **6.23** DEEP NERVES OF UPPER LIMB

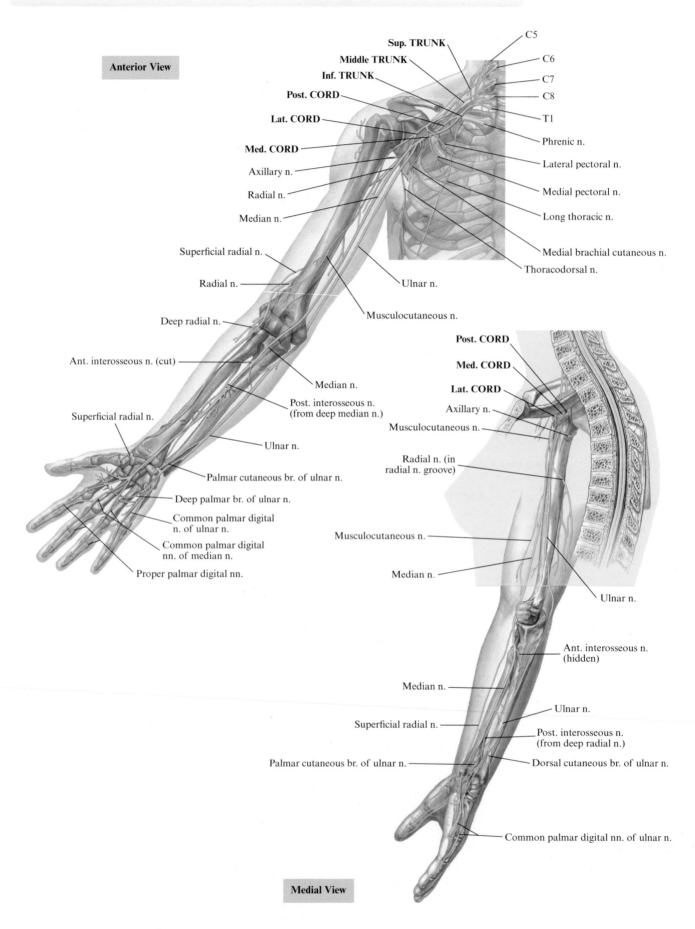

Anterior View

Sup. TRUNK

Middle TRUNK

Inf. TRUNK

Post. CORD

Lat. CORD

Med. CORD

Axillary n.

Radial n.

Median n.

Superficial radial n.

Radial n.

Deep radial n.

Ant. interosseous n. (cut)

Superficial radial n.

Median n.

Post. interosseous n. (from deep median n.)

Ulnar n.

Palmar cutaneous br. of ulnar n.

Deep palmar br. of ulnar n.

Common palmar digital n. of ulnar n.

Common palmar digital nn. of median n.

Proper palmar digital nn.

C5

C6

C7

C8

T1

Phrenic n.

Lateral pectoral n.

Medial pectoral n.

Long thoracic n.

Medial brachial cutaneous n.

Thoracodorsal n.

Ulnar n.

Musculocutaneous n.

Post. CORD

Med. CORD

Lat. CORD

Axillary n.

Musculocutaneous n.

Radial n. (in radial n. groove)

Musculocutaneous n.

Median n.

Ulnar n.

Ant. interosseous n. (hidden)

Median n.

Ulnar n.

Superficial radial n.

Post. interosseous n. (from deep radial n.)

Palmar cutaneous br. of ulnar n.

Dorsal cutaneous br. of ulnar n.

Common palmar digital nn. of ulnar n.

Medial View

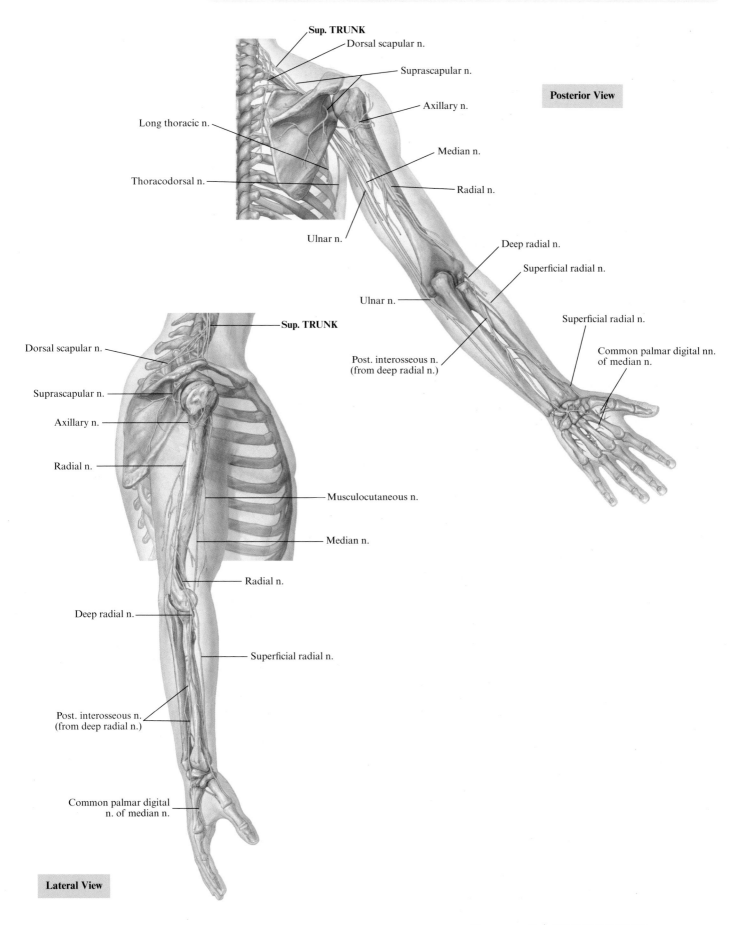

Sup. TRUNK

Dorsal scapular n.

Suprascapular n.

Posterior View

Axillary n.

Long thoracic n.

Median n.

Thoracodorsal n.

Radial n.

Ulnar n.

Deep radial n.

Superficial radial n.

Ulnar n.

Superficial radial n.

Post. interosseous n.
(from deep radial n.)

Common palmar digital nn.
of median n.

Sup. TRUNK

Dorsal scapular n.

Suprascapular n.

Axillary n.

Radial n.

Musculocutaneous n.

Median n.

Radial n.

Deep radial n.

Superficial radial n.

Post. interosseous n.
(from deep radial n.)

Common palmar digital
n. of median n.

Lateral View

PLATE 6.25   SUPERFICIAL & DEEP LYMPHATICS

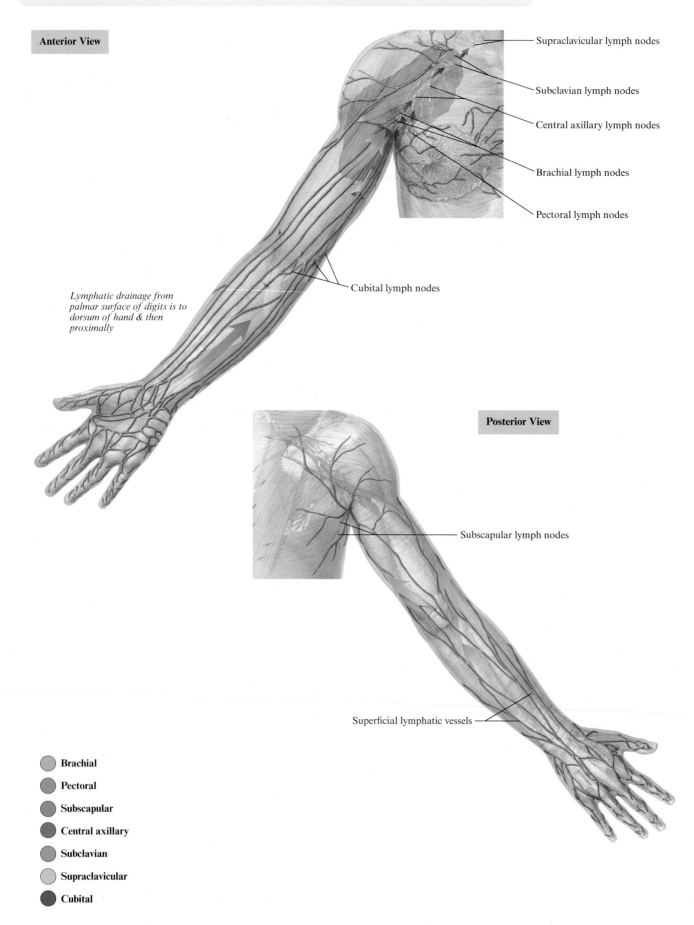

Anterior View

Supraclavicular lymph nodes

Subclavian lymph nodes

Central axillary lymph nodes

Brachial lymph nodes

Pectoral lymph nodes

Cubital lymph nodes

Lymphatic drainage from palmar surface of digits is to dorsum of hand & then proximally

Posterior View

Subscapular lymph nodes

Superficial lymphatic vessels

- Brachial
- Pectoral
- Subscapular
- Central axillary
- Subclavian
- Supraclavicular
- Cubital

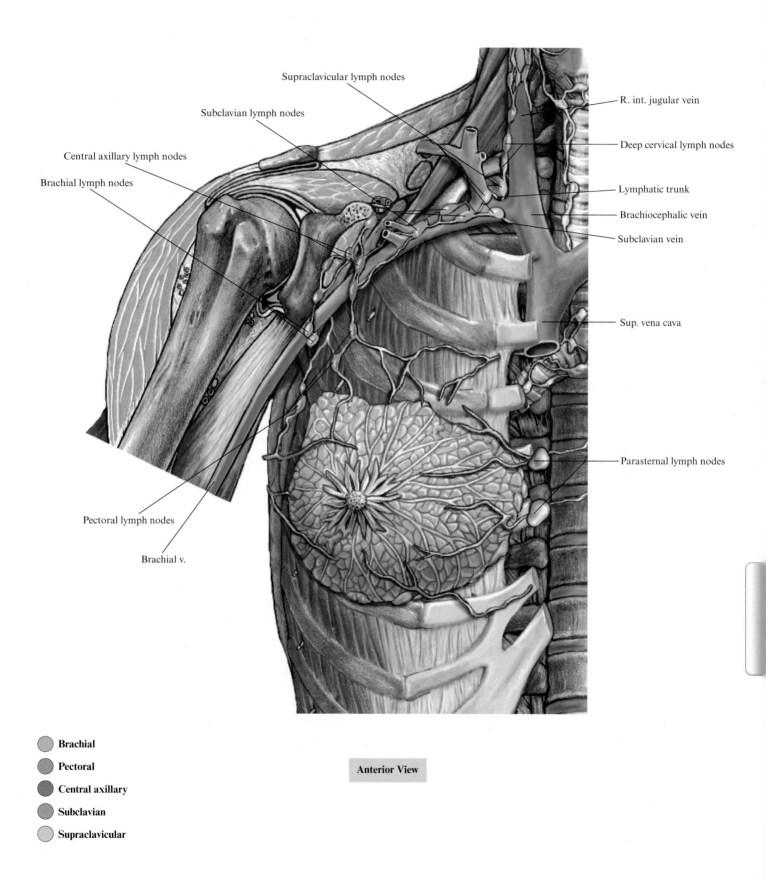

Supraclavicular lymph nodes

Subclavian lymph nodes

Central axillary lymph nodes

Brachial lymph nodes

R. int. jugular vein

Deep cervical lymph nodes

Lymphatic trunk

Brachiocephalic vein

Subclavian vein

Sup. vena cava

Parasternal lymph nodes

Pectoral lymph nodes

Brachial v.

Anterior View

● **Brachial**

● **Pectoral**

● **Central axillary**

● **Subclavian**

● **Supraclavicular**

PLATE 6.27   POSTERIOR SHOULDER MUSCLES

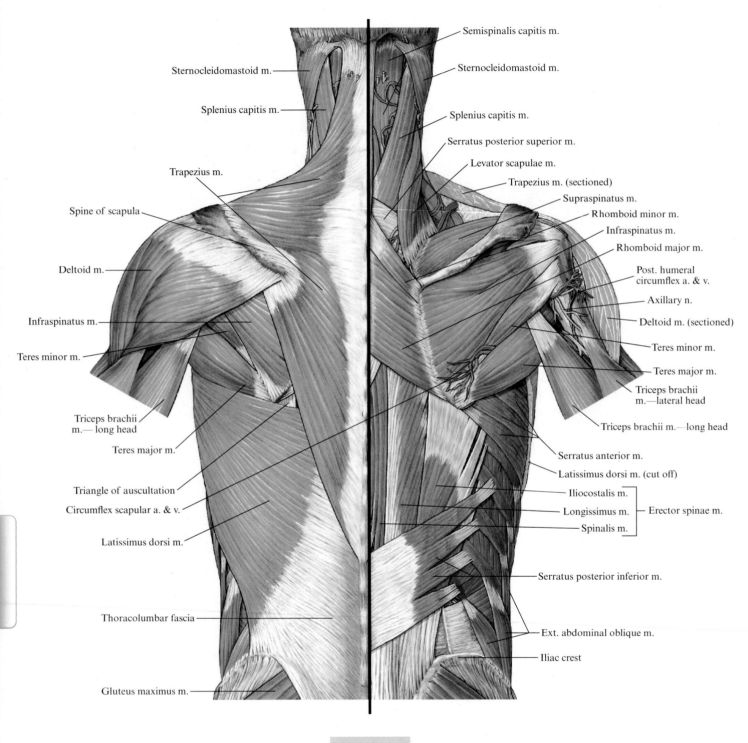

Semispinalis capitis m.

Sternocleidomastoid m.

Splenius capitis m.

Sternocleidomastoid m.

Splenius capitis m.

Serratus posterior superior m.

Levator scapulae m.

Trapezius m.

Trapezius m. (sectioned)

Spine of scapula

Supraspinatus m.

Rhomboid minor m.

Infraspinatus m.

Rhomboid major m.

Deltoid m.

Post. humeral circumflex a. & v.

Axillary n.

Infraspinatus m.

Deltoid m. (sectioned)

Teres minor m.

Teres minor m.

Teres major m.

Triceps brachii m.—lateral head

Triceps brachii m.— long head

Triceps brachii m.— long head

Teres major m.

Serratus anterior m.

Latissimus dorsi m. (cut off)

Triangle of auscultation

Iliocostalis m.

Circumflex scapular a. & v.

Longissimus m.

Erector spinae m.

Spinalis m.

Latissimus dorsi m.

Serratus posterior inferior m.

Thoracolumbar fascia

Ext. abdominal oblique m.

Iliac crest

Gluteus maximus m.

Posterior View

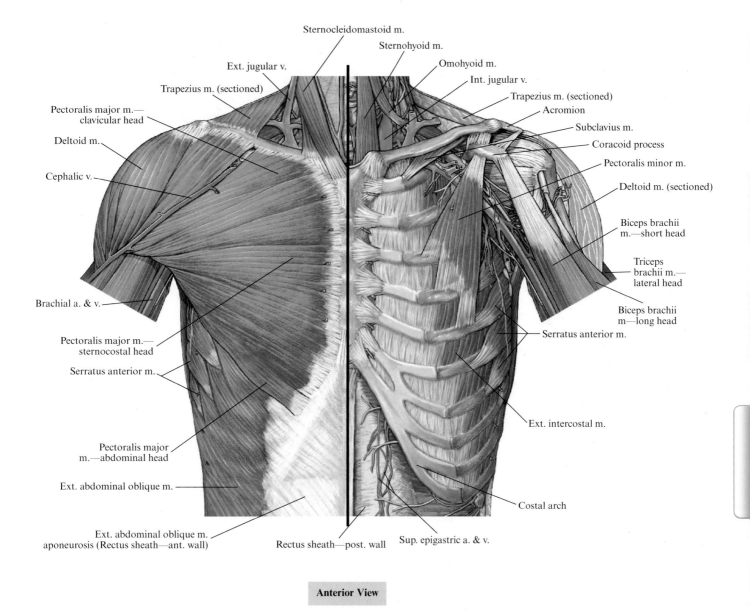

Sternocleidomastoid m.

Sternohyoid m.

Ext. jugular v.

Omohyoid m.

Trapezius m. (sectioned)

Int. jugular v.

Pectoralis major m.—
clavicular head

Trapezius m. (sectioned)

Acromion

Deltoid m.

Subclavius m.

Coracoid process

Cephalic v.

Pectoralis minor m.

Deltoid m. (sectioned)

Biceps brachii
m.—short head

Triceps
brachii m.—
lateral head

Brachial a. & v.

Biceps brachii
m—long head

Pectoralis major m.—
sternocostal head

Serratus anterior m.

Serratus anterior m.

Pectoralis major
m.—abdominal head

Ext. intercostal m.

Ext. abdominal oblique m.

Costal arch

Ext. abdominal oblique m.
aponeurosis (Rectus sheath—ant. wall)

Rectus sheath—post. wall

Sup. epigastric a. & v.

Anterior View

PLATE 6.29 **AXILLA—VASCULATURE**

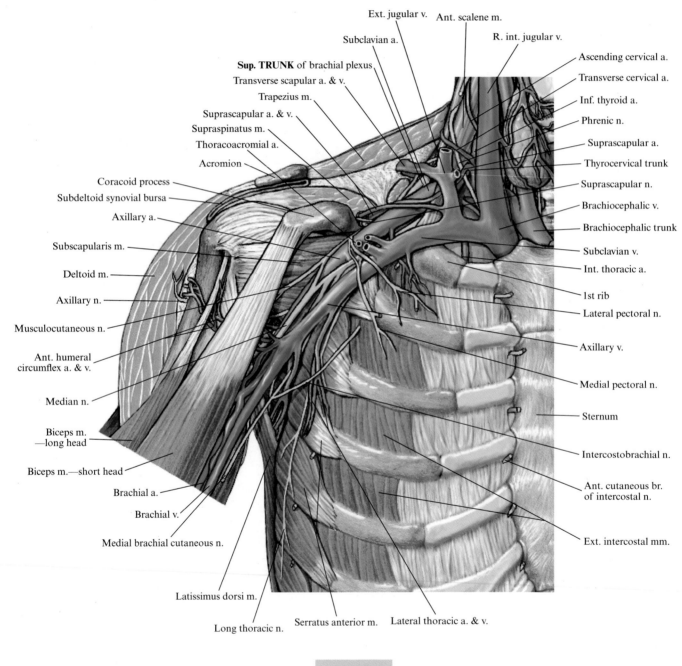

Ext. jugular v. Ant. scalene m.

Subclavian a.

R. int. jugular v.

Sup. TRUNK of brachial plexus

Transverse scapular a. & v.

Trapezius m.

Suprascapular a. & v.

Supraspinatus m.

Thoracoacromial a.

Acromion

Coracoid process

Subdeltoid synovial bursa

Axillary a.

Subscapularis m.

Deltoid m.

Axillary n.

Musculocutaneous n.

Ant. humeral
circumflex a. & v.

Median n.

Biceps m.
—long head

Biceps m.—short head

Brachial a.

Brachial v.

Medial brachial cutaneous n.

Latissimus dorsi m.

Long thoracic n.

Serratus anterior m. Lateral thoracic a. & v.

Ascending cervical a.

Transverse cervical a.

Inf. thyroid a.

Phrenic n.

Suprascapular a.

Thyrocervical trunk

Suprascapular n.

Brachiocephalic v.

Brachiocephalic trunk

Subclavian v.

Int. thoracic a.

1st rib

Lateral pectoral n.

Axillary v.

Medial pectoral n.

Sternum

Intercostobrachial n.

Ant. cutaneous br.
of intercostal n.

Ext. intercostal mm.

Anterior View

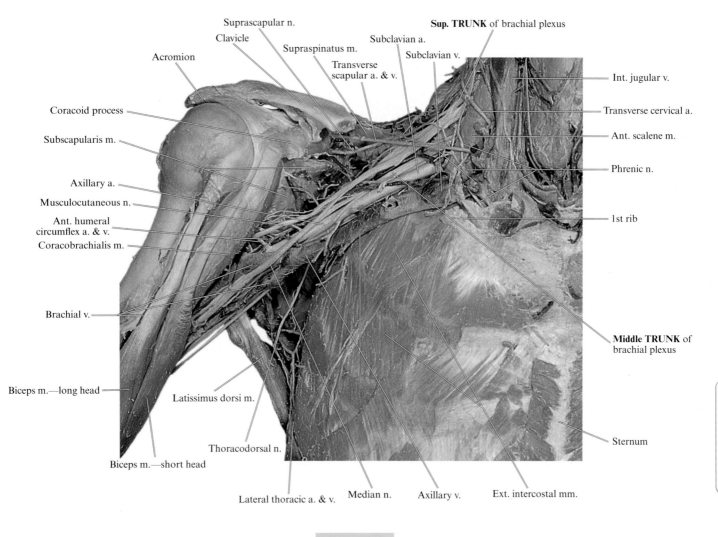

Suprascapular n.

Clavicle

Supraspinatus m.

Acromion

Transverse
scapular a. & v.

Subclavian a.

Subclavian v.

Sup. TRUNK of brachial plexus

Coracoid process

Int. jugular v.

Transverse cervical a.

Subscapularis m.

Ant. scalene m.

Axillary a.

Phrenic n.

Musculocutaneous n.

Ant. humeral
circumflex a. & v.

1st rib

Coracobrachialis m.

Brachial v.

Middle TRUNK of
brachial plexus

Biceps m.—long head

Latissimus dorsi m.

Biceps m.—short head

Sternum

Thoracodorsal n.

Lateral thoracic a. & v.   Median n.   Axillary v.   Ext. intercostal mm.

Anterior View

PLATE 6.31   AXILLA—BRACHIAL PLEXUS

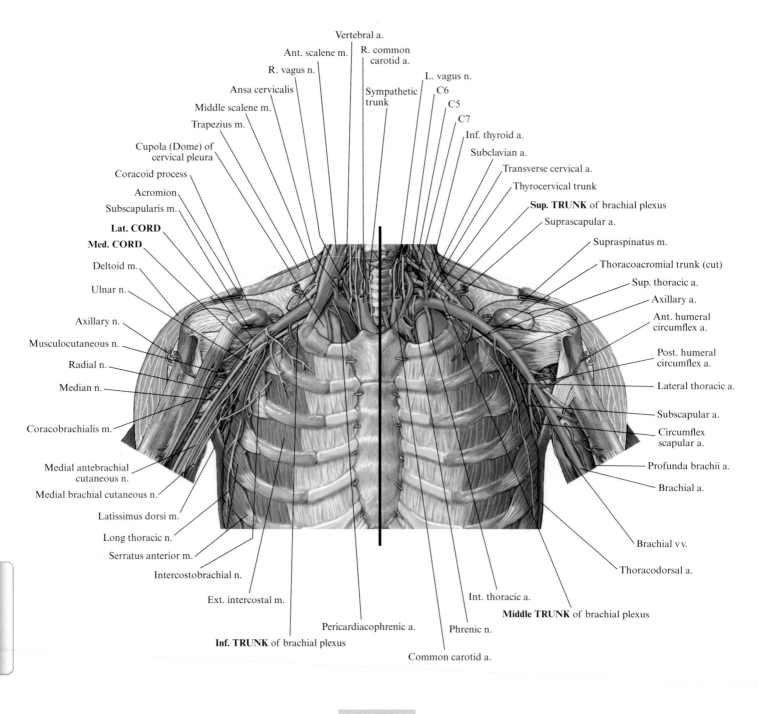

Vertebral a.
Ant. scalene m.
R. common carotid a.
R. vagus n.
Ansa cervicalis
L. vagus n.
Middle scalene m.
Sympathetic trunk
C6
Trapezius m.
C5
C7
Cupola (Dome) of cervical pleura
Inf. thyroid a.
Coracoid process
Subclavian a.
Acromion
Transverse cervical a.
Subscapularis m.
Thyrocervical trunk
Lat. CORD
Sup. TRUNK of brachial plexus
Med. CORD
Suprascapular a.
Deltoid m.
Supraspinatus m.
Ulnar n.
Thoracoacromial trunk (cut)
Sup. thoracic a.
Axillary n.
Axillary a.
Musculocutaneous n.
Ant. humeral circumflex a.
Radial n.
Post. humeral circumflex a.
Median n.
Lateral thoracic a.
Coracobrachialis m.
Subscapular a.
Circumflex scapular a.
Medial antebrachial cutaneous n.
Profunda brachii a.
Medial brachial cutaneous n.
Brachial a.
Latissimus dorsi m.
Long thoracic n.
Serratus anterior m.
Brachial vv.
Intercostobrachial n.
Thoracodorsal a.
Ext. intercostal m.
Middle TRUNK of brachial plexus
Pericardiacophrenic a.
Phrenic n.
Int. thoracic a.
Inf. TRUNK of brachial plexus
Common carotid a.

Anterior View

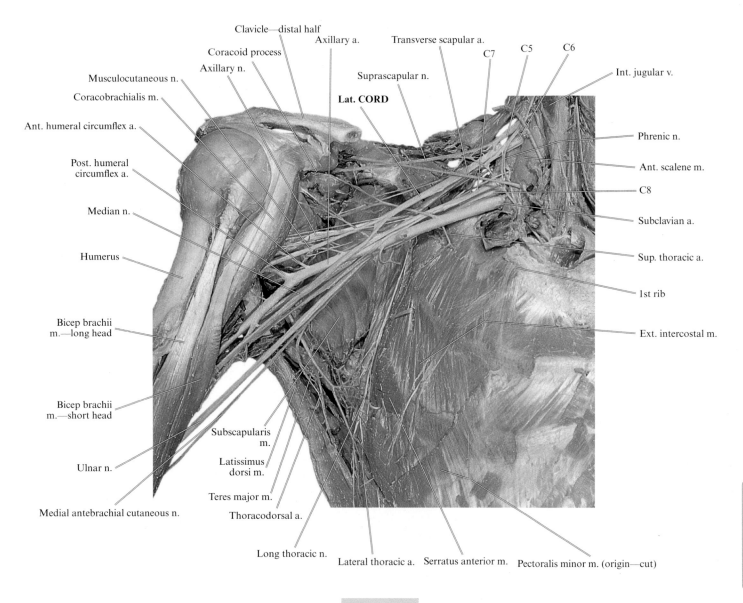

Clavicle—distal half

Coracoid process

Axillary n.

Axillary a.

Transverse scapular a.

C7

C5

C6

Suprascapular n.

Int. jugular v.

Musculocutaneous n.

Lat. CORD

Coracobrachialis m.

Phrenic n.

Ant. humeral circumflex a.

Ant. scalene m.

Post. humeral circumflex a.

C8

Median n.

Subclavian a.

Humerus

Sup. thoracic a.

1st rib

Bicep brachii m.—long head

Ext. intercostal m.

Bicep brachii m.—short head

Subscapularis m.

Ulnar n.

Latissimus dorsi m.

Medial antebrachial cutaneous n.

Teres major m.

Thoracodorsal a.

Long thoracic n.

Lateral thoracic a.

Serratus anterior m.

Pectoralis minor m. (origin—cut)

Anterior View

PLATE 6.33   ROTATOR CUFF MUSCLES

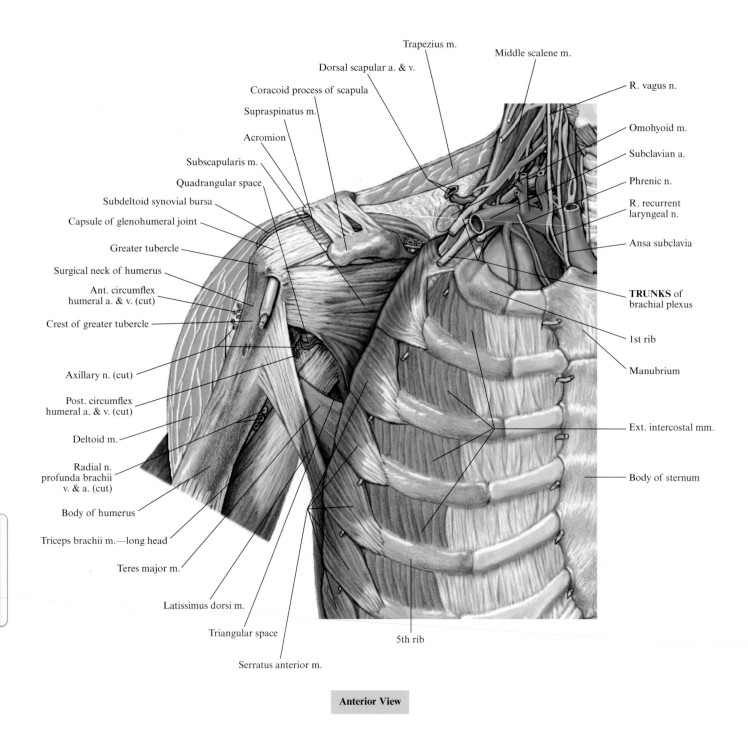

Trapezius m.

Middle scalene m.

Dorsal scapular a. & v.

Coracoid process of scapula

R. vagus n.

Supraspinatus m.

Omohyoid m.

Acromion

Subclavian a.

Subscapularis m.

Phrenic n.

Quadrangular space

R. recurrent
laryngeal n.

Subdeltoid synovial bursa

Capsule of glenohumeral joint

Ansa subclavia

Greater tubercle

Surgical neck of humerus

TRUNKS of
brachial plexus

Ant. circumflex
humeral a. & v. (cut)

Crest of greater tubercle

1st rib

Manubrium

Axillary n. (cut)

Post. circumflex
humeral a. & v. (cut)

Deltoid m.

Ext. intercostal mm.

Radial n.
profunda brachii
v. & a. (cut)

Body of humerus

Body of sternum

Triceps brachii m.—long head

Teres major m.

Latissimus dorsi m.

Triangular space

5th rib

Serratus anterior m.

Anterior View

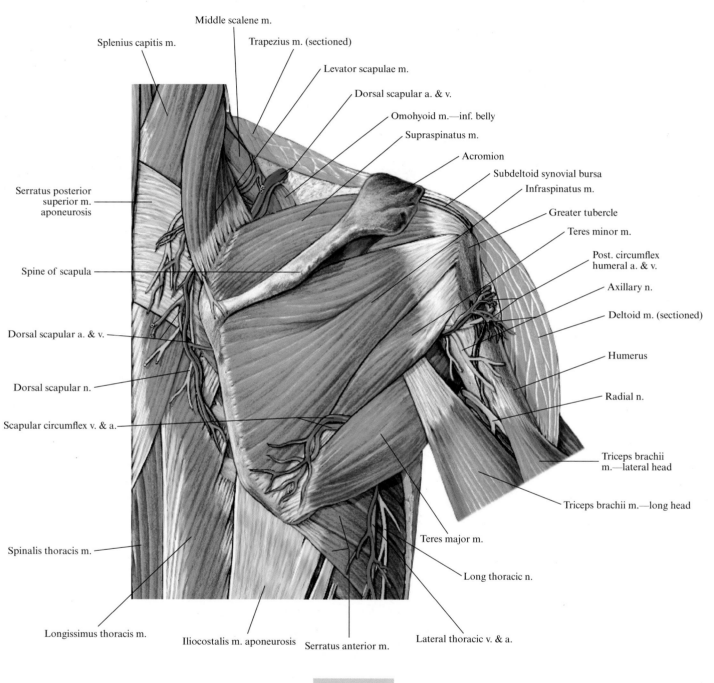

Middle scalene m.

Splenius capitis m.

Trapezius m. (sectioned)

Levator scapulae m.

Dorsal scapular a. & v.

Omohyoid m.—inf. belly

Supraspinatus m.

Acromion

Subdeltoid synovial bursa

Infraspinatus m.

Serratus posterior
superior m.
aponeurosis

Greater tubercle

Teres minor m.

Spine of scapula

Post. circumflex
humeral a. & v.

Axillary n.

Dorsal scapular a. & v.

Deltoid m. (sectioned)

Humerus

Dorsal scapular n.

Radial n.

Scapular circumflex v. & a.

Triceps brachii
m.—lateral head

Triceps brachii m.—long head

Spinalis thoracis m.

Teres major m.

Long thoracic n.

Longissimus thoracis m.

Iliocostalis m. aponeurosis   Serratus anterior m.

Lateral thoracic v. & a.

Posterior View

PLATE 6.35   SHOULDER—CORONAL SECTION

Medial View of Sagittally Sectioned Axilla

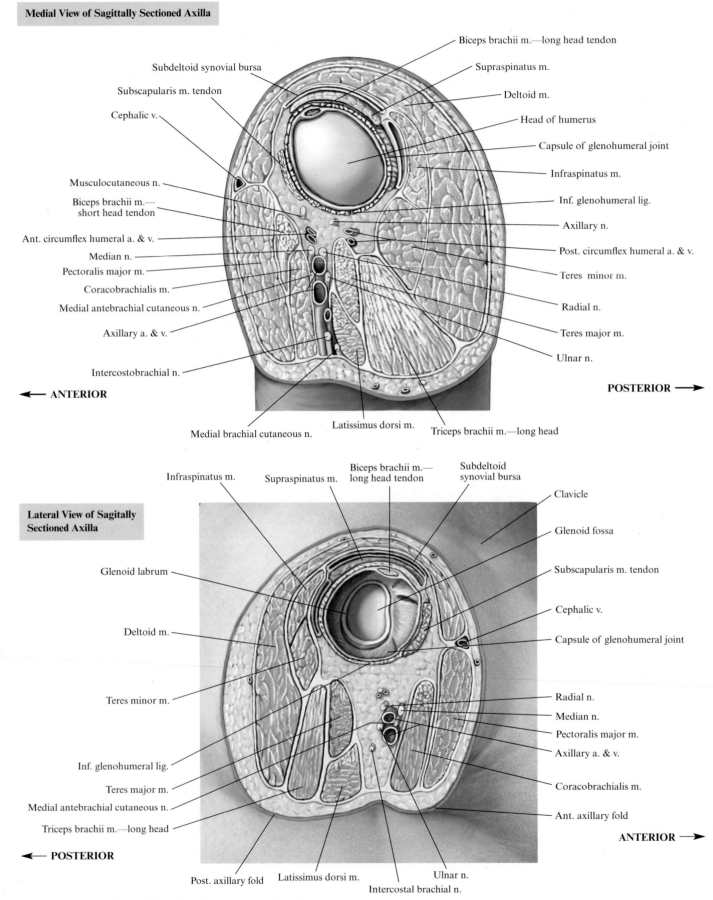

Biceps brachii m.—long head tendon

Subdeltoid synovial bursa

Supraspinatus m.

Subscapularis m. tendon

Deltoid m.

Cephalic v.

Head of humerus

Capsule of glenohumeral joint

Infraspinatus m.

Musculocutaneous n.

Inf. glenohumeral lig.

Biceps brachii m.—
short head tendon

Axillary n.

Ant. circumflex humeral a. & v.

Post. circumflex humeral a. & v.

Median n.

Pectoralis major m.

Teres minor m.

Coracobrachialis m.

Radial n.

Medial antebrachial cutaneous n.

Teres major m.

Axillary a. & v.

Ulnar n.

Intercostobrachial n.

← ANTERIOR   POSTERIOR →

Medial brachial cutaneous n.

Latissimus dorsi m.

Triceps brachii m.—long head

**Lateral View of Sagittally
Sectioned Axilla**

Infraspinatus m.

Supraspinatus m.

Biceps brachii m.—
long head tendon

Subdeltoid
synovial bursa

Clavicle

Glenoid fossa

Glenoid labrum

Subscapularis m. tendon

Deltoid m.

Cephalic v.

Capsule of glenohumeral joint

Teres minor m.

Radial n.

Median n.

Pectoralis major m.

Axillary a. & v.

Inf. glenohumeral lig.

Teres major m.

Coracobrachialis m.

Medial antebrachial cutaneous n.

Triceps brachii m.—long head

Ant. axillary fold

← POSTERIOR   ANTERIOR →

Post. axillary fold

Latissimus dorsi m.

Ulnar n.

Intercostal brachial n.

 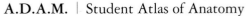

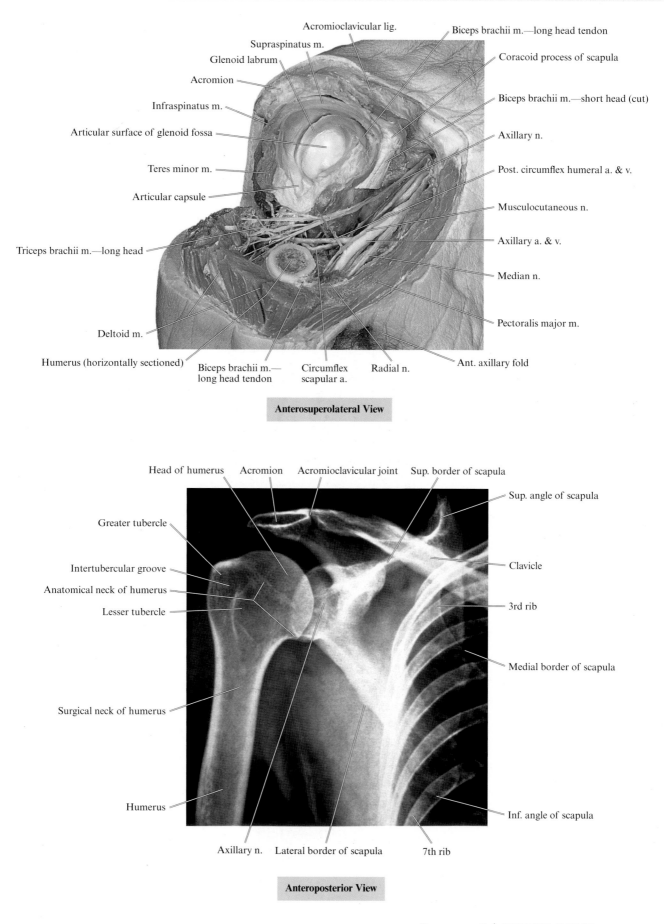

Acromioclavicular lig.

Supraspinatus m.

Biceps brachii m.—long head tendon

Glenoid labrum

Coracoid process of scapula

Acromion

Infraspinatus m.

Biceps brachii m.—short head (cut)

Articular surface of glenoid fossa

Axillary n.

Teres minor m.

Post. circumflex humeral a. & v.

Articular capsule

Musculocutaneous n.

Triceps brachii m.—long head

Axillary a. & v.

Median n.

Deltoid m.

Pectoralis major m.

Humerus (horizontally sectioned)

Biceps brachii m.—long head tendon

Circumflex scapular a.

Radial n.

Ant. axillary fold

Anterosuperolateral View

Head of humerus   Acromion   Acromioclavicular joint   Sup. border of scapula

Sup. angle of scapula

Greater tubercle

Intertubercular groove

Clavicle

Anatomical neck of humerus

3rd rib

Lesser tubercle

Medial border of scapula

Surgical neck of humerus

Humerus

Inf. angle of scapula

Axillary n.   Lateral border of scapula   7th rib

Anteroposterior View

PLATE 6.37   ANTEROMEDIAL ARM

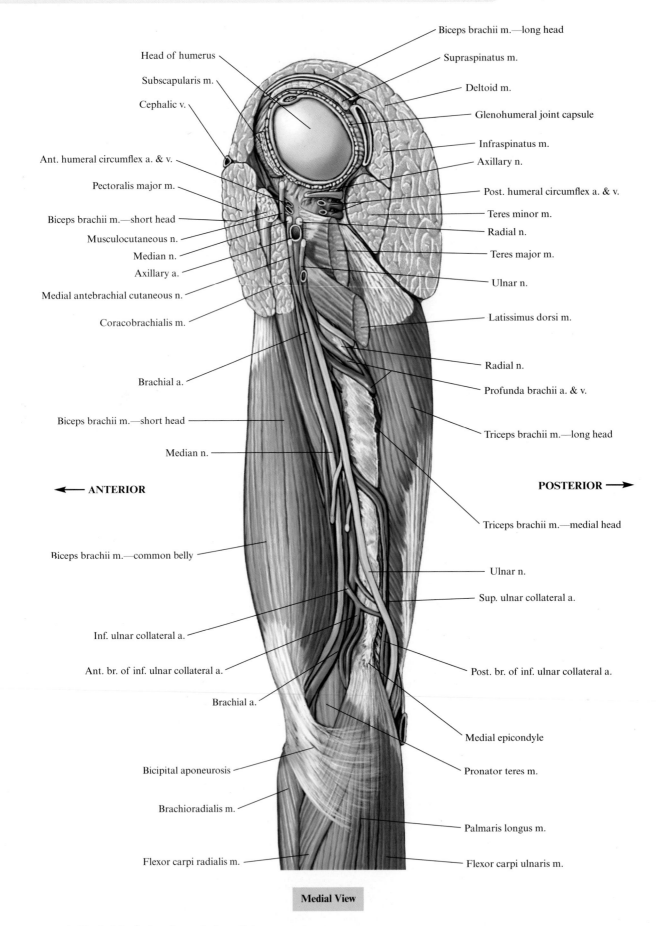

Head of humerus

Subscapularis m.

Cephalic v.

Ant. humeral circumflex a. & v.

Pectoralis major m.

Biceps brachii m.—short head

Musculocutaneous n.

Median n.

Axillary a.

Medial antebrachial cutaneous n.

Coracobrachialis m.

Brachial a.

Biceps brachii m.—short head

Median n.

← ANTERIOR

Biceps brachii m.—common belly

Inf. ulnar collateral a.

Ant. br. of inf. ulnar collateral a.

Brachial a.

Bicipital aponeurosis

Brachioradialis m.

Flexor carpi radialis m.

Biceps brachii m.—long head

Supraspinatus m.

Deltoid m.

Glenohumeral joint capsule

Infraspinatus m.

Axillary n.

Post. humeral circumflex a. & v.

Teres minor m.

Radial n.

Teres major m.

Ulnar n.

Latissimus dorsi m.

Radial n.

Profunda brachii a. & v.

Triceps brachii m.—long head

POSTERIOR →

Triceps brachii m.—medial head

Ulnar n.

Sup. ulnar collateral a.

Post. br. of inf. ulnar collateral a.

Medial epicondyle

Pronator teres m.

Palmaris longus m.

Flexor carpi ulnaris m.

Medial View

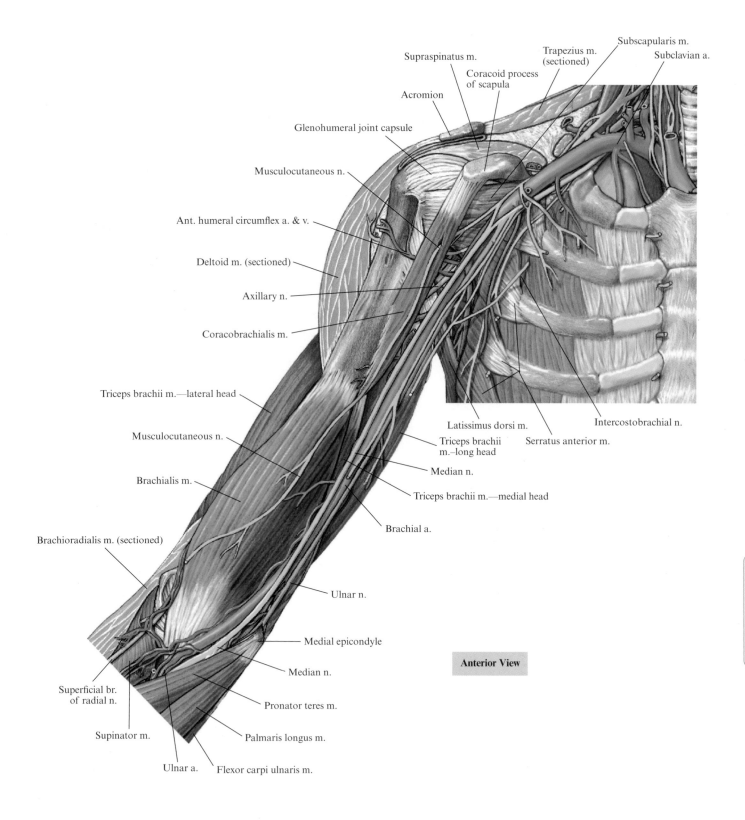

Supraspinatus m.

Coracoid process
of scapula

Trapezius m.
(sectioned)

Subscapularis m.

Subclavian a.

Acromion

Glenohumeral joint capsule

Musculocutaneous n.

Ant. humeral circumflex a. & v.

Deltoid m. (sectioned)

Axillary n.

Coracobrachialis m.

Triceps brachii m.—lateral head

Musculocutaneous n.

Brachialis m.

Brachioradialis m. (sectioned)

Superficial br.
of radial n.

Supinator m.

Ulnar a.

Flexor carpi ulnaris m.

Palmaris longus m.

Pronator teres m.

Median n.

Medial epicondyle

Ulnar n.

Brachial a.

Triceps brachii m.—medial head

Median n.

Triceps brachii
m.–long head

Latissimus dorsi m.

Serratus anterior m.

Intercostobrachial n.

Anterior View

PLATE 6.39   ANTERIOR ARM

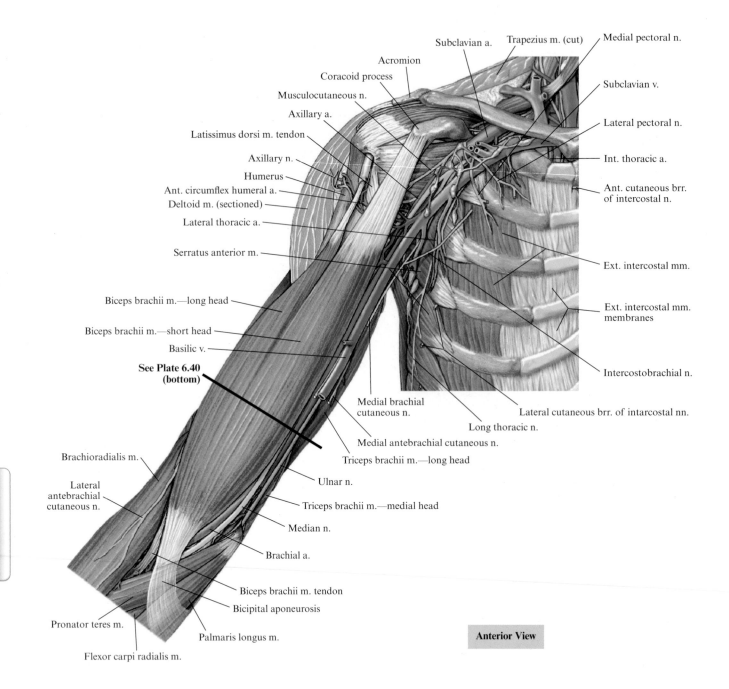

Subclavian a.

Trapezius m. (cut)

Medial pectoral n.

Acromion

Coracoid process

Musculocutaneous n.

Axillary a.

Latissimus dorsi m. tendon

Subclavian v.

Lateral pectoral n.

Int. thoracic a.

Ant. cutaneous brr.
of intercostal n.

Axillary n.

Humerus

Ant. circumflex humeral a.

Deltoid m. (sectioned)

Lateral thoracic a.

Serratus anterior m.

Ext. intercostal mm.

Biceps brachii m.—long head

Ext. intercostal mm.
membranes

Biceps brachii m.—short head

Basilic v.

**See Plate 6.40
(bottom)**

Intercostobrachial n.

Medial brachial
cutaneous n.

Lateral cutaneous brr. of intarcostal nn.

Long thoracic n.

Medial antebrachial cutaneous n.

Brachioradialis m.

Triceps brachii m.—long head

Lateral
antebrachial
cutaneous n.

Ulnar n.

Triceps brachii m.—medial head

Median n.

Brachial a.

Biceps brachii m. tendon

Bicipital aponeurosis

Anterior View

Pronator teres m.

Palmaris longus m.

Flexor carpi radialis m.

Anterior View

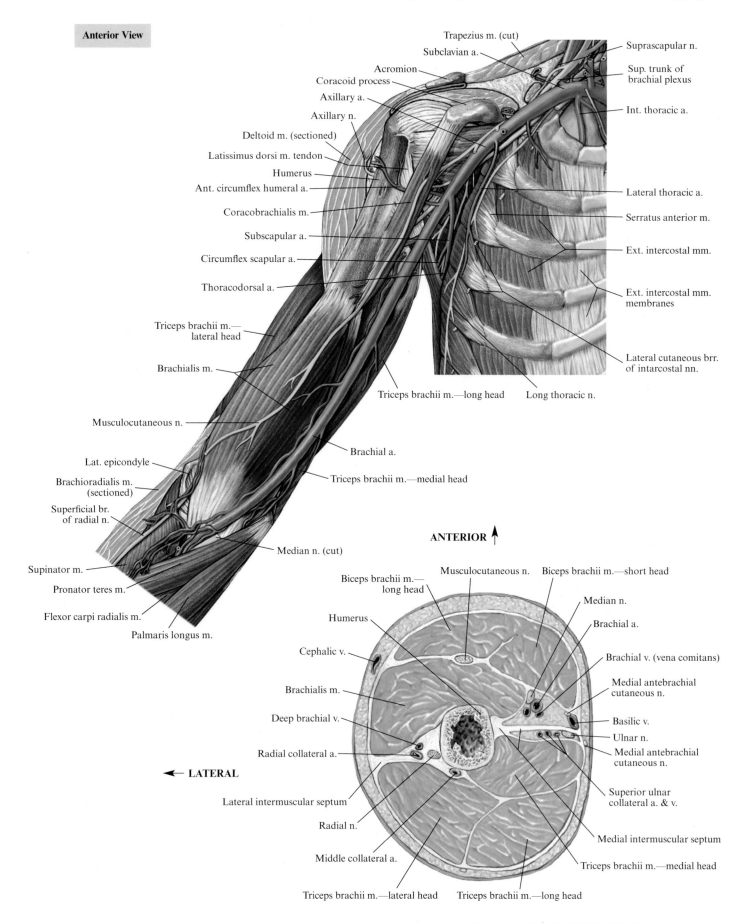

Trapezius m. (cut)

Subclavian a.

Acromion

Coracoid process

Axillary a.

Axillary n.

Deltoid m. (sectioned)

Latissimus dorsi m. tendon

Humerus

Ant. circumflex humeral a.

Coracobrachialis m.

Subscapular a.

Circumflex scapular a.

Thoracodorsal a.

Triceps brachii m.—
lateral head

Brachialis m.

Musculocutaneous n.

Lat. epicondyle

Brachioradialis m.
(sectioned)

Superficial br.
of radial n.

Supinator m.

Pronator teres m.

Flexor carpi radialis m.

Palmaris longus m.

Suprascapular n.

Sup. trunk of
brachial plexus

Int. thoracic a.

Lateral thoracic a.

Serratus anterior m.

Ext. intercostal mm.

Ext. intercostal mm.
membranes

Lateral cutaneous brr.
of intarcostal nn.

Triceps brachii m.—long head

Long thoracic n.

Brachial a.

Triceps brachii m.—medial head

Median n. (cut)

ANTERIOR ↑

Biceps brachii m.—
long head

Musculocutaneous n.

Biceps brachii m.—short head

Humerus

Median n.

Brachial a.

Cephalic v.

Brachial v. (vena comitans)

Brachialis m.

Medial antebrachial
cutaneous n.

Deep brachial v.

Basilic v.

Ulnar n.

Radial collateral a.

Medial antebrachial
cutaneous n.

◄ **LATERAL**

Superior ulnar
collateral a. & v.

Lateral intermuscular septum

Radial n.

Medial intermuscular septum

Middle collateral a.

Triceps brachii m.—medial head

Triceps brachii m.—lateral head

Triceps brachii m.—long head

PLATE 6.41   ANTERIOR FOREARM—SUPERFICIAL

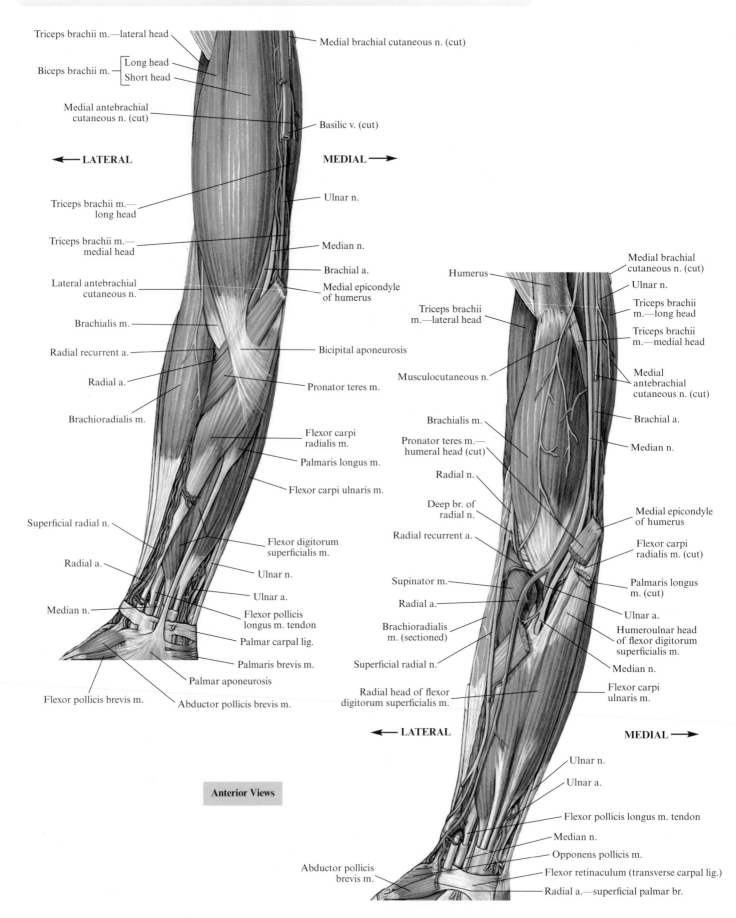

Triceps brachii m.—lateral head

Biceps brachii m. — Long head / Short head

Medial antebrachial cutaneous n. (cut)

Medial brachial cutaneous n. (cut)

Basilic v. (cut)

← LATERAL   MEDIAL →

Triceps brachii m.—long head

Triceps brachii m.—medial head

Lateral antebrachial cutaneous n.

Brachialis m.

Radial recurrent a.

Radial a.

Brachioradialis m.

Ulnar n.

Median n.

Brachial a.

Medial epicondyle of humerus

Bicipital aponeurosis

Pronator teres m.

Flexor carpi radialis m.

Palmaris longus m.

Flexor carpi ulnaris m.

Superficial radial n.

Radial a.

Median n.

Flexor digitorum superficialis m.

Ulnar n.

Ulnar a.

Flexor pollicis longus m. tendon

Palmar carpal lig.

Palmaris brevis m.

Palmar aponeurosis

Flexor pollicis brevis m.

Abductor pollicis brevis m.

Anterior Views

Humerus

Triceps brachii m.—lateral head

Musculocutaneous n.

Brachialis m.

Pronator teres m.—humeral head (cut)

Radial n.

Deep br. of radial n.

Radial recurrent a.

Supinator m.

Radial a.

Brachioradialis m. (sectioned)

Superficial radial n.

Radial head of flexor digitorum superficialis m.

Medial brachial cutaneous n. (cut)

Ulnar n.

Triceps brachii m.—long head

Triceps brachii m.—medial head

Medial antebrachial cutaneous n. (cut)

Brachial a.

Median n.

Medial epicondyle of humerus

Flexor carpi radialis m. (cut)

Palmaris longus m. (cut)

Ulnar a.

Humeroulnar head of flexor digitorum superficialis m.

Median n.

Flexor carpi ulnaris m.

← LATERAL   MEDIAL →

Ulnar n.

Ulnar a.

Flexor pollicis longus m. tendon

Median n.

Opponens pollicis m.

Flexor retinaculum (transverse carpal lig.)

Radial a.—superficial palmar br.

Abductor pollicis brevis m.

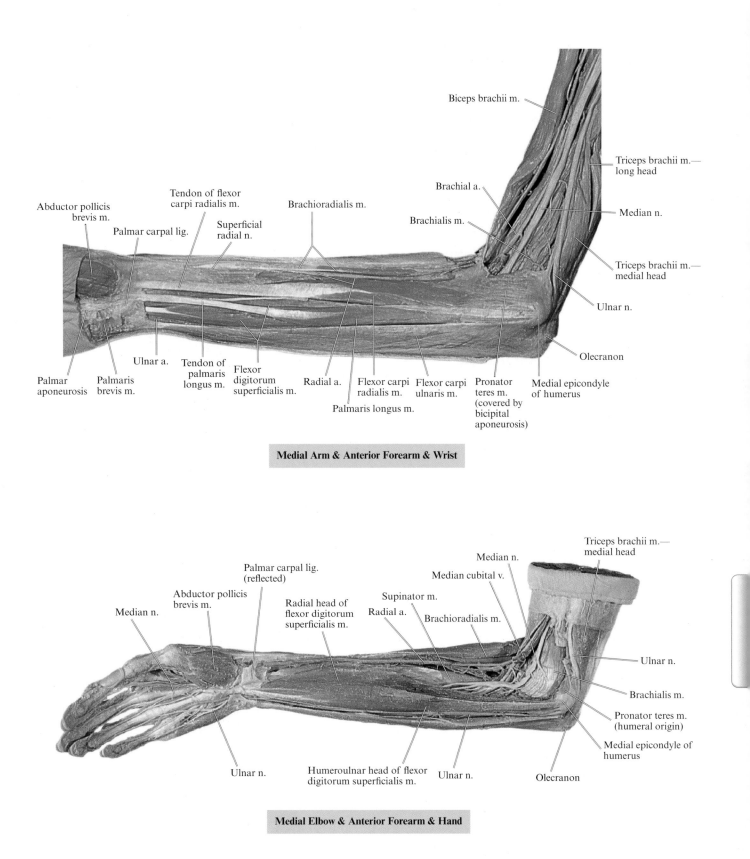

Biceps brachii m.

Triceps brachii m.—long head

Brachial a.

Median n.

Brachialis m.

Triceps brachii m.—medial head

Ulnar n.

Olecranon

Abductor pollicis brevis m.

Tendon of flexor carpi radialis m.

Brachioradialis m.

Palmar carpal lig.

Superficial radial n.

Palmar aponeurosis

Palmaris brevis m.

Ulnar a.

Tendon of palmaris longus m.

Flexor digitorum superficialis m.

Radial a.

Flexor carpi radialis m.

Flexor carpi ulnaris m.

Pronator teres m. (covered by bicipital aponeurosis)

Medial epicondyle of humerus

Palmaris longus m.

Medial Arm & Anterior Forearm & Wrist

Median n.

Abductor pollicis brevis m.

Palmar carpal lig. (reflected)

Radial head of flexor digitorum superficialis m.

Supinator m.

Radial a.

Brachioradialis m.

Median cubital v.

Median n.

Triceps brachii m.—medial head

Ulnar n.

Brachialis m.

Pronator teres m. (humeral origin)

Medial epicondyle of humerus

Ulnar n.

Humeroulnar head of flexor digitorum superficialis m.

Ulnar n.

Olecranon

Medial Elbow & Anterior Forearm & Hand

PLATE 6.43   ANTERIOR FOREARM—DEEP

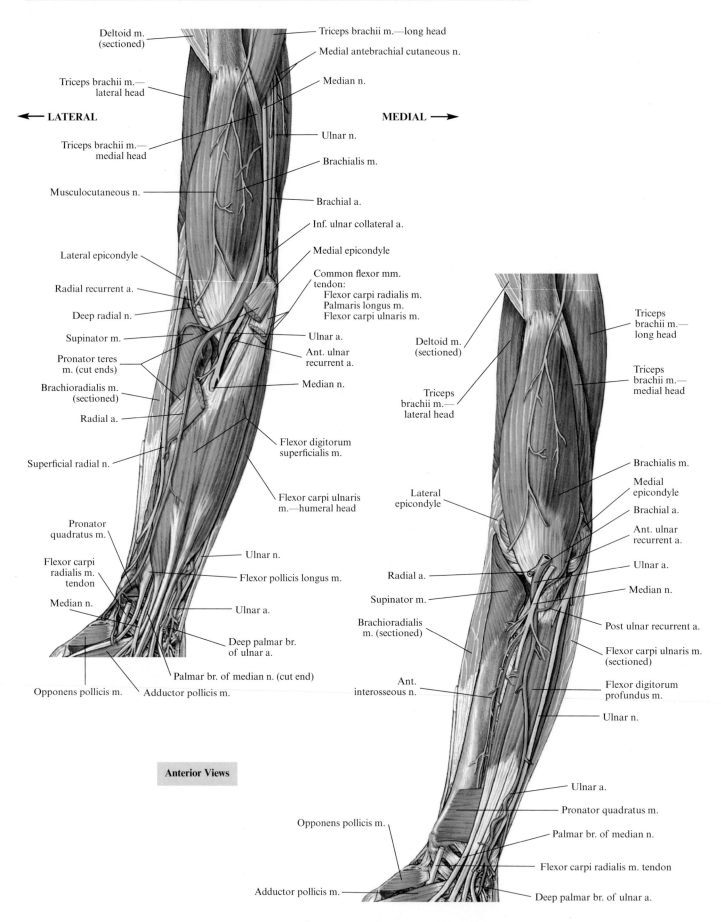

Deltoid m.
(sectioned)

Triceps brachii m.—long head

Medial antebrachial cutaneous n.

Triceps brachii m.—
lateral head

Median n.

← LATERAL

MEDIAL →

Triceps brachii m.—
medial head

Ulnar n.

Brachialis m.

Musculocutaneous n.

Brachial a.

Inf. ulnar collateral a.

Lateral epicondyle

Medial epicondyle

Radial recurrent a.

Common flexor mm.
tendon:
    Flexor carpi radialis m.
    Palmaris longus m.
    Flexor carpi ulnaris m.

Deep radial n.

Supinator m.

Ulnar a.

Pronator teres
m. (cut ends)

Ant. ulnar
recurrent a.

Brachioradialis m.
(sectioned)

Median n.

Radial a.

Superficial radial n.

Flexor digitorum
superficialis m.

Pronator
quadratus m.

Flexor carpi ulnaris
m.—humeral head

Flexor carpi
radialis m.
tendon

Ulnar n.

Flexor pollicis longus m.

Median n.

Ulnar a.

Deep palmar br.
of ulnar a.

Palmar br. of median n. (cut end)

Opponens pollicis m.   Adductor pollicis m.

Deltoid m.
(sectioned)

Triceps
brachii m.—
long head

Triceps
brachii m.—
medial head

Triceps
brachii m.—
lateral head

Brachialis m.

Medial
epicondyle

Brachial a.

Ant. ulnar
recurrent a.

Lateral
epicondyle

Ulnar a.

Radial a.

Median n.

Supinator m.

Post ulnar recurrent a.

Brachioradialis
m. (sectioned)

Flexor carpi ulnaris m.
(sectioned)

Ant.
interosseous n.

Flexor digitorum
profundus m.

Ulnar n.

Ulnar a.

Pronator quadratus m.

Opponens pollicis m.

Palmar br. of median n.

Flexor carpi radialis m. tendon

Adductor pollicis m.

Deep palmar br. of ulnar a.

Anterior Views

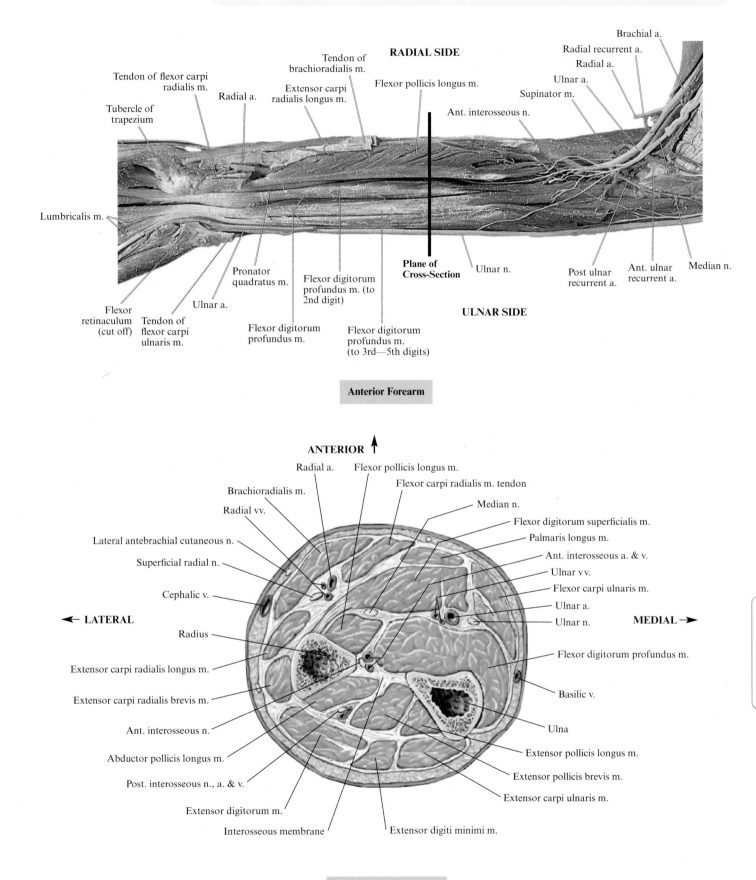

RADIAL SIDE

Tendon of flexor carpi radialis m.

Radial a.

Extensor carpi radialis longus m.

Tendon of brachioradialis m.

Flexor pollicis longus m.

Tubercle of trapezium

Ant. interosseous n.

Brachial a.

Radial recurrent a.

Radial a.

Ulnar a.

Supinator m.

Lumbricalis m.

Flexor retinaculum (cut off)

Tendon of flexor carpi ulnaris m.

Ulnar a.

Pronator quadratus m.

Flexor digitorum profundus m.

Flexor digitorum profundus m. (to 2nd digit)

Flexor digitorum profundus m. (to 3rd—5th digits)

Plane of Cross-Section

Ulnar n.

ULNAR SIDE

Post ulnar recurrent a.

Ant. ulnar recurrent a.

Median n.

Anterior Forearm

ANTERIOR ↑

Radial a.

Flexor pollicis longus m.

Brachioradialis m.

Flexor carpi radialis m. tendon

Radial vv.

Median n.

Lateral antebrachial cutaneous n.

Flexor digitorum superficialis m.

Superficial radial n.

Palmaris longus m.

Ant. interosseous a. & v.

Cephalic v.

Ulnar vv.

Flexor carpi ulnaris m.

Ulnar a.

← LATERAL

Ulnar n.

MEDIAL →

Radius

Extensor carpi radialis longus m.

Flexor digitorum profundus m.

Extensor carpi radialis brevis m.

Basilic v.

Ant. interosseous n.

Ulna

Abductor pollicis longus m.

Extensor pollicis longus m.

Post. interosseous n., a. & v.

Extensor pollicis brevis m.

Extensor carpi ulnaris m.

Extensor digitorum m.

Interosseous membrane

Extensor digiti minimi m.

Section at Mid-Forearm

PLATE 6.45   ELBOW & WRIST JOINTS

Lateral View—Muscles Sectioned

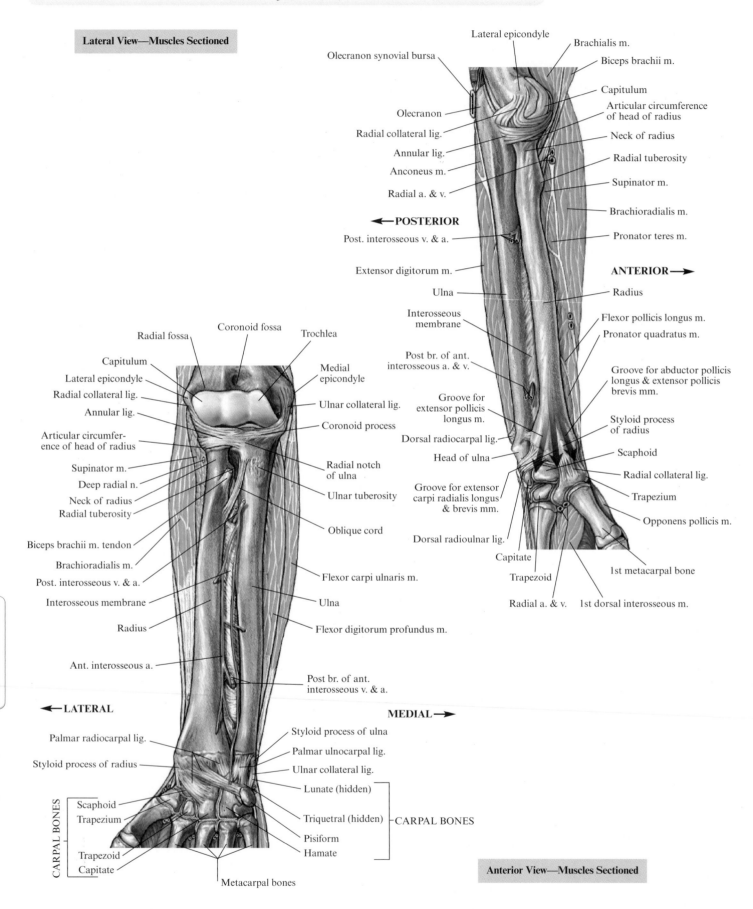

Olecranon synovial bursa

Lateral epicondyle

Brachialis m.

Biceps brachii m.

Olecranon

Capitulum

Articular circumference of head of radius

Radial collateral lig.

Annular lig.

Neck of radius

Anconeus m.

Radial tuberosity

Radial a. & v.

Supinator m.

Brachioradialis m.

← POSTERIOR

Pronator teres m.

Post. interosseous v. & a.

ANTERIOR →

Extensor digitorum m.

Ulna

Radius

Interosseous membrane

Flexor pollicis longus m.

Pronator quadratus m.

Post br. of ant. interosseous a. & v.

Groove for abductor pollicis longus & extensor pollicis brevis mm.

Groove for extensor pollicis longus m.

Styloid process of radius

Dorsal radiocarpal lig.

Scaphoid

Head of ulna

Radial collateral lig.

Groove for extensor carpi radialis longus & brevis mm.

Trapezium

Opponens pollicis m.

Dorsal radioulnar lig.

Capitate

1st metacarpal bone

Trapezoid

Radial a. & v.   1st dorsal interosseous m.

Radial fossa

Coronoid fossa

Trochlea

Capitulum

Medial epicondyle

Lateral epicondyle

Radial collateral lig.

Ulnar collateral lig.

Annular lig.

Coronoid process

Articular circumference of head of radius

Radial notch of ulna

Supinator m.

Deep radial n.

Ulnar tuberosity

Neck of radius

Radial tuberosity

Oblique cord

Biceps brachii m. tendon

Brachioradialis m.

Flexor carpi ulnaris m.

Post. interosseous v. & a.

Ulna

Interosseous membrane

Radius

Flexor digitorum profundus m.

Ant. interosseous a.

Post br. of ant. interosseous v. & a.

← LATERAL

MEDIAL →

Palmar radiocarpal lig.

Styloid process of ulna

Palmar ulnocarpal lig.

Styloid process of radius

Ulnar collateral lig.

CARPAL BONES

Scaphoid

Lunate (hidden)

Trapezium

Triquetral (hidden)   CARPAL BONES

Trapezoid

Pisiform

Capitate

Hamate

Metacarpal bones

Anterior View—Muscles Sectioned

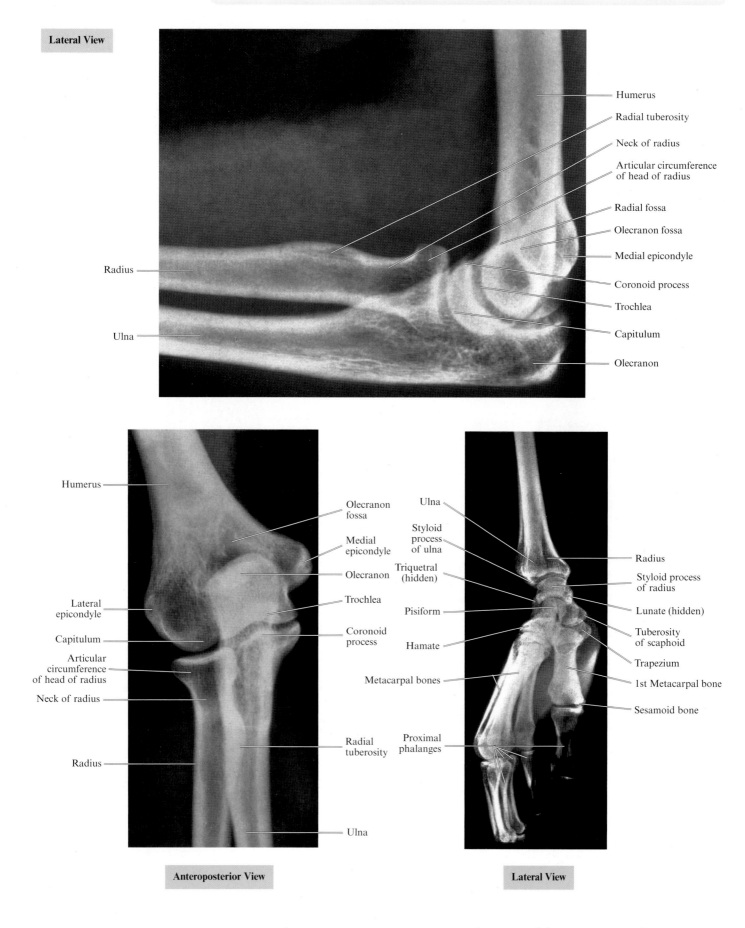

Lateral View

Humerus

Radial tuberosity

Neck of radius

Articular circumference of head of radius

Radial fossa

Olecranon fossa

Medial epicondyle

Coronoid process

Trochlea

Capitulum

Olecranon

Radius

Ulna

Humerus

Olecranon fossa

Medial epicondyle

Olecranon

Trochlea

Coronoid process

Lateral epicondyle

Capitulum

Articular circumference of head of radius

Neck of radius

Radius

Radial tuberosity

Ulna

Anteroposterior View

Ulna

Styloid process of ulna

Triquetral (hidden)

Pisiform

Hamate

Metacarpal bones

Proximal phalanges

Radius

Styloid process of radius

Lunate (hidden)

Tuberosity of scaphoid

Trapezium

1st Metacarpal bone

Sesamoid bone

Lateral View

PLATE 6.47   LATERAL FOREARM & HAND

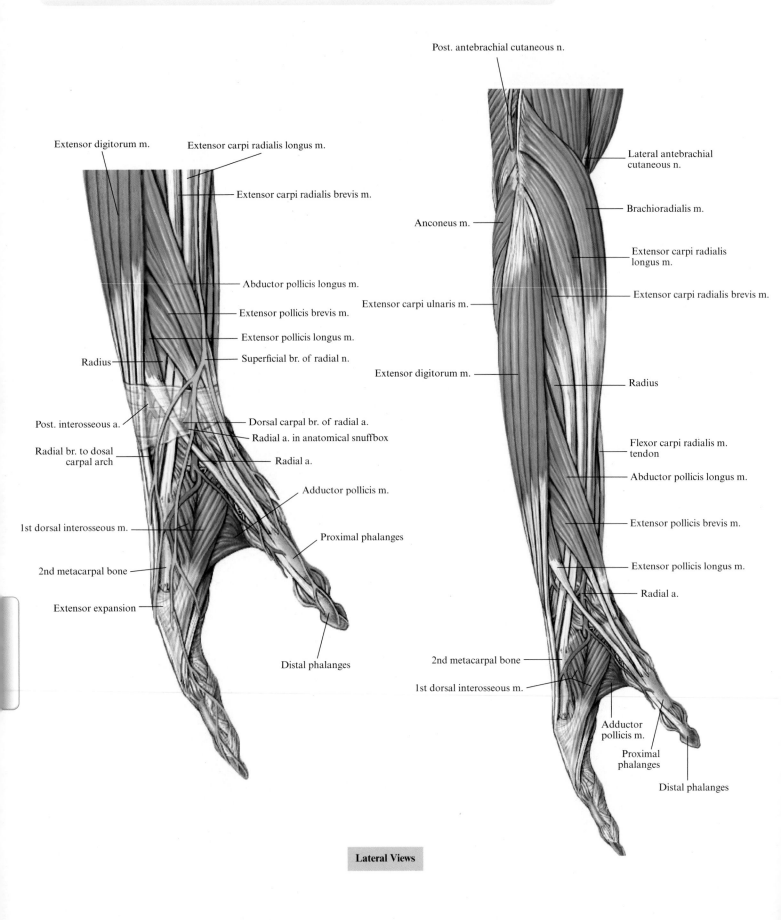

Post. antebrachial cutaneous n.

Extensor digitorum m.

Extensor carpi radialis longus m.

Extensor carpi radialis brevis m.

Lateral antebrachial cutaneous n.

Brachioradialis m.

Anconeus m.

Extensor carpi radialis longus m.

Extensor carpi radialis brevis m.

Abductor pollicis longus m.

Extensor carpi ulnaris m.

Extensor pollicis brevis m.

Extensor pollicis longus m.

Superficial br. of radial n.

Radius

Extensor digitorum m.

Radius

Post. interosseous a.

Dorsal carpal br. of radial a.

Radial a. in anatomical snuffbox

Flexor carpi radialis m. tendon

Radial br. to dosal carpal arch

Radial a.

Abductor pollicis longus m.

Adductor pollicis m.

Extensor pollicis brevis m.

1st dorsal interosseous m.

Proximal phalanges

Extensor pollicis longus m.

2nd metacarpal bone

Radial a.

Extensor expansion

2nd metacarpal bone

1st dorsal interosseous m.

Distal phalanges

Adductor pollicis m.

Proximal phalanges

Distal phalanges

Lateral Views

A.D.A.M. | Student Atlas of Anatomy

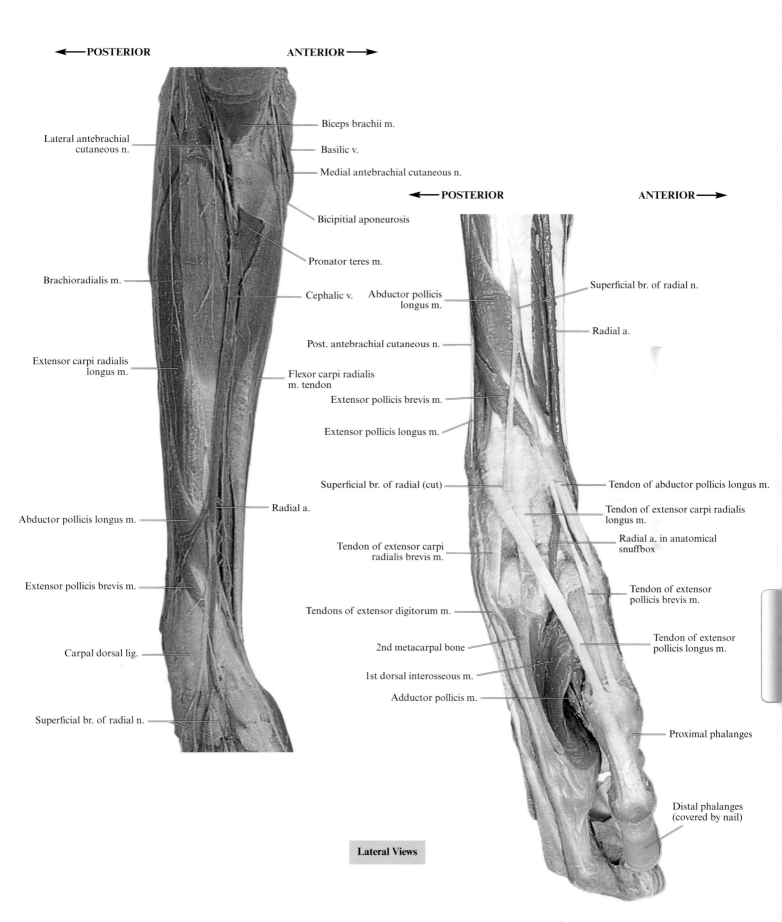

←POSTERIOR   ANTERIOR→

Lateral antebrachial
cutaneous n.

Biceps brachii m.

Basilic v.

Medial antebrachial cutaneous n.

Bicipitial aponeurosis

Pronator teres m.

Brachioradialis m.

Cephalic v.   Abductor pollicis
longus m.

Post. antebrachial cutaneous n.

Extensor carpi radialis
longus m.

Flexor carpi radialis
m. tendon

Extensor pollicis brevis m.

Extensor pollicis longus m.

Abductor pollicis longus m.

Radial a.

Superficial br. of radial (cut)

Extensor pollicis brevis m.

Tendon of extensor carpi
radialis brevis m.

Carpal dorsal lig.

Tendons of extensor digitorum m.

2nd metacarpal bone

1st dorsal interosseous m.

Superficial br. of radial n.

Adductor pollicis m.

←POSTERIOR   ANTERIOR→

Superficial br. of radial n.

Radial a.

Tendon of abductor pollicis longus m.

Tendon of extensor carpi radialis
longus m.

Radial a. in anatomical
snuffbox

Tendon of extensor
pollicis brevis m.

Tendon of extensor
pollicis longus m.

Proximal phalanges

Distal phalanges
(covered by nail)

Lateral Views

PLATE 6.49   POSTERIOR ARM

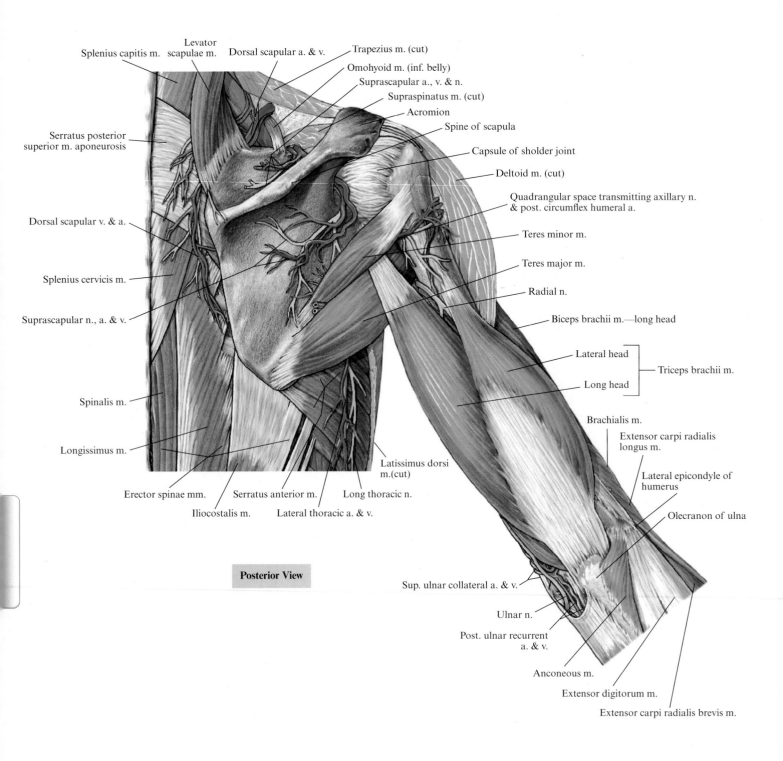

Splenius capitis m.

Levator scapulae m.

Dorsal scapular a. & v.

Trapezius m. (cut)

Omohyoid m. (inf. belly)

Suprascapular a., v. & n.

Supraspinatus m. (cut)

Acromion

Spine of scapula

Capsule of sholder joint

Deltoid m. (cut)

Quadrangular space transmitting axillary n. & post. circumflex humeral a.

Serratus posterior superior m. aponeurosis

Dorsal scapular v. & a.

Splenius cervicis m.

Suprascapular n., a. & v.

Teres minor m.

Teres major m.

Radial n.

Biceps brachii m.—long head

Lateral head

Long head

Triceps brachii m.

Spinalis m.

Longissimus m.

Brachialis m.

Extensor carpi radialis longus m.

Lateral epicondyle of humerus

Olecranon of ulna

Erector spinae mm.

Serratus anterior m.

Long thoracic n.

Iliocostalis m.

Lateral thoracic a. & v.

Latissimus dorsi m.(cut)

Posterior View

Sup. ulnar collateral a. & v.

Ulnar n.

Post. ulnar recurrent a. & v.

Anconeous m.

Extensor digitorum m.

Extensor carpi radialis brevis m.

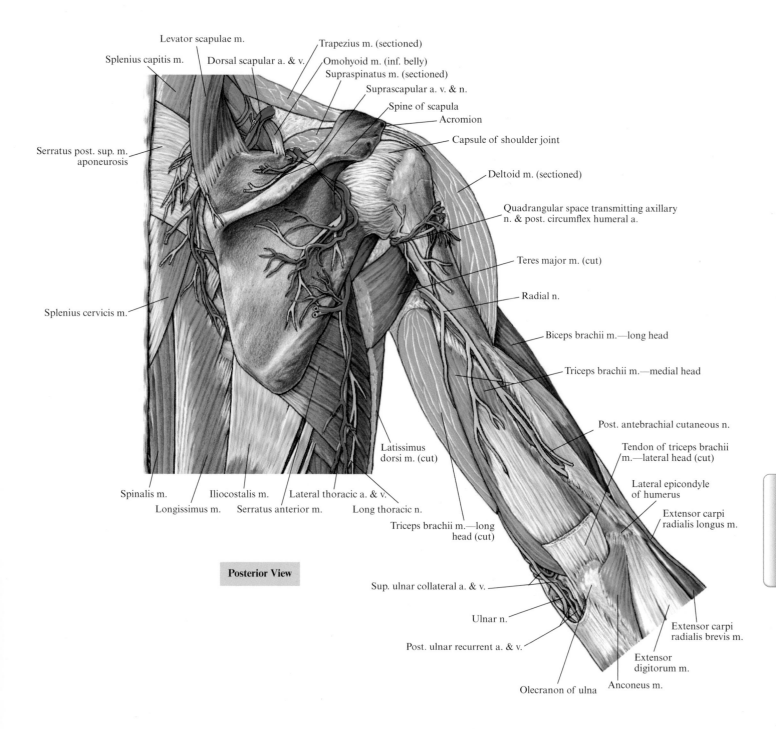

Levator scapulae m.

Splenius capitis m.

Dorsal scapular a. & v.

Trapezius m. (sectioned)

Omohyoid m. (inf. belly)

Supraspinatus m. (sectioned)

Suprascapular a. v. & n.

Spine of scapula

Acromion

Serratus post. sup. m.
aponeurosis

Capsule of shoulder joint

Deltoid m. (sectioned)

Quadrangular space transmitting axillary
n. & post. circumflex humeral a.

Teres major m. (cut)

Radial n.

Splenius cervicis m.

Biceps brachii m.—long head

Triceps brachii m.—medial head

Post. antebrachial cutaneous n.

Tendon of triceps brachii
m.—lateral head (cut)

Lateral epicondyle
of humerus

Latissimus
dorsi m. (cut)

Extensor carpi
radialis longus m.

Spinalis m.

Iliocostalis m.

Lateral thoracic a. & v.

Longissimus m.

Serratus anterior m.

Long thoracic n.

Triceps brachii m.—long
head (cut)

Posterior View

Sup. ulnar collateral a. & v.

Ulnar n.

Extensor carpi
radialis brevis m.

Post. ulnar recurrent a. & v.

Extensor
digitorum m.

Olecranon of ulna

Anconeus m.

PLATE 6.51   SUPERFICIAL DORSUM OF HAND

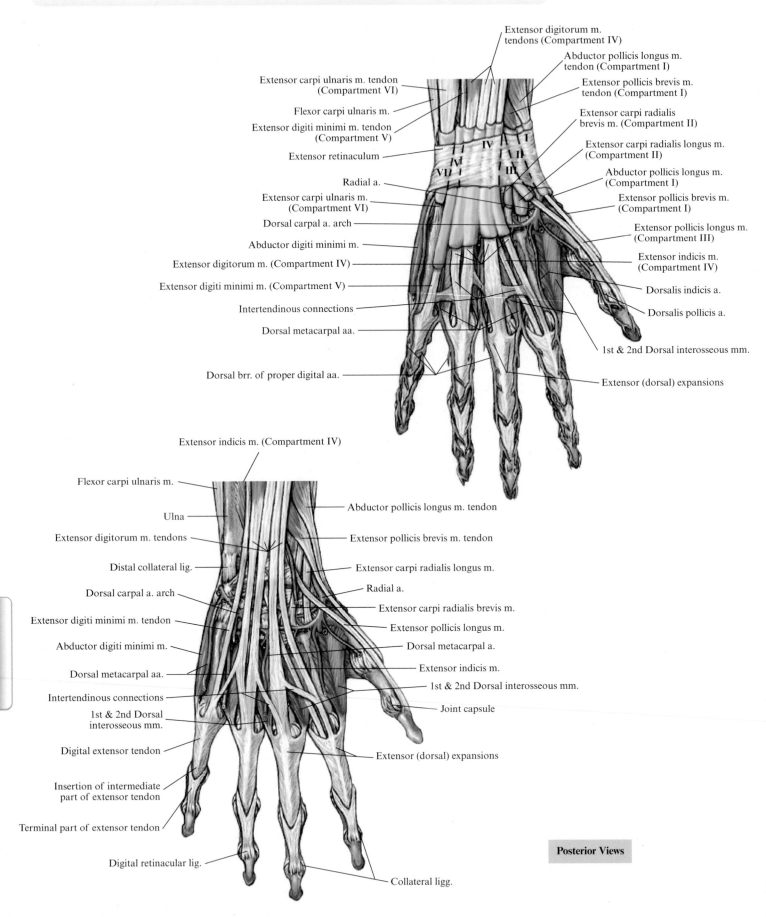

Extensor digitorum m.
tendons (Compartment IV)

Abductor pollicis longus m.
tendon (Compartment I)

Extensor pollicis brevis m.
tendon (Compartment I)

Extensor carpi ulnaris m. tendon
(Compartment VI)

Extensor carpi radialis
brevis m. (Compartment II)

Flexor carpi ulnaris m.

Extensor digiti minimi m. tendon
(Compartment V)

Extensor carpi radialis longus m.
(Compartment II)

Extensor retinaculum

Abductor pollicis longus m.
(Compartment I)

Radial a.

Extensor pollicis brevis m.
(Compartment I)

Extensor carpi ulnaris m.
(Compartment VI)

Extensor pollicis longus m.
(Compartment III)

Dorsal carpal a. arch

Extensor indicis m.
(Compartment IV)

Abductor digiti minimi m.

Extensor digitorum m. (Compartment IV)

Dorsalis indicis a.

Extensor digiti minimi m. (Compartment V)

Dorsalis pollicis a.

Intertendinous connections

Dorsal metacarpal aa.

1st & 2nd Dorsal interosseous mm.

Dorsal brr. of proper digital aa.

Extensor (dorsal) expansions

Extensor indicis m. (Compartment IV)

Flexor carpi ulnaris m.

Abductor pollicis longus m. tendon

Ulna

Extensor pollicis brevis m. tendon

Extensor digitorum m. tendons

Extensor carpi radialis longus m.

Distal collateral lig.

Radial a.

Dorsal carpal a. arch

Extensor carpi radialis brevis m.

Extensor digiti minimi m. tendon

Extensor pollicis longus m.

Abductor digiti minimi m.

Dorsal metacarpal a.

Dorsal metacarpal aa.

Extensor indicis m.

Intertendinous connections

1st & 2nd Dorsal interosseous mm.

1st & 2nd Dorsal
interosseous mm.

Joint capsule

Digital extensor tendon

Extensor (dorsal) expansions

Insertion of intermediate
part of extensor tendon

Terminal part of extensor tendon

Digital retinacular lig.

Collateral ligg.

Posterior Views

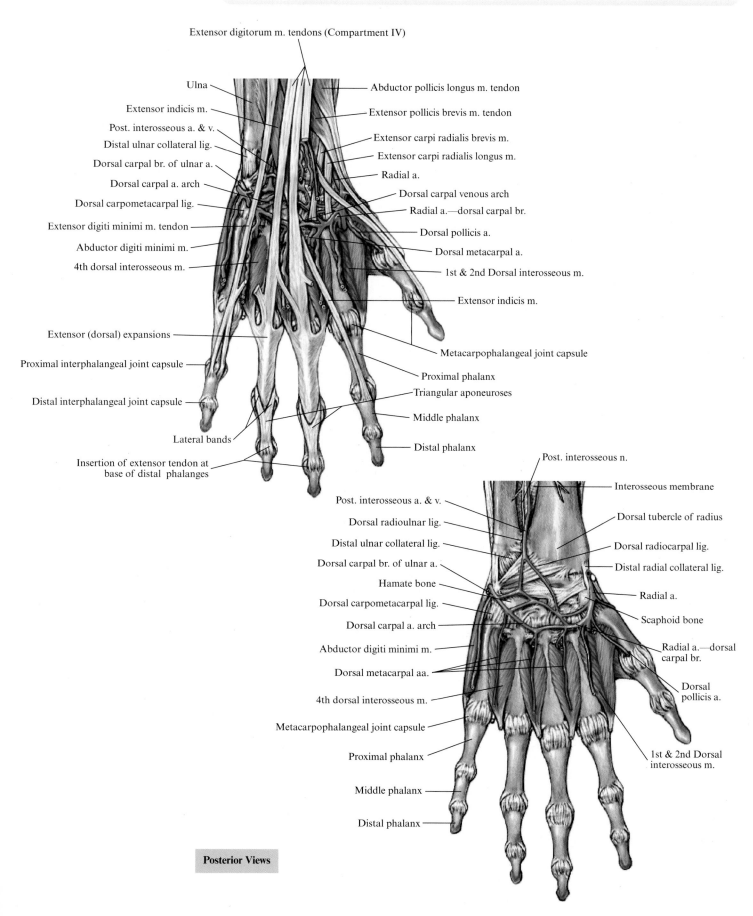

Extensor digitorum m. tendons (Compartment IV)

Ulna

Extensor indicis m.

Post. interosseous a. & v.

Distal ulnar collateral lig.

Dorsal carpal br. of ulnar a.

Dorsal carpal a. arch

Dorsal carpometacarpal lig.

Extensor digiti minimi m. tendon

Abductor digiti minimi m.

4th dorsal interosseous m.

Extensor (dorsal) expansions

Proximal interphalangeal joint capsule

Distal interphalangeal joint capsule

Lateral bands

Insertion of extensor tendon at
base of distal phalanges

Abductor pollicis longus m. tendon

Extensor pollicis brevis m. tendon

Extensor carpi radialis brevis m.

Extensor carpi radialis longus m.

Radial a.

Dorsal carpal venous arch

Radial a.—dorsal carpal br.

Dorsal pollicis a.

Dorsal metacarpal a.

1st & 2nd Dorsal interosseous m.

Extensor indicis m.

Metacarpophalangeal joint capsule

Proximal phalanx

Triangular aponeuroses

Middle phalanx

Distal phalanx

Post. interosseous n.

Post. interosseous a. & v.

Dorsal radioulnar lig.

Distal ulnar collateral lig.

Dorsal carpal br. of ulnar a.

Hamate bone

Dorsal carpometacarpal lig.

Dorsal carpal a. arch

Abductor digiti minimi m.

Dorsal metacarpal aa.

4th dorsal interosseous m.

Metacarpophalangeal joint capsule

Proximal phalanx

Middle phalanx

Distal phalanx

Interosseous membrane

Dorsal tubercle of radius

Dorsal radiocarpal lig.

Distal radial collateral lig.

Radial a.

Scaphoid bone

Radial a.—dorsal
carpal br.

Dorsal
pollicis a.

1st & 2nd Dorsal
interosseous m.

Posterior Views

PLATE **6.53**   MEDIAL FOREARM & HAND

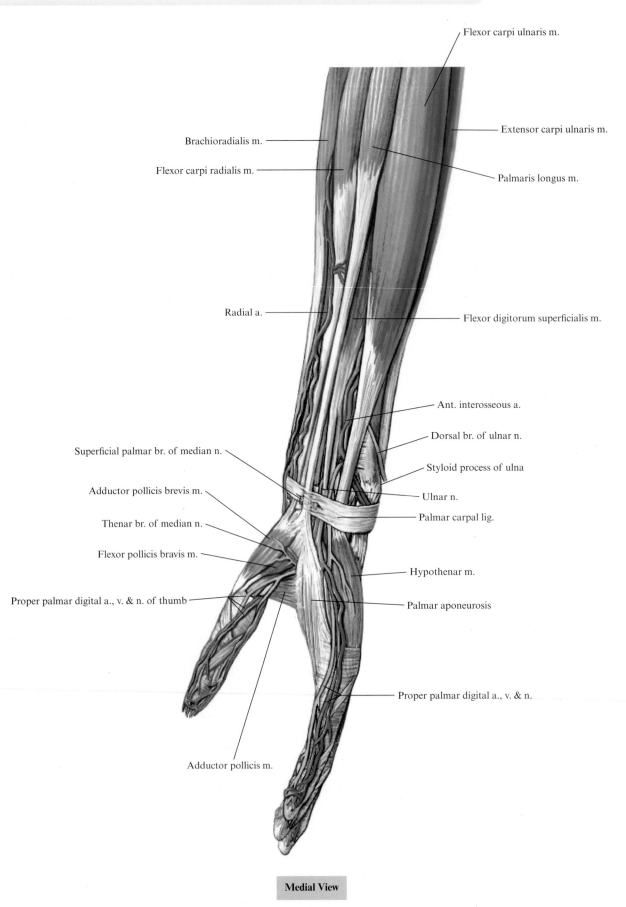

Flexor carpi ulnaris m.

Extensor carpi ulnaris m.

Brachioradialis m. ———

Palmaris longus m.

Flexor carpi radialis m. ———

Radial a. ———

Flexor digitorum superficialis m.

Ant. interosseous a.

Dorsal br. of ulnar n.

Superficial palmar br. of median n. ———

Styloid process of ulna

Adductor pollicis brevis m. ———

Ulnar n.

Thenar br. of median n. ———

Palmar carpal lig.

Flexor pollicis bravis m. ———

Hypothenar m.

Proper palmar digital a., v. & n. of thumb ———

Palmar aponeurosis

Proper palmar digital a., v. & n.

Adductor pollicis m.

Medial View

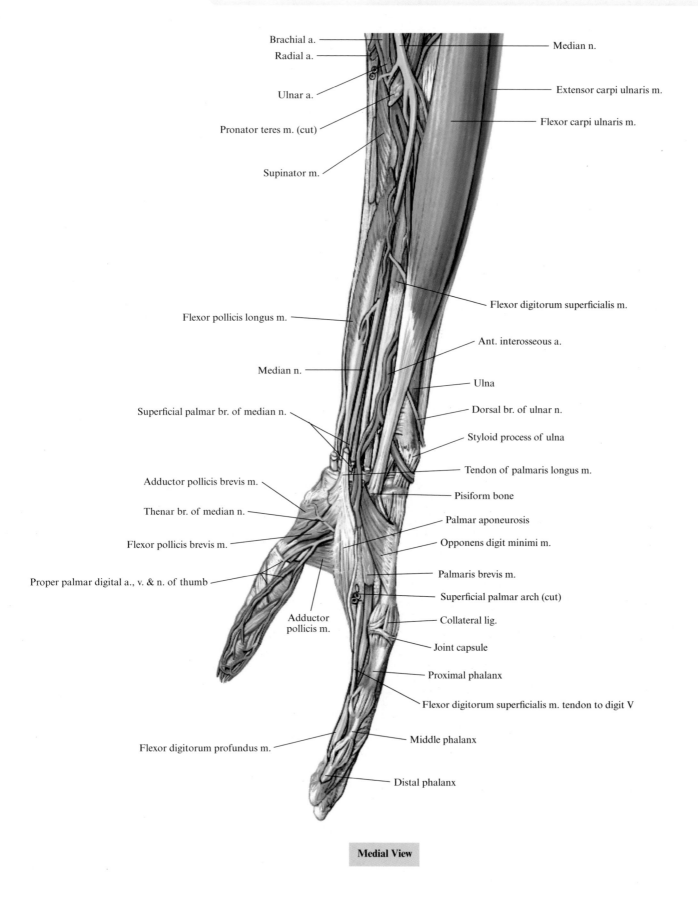

Brachial a.

Radial a.

Ulnar a.

Pronator teres m. (cut)

Supinator m.

Median n.

Extensor carpi ulnaris m.

Flexor carpi ulnaris m.

Flexor digitorum superficialis m.

Flexor pollicis longus m.

Ant. interosseous a.

Median n.

Ulna

Superficial palmar br. of median n.

Dorsal br. of ulnar n.

Styloid process of ulna

Adductor pollicis brevis m.

Tendon of palmaris longus m.

Pisiform bone

Thenar br. of median n.

Palmar aponeurosis

Flexor pollicis brevis m.

Opponens digit minimi m.

Proper palmar digital a., v. & n. of thumb

Palmaris brevis m.

Superficial palmar arch (cut)

Adductor
pollicis m.

Collateral lig.

Joint capsule

Proximal phalanx

Flexor digitorum superficialis m. tendon to digit V

Middle phalanx

Flexor digitorum profundus m.

Distal phalanx

Medial View

PLATE 6.55   SUPERFICIAL PALM OF HAND

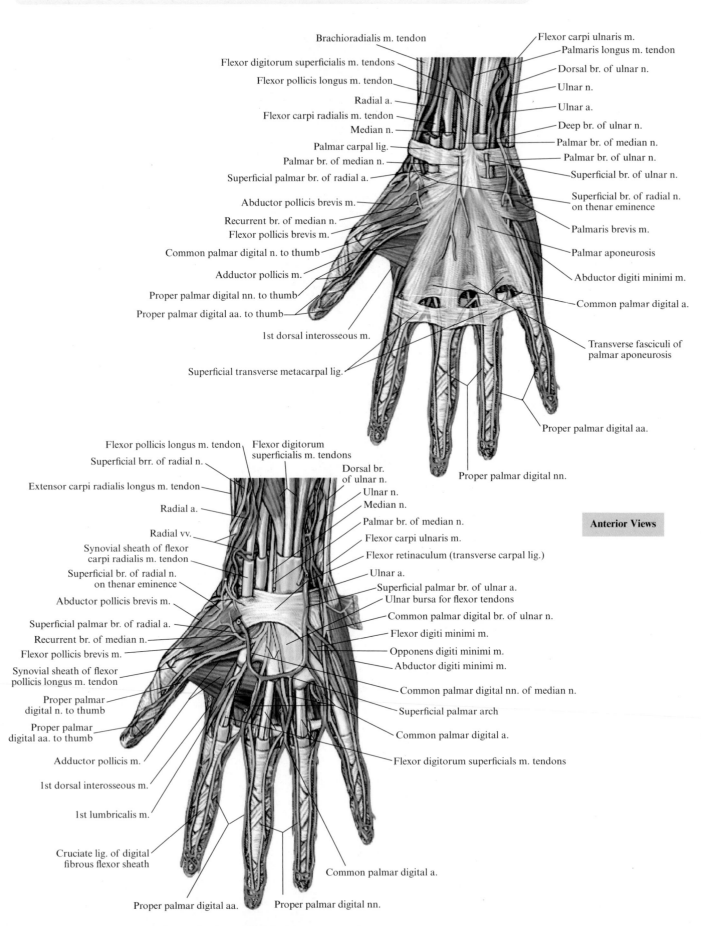

Brachioradialis m. tendon

Flexor carpi ulnaris m.

Palmaris longus m. tendon

Flexor digitorum superficialis m. tendons

Flexor pollicis longus m. tendon

Dorsal br. of ulnar n.

Radial a.

Ulnar n.

Flexor carpi radialis m. tendon

Ulnar a.

Median n.

Deep br. of ulnar n.

Palmar carpal lig.

Palmar br. of median n.

Palmar br. of median n.

Palmar br. of ulnar n.

Superficial palmar br. of radial a.

Superficial br. of ulnar n.

Abductor pollicis brevis m.

Superficial br. of radial n.
on thenar eminence

Recurrent br. of median n.

Palmaris brevis m.

Flexor pollicis brevis m.

Common palmar digital n. to thumb

Palmar aponeurosis

Adductor pollicis m.

Abductor digiti minimi m.

Proper palmar digital nn. to thumb

Common palmar digital a.

Proper palmar digital aa. to thumb

1st dorsal interosseous m.

Transverse fasciculi of
palmar aponeurosis

Superficial transverse metacarpal lig.

Proper palmar digital aa.

Proper palmar digital nn.

Flexor pollicis longus m. tendon

Flexor digitorum
superficialis m. tendons

Superficial brr. of radial n.

Dorsal br.
of ulnar n.

Extensor carpi radialis longus m. tendon

Ulnar n.

Radial a.

Median n.

Palmar br. of median n.

Radial vv.

Flexor carpi ulnaris m.

Synovial sheath of flexor
carpi radialis m. tendon

Flexor retinaculum (transverse carpal lig.)

Superficial br. of radial n.
on thenar eminence

Ulnar a.

Superficial palmar br. of ulnar a.

Abductor pollicis brevis m.

Ulnar bursa for flexor tendons

Superficial palmar br. of radial a.

Common palmar digital br. of ulnar n.

Recurrent br. of median n.

Flexor digiti minimi m.

Flexor pollicis brevis m.

Opponens digiti minimi m.

Synovial sheath of flexor
pollicis longus m. tendon

Abductor digiti minimi m.

Proper palmar
digital n. to thumb

Common palmar digital nn. of median n.

Proper palmar
digital aa. to thumb

Superficial palmar arch

Adductor pollicis m.

Common palmar digital a.

1st dorsal interosseous m.

Flexor digitorum superficials m. tendons

1st lumbricalis m.

Cruciate lig. of digital
fibrous flexor sheath

Common palmar digital a.

Proper palmar digital aa.

Proper palmar digital nn.

Anterior Views

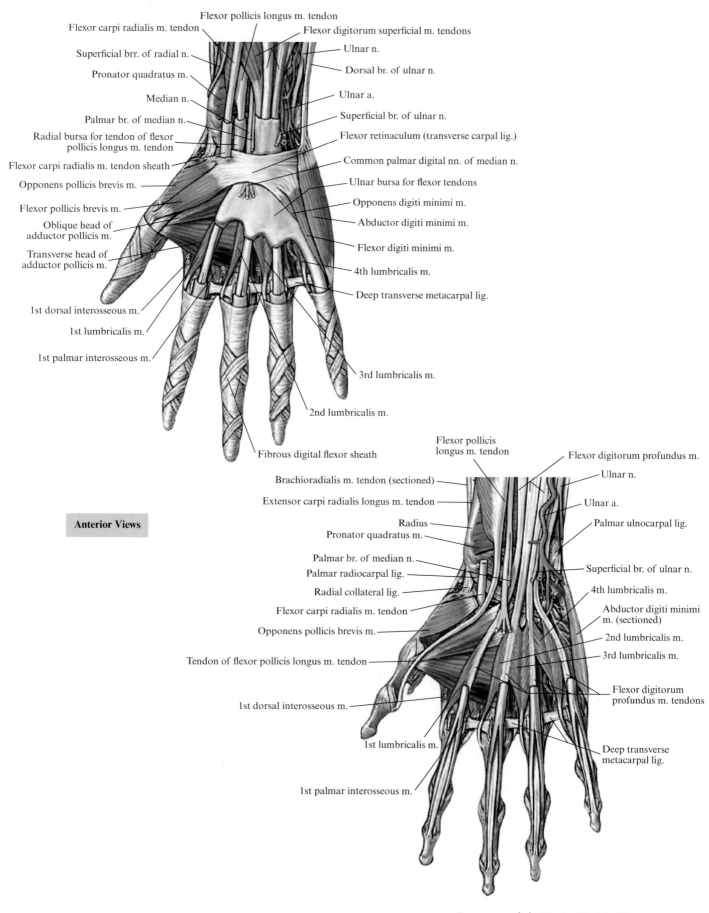

Flexor pollicis longus m. tendon

Flexor carpi radialis m. tendon

Flexor digitorum superficial m. tendons

Superficial brr. of radial n.

Ulnar n.

Pronator quadratus m.

Dorsal br. of ulnar n.

Median n.

Ulnar a.

Palmar br. of median n.

Superficial br. of ulnar n.

Radial bursa for tendon of flexor pollicis longus m. tendon

Flexor retinaculum (transverse carpal lig.)

Flexor carpi radialis m. tendon sheath

Common palmar digital nn. of median n.

Opponens pollicis brevis m.

Ulnar bursa for flexor tendons

Flexor pollicis brevis m.

Opponens digiti minimi m.

Oblique head of adductor pollicis m.

Abductor digiti minimi m.

Transverse head of adductor pollicis m.

Flexor digiti minimi m.

4th lumbricalis m.

1st dorsal interosseous m.

Deep transverse metacarpal lig.

1st lumbricalis m.

1st palmar interosseous m.

3rd lumbricalis m.

2nd lumbricalis m.

Fibrous digital flexor sheath

Flexor pollicis longus m. tendon

Flexor digitorum profundus m.

Brachioradialis m. tendon (sectioned)

Ulnar n.

Extensor carpi radialis longus m. tendon

Ulnar a.

Anterior Views

Radius

Palmar ulnocarpal lig.

Pronator quadratus m.

Palmar br. of median n.

Palmar radiocarpal lig.

Superficial br. of ulnar n.

Radial collateral lig.

4th lumbricalis m.

Flexor carpi radialis m. tendon

Abductor digiti minimi m. (sectioned)

Opponens pollicis brevis m.

2nd lumbricalis m.

Tendon of flexor pollicis longus m. tendon

3rd lumbricalis m.

Flexor digitorum profundus m. tendons

1st dorsal interosseous m.

1st lumbricalis m.

Deep transverse metacarpal lig.

1st palmar interosseous m.

PLATE 6.57   DEEP PALM OF HAND

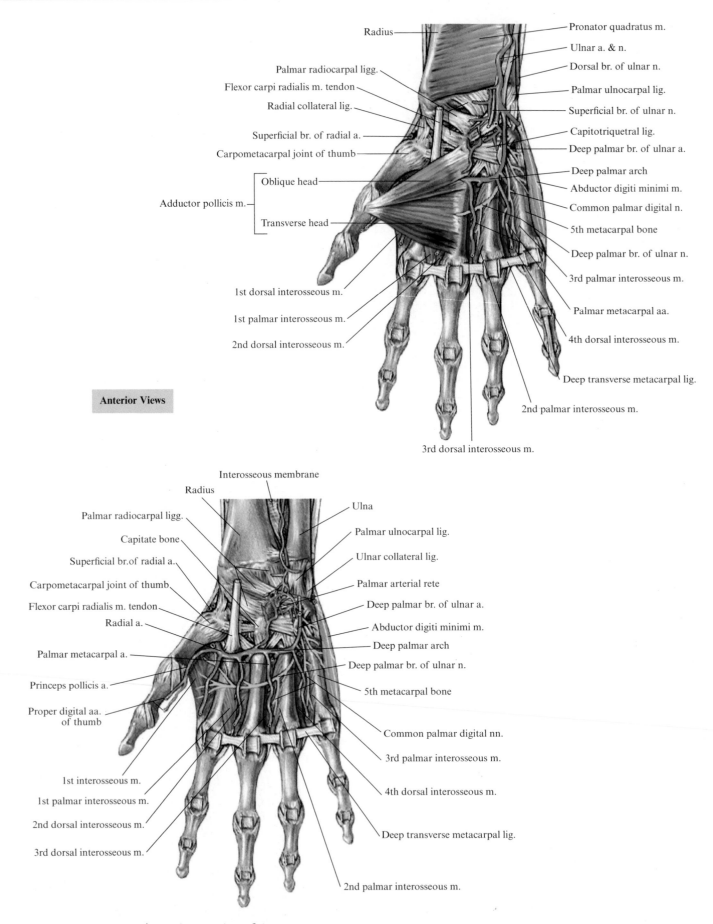

Radius

Pronator quadratus m.

Ulnar a. & n.

Palmar radiocarpal ligg.

Dorsal br. of ulnar n.

Flexor carpi radialis m. tendon

Palmar ulnocarpal lig.

Radial collateral lig.

Superficial br. of ulnar n.

Superficial br. of radial a.

Capitotriquetral lig.

Carpometacarpal joint of thumb

Deep palmar br. of ulnar a.

Oblique head

Deep palmar arch

Abductor digiti minimi m.

Adductor pollicis m.

Common palmar digital n.

Transverse head

5th metacarpal bone

Deep palmar br. of ulnar n.

3rd palmar interosseous m.

1st dorsal interosseous m.

Palmar metacarpal aa.

1st palmar interosseous m.

4th dorsal interosseous m.

2nd dorsal interosseous m.

Deep transverse metacarpal lig.

2nd palmar interosseous m.

Anterior Views

3rd dorsal interosseous m.

Interosseous membrane

Radius

Ulna

Palmar radiocarpal ligg.

Palmar ulnocarpal lig.

Capitate bone

Ulnar collateral lig.

Superficial br. of radial a.

Palmar arterial rete

Carpometacarpal joint of thumb

Deep palmar br. of ulnar a.

Flexor carpi radialis m. tendon

Abductor digiti minimi m.

Radial a.

Deep palmar arch

Palmar metacarpal a.

Deep palmar br. of ulnar n.

Princeps pollicis a.

5th metacarpal bone

Proper digital aa.
of thumb

Common palmar digital nn.

3rd palmar interosseous m.

1st interosseous m.

4th dorsal interosseous m.

1st palmar interosseous m.

2nd dorsal interosseous m.

Deep transverse metacarpal lig.

3rd dorsal interosseous m.

2nd palmar interosseous m.

A.D.A.M. | Student Atlas of Anatomy

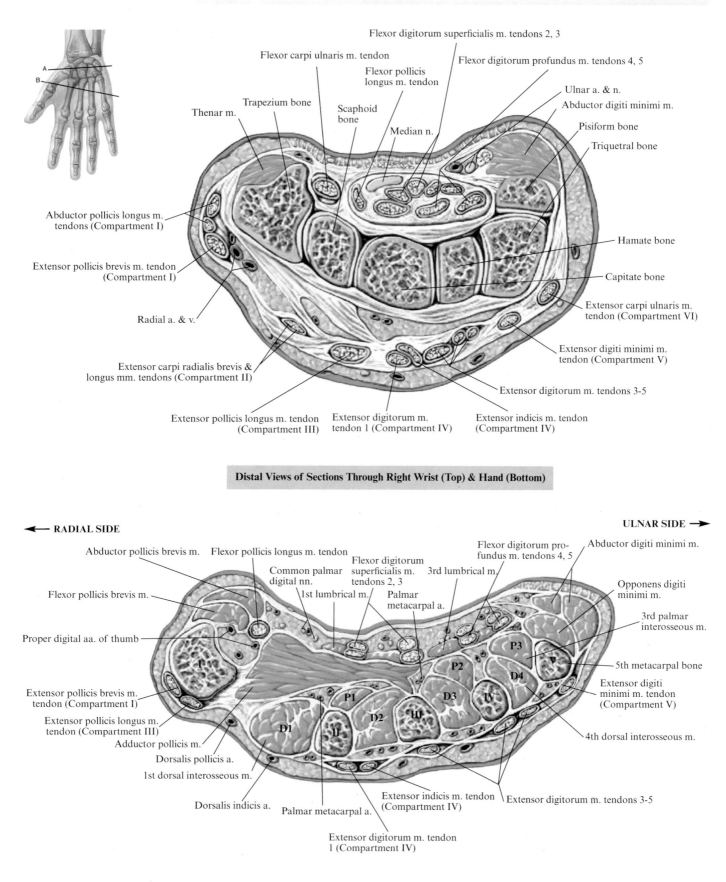

Flexor digitorum superficialis m. tendons 2, 3

Flexor carpi ulnaris m. tendon

Flexor digitorum profundus m. tendons 4, 5

Flexor pollicis longus m. tendon

Ulnar a. & n.

Abductor digiti minimi m.

Trapezium bone

Scaphoid bone

Pisiform bone

Thenar m.

Triquetral bone

Median n.

Abductor pollicis longus m. tendons (Compartment I)

Extensor pollicis brevis m. tendon (Compartment I)

Hamate bone

Capitate bone

Radial a. & v.

Extensor carpi ulnaris m. tendon (Compartment VI)

Extensor carpi radialis brevis & longus mm. tendons (Compartment II)

Extensor digiti minimi m. tendon (Compartment V)

Extensor pollicis longus m. tendon (Compartment III)

Extensor digitorum m. tendon 1 (Compartment IV)

Extensor indicis m. tendon (Compartment IV)

Extensor digitorum m. tendons 3-5

Distal Views of Sections Through Right Wrist (Top) & Hand (Bottom)

◄— **RADIAL SIDE**

ULNAR SIDE —►

Abductor pollicis brevis m.

Flexor pollicis longus m. tendon

Flexor digitorum profundus m. tendons 4, 5

Abductor digiti minimi m.

Common palmar digital nn.

Flexor digitorum superficialis m. tendons 2, 3

3rd lumbrical m.

Flexor pollicis brevis m.

1st lumbrical m.

Palmar metacarpal a.

Opponens digiti minimi m.

3rd palmar interosseous m.

Proper digital aa. of thumb

P3

V

5th metacarpal bone

P2

D4

Extensor digiti minimi m. tendon (Compartment V)

Extensor pollicis brevis m. tendon (Compartment I)

P1

D3

IV

Extensor pollicis longus m. tendon (Compartment III)

D2

III

Adductor pollicis m.

D1

II

4th dorsal interosseous m.

Dorsalis pollicis a.

1st dorsal interosseous m.

Dorsalis indicis a.

Palmar metacarpal a.

Extensor indicis m. tendon (Compartment IV)

Extensor digitorum m. tendons 3-5

Extensor digitorum m. tendon 1 (Compartment IV)

PLATE 6.59 LIGAMENTS & TENDONS OF HAND

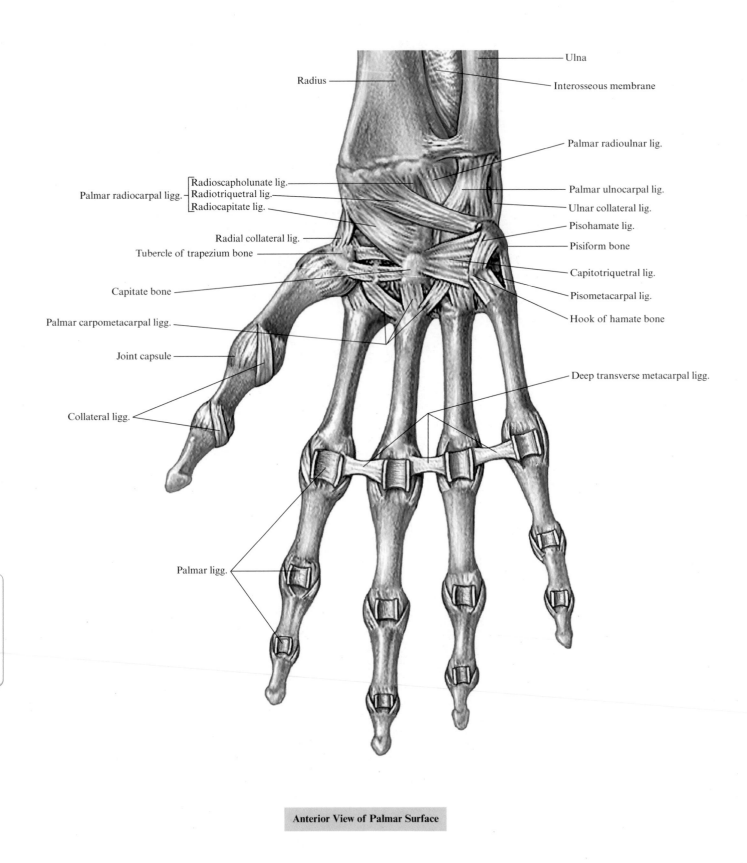

Radius

Ulna

Interosseous membrane

Palmar radioulnar lig.

Radioscapholunate lig.

Palmar radiocarpal ligg.

Radiotriquetral lig.

Radiocapitate lig.

Palmar ulnocarpal lig.

Ulnar collateral lig.

Radial collateral lig.

Pisohamate lig.

Tubercle of trapezium bone

Pisiform bone

Capitate bone

Capitotriquetral lig.

Pisometacarpal lig.

Palmar carpometacarpal ligg.

Hook of hamate bone

Joint capsule

Deep transverse metacarpal ligg.

Collateral ligg.

Palmar ligg.

Anterior View of Palmar Surface

A.D.A.M. | Student Atlas of Anatomy

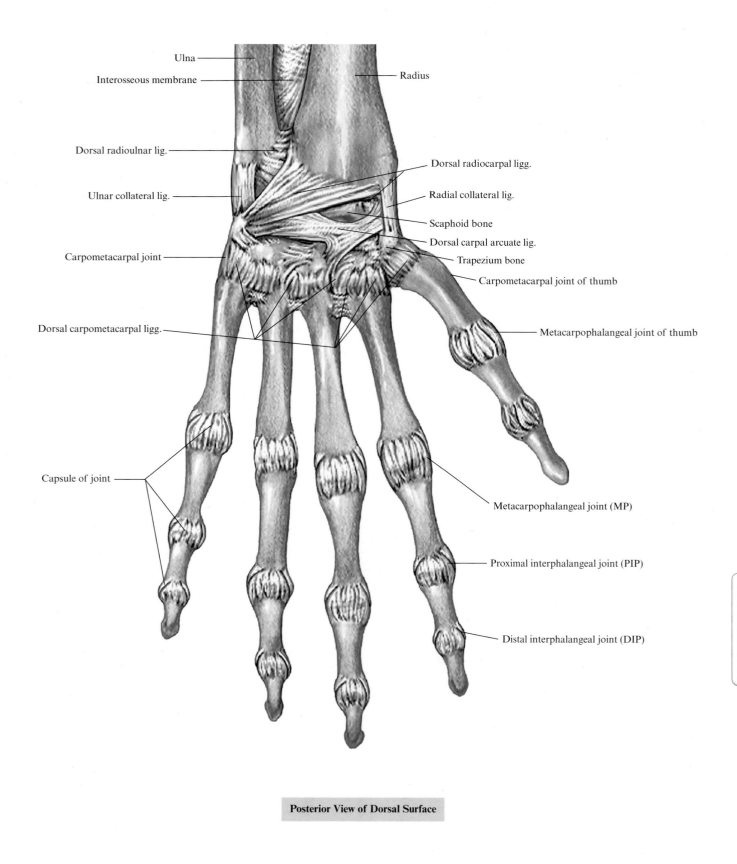

Ulna

Interosseous membrane

Radius

Dorsal radioulnar lig.

Dorsal radiocarpal ligg.

Ulnar collateral lig.

Radial collateral lig.

Scaphoid bone

Dorsal carpal arcuate lig.

Carpometacarpal joint

Trapezium bone

Carpometacarpal joint of thumb

Dorsal carpometacarpal ligg.

Metacarpophalangeal joint of thumb

Metacarpophalangeal joint (MP)

Capsule of joint

Proximal interphalangeal joint (PIP)

Distal interphalangeal joint (DIP)

Posterior View of Dorsal Surface

PLATE 6.61   BONES OF WRIST & HAND

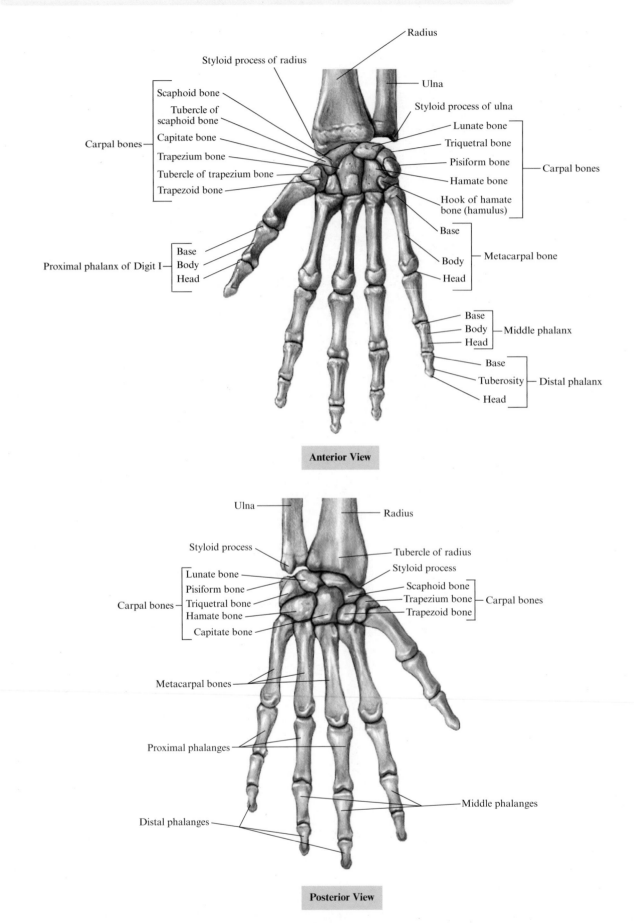

Radius

Styloid process of radius

Ulna

Styloid process of ulna

Scaphoid bone

Tubercle of
scaphoid bone

Capitate bone

Trapezium bone

Tubercle of trapezium bone

Trapezoid bone

Carpal bones

Lunate bone

Triquetral bone

Pisiform bone

Hamate bone

Hook of hamate
bone (hamulus)

Carpal bones

Base

Body

Head

Metacarpal bone

Proximal phalanx of Digit I

Base

Body

Head

Base

Body

Head

Middle phalanx

Base

Tuberosity

Head

Distal phalanx

Anterior View

Ulna

Radius

Styloid process

Tubercle of radius

Styloid process

Lunate bone

Pisiform bone

Triquetral bone

Hamate bone

Capitate bone

Carpal bones

Scaphoid bone

Trapezium bone

Trapezoid bone

Carpal bones

Metacarpal bones

Proximal phalanges

Middle phalanges

Distal phalanges

Posterior View

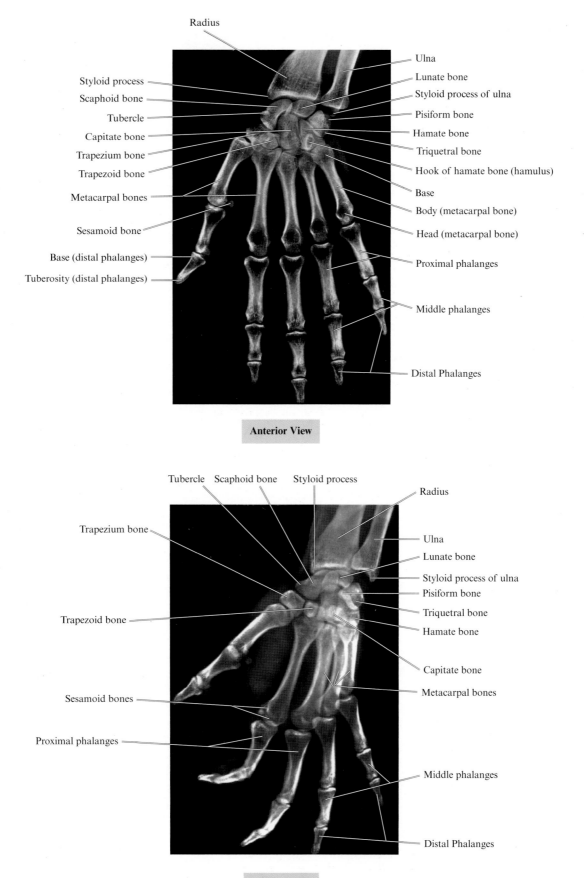

Radius

Styloid process
Scaphoid bone
Tubercle
Capitate bone
Trapezium bone
Trapezoid bone

Metacarpal bones

Sesamoid bone

Base (distal phalanges)
Tuberosity (distal phalanges)

Ulna
Lunate bone
Styloid process of ulna
Pisiform bone
Hamate bone
Triquetral bone
Hook of hamate bone (hamulus)
Base
Body (metacarpal bone)
Head (metacarpal bone)
Proximal phalanges

Middle phalanges

Distal Phalanges

Anterior View

Tubercle   Scaphoid bone   Styloid process

Trapezium bone

Trapezoid bone

Sesamoid bones

Proximal phalanges

Radius

Ulna
Lunate bone
Styloid process of ulna
Pisiform bone
Triquetral bone
Hamate bone

Capitate bone

Metacarpal bones

Middle phalanges

Distal Phalanges

Oblique View

7 HEAD AND NECK

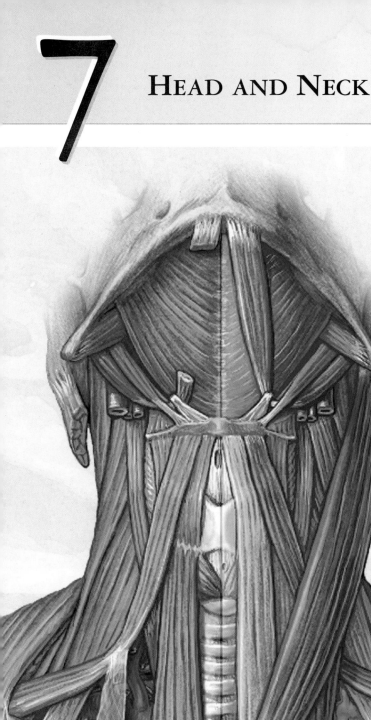

TOPOGRAPHY

SKELETON

MUSCLES

CERVICAL FASCIAL
PLANES

ARTERIES

VEINS

DERMATOMES &
CUTANEOUS
INNERVATION

BRAIN

LYMPHATICS

GLANDS

SUPERFICIAL FACE
& NECK

DEEP CERVICAL
STRUCTURES

LARYNX

PHARYNX

ORAL & NASAL
CAVITIES

ORBIT & EYE

INFRATEMPORAL FOSSA

PTERYGOPALATINE FOSSA

POSTERIOR CRANIAL
FOSSA

EAR

PLATE 7.1   TOPOGRAPHY

Anterior View

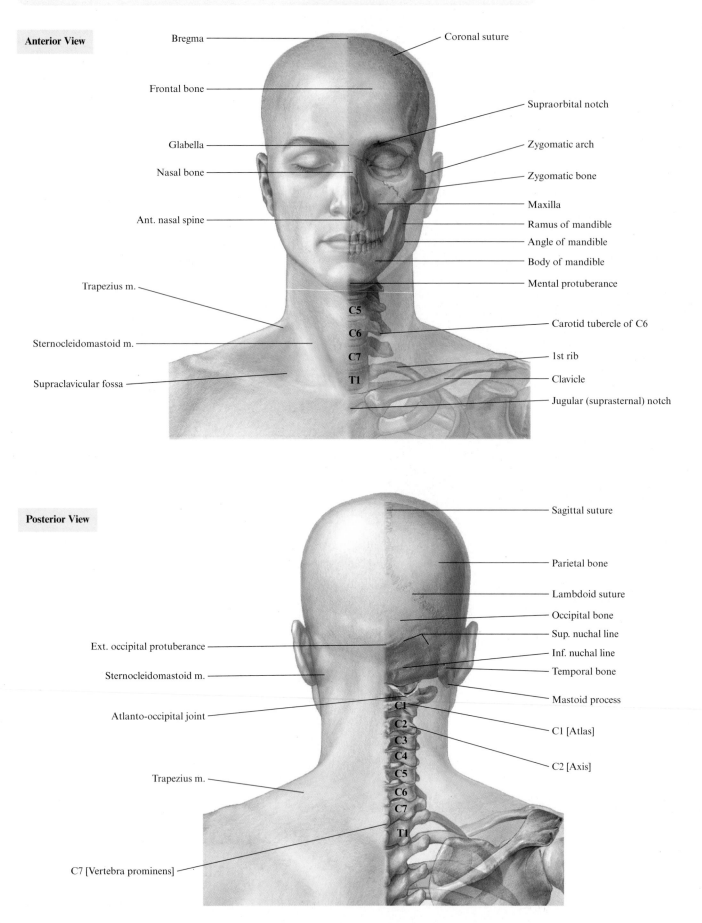

Bregma

Coronal suture

Frontal bone

Supraorbital notch

Glabella

Zygomatic arch

Nasal bone

Zygomatic bone

Maxilla

Ant. nasal spine

Ramus of mandible

Angle of mandible

Body of mandible

Mental protuberance

Trapezius m.

C5

C6

Carotid tubercle of C6

Sternocleidomastoid m.

C7

1st rib

Supraclavicular fossa

T1

Clavicle

Jugular (suprasternal) notch

Posterior View

Sagittal suture

Parietal bone

Lambdoid suture

Occipital bone

Sup. nuchal line

Ext. occipital protuberance

Inf. nuchal line

Sternocleidomastoid m.

Temporal bone

Mastoid process

C1

Atlanto-occipital joint

C2

C1 [Atlas]

C3

C4

C2 [Axis]

C5

Trapezius m.

C6

C7

T1

C7 [Vertebra prominens]

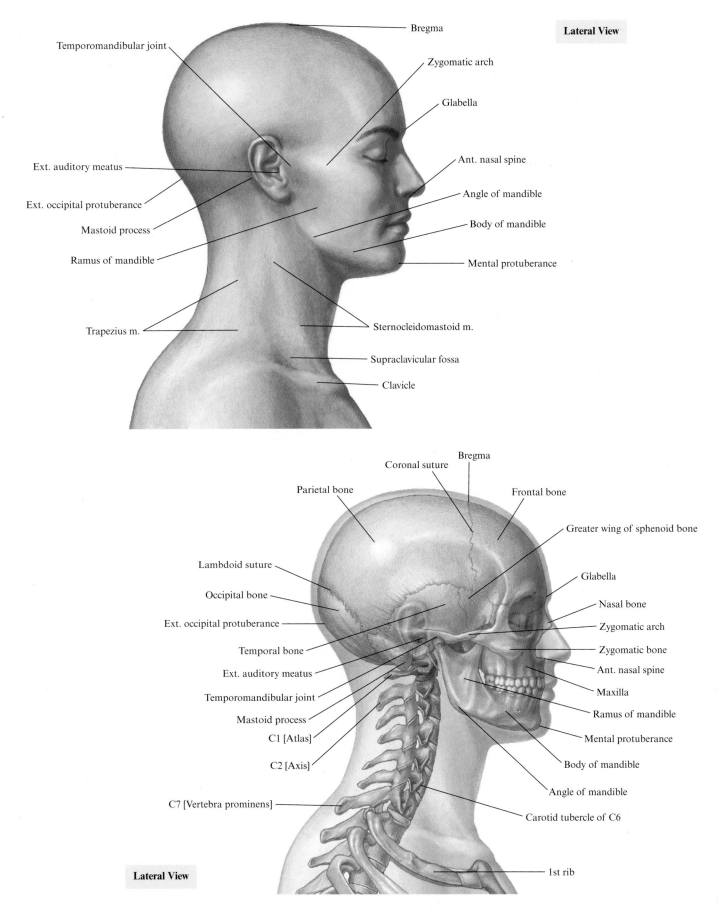

Lateral View

Bregma

Temporomandibular joint

Zygomatic arch

Glabella

Ant. nasal spine

Ext. auditory meatus

Angle of mandible

Ext. occipital protuberance

Body of mandible

Mastoid process

Mental protuberance

Ramus of mandible

Trapezius m.

Sternocleidomastoid m.

Supraclavicular fossa

Clavicle

Coronal suture

Bregma

Parietal bone

Frontal bone

Greater wing of sphenoid bone

Lambdoid suture

Glabella

Occipital bone

Nasal bone

Ext. occipital protuberance

Zygomatic arch

Temporal bone

Zygomatic bone

Ext. auditory meatus

Ant. nasal spine

Temporomandibular joint

Maxilla

Mastoid process

Ramus of mandible

C1 [Atlas]

Mental protuberance

C2 [Axis]

Body of mandible

Angle of mandible

C7 [Vertebra prominens]

Carotid tubercle of C6

Lateral View

1st rib

PLATE 7.3   TOPOGRAPHY

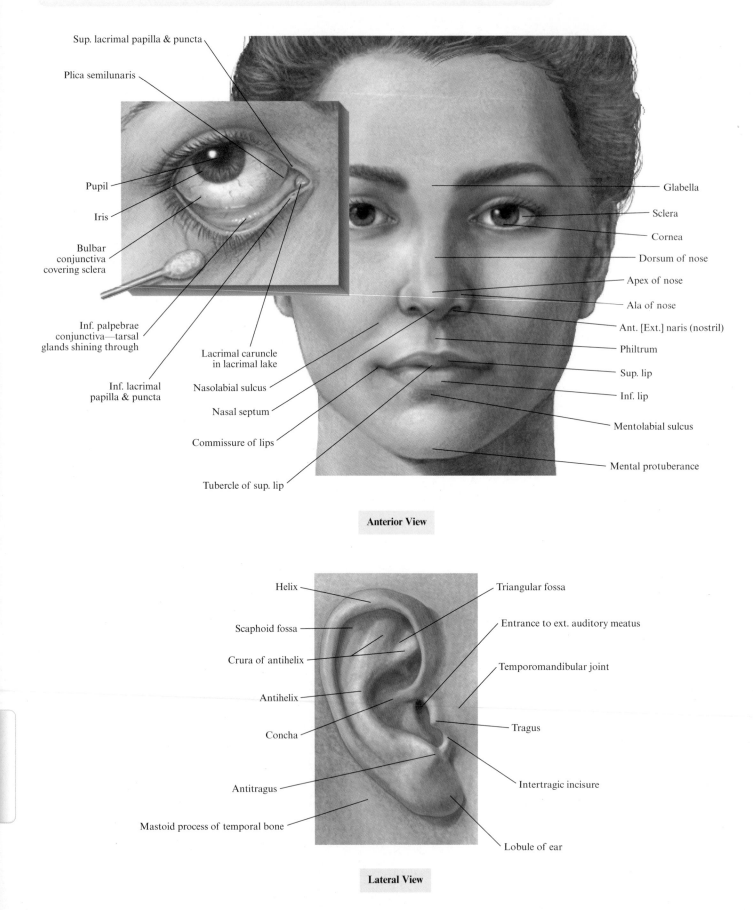

Sup. lacrimal papilla & puncta

Plica semilunaris

Pupil

Iris

Bulbar
conjunctiva
covering sclera

Inf. palpebrae
conjunctiva—tarsal
glands shining through

Inf. lacrimal
papilla & puncta

Lacrimal caruncle
in lacrimal lake

Nasolabial sulcus

Nasal septum

Commissure of lips

Tubercle of sup. lip

Glabella

Sclera

Cornea

Dorsum of nose

Apex of nose

Ala of nose

Ant. [Ext.] naris (nostril)

Philtrum

Sup. lip

Inf. lip

Mentolabial sulcus

Mental protuberance

Anterior View

Helix

Scaphoid fossa

Crura of antihelix

Antihelix

Concha

Antitragus

Mastoid process of temporal bone

Triangular fossa

Entrance to ext. auditory meatus

Temporomandibular joint

Tragus

Intertragic incisure

Lobule of ear

Lateral View

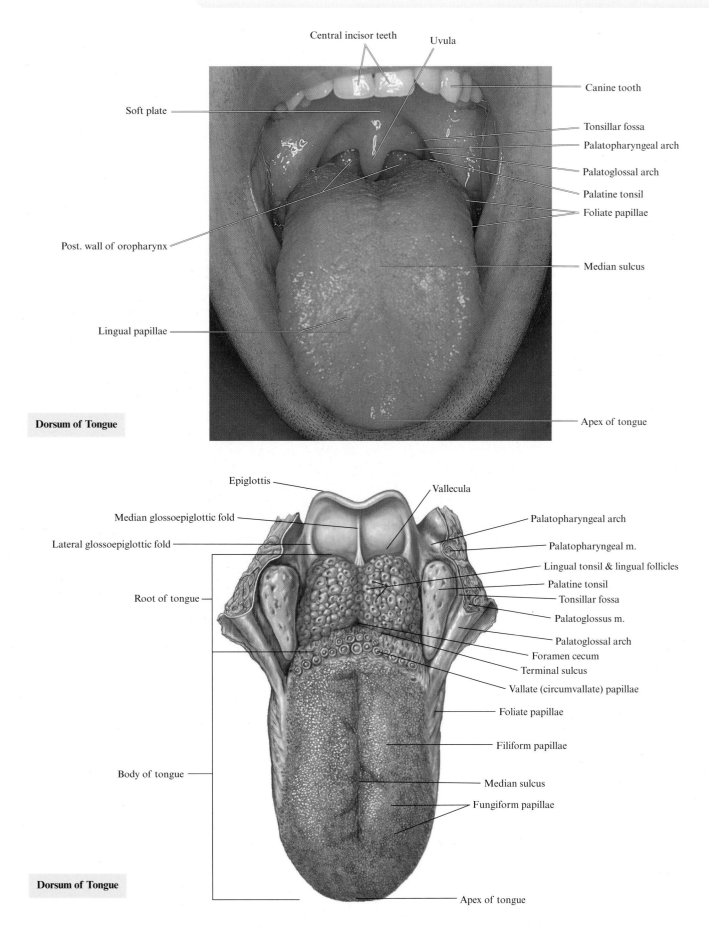

Central incisor teeth

Uvula

Canine tooth

Soft plate

Tonsillar fossa

Palatopharyngeal arch

Palatoglossal arch

Palatine tonsil

Foliate papillae

Post. wall of oropharynx

Median sulcus

Lingual papillae

Apex of tongue

Dorsum of Tongue

Epiglottis

Vallecula

Median glossoepiglottic fold

Palatopharyngeal arch

Lateral glossoepiglottic fold

Palatopharyngeal m.

Lingual tonsil & lingual follicles

Palatine tonsil

Root of tongue

Tonsillar fossa

Palatoglossus m.

Palatoglossal arch

Foramen cecum

Terminal sulcus

Vallate (circumvallate) papillae

Foliate papillae

Filiform papillae

Body of tongue

Median sulcus

Fungiform papillae

Dorsum of Tongue

Apex of tongue

PLATE 7.5   CRANIUM—ANTERIOR

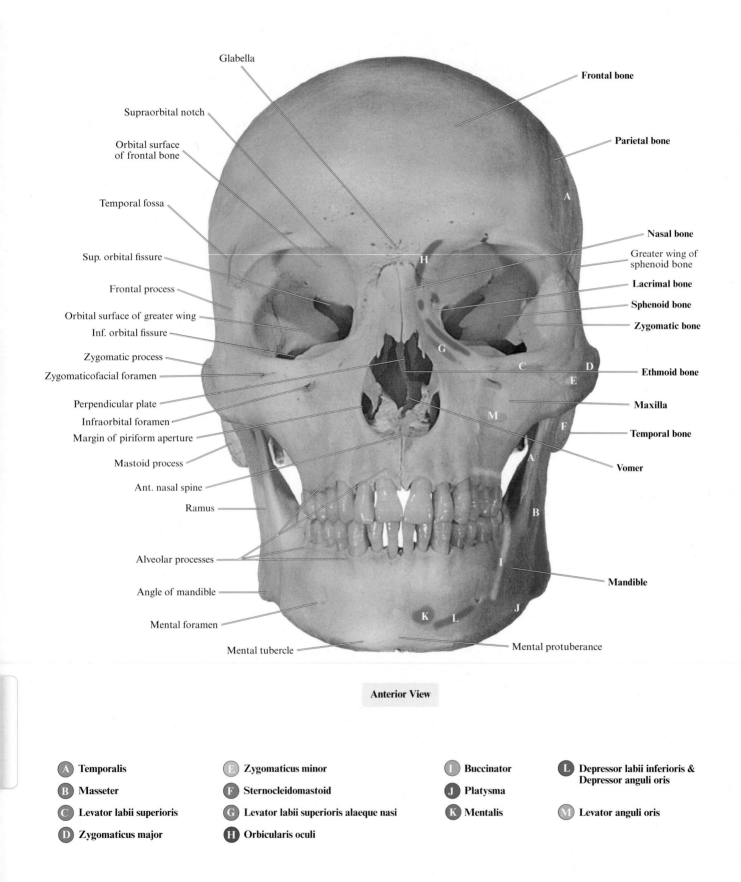

Glabella

Frontal bone

Supraorbital notch

Orbital surface
of frontal bone

Parietal bone

Temporal fossa

Sup. orbital fissure

Nasal bone

Greater wing of
sphenoid bone

Frontal process

Lacrimal bone

Orbital surface of greater wing

Sphenoid bone

Inf. orbital fissure

Zygomatic bone

Zygomatic process

Zygomaticofacial foramen

Ethmoid bone

Perpendicular plate

Maxilla

Infraorbital foramen

Margin of piriform aperture

Temporal bone

Mastoid process

Vomer

Ant. nasal spine

Ramus

Alveolar processes

Angle of mandible

Mandible

Mental foramen

Mental tubercle

Mental protuberance

Anterior View

(A) **Temporalis**

(B) **Masseter**

(C) **Levator labii superioris**

(D) **Zygomaticus major**

(E) **Zygomaticus minor**

(F) **Sternocleidomastoid**

(G) **Levator labii superioris alaeque nasi**

(H) **Orbicularis oculi**

(I) **Buccinator**

(J) **Platysma**

(K) **Mentalis**

(L) **Depressor labii inferioris &
Depressor anguli oris**

(M) **Levator anguli oris**

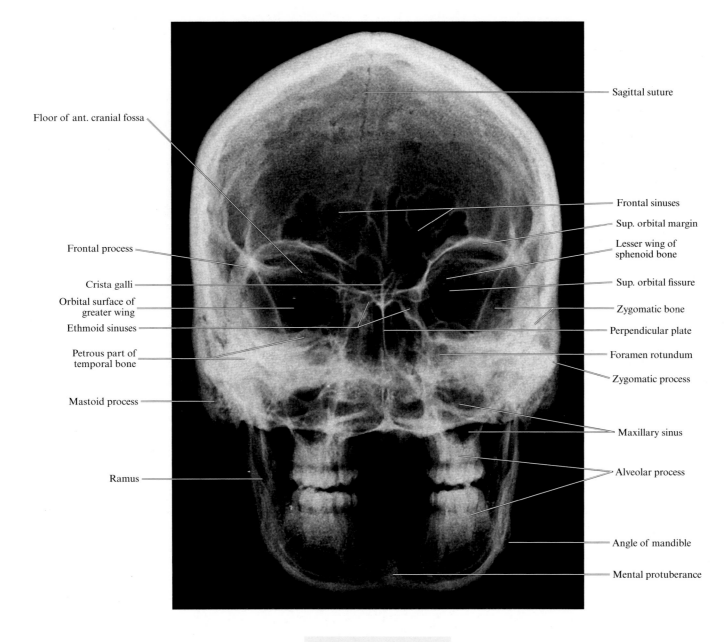

Sagittal suture

Floor of ant. cranial fossa

Frontal sinuses

Sup. orbital margin

Lesser wing of
sphenoid bone

Frontal process

Sup. orbital fissure

Crista galli

Orbital surface of
greater wing

Zygomatic bone

Ethmoid sinuses

Perpendicular plate

Petrous part of
temporal bone

Foramen rotundum

Zygomatic process

Mastoid process

Maxillary sinus

Ramus

Alveolar process

Angle of mandible

Mental protuberance

Anteroposterior View of Skull

PLATE 7.7   CRANIUM—MEDIAL

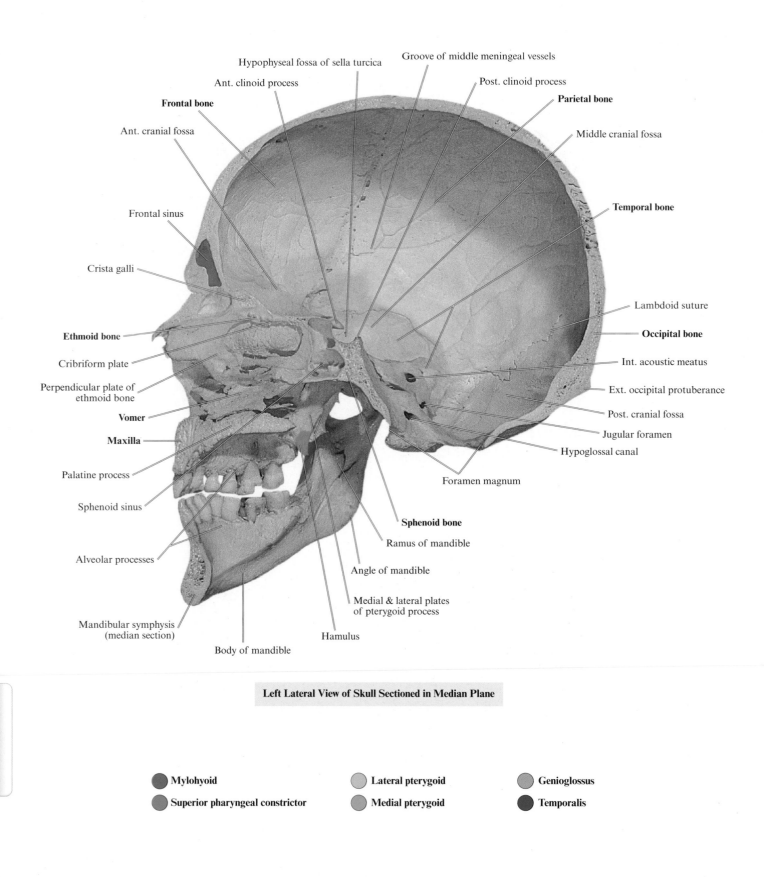

Hypophyseal fossa of sella turcica

Groove of middle meningeal vessels

Ant. clinoid process

Post. clinoid process

Frontal bone

Parietal bone

Ant. cranial fossa

Middle cranial fossa

Frontal sinus

Temporal bone

Crista galli

Lambdoid suture

Ethmoid bone

Occipital bone

Cribriform plate

Int. acoustic meatus

Perpendicular plate of
ethmoid bone

Ext. occipital protuberance

Vomer

Post. cranial fossa

Maxilla

Jugular foramen

Palatine process

Hypoglossal canal

Sphenoid sinus

Foramen magnum

Sphenoid bone

Alveolar processes

Ramus of mandible

Angle of mandible

Mandibular symphysis
(median section)

Medial & lateral plates
of pterygoid process

Hamulus

Body of mandible

Left Lateral View of Skull Sectioned in Median Plane

● Mylohyoid   ○ Lateral pterygoid   ● Genioglossus

● Superior pharyngeal constrictor   ● Medial pterygoid   ● Temporalis

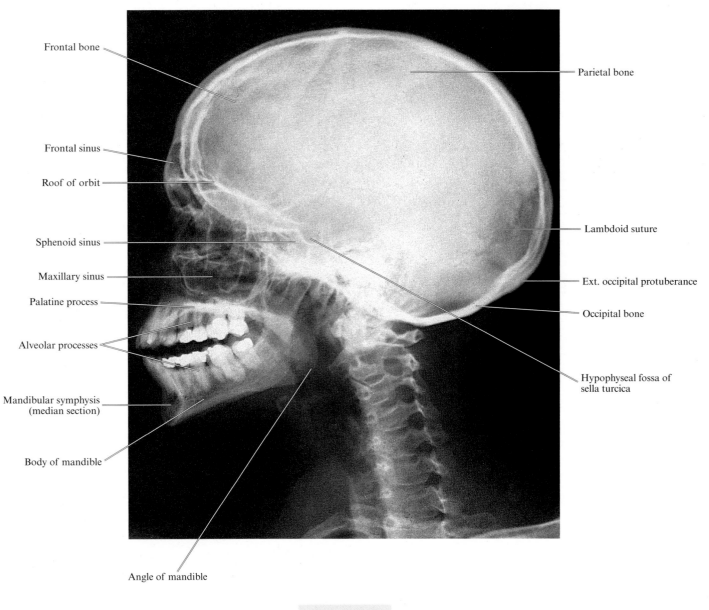

Frontal bone

Parietal bone

Frontal sinus

Roof of orbit

Sphenoid sinus

Lambdoid suture

Maxillary sinus

Ext. occipital protuberance

Palatine process

Occipital bone

Alveolar processes

Mandibular symphysis
(median section)

Hypophyseal fossa of
sella turcica

Body of mandible

Angle of mandible

Left Lateral View

PLATE 7.9   CRANIUM—LATERAL

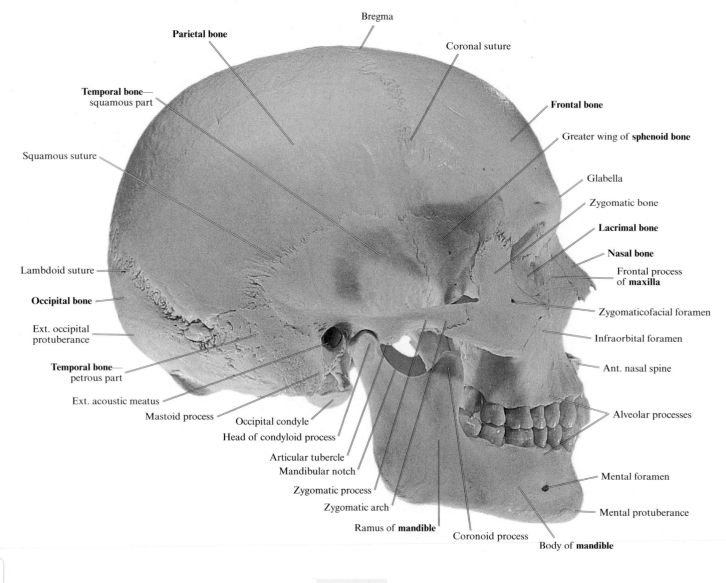

Bregma

Parietal bone

Coronal suture

Temporal bone—
squamous part

Frontal bone

Greater wing of sphenoid bone

Squamous suture

Glabella

Zygomatic bone

Lacrimal bone

Nasal bone

Lambdoid suture

Frontal process
of maxilla

Occipital bone

Zygomaticofacial foramen

Infraorbital foramen

Ext. occipital
protuberance

Ant. nasal spine

Temporal bone—
petrous part

Ext. acoustic meatus

Alveolar processes

Mastoid process

Occipital condyle

Head of condyloid process

Articular tubercle

Mandibular notch

Zygomatic process

Mental foramen

Zygomatic arch

Mental protuberance

Ramus of mandible

Coronoid process

Body of mandible

Lateral View

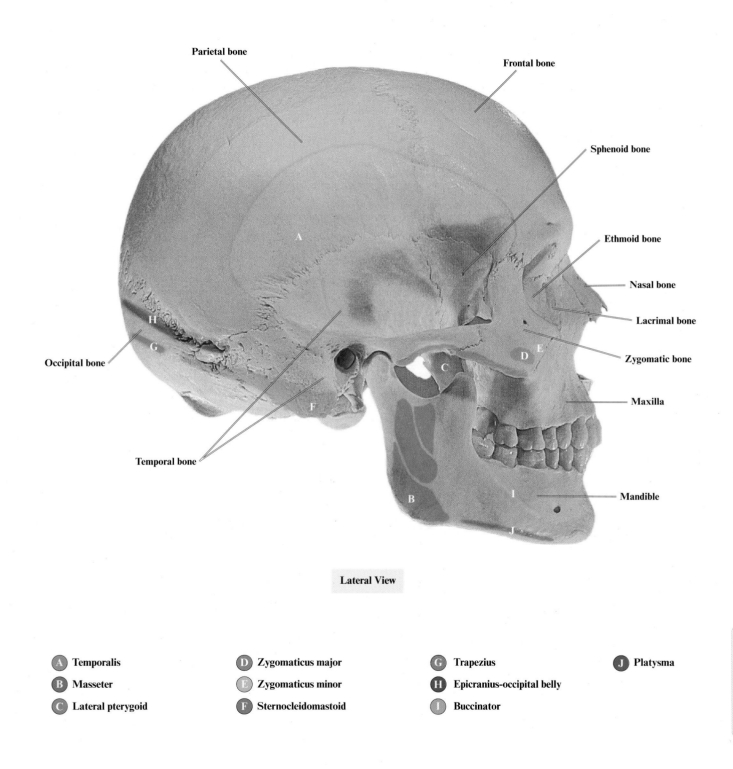

Parietal bone

Frontal bone

Sphenoid bone

Ethmoid bone

Nasal bone

Lacrimal bone

Zygomatic bone

Maxilla

Mandible

Occipital bone

Temporal bone

Lateral View

A Temporalis

B Masseter

C Lateral pterygoid

D Zygomaticus major

E Zygomaticus minor

F Sternocleidomastoid

G Trapezius

H Epicranius-occipital belly

I Buccinator

J Platysma

TABLE 7.1   CRANIAL FORAMINA, FISSURES & CANALS

Foramina/Openings	Contents
FACE	
Supraorbital notch/foramen	CN V^1 — supraorbital n. & vessels
Infraorbital notch/foramen	CN V^2 — infraorbital n. & vessels
Mental foramen	CN V^3 — mental n. & vessels
Zygomaticofacial foramen	CN V^2 — zygomaticofacial n. & vessels
ORBIT	
Superior orbital fissure	Passage between middle cranial fossa & orbit for CN III, IV, VI, V^1 — lacrimal n., V^1 — frontal n., V^1 — nasociliary n., postganglionic sympathetic n. fibers, & ophthalmic v.
Optic canal	CN II, & ophthalmic a.
Inferior orbital fissure	Passage between pterygopalatine fossa & orbit for CN V^2 — infraorbital n. & vessels, & nerves from pterygopalatine ganglion
Anterior ethmoidal foramen	CN V^1 — ant. ethmoidal br. of nasociliary n. & vessels
Posterior ethmoidal foramen	CN V^1 — post. ethmoidal br. of nasociliary n. & vessels
Nasolacrimal canal	Nasolacrimal duct
NASAL CAVITY	
Piriform aperture (anterior nasal aperture)	Anterior opening into nasal cavity
Incisive canals	CN V^1 — nasopalatine n. & greater palatine vessels
Foramina in cribriform plates	CN I — Sensory axons from olfactory epithelium that collectively constitute olfactory nn.
Sphenoethmoidal recess	Opening of sphenoid sinuses
Superior meatus	Duct from post. ethmoid sinuses
Middle meatus	Ducts from frontal sinus, ant. & middle ethmoidal sinuses, & opening of maxillary sinus through semilunar hiatus
Anterior meatus	Nasolacrimal duct
Sphenopalatine foramen	CN V^2 — nasopalatine n. & sphenopalatine vessels
Choana (posterior nasal aperture)	Opening between nasal cavity & nasopharynx
LATERAL CRANIAL SURFACE	
Zygomaticofacial foramen	CN V^2 — zygomaticofacial n. & vessels
Pterygomaxillary fissure	Passage between infratemporal & pterygopalatine fossae for CN V^2 — post. sup. alveolar nn. & vessels, & 3rd part of maxillary a.
External acoustic meatus—bony part	Opening in temporal bone leading to tympanic membrane
Mastoid foramen	Mastoid br. or occipital a. & mastoid emissary v. to sigmoid sinus & diploic vv.
CRANIAL BASE	
Incisive fossa & canals	CN V^2 — nasopalatine n., & greater palatine vessels
Greater palatine foramen/canal	Passage between oral cavity & pterygopalatine fossa for CN V^2 — greater palatine n. & vessels
Lesser palatine foramina	Passages between greater palatine canal & oral cavity for CN V^2 — lesser palatine n. & vessels
Mandibular canal	CN V^3 — inf. alveolar n. & vessels
Foramen lacerum	Closed inferoexternally by fibrocartilage
Auditory tube—bony portion	Passage between nasopharynx & middle ear, tensor tympani m., & sup. tympanic a.
Pterygoid (Vidian) canal	Passage through base of median pterygoid process between foramen lacerum & pterygopalatine fossa for CN VII — n. & vessels of pterygoid (vidian) canal
Foramen ovale	CN V^3 — mandibular n., CN IX — lesser petrosal n. & accessory meningeal a.
Foramen spinosum	CN V^3 — meningeal br. & middle meningeal vessels
Carotid canal	Internal carotid a. & sympathetic n. plexus
Stylomastoid foramen	CN VII — facial n., & stylomastoid vessels
Petrotympanic fissure	CN VII — chorda tympani n., & ant. tympanic a.
Mastoid canaliculus	CN X — auricular br.
Tympanic canaliculus	CN IX — tympanic br., & inf. tympanic a.
Jugular fossa & foramen	CN IX, X & XI, sup. bulb of internal jugular v., inferior petrosal & sigmoid sinuses, & meningeal brr. of ascending pharyngeal & occipital aa.
Condylar fossa & canal	*Inconsistent* passage for condylar emissary v. between sigmoid sinus & vertebral venous plexi
Hypoglossal canal	CN XII — hypoglossal n., meningeal br. of ascending pharyngeal a.
Foramen magnum	Medulla & meninges of spinal cord, CN XI, vertebral aa., ant. & post. spinal aa., & brr. of internal vertebral venous plexus

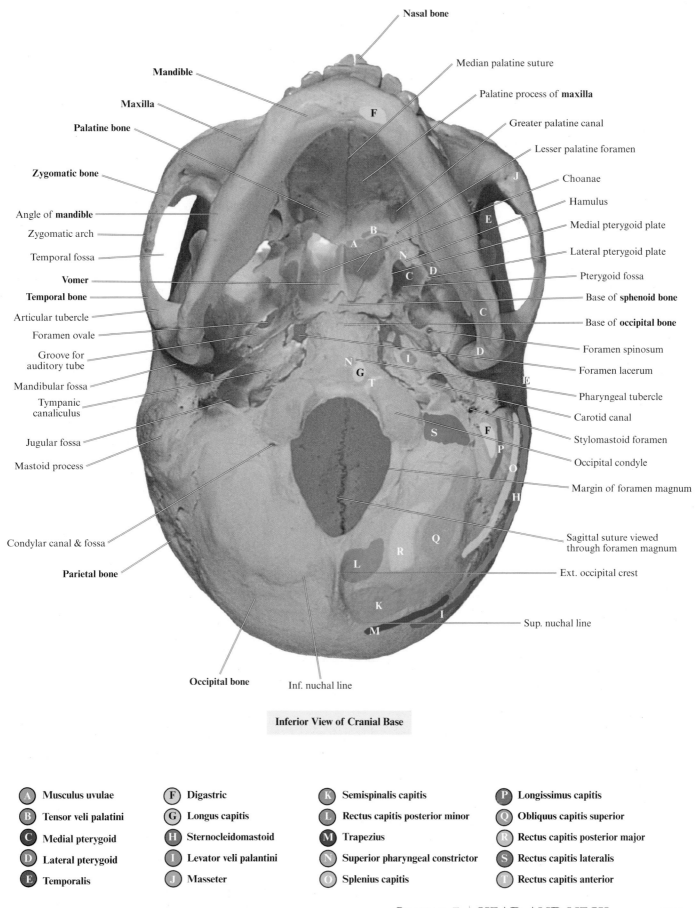

Nasal bone

Median palatine suture

Palatine process of **maxilla**

Greater palatine canal

Lesser palatine foramen

Choanae

Hamulus

Medial pterygoid plate

Lateral pterygoid plate

Pterygoid fossa

Base of **sphenoid bone**

Base of **occipital bone**

Foramen spinosum

Foramen lacerum

Pharyngeal tubercle

Carotid canal

Stylomastoid foramen

Occipital condyle

Margin of foramen magnum

Sagittal suture viewed
through foramen magnum

Ext. occipital crest

Sup. nuchal line

Mandible

Maxilla

Palatine bone

Zygomatic bone

Angle of **mandible**

Zygomatic arch

Temporal fossa

Vomer

Temporal bone

Articular tubercle

Foramen ovale

Groove for
auditory tube

Mandibular fossa

Tympanic
canaliculus

Jugular fossa

Mastoid process

Condylar canal & fossa

Parietal bone

Occipital bone   Inf. nuchal line

Inferior View of Cranial Base

A Musculus uvulae	**F** Digastric	**K** Semispinalis capitis	**P** Longissimus capitis
B Tensor veli palatini	**G** Longus capitis	**L** Rectus capitis posterior minor	**Q** Obliquus capitis superior
C Medial pterygoid	**H** Sternocleidomastoid	**M** Trapezius	**R** Rectus capitis posterior major
D Lateral pterygoid	**I** Levator veli palantini	**N** Superior pharyngeal constrictor	**S** Rectus capitis lateralis
E Temporalis	**J** Masseter	**O** Splenius capitis	**T** Rectus capitis anterior

TABLE 7.2 INTERNAL NEUROCRANIAL FORAMINA, FISSURES & CANALS

Foramina/Openings	Contents
ANTERIOR CRANIAL FOSSA	
Foramen cecum	Inconsistent passage for nasal emissary vv. tributaries of superior sagittal sinus
Foramina in cribriform plates	CN I — Sensory axons from olfactory epithelium that collectively constitute the olfactory nn.
Anterior ethmoidal foramen	CN V^1 — anterior ethmoidal br. of nasociliary n. & vessels
Posterior ethmoidal foramen	CN V^1 — posterior ethmoidal br. of nasociliary n. & vessels
MIDDLE CRANIAL FOSSA	
Optic canal	CN II, & ophthalmic a.
Superior orbital fissure	Passage between middle cranial fossa & orbit for CN III, IV, VI, V1 — lacrimal n., V1 — frontal n., V^1 — nasociliary n., postganglionic sympathetic n. fibers, & ophthalmic v.
Foramen rotundum	CN V^2 — maxillary n.
Foramen ovale	CN V^3 — mandibular n., CN IX - lesser petrosal n. & accessory meningeal a.
Foramen spinosum	CN V^3 — meningeal br. & middle meningeal vessels
Foramen lacerum	Internal carotid a., sympathetic nn. & venous plexi from carotid canal, & CN VII — greater petrosal n. Closed inferoexternally by fibrocartilage
Hiatus for greater petrosal n. (Facial hiatus)	CN VII — greater petrosal n., & petrosal br. of middle meningeal a.
Hiatus for lesser petrosal n.	CN IX — lesser petrosal n.
POSTERIOR CRANIAL FOSSA	
Internal acoustic meatus	CN VII & VIII, labyrinthine a.
Jugular fossa & foramen	CN IX, X & XI, superior bulb of internal jugular v., inferior petrosal & sigmoid sinuses, & meningeal brr. of ascending pharyngeal & occipital aa.
Condylar fossa & canal	*Inconsistent* passage for condylar emissary v. between sigmoid sinus & vertebral venous plexi
Mastoid foramen	Mastoid br. of occipital a. & mastoid emissary v. to sigmoid sinus & diploic vv.
Hypoglossal canal	CN XII — hypoglossal n.
Foramen magnum	Medulla & meninges of spinal cord, CN XI, vertebral aa., ant. & post. spinal aa., & brr. of internal vertebral venous plexus

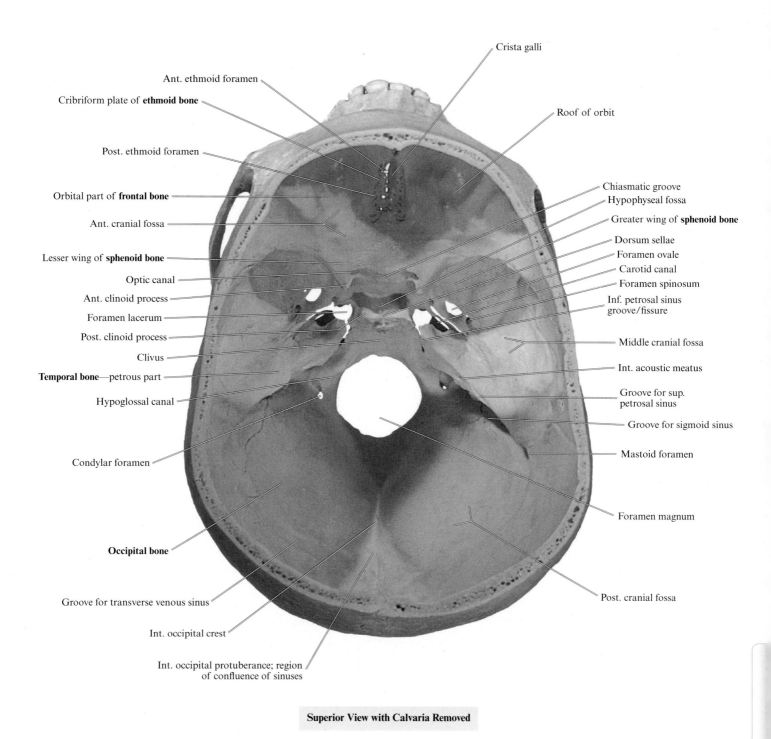

Crista galli

Ant. ethmoid foramen

Cribriform plate of **ethmoid bone**

Roof of orbit

Post. ethmoid foramen

Orbital part of **frontal bone**

Chiasmatic groove
Hypophyseal fossa

Ant. cranial fossa

Greater wing of **sphenoid bone**

Lesser wing of **sphenoid bone**

Dorsum sellae
Foramen ovale

Optic canal

Carotid canal

Ant. clinoid process

Foramen spinosum

Foramen lacerum

Inf. petrosal sinus
groove/fissure

Post. clinoid process

Middle cranial fossa

Clivus

Int. acoustic meatus

Temporal bone—petrous part

Groove for sup.
petrosal sinus

Hypoglossal canal

Groove for sigmoid sinus

Condylar foramen

Mastoid foramen

Foramen magnum

Occipital bone

Post. cranial fossa

Groove for transverse venous sinus

Int. occipital crest

Int. occipital protuberance; region
of confluence of sinuses

Superior View with Calvaria Removed

PLATE 7.13   CRANIUM—SPHENOID BONE

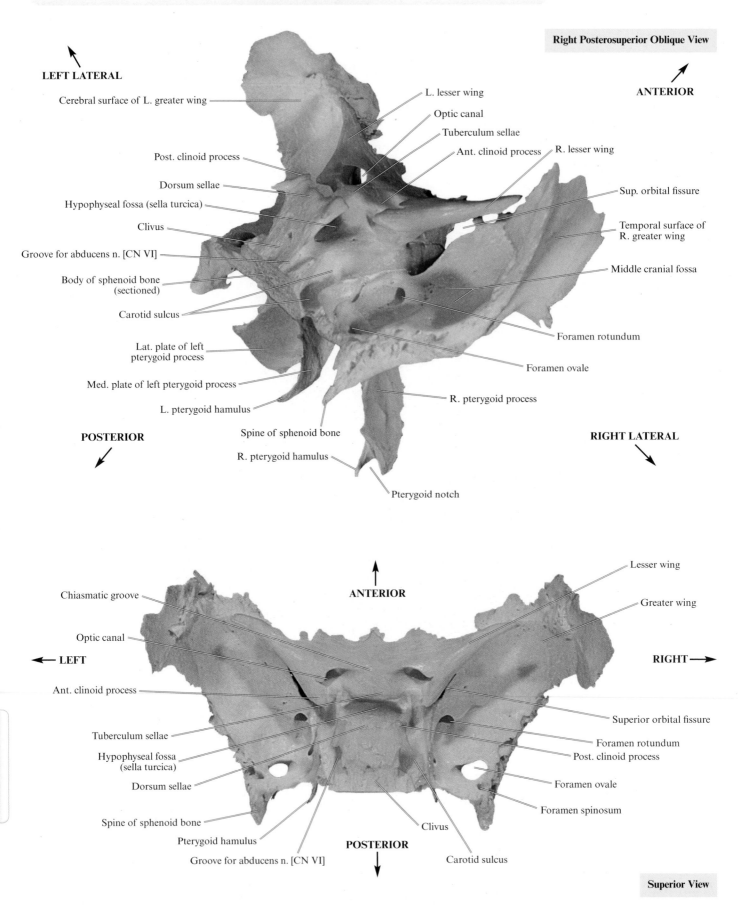

LEFT LATERAL

Cerebral surface of L. greater wing

L. lesser wing
Optic canal
Tuberculum sellae
Ant. clinoid process
R. lesser wing

ANTERIOR

Post. clinoid process
Dorsum sellae
Hypophyseal fossa (sella turcica)
Clivus
Groove for abducens n. [CN VI]
Body of sphenoid bone (sectioned)
Carotid sulcus
Lat. plate of left pterygoid process
Med. plate of left pterygoid process
L. pterygoid hamulus

Sup. orbital fissure
Temporal surface of R. greater wing
Middle cranial fossa
Foramen rotundum
Foramen ovale
R. pterygoid process

POSTERIOR

Spine of sphenoid bone
R. pterygoid hamulus
Pterygoid notch

RIGHT LATERAL

Chiasmatic groove

Optic canal

ANTERIOR

Lesser wing

Greater wing

LEFT

RIGHT

Ant. clinoid process

Tuberculum sellae
Hypophyseal fossa (sella turcica)
Dorsum sellae

Spine of sphenoid bone
Pterygoid hamulus
Groove for abducens n. [CN VI]

Superior orbital fissure
Foramen rotundum
Post. clinoid process
Foramen ovale
Foramen spinosum

Clivus
Carotid sulcus

POSTERIOR

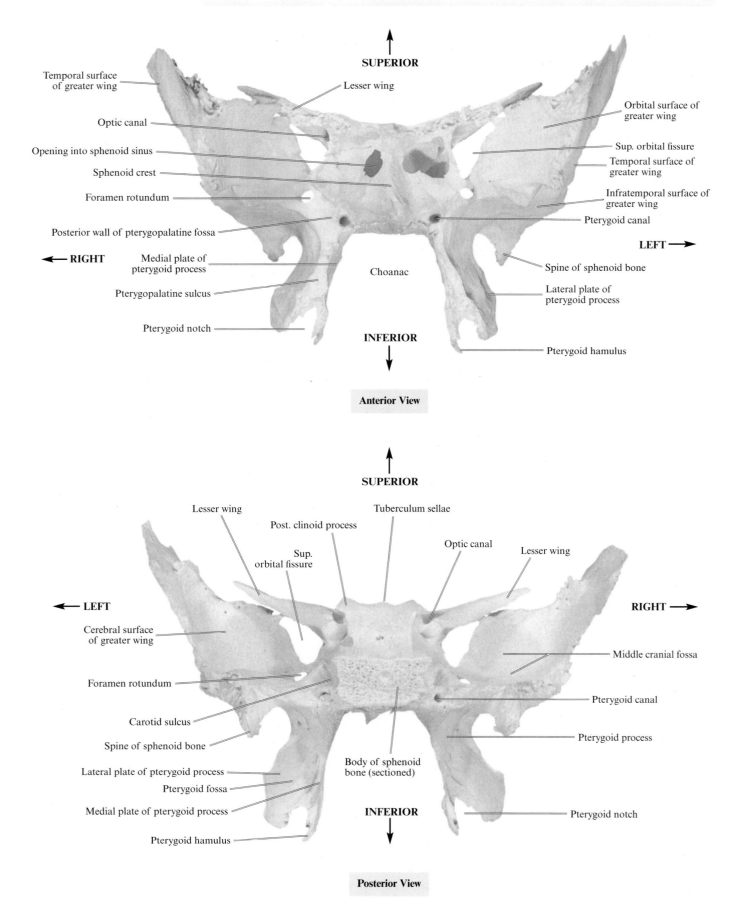

SUPERIOR

Temporal surface
of greater wing

Lesser wing

Orbital surface of
greater wing

Optic canal

Opening into sphenoid sinus

Sup. orbital fissure

Temporal surface of
greater wing

Sphenoid crest

Foramen rotundum

Infratemporal surface of
greater wing

Posterior wall of pterygopalatine fossa

Pterygoid canal

◄— RIGHT

LEFT —►

Medial plate of
pterygoid process

Choanac

Spine of sphenoid bone

Pterygopalatine sulcus

Lateral plate of
pterygoid process

Pterygoid notch

INFERIOR

Pterygoid hamulus

Anterior View

SUPERIOR

Lesser wing

Tuberculum sellae

Post. clinoid process

Sup.
orbital fissure

Optic canal

Lesser wing

◄— LEFT

RIGHT —►

Cerebral surface
of greater wing

Middle cranial fossa

Foramen rotundum

Pterygoid canal

Carotid sulcus

Spine of sphenoid bone

Pterygoid process

Lateral plate of pterygoid process

Body of sphenoid
bone (sectioned)

Pterygoid fossa

Medial plate of pterygoid process

Pterygoid notch

Pterygoid hamulus

INFERIOR

Posterior View

PLATE 7.15 CRANIUM—ORBITAL & NASAL WALLS

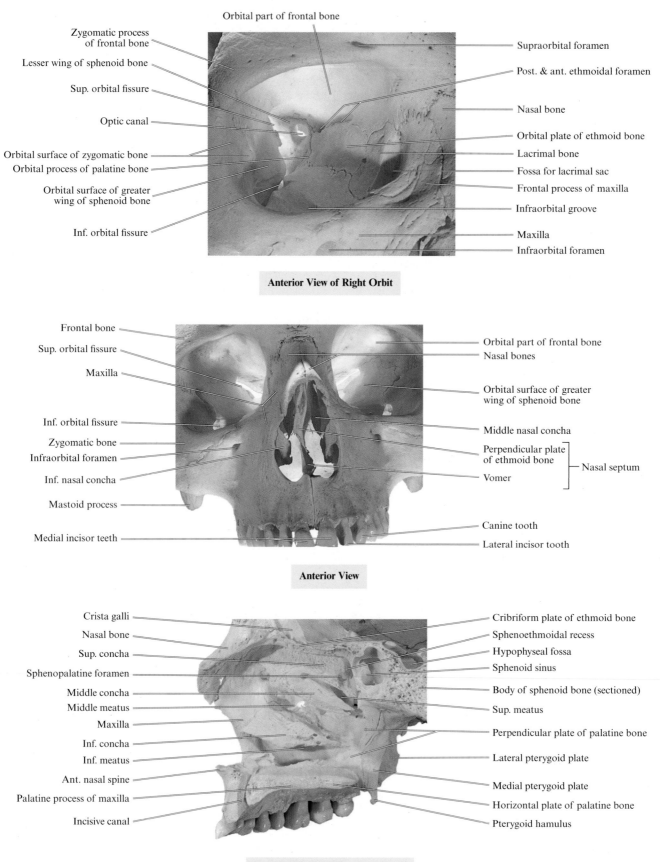

Orbital part of frontal bone

Zygomatic process
of frontal bone

Lesser wing of sphenoid bone

Sup. orbital fissure

Optic canal

Orbital surface of zygomatic bone

Orbital process of palatine bone

Orbital surface of greater
wing of sphenoid bone

Inf. orbital fissure

Supraorbital foramen

Post. & ant. ethmoidal foramen

Nasal bone

Orbital plate of ethmoid bone

Lacrimal bone

Fossa for lacrimal sac

Frontal process of maxilla

Infraorbital groove

Maxilla

Infraorbital foramen

Anterior View of Right Orbit

Frontal bone

Sup. orbital fissure

Maxilla

Inf. orbital fissure

Zygomatic bone

Infraorbital foramen

Inf. nasal concha

Mastoid process

Medial incisor teeth

Orbital part of frontal bone

Nasal bones

Orbital surface of greater
wing of sphenoid bone

Middle nasal concha

Perpendicular plate
of ethmoid bone

Vomer

Nasal septum

Canine tooth

Lateral incisor tooth

Anterior View

Crista galli

Nasal bone

Sup. concha

Sphenopalatine foramen

Middle concha

Middle meatus

Maxilla

Inf. concha

Inf. meatus

Ant. nasal spine

Palatine process of maxilla

Incisive canal

Cribriform plate of ethmoid bone

Sphenoethmoidal recess

Hypophyseal fossa

Sphenoid sinus

Body of sphenoid bone (sectioned)

Sup. meatus

Perpendicular plate of palatine bone

Lateral pterygoid plate

Medial pterygoid plate

Horizontal plate of palatine bone

Pterygoid hamulus

Medial View of Right Nasal Cavity

A.D.A.M. | Student Atlas of Anatomy

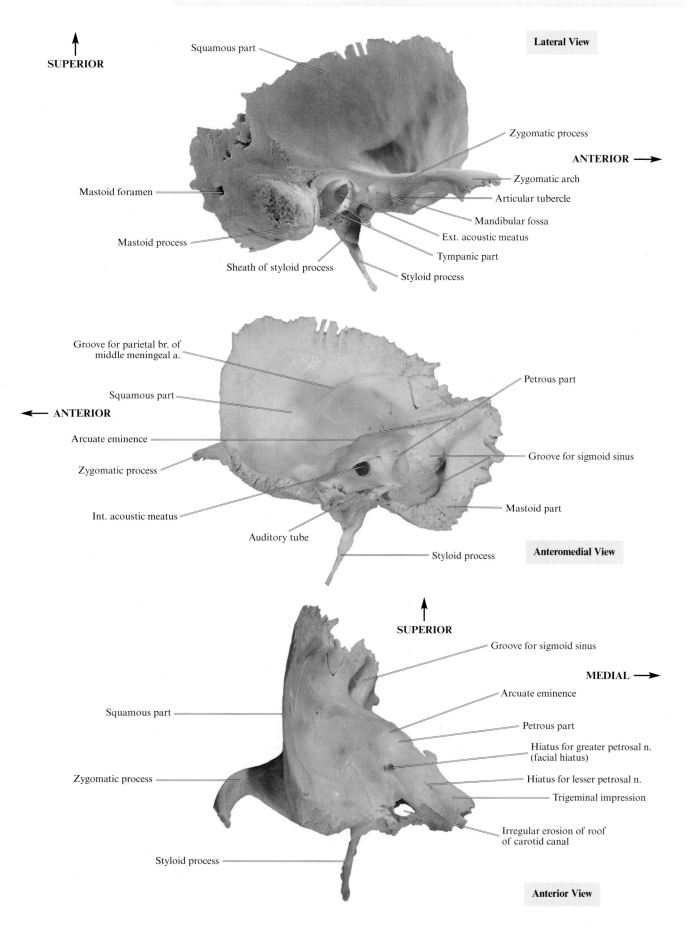

Lateral View

SUPERIOR

Squamous part

Zygomatic process

ANTERIOR →

Zygomatic arch

Mastoid foramen

Articular tubercle

Mandibular fossa

Ext. acoustic meatus

Mastoid process

Tympanic part

Sheath of styloid process

Styloid process

Groove for parietal br. of
middle meningeal a.

Petrous part

Squamous part

← ANTERIOR

Arcuate eminence

Zygomatic process

Groove for sigmoid sinus

Int. acoustic meatus

Mastoid part

Auditory tube

Styloid process

Anteromedial View

SUPERIOR

Groove for sigmoid sinus

MEDIAL →

Arcuate eminence

Squamous part

Petrous part

Hiatus for greater petrosal n.
(facial hiatus)

Zygomatic process

Hiatus for lesser petrosal n.

Trigeminal impression

Irregular erosion of roof
of carotid canal

Styloid process

Anterior View

PLATE 7.17   PALATE & PHARYNGEAL REGION

Oblique Basal View of Choanae

← RIGHT   ANTERIOR   LEFT →

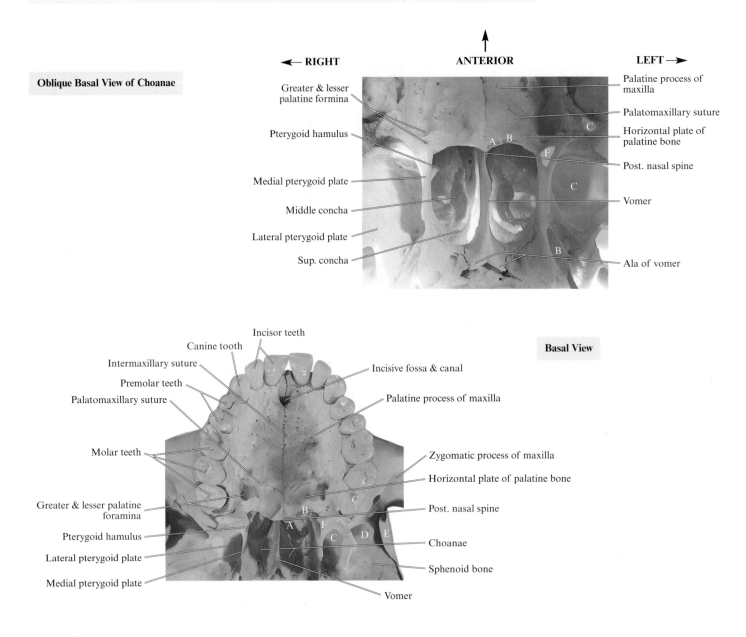

Greater & lesser palatine formina
Pterygoid hamulus
Medial pterygoid plate
Middle concha
Lateral pterygoid plate
Sup. concha

Palatine process of maxilla
Palatomaxillary suture
Horizontal plate of palatine bone
Post. nasal spine
Vomer
Ala of vomer

Basal View

Incisor teeth
Canine tooth
Intermaxillary suture
Premolar teeth
Palatomaxillary suture
Molar teeth
Greater & lesser palatine foramina
Pterygoid hamulus
Lateral pterygoid plate
Medial pterygoid plate
Vomer

Incisive fossa & canal
Palatine process of maxilla
Zygomatic process of maxilla
Horizontal plate of palatine bone
Post. nasal spine
Choanae
Sphenoid bone

Basal View of Left Mandibular Fossa

Ⓐ **Musculus uvulae**

Ⓑ **Tensor veli palatini**

Ⓒ **Medial pterygoid**

Ⓓ **Lateral pterygoid**

Ⓔ **Temporalis**

Ⓕ **Superior pharyngeal constrictor**

Ⓖ **Tensor tympani**

Ⓗ **Levator veli palatini**

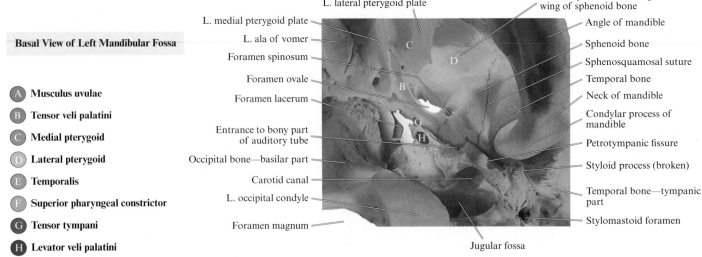

L. lateral pterygoid plate
L. medial pterygoid plate
L. ala of vomer
Foramen spinosum
Foramen ovale
Foramen lacerum
Entrance to bony part of auditory tube
Occipital bone—basilar part
Carotid canal
L. occipital condyle
Foramen magnum
Jugular fossa

Infratemporal surface of greater wing of sphenoid bone
Angle of mandible
Sphenoid bone
Sphenosquamosal suture
Temporal bone
Neck of mandible
Condylar process of mandible
Petrotympanic fissure
Styloid process (broken)
Temporal bone—tympanic part
Stylomastoid foramen

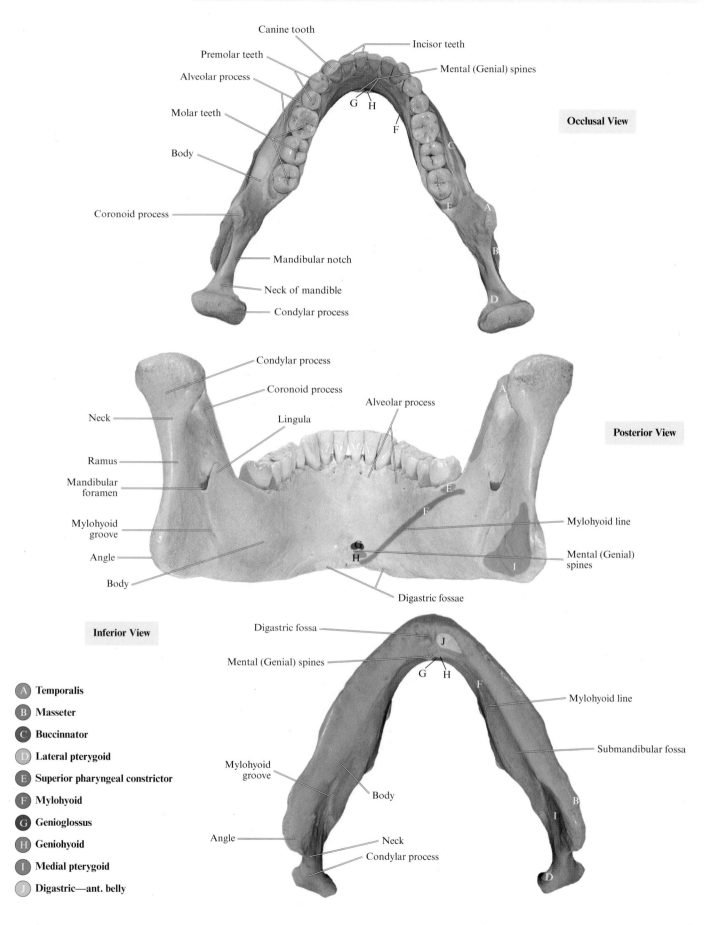

Canine tooth

Incisor teeth

Premolar teeth

Mental (Genial) spines

Alveolar process

Occlusal View

Molar teeth

G H

Body

F

C

Coronoid process

E A

B

Mandibular notch

Neck of mandible

D

Condylar process

Condylar process

Coronoid process

Alveolar process

A

Neck

Lingula

Posterior View

Ramus

Mandibular
foramen

E

Mylohyoid
groove

F

Mylohyoid line

Angle

G

Mental (Genial)
spines

H

I

Body

Digastric fossae

Digastric fossa

Inferior View

J

Mental (Genial) spines

G H

F

Mylohyoid line

A **Temporalis**

B **Masseter**

Submandibular fossa

C **Buccinnator**

D **Lateral pterygoid**

Mylohyoid
groove

E **Superior pharyngeal constrictor**

B

F **Mylohyoid**

I

Body

G **Genioglossus**

H **Geniohyoid**

Angle

Neck

I **Medial pterygoid**

Condylar process

D

J **Digastric—ant. belly**

PLATE 7.19   SKELETON—LARYNGEAL

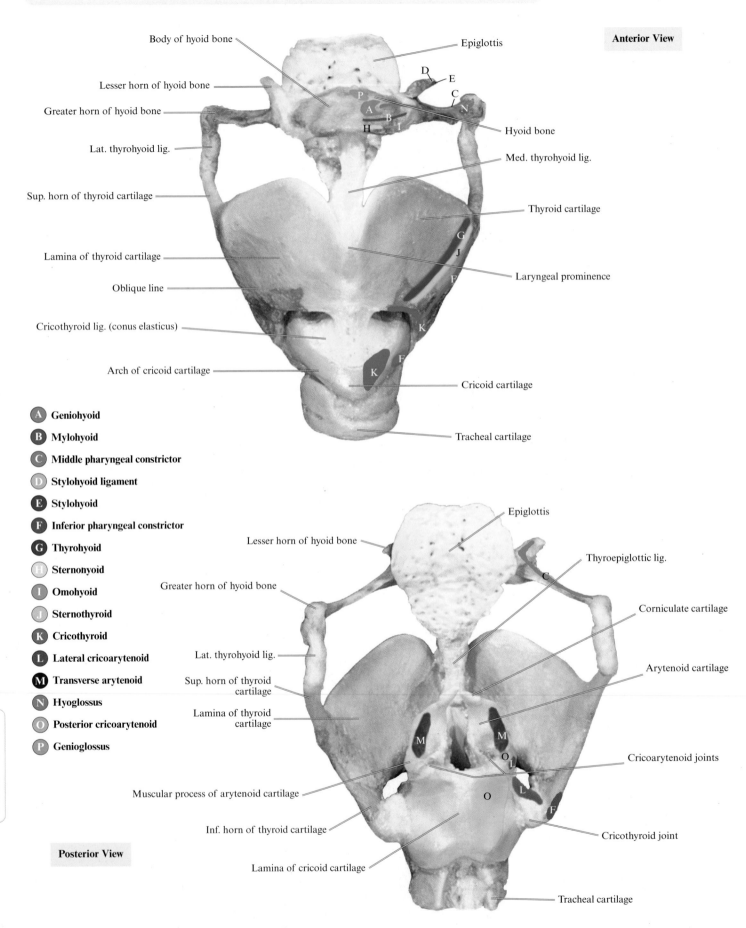

Anterior View

Body of hyoid bone

Lesser horn of hyoid bone

Greater horn of hyoid bone

Lat. thyrohyoid lig.

Sup. horn of thyroid cartilage

Lamina of thyroid cartilage

Oblique line

Cricothyroid lig. (conus elasticus)

Arch of cricoid cartilage

Epiglottis

D
E
C
P
A
B
N
H
I

Hyoid bone

Med. thyrohyoid lig.

Thyroid cartilage

G
J

Laryngeal prominence

K
F
K

Cricoid cartilage

Tracheal cartilage

A Geniohyoid

B Mylohyoid

C Middle pharyngeal constrictor

D Stylohyoid ligament

E Stylohyoid

F Inferior pharyngeal constrictor

G Thyrohyoid

H Sternonyoid

I Omohyoid

J Sternothyroid

K Cricothyroid

L Lateral cricoarytenoid

M Transverse arytenoid

N Hyoglossus

O Posterior cricoarytenoid

P Genioglossus

Lesser horn of hyoid bone

Greater horn of hyoid bone

Lat. thyrohyoid lig.

Sup. horn of thyroid cartilage

Lamina of thyroid cartilage

Muscular process of arytenoid cartilage

Inf. horn of thyroid cartilage

Posterior View

Lamina of cricoid cartilage

Epiglottis

Thyroepiglottic lig.

C

Corniculate cartilage

Arytenoid cartilage

M   M

O   L
L

Cricoarytenoid joints

O

L

F

Cricothyroid joint

Tracheal cartilage

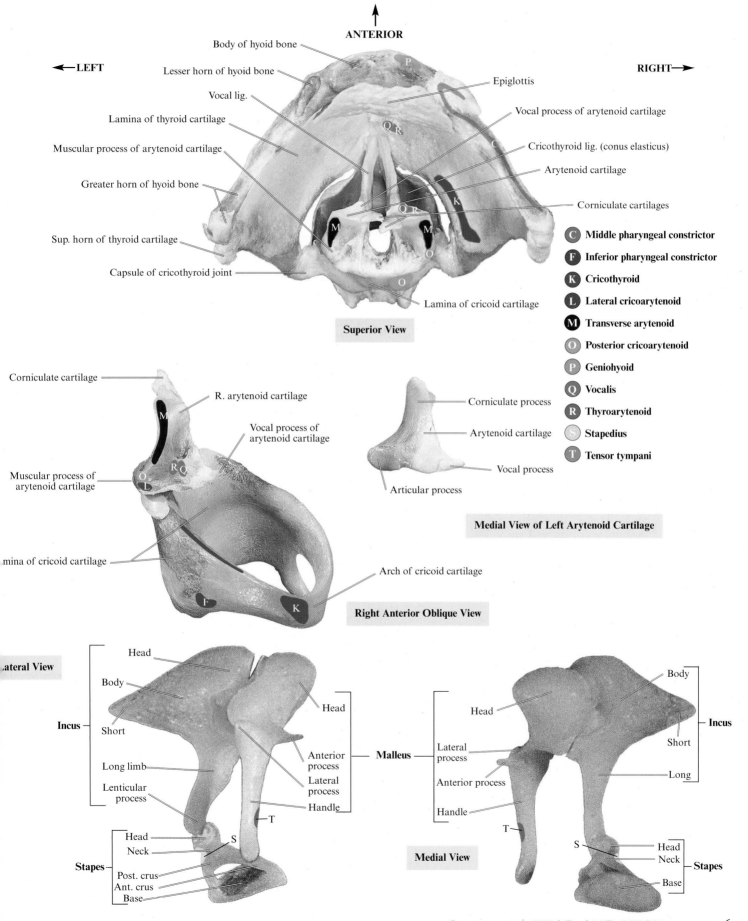

ANTERIOR

←LEFT

RIGHT→

Body of hyoid bone

Lesser horn of hyoid bone

Vocal lig.

Lamina of thyroid cartilage

Muscular process of arytenoid cartilage

Greater horn of hyoid bone

Sup. horn of thyroid cartilage

Capsule of cricothyroid joint

Epiglottis

Vocal process of arytenoid cartilage

Cricothyroid lig. (conus elasticus)

Arytenoid cartilage

Corniculate cartilages

Lamina of cricoid cartilage

Superior View

C Middle pharyngeal constrictor
F Inferior pharyngeal constrictor
K Cricothyroid
L Lateral cricoarytenoid
M Transverse arytenoid
O Posterior cricoarytenoid
P Geniohyoid
Q Vocalis
R Thyroarytenoid
S Stapedius
T Tensor tympani

Corniculate cartilage

Muscular process of arytenoid cartilage

mina of cricoid cartilage

R. arytenoid cartilage

Vocal process of arytenoid cartilage

Arch of cricoid cartilage

Right Anterior Oblique View

Corniculate process

Arytenoid cartilage

Vocal process

Articular process

Medial View of Left Arytenoid Cartilage

.ateral View

Head

Body

Incus

Short

Long limb

Lenticular process

Head

Neck

Stapes

Post. crus

Ant. crus

Base

Head

Anterior process

Lateral process

Handle

T

S

Medial View

Body

Head

Incus

Short

Long

Lateral process

Anterior process

Handle

T

S

Head

Neck

Base

Stapes

Malleus

PLATE 7.21   MUSCLES—SUPERFICIAL

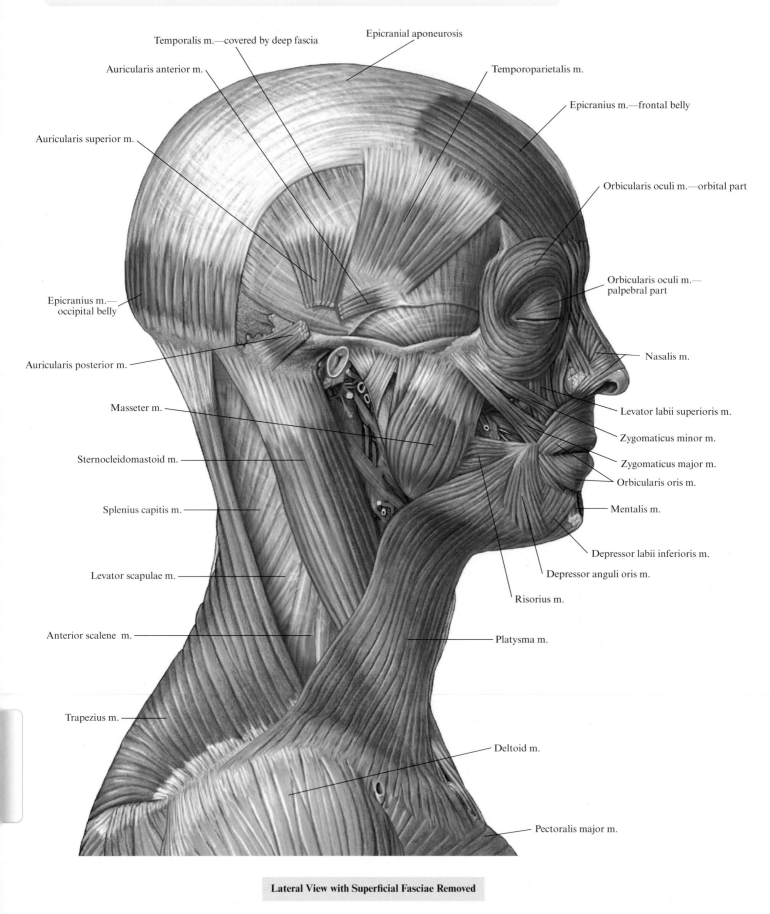

Temporalis m.—covered by deep fascia

Epicranial aponeurosis

Auricularis anterior m.

Temporoparietalis m.

Auricularis superior m.

Epicranius m.—frontal belly

Orbicularis oculi m.—orbital part

Epicranius m.—
occipital belly

Orbicularis oculi m.—
palpebral part

Auricularis posterior m.

Nasalis m.

Masseter m.

Levator labii superioris m.

Sternocleidomastoid m.

Zygomaticus minor m.

Zygomaticus major m.

Orbicularis oris m.

Splenius capitis m.

Mentalis m.

Levator scapulae m.

Depressor labii inferioris m.

Depressor anguli oris m.

Anterior scalene m.

Risorius m.

Platysma m.

Trapezius m.

Deltoid m.

Pectoralis major m.

Lateral View with Superficial Fasciae Removed

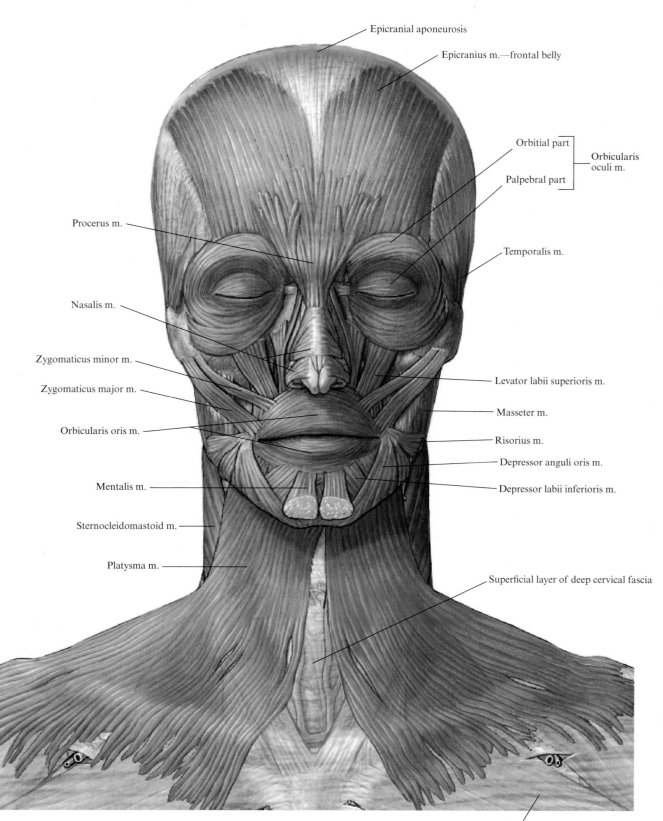

Epicranial aponeurosis

Epicranius m.—frontal belly

Orbitial part

Orbicularis oculi m.

Palpebral part

Procerus m.

Temporalis m.

Nasalis m.

Zygomaticus minor m.

Levator labii superioris m.

Zygomaticus major m.

Masseter m.

Orbicularis oris m.

Risorius m.

Depressor anguli oris m.

Mentalis m.

Depressor labii inferioris m.

Sternocleidomastoid m.

Platysma m.

Superficial layer of deep cervical fascia

Deep layer of superficial fascia

Anterior View

TABLE 7.3   MUSCLES—MASTICATORY

Muscles Acting on the Temporomandibular Joint

Muscle	Stable Attachment	Mobile Attachment	Innervation	Main Actions
Temporalis	Floor of temporal fossa & deep surface of temporal fascia	Tip & medial surface of coronoid process & ant. border of ramus of mandible	Deep temporal br. of mandibular n. (CN V³)	Elevates mandible, closing jaws; its posterior fibers retrude mandible after protrusion
Masseter	Inf. border & medial surface of zygomatic arch	Lateral surface of ramus of mandible & its coronoid process	Mandibular n. (CN V³) via masseteric nerve that enters its deep surface	Elevates & protrudes mandible, thus closing jaws
Lateral pterygoid	*Superior head:* Infratemporal surface & infratemporal crest of greater wing of sphenoid bone *Inferior head:* Lateral surface of lateral pterygoid plate	Articular disc & capsule of temporomandibular joint Neck of mandible	Mandibular n. (CN V³) via lateral petrygoid n. from ant. trunk, which enters it unilaterally deep surface	*Acting bilaterally,* they protrude mandible & depress chin *Acting unilaterally* & alternately, they produce side-to-side movements of mandible
Medial pterygoid	*Deep head:* Medial surface of lateral pterygoid plate & pyramidal process of palatine bone *Superficial head:* Tuberosity of maxilla	Medial surface of ramus of mandible, inf. to mandibular foramen	Mandibular n. (CN V³) via medial pterygoid n.	Helps to elevate mandible, closing jaws *Acting bilaterally,* they help to protrude mandible *Acting unilaterally,* it protrudes side of jaw *Acting alternately,* they produce a grinding motion

Actions and Nerve Supply of the Ocular Muscles

Muscle	Abbreviations	Action(s) on the Eyeball	Nerve Supply
Medial rectus[a]	MR	Adducts	CN III
Lateral rectus[a]	LR	Abducts	CN VI[b]
Superior rectus	SR	Elevates, adducts & rotate medially	CN III
Inferior rectus	IR	Depresses, adducts & rotates laterally	CN III
Superior oblique[c]	SO	Abducts, depresses & rotates eye medially (intorsion), depresses adducted eye	CN IV[b]
Inferior oblique[c]	IO	Abducts, elevates & rotates eye laterally (extorsion), elevates adducted eye	CN III

[a]The medial and lateral rectus muscles move the eyeball in one axis only, whereas each of the other four muscles moves it in all three axes.
[b]CN IV and VI each supply one muscle, whereas CN III supplies the other four muscles.
[c]The superior and inferior oblique muscles are used with the medial rectus muscle in adducting both eyes medially for near vision. This movement, accompanied by pupillary construction, is known as accommodation.

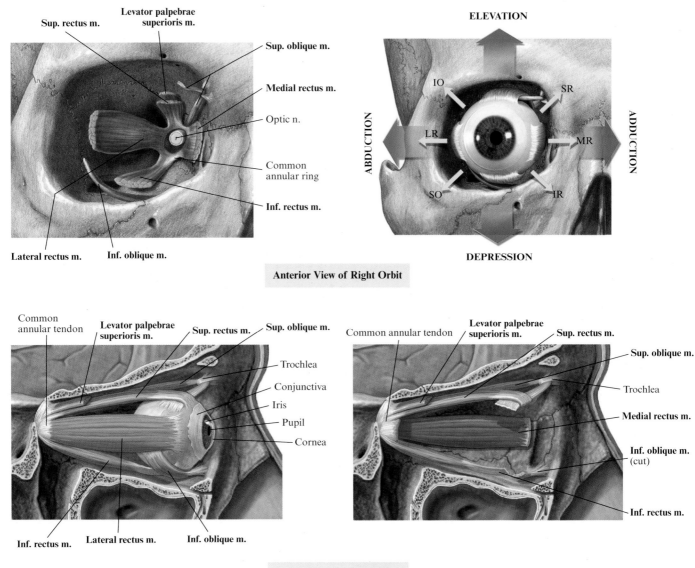

Anterior View of Right Orbit

Lateral View of Right Orbit

TABLE 7.5   MUSCLES—SOFT PALATE & TONGUE

Muscles of the Soft Palate

Muscle	Superior Attachment	Inferior Attachment	Innervation	Main Actions
Levator veli palatini	Cartilage of auditory tube & petrous part of temporal bone	Palatine aponeurosis	Pharyngeal br. of vagus n. via pharyngeal plexus (CN X)	Elevates soft palate during swallowing & yawning
Tensor veli palatini	Scaphoid fossa of medial pterygoid plate, spine of sphenoid bone & cartilage of auditory tube		Medial pterygoid n. (a br. of the mandibular n.) via otic ganglion (CN V³)	Tenses soft palate & opens cartilagenous part of auditory tube during swallowing & yawning
Palatoglossus	Palatine aponeurosis	Side of tongue	Pharyngeal br. of vagus n. (CN X) via pharyngeal plexus	Elevates posterior part of tongue & draws soft palate onto tongue
Palatopharyngeus	Hard palate & palatine aponeurosis	Lateral wall of pharynx		Tenses soft palate & pulls walls of pharynx superiorly, anteriorly, and medially during swallowing
Musculus uvulae	Posterior nasal spine & palatine aponeurosis	Mucosa of uvula		Shortens uvula & pulls it superiorly

Extrinsic Muscles of the Tongue

Muscle	Stable Attachment	Mobile Attachment	Innervation	Actions
Genioglossus	Sup. part of mental spine of mandible	Dorsum of tongue & body of hyoid bone	Hypoglossal n. CN XII	Protrudes, retracts & depresses tongue; its post, part protrudes tongue
Hyoglossus	Body & greater horn of hyoid bone	Side of tongue		Depresses & retracts tongue
Styloglossus	Styloid process & stylohyoid lig.	Side & inf. aspect of tongue		Retracts tongue & draws it up to create a trough for swallowing
Palatoglossus	Palatine aponeurosis of soft palate	Side of tongue	Pharyngeal br. CN X & pharyngeal plexus	Elevates post. part of tongue

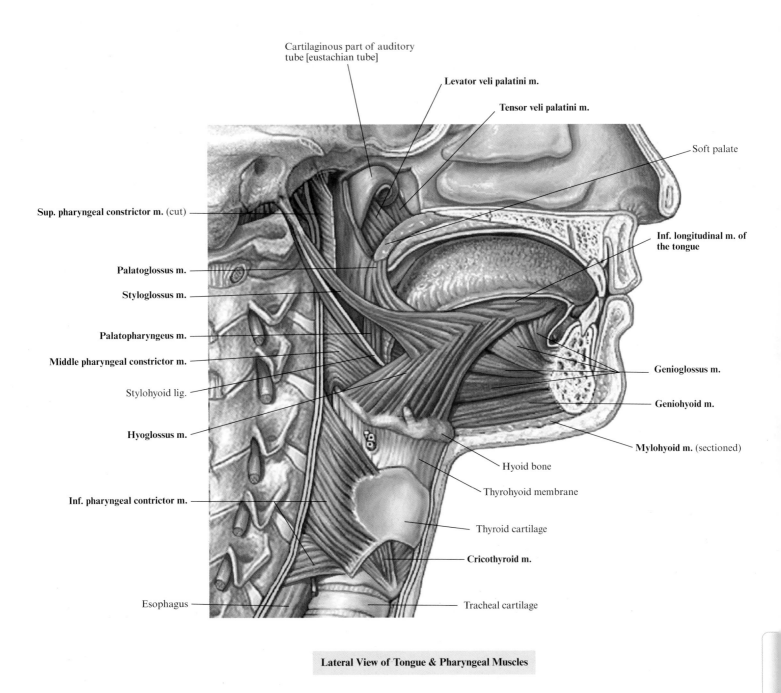

Cartilaginous part of auditory tube [eustachian tube]

Levator veli palatini m.

Tensor veli palatini m.

Soft palate

Sup. pharyngeal constrictor m. (cut)

Inf. longitudinal m. of the tongue

Palatoglossus m.

Styloglossus m.

Palatopharyngeus m.

Middle pharyngeal constrictor m.

Stylohyoid lig.

Hyoglossus m.

Inf. pharyngeal contrictor m.

Esophagus

Genioglossus m.

Geniohyoid m.

Mylohyoid m. (sectioned)

Hyoid bone

Thyrohyoid membrane

Thyroid cartilage

Cricothyroid m.

Tracheal cartilage

Lateral View of Tongue & Pharyngeal Muscles

TABLE 7.6   MUSCLES—HYOID

Suprahyoid Muscles[a]

Muscle	Superior Attachment	Inferior Attachment	Innervation	Main Actions
Mylohyoid	Mylohyoid line of mandible	Oral raphe & body of hyoid bone	Mylohyoid n., a br. of inf. alveolar n. (CN V³)	Elevates hyoid bone, floor of mouth & tongue during swallowing & speaking
Geniohyoid	Inf. mental spine of mandible	Body of hyoid bone	C1 via the hypoglossal n. (CN XII)	Pulls hyoid bone anterosuperiorly, shortens floor of mouth & widens pharynx
Stylohyoid	Styloid process of temporal bone		Facial n. (CN VII)	Elevates & retracts hyoid bone, thereby elongating floor of mouth
Digastric	*Anterior belly:* Digastric fossa of mandible *Posterior belly:* Mastoid notch of temporal bone	Intermediate tendon to body & greater horn of hyoid bone	*Anterior belly:* Mylohyoid n., a br. of inf. alveolar n. (CN V³) *Posterior belly:* Facial n. (CN VII)	Depresses mandible, raises hyoid bone & steadies it during swallowing & speaking

[a]These muscles connect the hyoid bone to the skull.

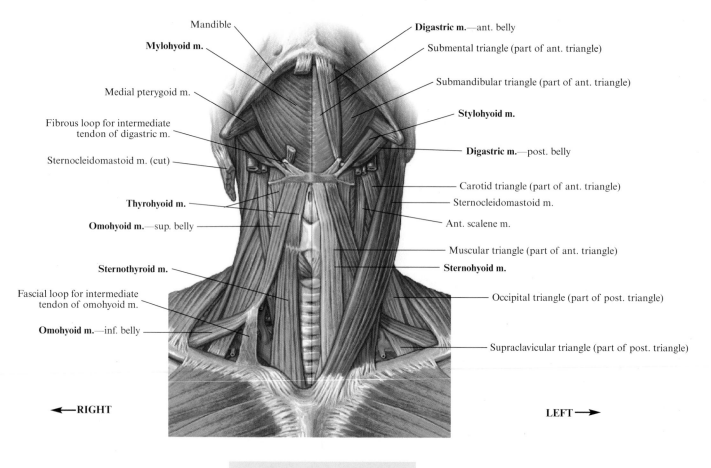

Mandible

Mylohyoid m.

Medial pterygoid m.

Fibrous loop for intermediate tendon of digastric m.

Sternocleidomastoid m. (cut)

Thyrohyoid m.

Omohyoid m.—sup. belly

Sternothyroid m.

Fascial loop for intermediate tendon of omohyoid m.

Omohyoid m.—inf. belly

Digastric m.—ant. belly

Submental triangle (part of ant. triangle)

Submandibular triangle (part of ant. triangle)

Stylohyoid m.

Digastric m.—post. belly

Carotid triangle (part of ant. triangle)

Sternocleidomastoid m.

Ant. scalene m.

Muscular triangle (part of ant. triangle)

Sternohyoid m.

Occipital triangle (part of post. triangle)

Supraclavicular triangle (part of post. triangle)

←—**RIGHT**   **LEFT**—→

Anterior View with Superficial Muscles on Left & Deeper Muscles on Right

Infrahyoid Muscles[a]

Muscle	Origin	Insertion	Innervation	Actions
Sternohyoid	Manubrium of sternum & medial end of clavicle	Body of hyoid bone	C1, C2 & C3 from ansa cervicalis	Depresses hyoid bone after it has been elevated during swallowing
Sternothyroid	Post. surface of manubrium of sternum	Oblique line of thyroid cartilage	C2 & C3 by a br. of ansa cervicalis	Depresses hyoid bone & larynx
Thyrohyoid	Oblique line of thyroid cartilage	Inf. border of body & greater horn of hyoid bone	C1 via hypoglossal n. (CN XII)	Depresses hyoid bone & elevates larynx
Omohyoid	Sup. border of scapula near suprascapular notch	Inf. border of hyoid bone	C1, C2 & C3 by a br. of ansa cervicalis	Depresses, retracts & steadies hyoid bone

[a]These four step-like muscles anchor the hyoid bone (*ie.,* they fix and steady it). They are concerned with the suprahyoid muscles in movements of the tongue, hyoid bone, and larynx in both swallowing and speaking.

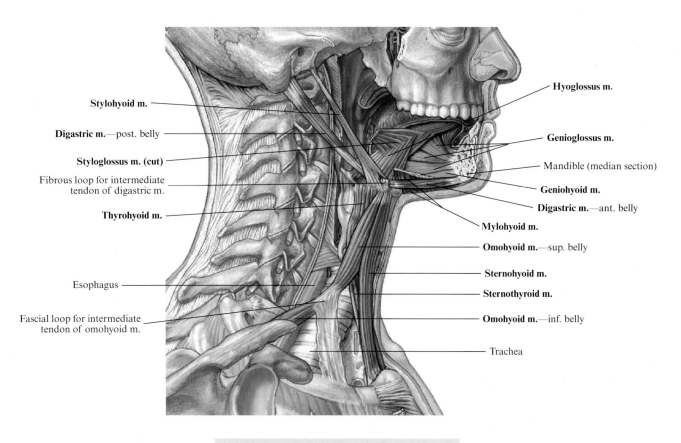

Stylohyoid m.

Digastric m.—post. belly

Styloglossus m. (cut)

Fibrous loop for intermediate tendon of digastric m.

Thyrohyoid m.

Esophagus

Fascial loop for intermediate tendon of omohyoid m.

Hyoglossus m.

Genioglossus m.

Mandible (median section)

Geniohyoid m.

Digastric m.—ant. belly

Mylohyoid m.

Omohyoid m.—sup. belly

Sternohyoid m.

Sternothyroid m.

Omohyoid m.—inf. belly

Trachea

Lateral View with Right Half of Mandible Removed

TABLE 7.8   MUSCLES—PHARYNGEAL

Muscle	Lateral Attachments	Medial Attachments	Innervation	Main Actions
CIRCULAR PHARYNGEAL MUSCLES				
Superior constrictor	Pterygoid hamulus, ptergomandibular raphe, post. end of mylohyoid line of mandible & side of tongue	Median raphe of pharynx & pharyngeal tubercle	Pharyngeal & sup. laryngeal brr. of vagus n. [CN X] through pharyngeal plexus	Constrict wall of pharynx during swallowing
Middle constrictor	Stylohyoid lig. and greater & lesser horns of hyoid bone	Median raphe of pharynx		
Inferior constrictor	Oblique line of thyroid cartilage & side of cricoid cartilage			
LONGITUDINAL PHARYNGEAL MUSCLES				
Palatopharyngeus	Hard palate & palatine aponeurosis	Post. border of lamina of thyroid cartilage & side of pharynx & esophagus		Elevate pharynx & larynx during swallowing speaking[a]
Salpingopharynegeus	Cartilaginous part of auditory tube	Blends with palatopharynegeus		
Stylopharyngeus	Styloid process of temporal bone	Post. & sup. borders of thyroid cartilage with palatopharynegus m.	Glossopharyngeal n. [CN IX]	

[a]The salpingopharyngeus muscle also opens the auditory tube.

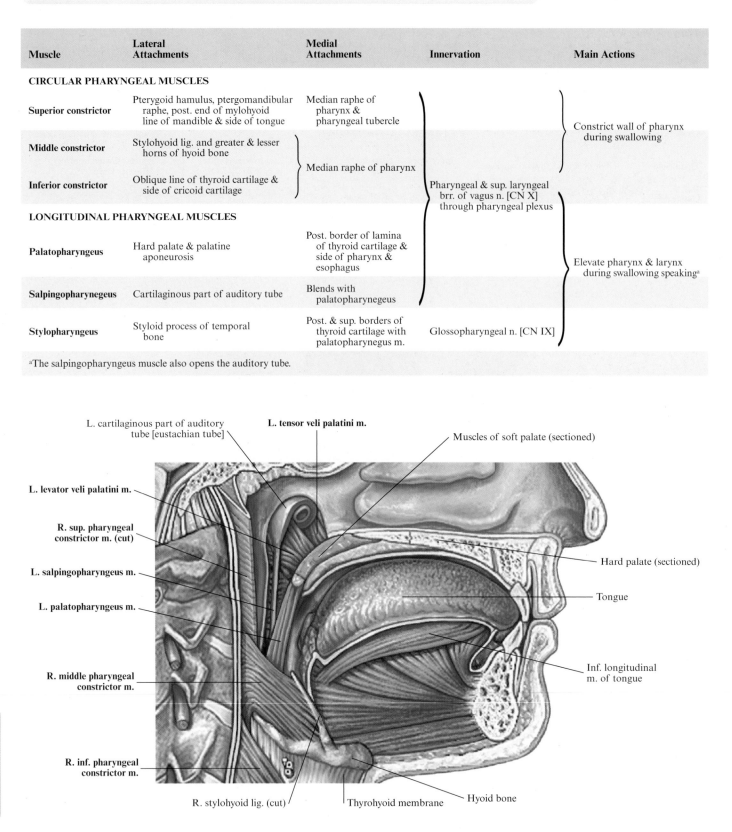

Lateral View of Neck & Median Sectioned Skull

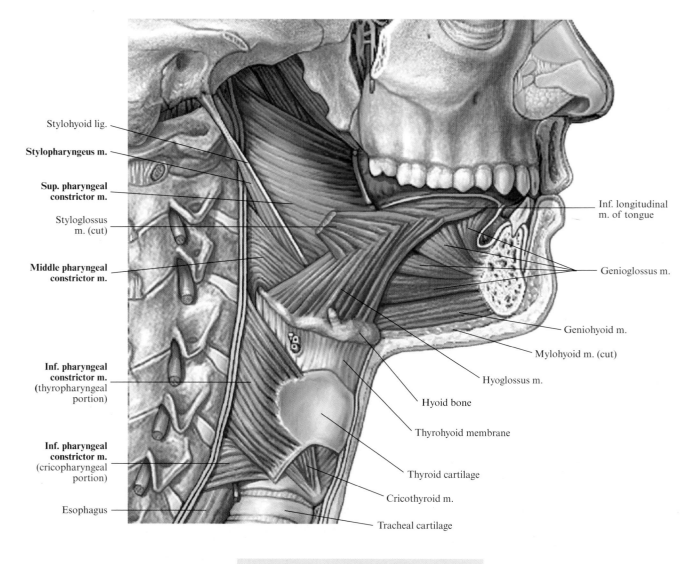

Stylohyoid lig.

Stylopharyngeus m.

Sup. pharyngeal constrictor m.

Styloglossus m. (cut)

Middle pharyngeal constrictor m.

Inf. pharyngeal constrictor m. (thyropharyngeal portion)

Inf. pharyngeal constrictor m. (cricopharyngeal portion)

Esophagus

Inf. longitudinal m. of tongue

Genioglossus m.

Geniohyoid m.

Mylohyoid m. (cut)

Hyoglossus m.

Hyoid bone

Thyrohyoid membrane

Thyroid cartilage

Cricothyroid m.

Tracheal cartilage

Lateral View with Right Half of Mandible Removed

TABLE 7.9   MUSCLES—LARYNGEAL

Muscles of the Larynx

Muscle	Origin	Insertion	Innervation	Main Actions
Cricothyroid	Anterolateral part of cricoid cartilage	Inf. margin & inf. horn of thyroid cartilage	Sup. larnyngeal n. [CN X]	Stretches & tenses the vocal fold
Posterior cricoarytenoid	Post. surface of laminae of cricoid cartilage	Muscular process of arytenoid cartilage	Recurrent laryngeal n. [CN X]	Abducts vocal fold
Lateral cricoarytenoid	Arch of cricoid cartilage			Adducts vocal fold
Thyroarytenoid[a]	Post. surface of thyroid cartilage	Muscular process of arytenoid process		Relaxes vocal fold
Transverse & oblique arytenoids	One arytenoid cartilage	Opposition arytenoid cartilage		Close laryngeal aditus by approximating arytenoid cartilages
Vocalis[b]	Angle between laminae of thyroid cartilage	Vocal process of arytenoid cartilage		Alters vocal fold during phonation

[a]The superior fibers of the thyroarytenoid muscle pass into the aryepiglottic fold, and some of them reach the epiglottic cartilage. These fibers constitute the *thyroepiglottic muscle*, which widens the inlet of the larynx.
[b]These short fine muscular slips are derived from the most medial fibers of the thyroarytenoid muscle.

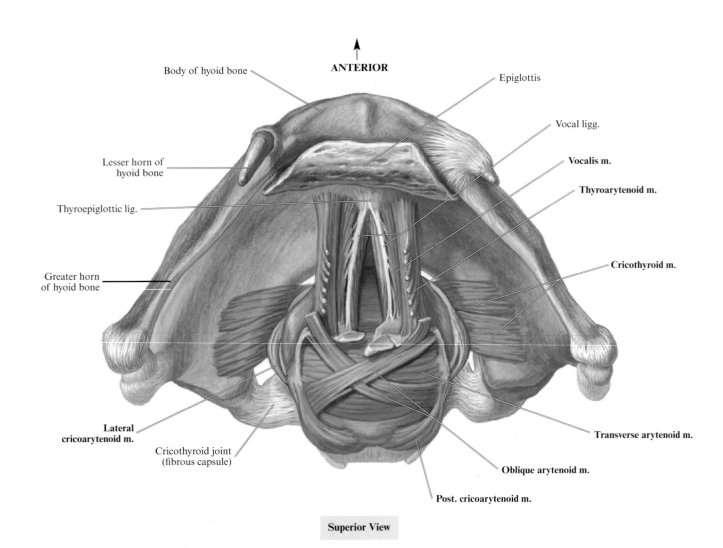

Superior View

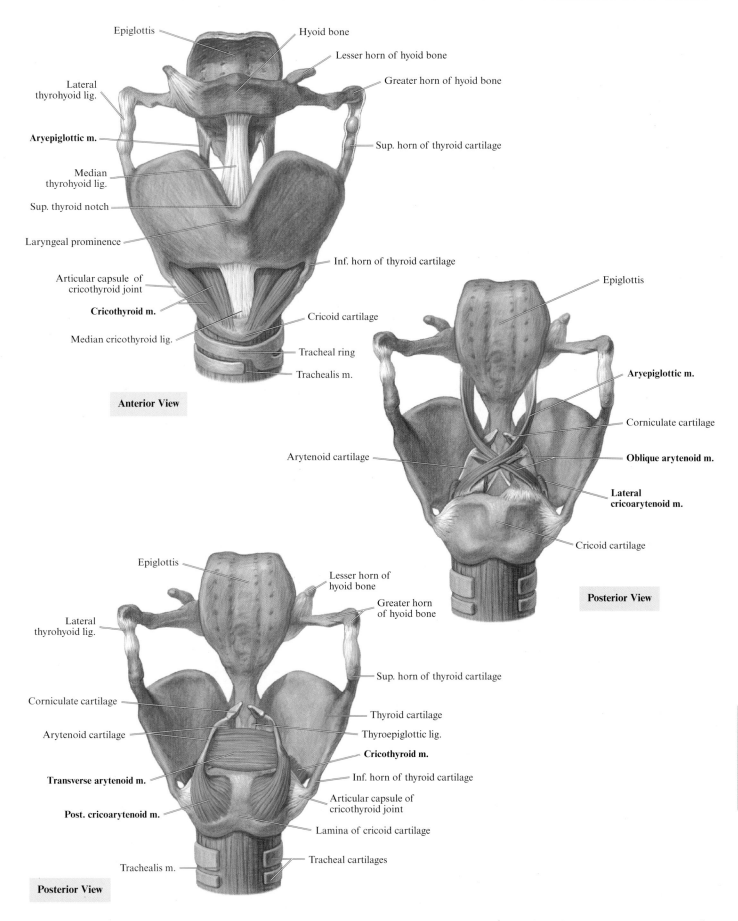

Epiglottis

Hyoid bone

Lesser horn of hyoid bone

Greater horn of hyoid bone

Lateral thyrohyoid lig.

Aryepiglottic m.

Sup. horn of thyroid cartilage

Median thyrohyoid lig.

Sup. thyroid notch

Laryngeal prominence

Inf. horn of thyroid cartilage

Articular capsule of cricothyroid joint

Cricothyroid m.

Cricoid cartilage

Median cricothyroid lig.

Tracheal ring

Trachealis m.

Anterior View

Epiglottis

Aryepiglottic m.

Corniculate cartilage

Arytenoid cartilage

Oblique arytenoid m.

Lateral cricoarytenoid m.

Cricoid cartilage

Posterior View

Epiglottis

Lesser horn of hyoid bone

Greater horn of hyoid bone

Lateral thyrohyoid lig.

Sup. horn of thyroid cartilage

Corniculate cartilage

Thyroid cartilage

Arytenoid cartilage

Thyroepiglottic lig.

Cricothyroid m.

Transverse arytenoid m.

Inf. horn of thyroid cartilage

Articular capsule of cricothyroid joint

Post. cricoarytenoid m.

Lamina of cricoid cartilage

Trachealis m.

Tracheal cartilages

Posterior View

TABLE 7.10   MUSCLES—LATERAL & PREVERTEBRAL

Muscle	Inferior Attachment	Superior Attachment	Innervation	Main Actions
Sternocleidomastoid				
Sternal head	Ventral surface of the manubrium sterni	Lateral surface of mastoid process; sup. nuchal line of occipital bone	Accessory n. [CN XI] (motor); sensory fibers of C2 cervical spinal n.	Various: both sides together support head, move chin upward, and pull back of head down. One side alone turns chin upward and to opposite side.
Clavicular head	Cranial surface of medial third of clavicle			
Splenius capitis	Inf. half of ligamentum nuchae & spinous process of sup. six thoracic vertebrae	Lateral aspect of mastoid process & lateral third of sup. nuchal line	Dorsal rami of middle cervical spinal nn.	Laterally flexes & rotates head & neck to same side; acting bilaterally, they extend head & neck
Splenius cervicis	Spines of 3rd (or 4th) to 6th thoracic vertebrae	Posterior tubercles of the transverse process of the upper three cervical vertebrae	Dorsal rami of nn. (C2-C5) lateral brr. (same as splenius capitis m.)	
Posterior scalene	Post. tubercles of transverse processes of C4-C6	Ext. border of second rib	Ventral rami of cervical spinal nn. (C7 & C8)	Flexes neck laterally; elevates second rib during forced inspiration
Middle scalene	Posterior tubercles of transverse processes of C2-C7	Sup. surface of first rib, posterior to groove for subclavian a.	Ventral rami of cervical spinal nn. (C3-C8)	Flexes neck laterally; elevates first rib during forced inspiration
Anterior scalene	Ant. tubercles of transverse processes of C3-C6	Scalene tubercle of 1st rib	Long thoracic n. (C5-C7)	
Longus colli				
Vertical portion	Body of first three thoracic & last three cervical vertebrae	Bodies of C2-C4	Ventral rami of cervical spinal nn. (C2-C6)	Bilaterally acting to flex neck and head anteriorly, unilaterally to flex head and neck laterally and to rotate the head toward the same side
Superior oblique	Ant. tubercles of transverse process of C3-C5	Tubercle on ant. arch of the atlas & body axis		
Inferior oblique	Ant. surface of bodies of first two or three thoracic vertebrae	Ant. tubercles of the transverse processes of C5 & C6	Ventral rami of cervical spinal nn. (C1-C4)	
Longus capitis	Ant. tubercle of transverse processes of C3-C6	Inf. border of basilar part of occipital		

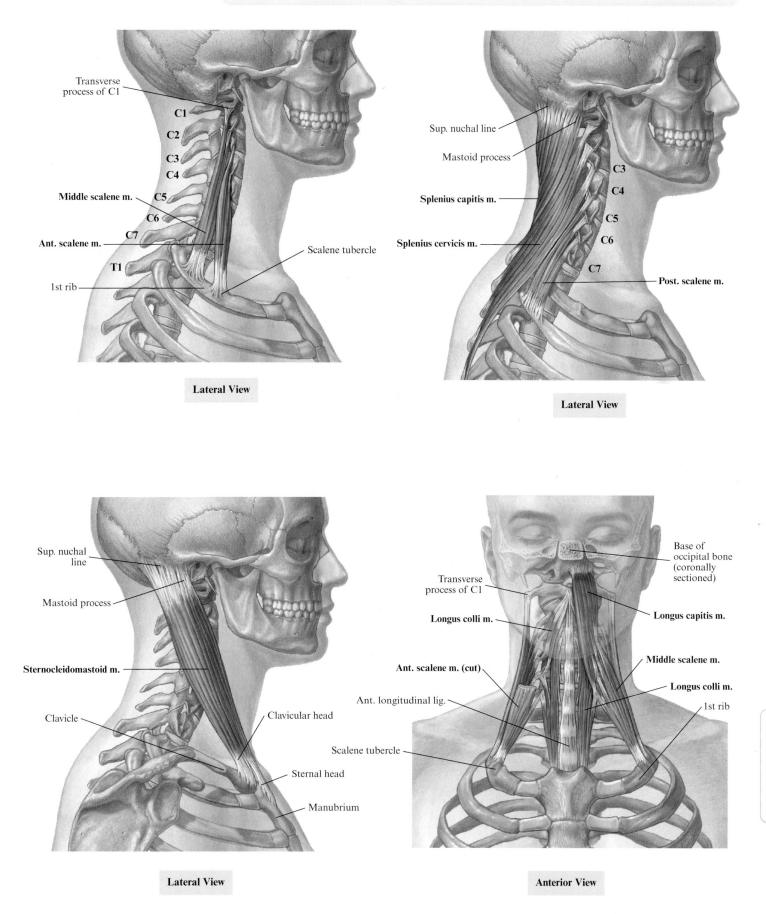

Transverse process of C1

C1
C2
C3
C4
Middle scalene m. C5
C6
Ant. scalene m. C7

T1

1st rib

Scalene tubercle

Lateral View

Sup. nuchal line

Mastoid process

Splenius capitis m.

Splenius cervicis m.

C3
C4
C5
C6
C7

Post. scalene m.

Lateral View

Sup. nuchal line

Mastoid process

Sternocleidomastoid m.

Clavicle

Clavicular head

Sternal head

Manubrium

Lateral View

Base of occipital bone (coronally sectioned)

Transverse process of C1

Longus colli m.

Longus capitis m.

Ant. scalene m. (cut)

Middle scalene m.

Ant. longitudinal lig.

Longus colli m.

1st rib

Scalene tubercle

Anterior View

PLATE 7.27 CERVICAL FASCIAL PLANES

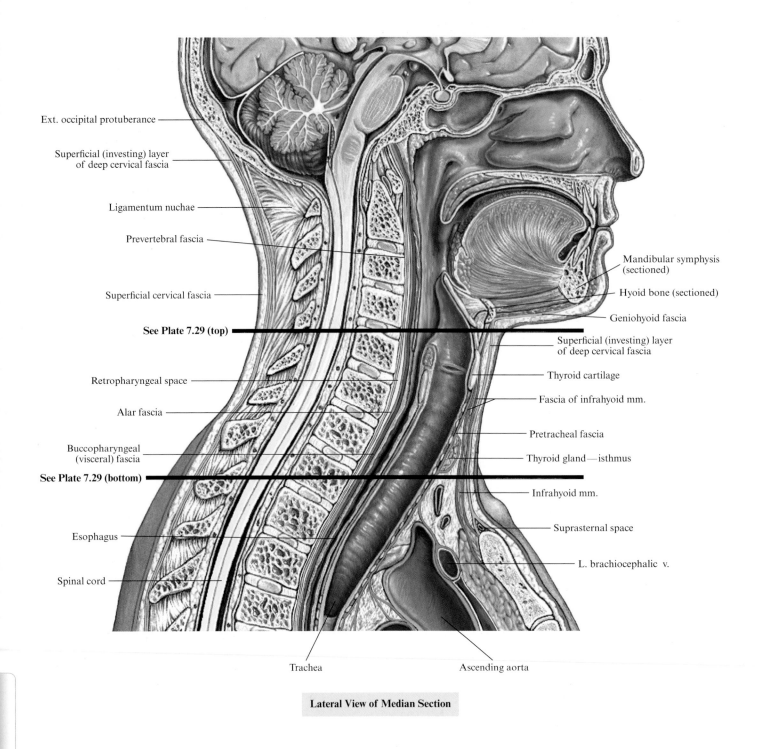

Ext. occipital protuberance

Superficial (investing) layer of deep cervical fascia

Ligamentum nuchae

Prevertebral fascia

Superficial cervical fascia

See Plate 7.29 (top)

Retropharyngeal space

Alar fascia

Buccopharyngeal (visceral) fascia

See Plate 7.29 (bottom)

Esophagus

Spinal cord

Mandibular symphysis (sectioned)

Hyoid bone (sectioned)

Geniohyoid fascia

Superficial (investing) layer of deep cervical fascia

Thyroid cartilage

Fascia of infrahyoid mm.

Pretracheal fascia

Thyroid gland—isthmus

Infrahyoid mm.

Suprasternal space

L. brachiocephalic v.

Trachea

Ascending aorta

Lateral View of Median Section

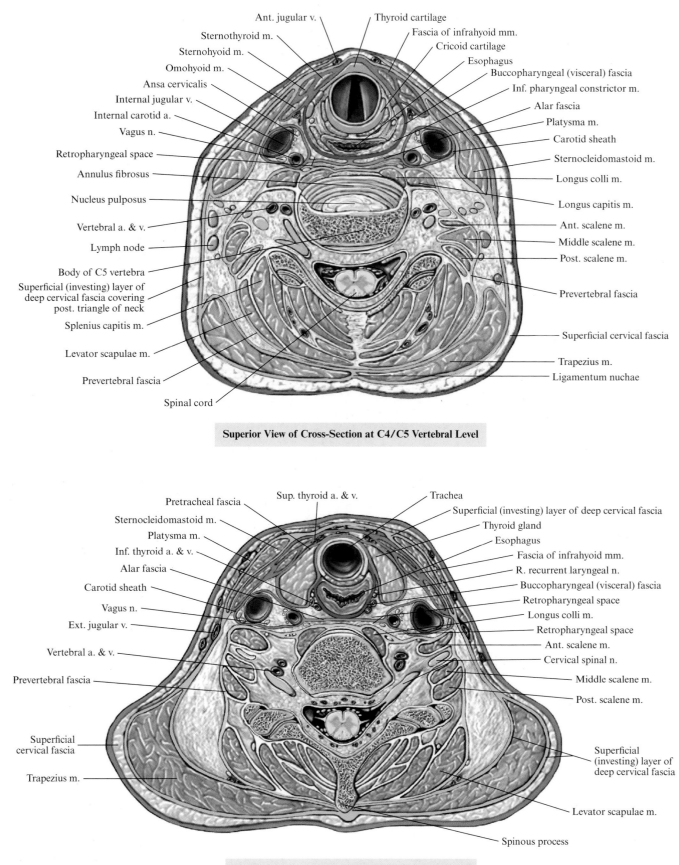

Ant. jugular v.
Thyroid cartilage
Sternothyroid m.
Fascia of infrahyoid mm.
Sternohyoid m.
Cricoid cartilage
Omohyoid m.
Esophagus
Ansa cervicalis
Buccopharyngeal (visceral) fascia
Internal jugular v.
Inf. pharyngeal constrictor m.
Internal carotid a.
Alar fascia
Vagus n.
Platysma m.
Retropharyngeal space
Carotid sheath
Annulus fibrosus
Sternocleidomastoid m.
Nucleus pulposus
Longus colli m.
Vertebral a. & v.
Longus capitis m.
Lymph node
Ant. scalene m.
Body of C5 vertebra
Middle scalene m.
Superficial (investing) layer of
deep cervical fascia covering
post. triangle of neck
Post. scalene m.
Splenius capitis m.
Prevertebral fascia
Levator scapulae m.
Superficial cervical fascia
Prevertebral fascia
Trapezius m.
Spinal cord
Ligamentum nuchae

Superior View of Cross-Section at C4/C5 Vertebral Level

Pretracheal fascia
Sup. thyroid a. & v.
Trachea
Sternocleidomastoid m.
Superficial (investing) layer of deep cervical fascia
Platysma m.
Thyroid gland
Inf. thyroid a. & v.
Esophagus
Alar fascia
Fascia of infrahyoid mm.
Carotid sheath
R. recurrent laryngeal n.
Vagus n.
Buccopharyngeal (visceral) fascia
Ext. jugular v.
Retropharyngeal space
Vertebral a. & v.
Longus colli m.
Prevertebral fascia
Retropharyngeal space
Ant. scalene m.
Cervical spinal n.
Middle scalene m.
Post. scalene m.
Superficial
cervical fascia
Superficial
(investing) layer of
deep cervical fascia
Trapezius m.
Levator scapulae m.
Spinous process

Superior View of Cross-Section at T1 Vertebral Level

PLATE 7.29 ARTERIES—SUPERFICIAL

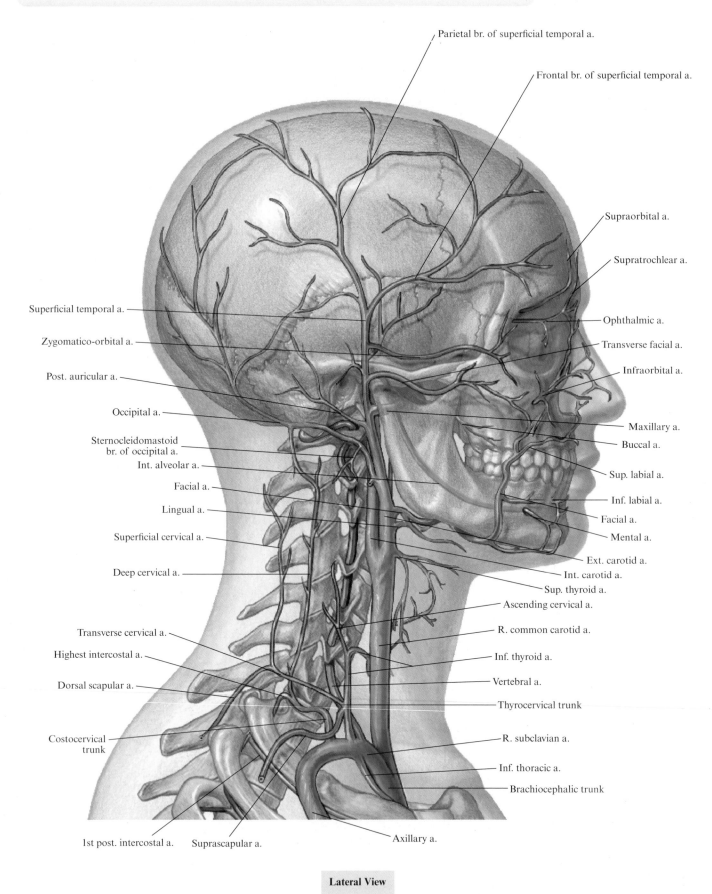

Parietal br. of superficial temporal a.

Frontal br. of superficial temporal a.

Supraorbital a.

Supratrochlear a.

Ophthalmic a.

Transverse facial a.

Infraorbital a.

Superficial temporal a.

Zygomatico-orbital a.

Post. auricular a.

Occipital a.

Maxillary a.

Buccal a.

Sternocleidomastoid
br. of occipital a.

Int. alveolar a.

Sup. labial a.

Facial a.

Inf. labial a.

Lingual a.

Facial a.

Superficial cervical a.

Mental a.

Deep cervical a.

Ext. carotid a.

Int. carotid a.

Sup. thyroid a.

Ascending cervical a.

R. common carotid a.

Transverse cervical a.

Highest intercostal a.

Inf. thyroid a.

Dorsal scapular a.

Vertebral a.

Thyrocervical trunk

Costocervical
trunk

R. subclavian a.

Inf. thoracic a.

Brachiocephalic trunk

1st post. intercostal a.   Suprascapular a.   Axillary a.

Lateral View

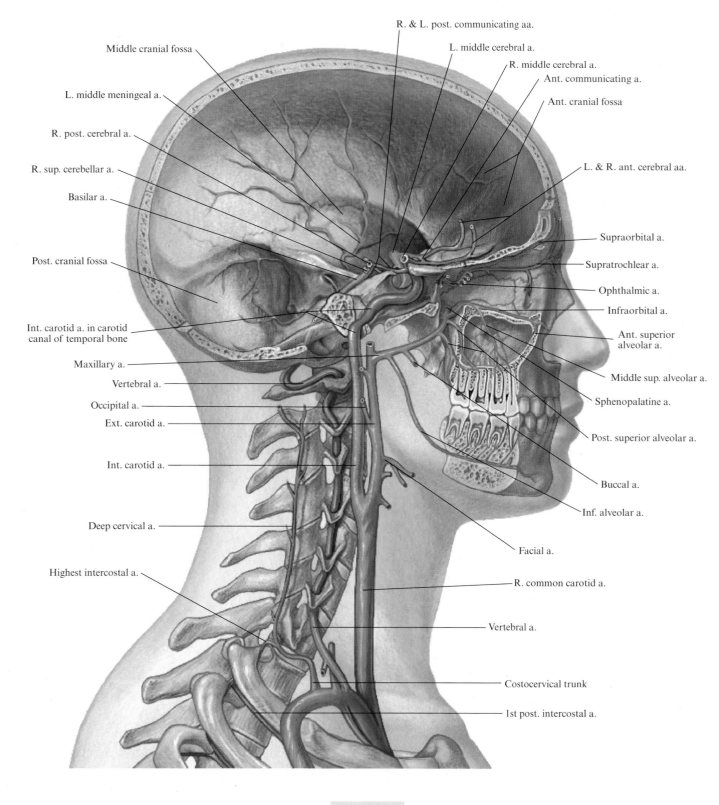

R. & L. post. communicating aa.

L. middle cerebral a.

R. middle cerebral a.

Ant. communicating a.

Ant. cranial fossa

Middle cranial fossa

L. middle meningeal a.

R. post. cerebral a.

R. sup. cerebellar a.

Basilar a.

Post. cranial fossa

Int. carotid a. in carotid
canal of temporal bone

Maxillary a.

Vertebral a.

Occipital a.

Ext. carotid a.

Int. carotid a.

Deep cervical a.

Highest intercostal a.

L. & R. ant. cerebral aa.

Supraorbital a.

Supratrochlear a.

Ophthalmic a.

Infraorbital a.

Ant. superior
alveolar a.

Middle sup. alveolar a.

Sphenopalatine a.

Post. superior alveolar a.

Buccal a.

Inf. alveolar a.

Facial a.

R. common carotid a.

Vertebral a.

Costocervical trunk

1st post. intercostal a.

Lateral View

PLATE 7.31   ARTERIES—BRAIN & BRAINSTEM

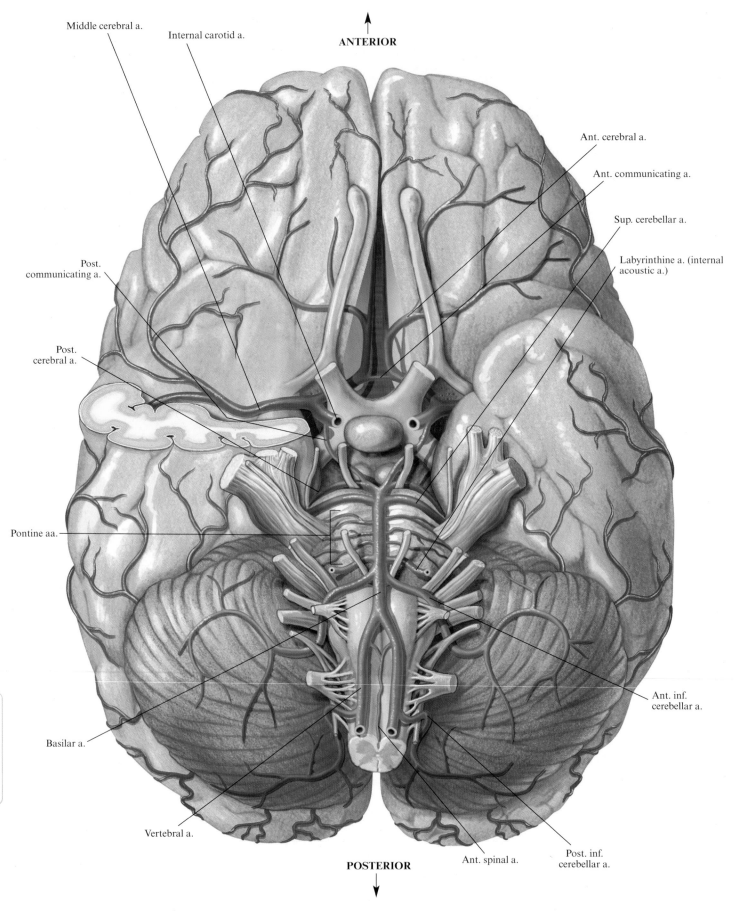

Middle cerebral a.

Internal carotid a.

ANTERIOR

Ant. cerebral a.

Ant. communicating a.

Sup. cerebellar a.

Labyrinthine a. (internal acoustic a.)

Post. communicating a.

Post. cerebral a.

Pontine aa.

Ant. inf. cerebellar a.

Basilar a.

Vertebral a.

Ant. spinal a.

Post. inf. cerebellar a.

POSTERIOR

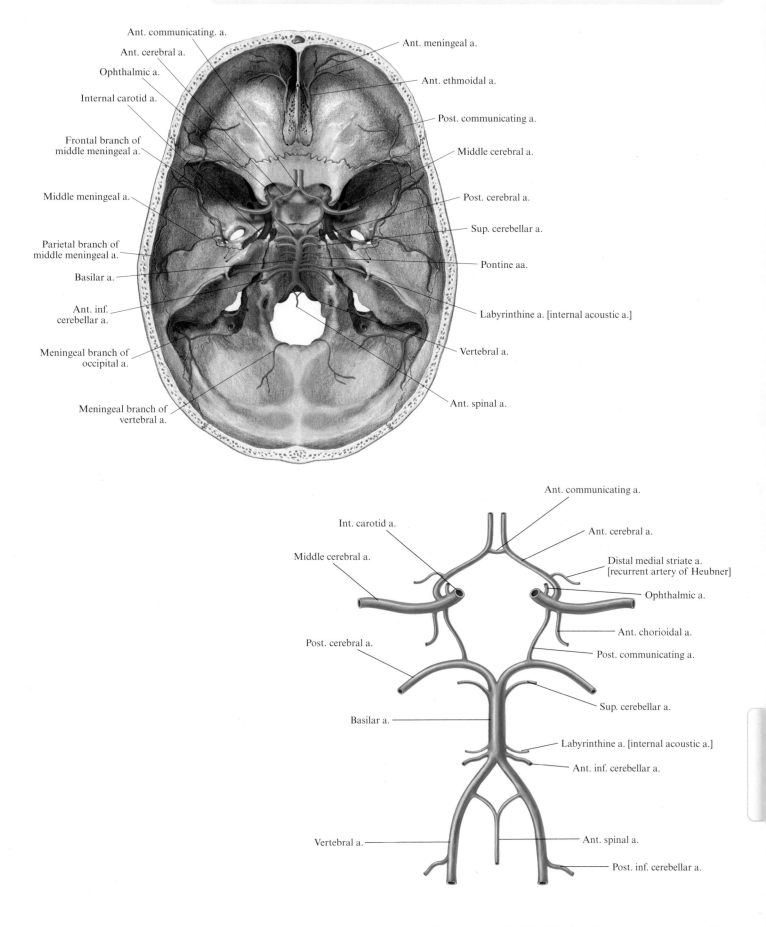

Ant. communicating. a.

Ant. cerebral a.

Ophthalmic a.

Internal carotid a.

Frontal branch of
middle meningeal a.

Middle meningeal a.

Parietal branch of
middle meningeal a.

Basilar a.

Ant. inf.
cerebellar a.

Meningeal branch of
occipital a.

Meningeal branch of
vertebral a.

Ant. meningeal a.

Ant. ethmoidal a.

Post. communicating a.

Middle cerebral a.

Post. cerebral a.

Sup. cerebellar a.

Pontine aa.

Labyrinthine a. [internal acoustic a.]

Vertebral a.

Ant. spinal a.

Ant. communicating a.

Int. carotid a.

Middle cerebral a.

Post. cerebral a.

Basilar a.

Vertebral a.

Ant. cerebral a.

Distal medial striate a.
[recurrent artery of Heubner]

Ophthalmic a.

Ant. chorioidal a.

Post. communicating a.

Sup. cerebellar a.

Labyrinthine a. [internal acoustic a.]

Ant. inf. cerebellar a.

Ant. spinal a.

Post. inf. cerebellar a.

PLATE 7.33   VEINS—SUPERFICIAL

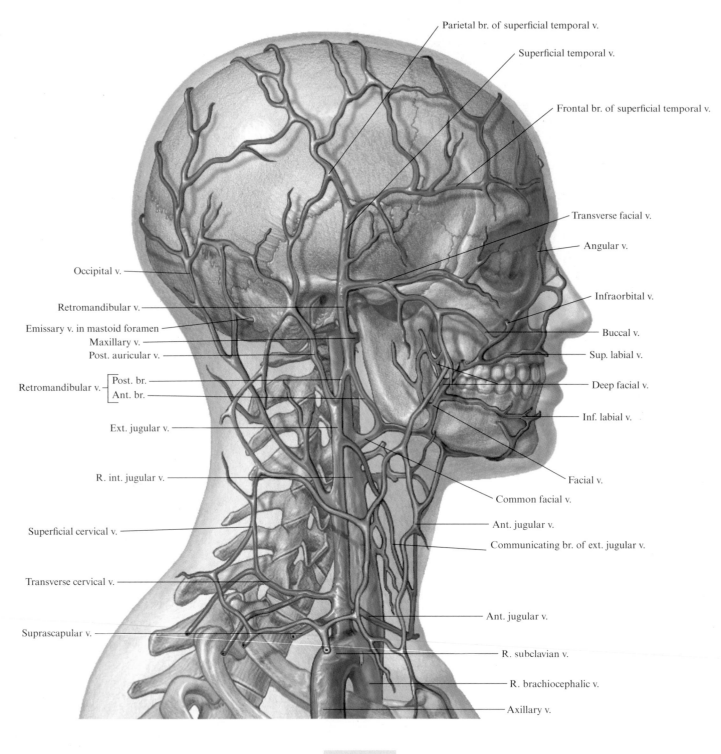

Parietal br. of superficial temporal v.

Superficial temporal v.

Frontal br. of superficial temporal v.

Transverse facial v.

Angular v.

Infraorbital v.

Buccal v.

Sup. labial v.

Deep facial v.

Inf. labial v.

Facial v.

Common facial v.

Ant. jugular v.

Communicating br. of ext. jugular v.

Ant. jugular v.

R. subclavian v.

R. brachiocephalic v.

Axillary v.

Occipital v.

Retromandibular v.

Emissary v. in mastoid foramen

Maxillary v.

Post. auricular v.

Retromandibular v. — ⌈ Post. br.
                      ⌊ Ant. br.

Ext. jugular v.

R. int. jugular v.

Superficial cervical v.

Transverse cervical v.

Suprascapular v.

Lateral View

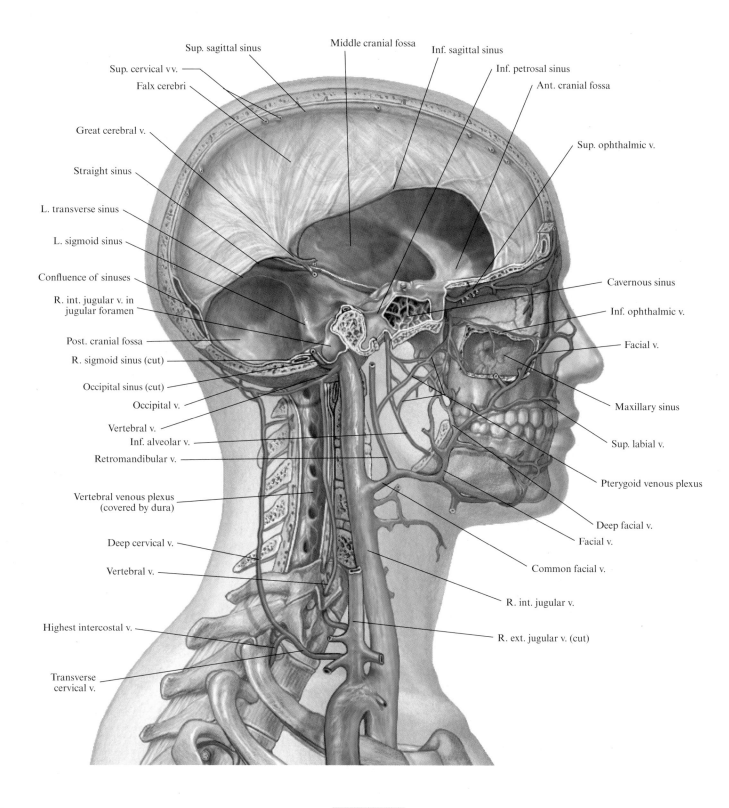

Sup. sagittal sinus

Sup. cervical vv.

Falx cerebri

Great cerebral v.

Straight sinus

L. transverse sinus

L. sigmoid sinus

Confluence of sinuses

R. int. jugular v. in jugular foramen

Post. cranial fossa

R. sigmoid sinus (cut)

Occipital sinus (cut)

Occipital v.

Vertebral v.

Inf. alveolar v.

Retromandibular v.

Vertebral venous plexus (covered by dura)

Deep cervical v.

Vertebral v.

Highest intercostal v.

Transverse cervical v.

Middle cranial fossa

Inf. sagittal sinus

Inf. petrosal sinus

Ant. cranial fossa

Sup. ophthalmic v.

Cavernous sinus

Inf. ophthalmic v.

Facial v.

Maxillary sinus

Sup. labial v.

Pterygoid venous plexus

Deep facial v.

Facial v.

Common facial v.

R. int. jugular v.

R. ext. jugular v. (cut)

Lateral View

PLATE 7.35   VEINS—DURAL & CAVERNOUS SINUSES

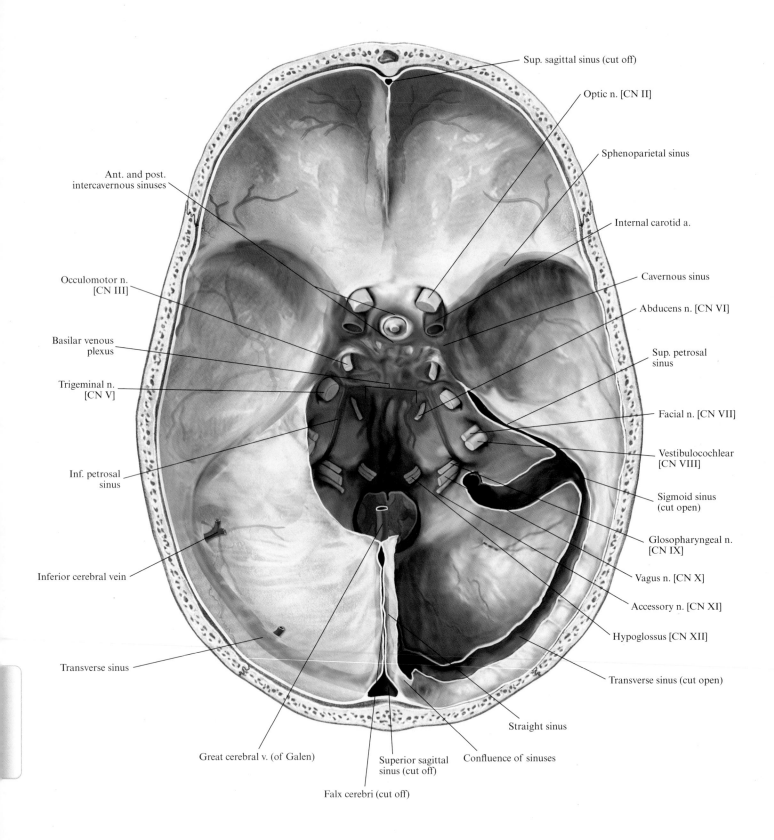

Sup. sagittal sinus (cut off)

Optic n. [CN II]

Sphenoparietal sinus

Internal carotid a.

Cavernous sinus

Abducens n. [CN VI]

Sup. petrosal sinus

Facial n. [CN VII]

Vestibulocochlear [CN VIII]

Sigmoid sinus (cut open)

Glosopharyngeal n. [CN IX]

Vagus n. [CN X]

Accessory n. [CN XI]

Hypoglossus [CN XII]

Transverse sinus (cut open)

Straight sinus

Confluence of sinuses

Superior sagittal sinus (cut off)

Great cerebral v. (of Galen)

Falx cerebri (cut off)

Transverse sinus

Inferior cerebral vein

Inf. petrosal sinus

Trigeminal n. [CN V]

Basilar venous plexus

Occulomotor n. [CN III]

Ant. and post. intercavernous sinuses

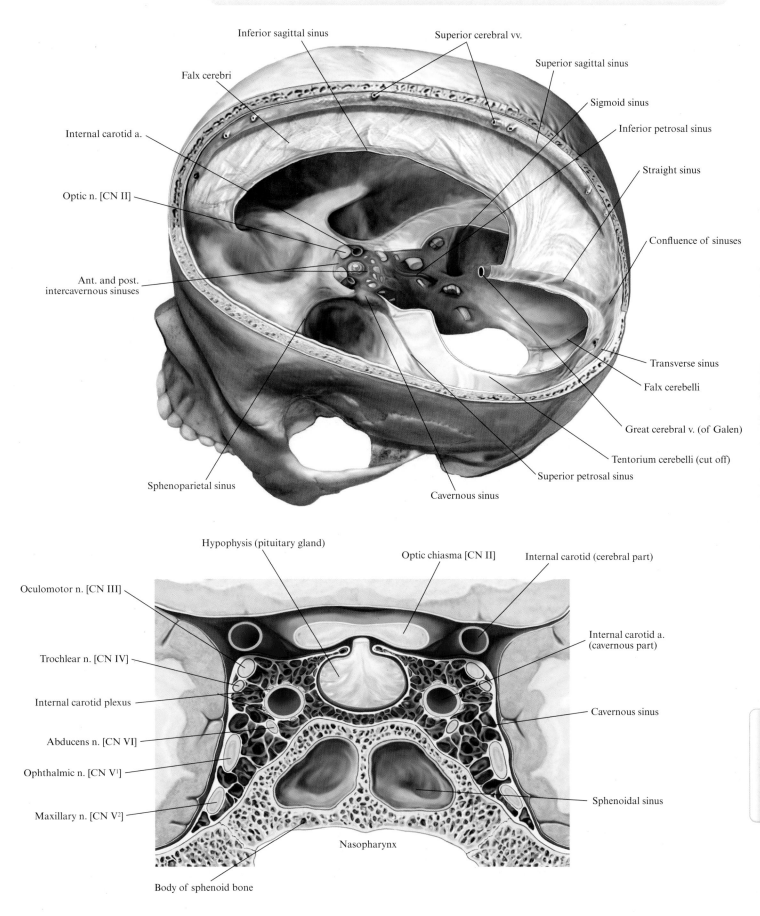

Inferior sagittal sinus

Superior cerebral vv.

Falx cerebri

Superior sagittal sinus

Sigmoid sinus

Internal carotid a.

Inferior petrosal sinus

Straight sinus

Optic n. [CN II]

Confluence of sinuses

Ant. and post.
intercavernous sinuses

Transverse sinus

Falx cerebelli

Great cerebral v. (of Galen)

Tentorium cerebelli (cut off)

Sphenoparietal sinus

Superior petrosal sinus

Cavernous sinus

Hypophysis (pituitary gland)

Optic chiasma [CN II]

Internal carotid (cerebral part)

Oculomotor n. [CN III]

Internal carotid a.
(cavernous part)

Trochlear n. [CN IV]

Internal carotid plexus

Cavernous sinus

Abducens n. [CN VI]

Ophthalmic n. [CN V¹]

Sphenoidal sinus

Maxillary n. [CN V²]

Nasopharynx

Body of sphenoid bone

PLATE 7.37   DERMATOMES & CUTANEOUS INNERVATION

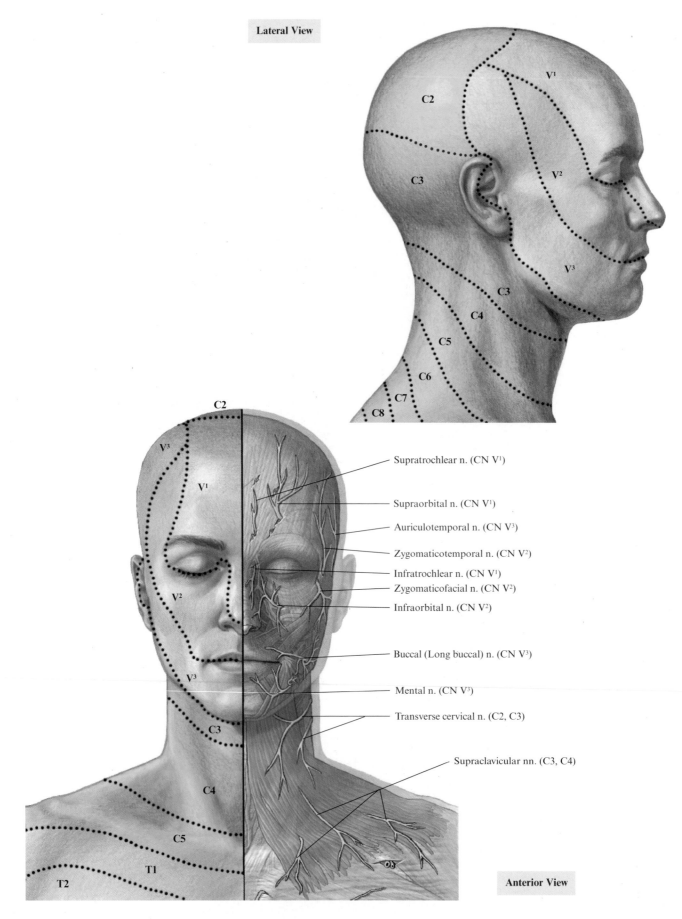

Lateral View

C2

V¹

C3

V²

V³

C3

C4

C5

C6

C7

C8

C2

V³

V¹

V²

V³

C3

C4

C5

T1

T2

Supratrochlear n. (CN V¹)

Supraorbital n. (CN V¹)

Auriculotemporal n. (CN V³)

Zygomaticotemporal n. (CN V²)

Infratrochlear n. (CN V¹)

Zygomaticofacial n. (CN V²)

Infraorbital n. (CN V²)

Buccal (Long buccal) n. (CN V³)

Mental n. (CN V³)

Transverse cervical n. (C2, C3)

Supraclavicular nn. (C3, C4)

Anterior View

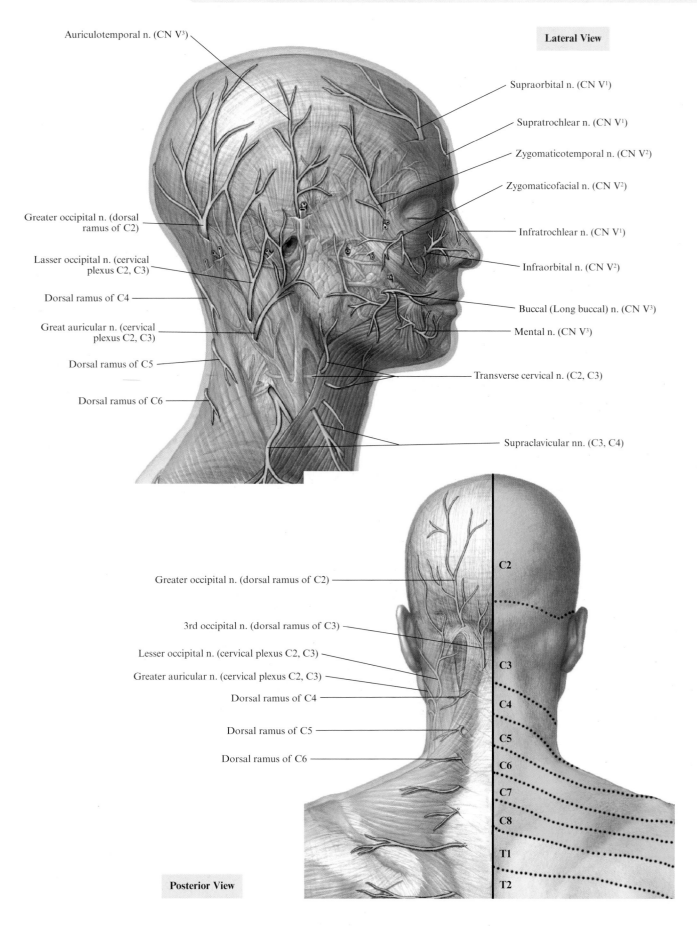

Lateral View

Auriculotemporal n. (CN V³)

Supraorbital n. (CN V¹)

Supratrochlear n. (CN V¹)

Zygomaticotemporal n. (CN V²)

Zygomaticofacial n. (CN V²)

Greater occipital n. (dorsal ramus of C2)

Infratrochlear n. (CN V¹)

Lasser occipital n. (cervical plexus C2, C3)

Infraorbital n. (CN V²)

Dorsal ramus of C4

Great auricular n. (cervical plexus C2, C3)

Buccal (Long buccal) n. (CN V³)

Mental n. (CN V³)

Dorsal ramus of C5

Dorsal ramus of C6

Transverse cervical n. (C2, C3)

Supraclavicular nn. (C3, C4)

Greater occipital n. (dorsal ramus of C2)

C2

3rd occipital n. (dorsal ramus of C3)

Lesser occipital n. (cervical plexus C2, C3)

C3

Greater auricular n. (cervical plexus C2, C3)

Dorsal ramus of C4

C4

Dorsal ramus of C5

C5

Dorsal ramus of C6

C6

C7

C8

T1

Posterior View

T2

PLATE 7.39   BRAIN

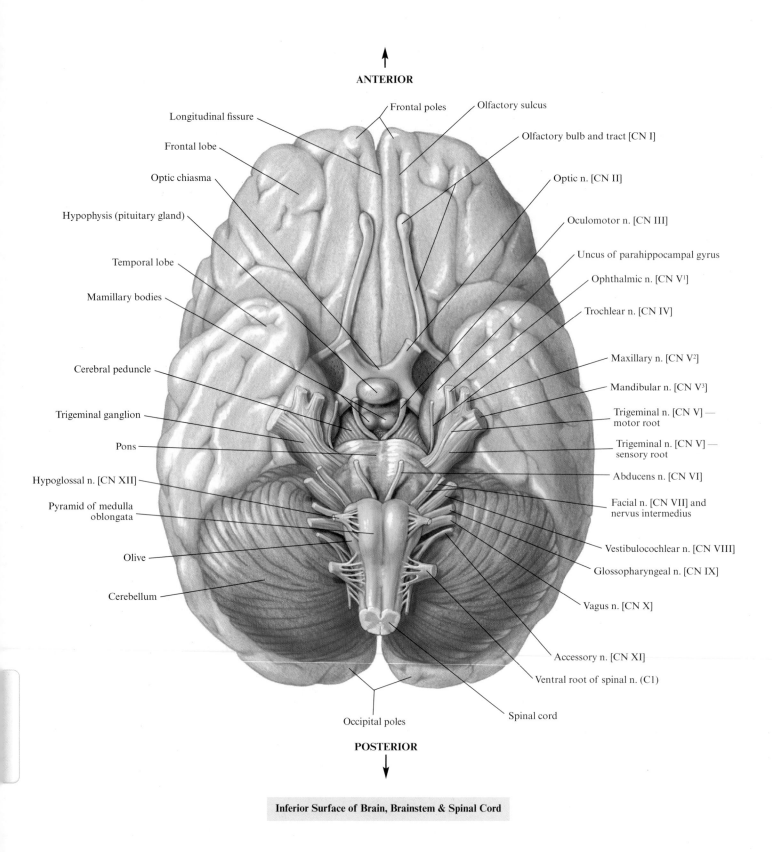

ANTERIOR

Longitudinal fissure

Frontal lobe

Optic chiasma

Hypophysis (pituitary gland)

Temporal lobe

Mamillary bodies

Cerebral peduncle

Trigeminal ganglion

Pons

Hypoglossal n. [CN XII]

Pyramid of medulla
oblongata

Olive

Cerebellum

Frontal poles

Olfactory sulcus

Olfactory bulb and tract [CN I]

Optic n. [CN II]

Oculomotor n. [CN III]

Uncus of parahippocampal gyrus

Ophthalmic n. [CN V¹]

Trochlear n. [CN IV]

Maxillary n. [CN V²]

Mandibular n. [CN V³]

Trigeminal n. [CN V] —
motor root

Trigeminal n. [CN V] —
sensory root

Abducens n. [CN VI]

Facial n. [CN VII] and
nervus intermedius

Vestibulocochlear n. [CN VIII]

Glossopharyngeal n. [CN IX]

Vagus n. [CN X]

Accessory n. [CN XI]

Ventral root of spinal n. (C1)

Spinal cord

Occipital poles

POSTERIOR

Inferior Surface of Brain, Brainstem & Spinal Cord

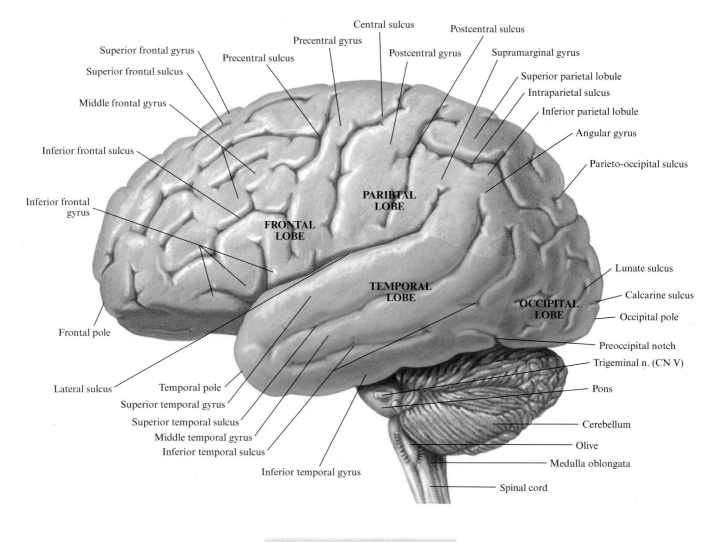

Central sulcus

Precentral gyrus

Superior frontal gyrus

Superior frontal sulcus

Precentral sulcus

Postcentral sulcus

Postcentral gyrus

Supramarginal gyrus

Middle frontal gyrus

Superior parietal lobule

Intraparietal sulcus

Inferior parietal lobule

Inferior frontal sulcus

Angular gyrus

Inferior frontal gyrus

Parieto-occipital sulcus

PARIBTAL LOBE

FRONTAL LOBE

Lunate sulcus

TEMPORAL LOBE

Calcarine sulcus

OCCIPITAL LOBE

Occipital pole

Frontal pole

Preoccipital notch

Trigeminal n. (CN V)

Pons

Lateral sulcus

Temporal pole

Cerebellum

Superior temporal gyrus

Olive

Superior temporal sulcus

Medulla oblongata

Middle temporal gyrus

Inferior temporal sulcus

Spinal cord

Inferior temporal gyrus

Left Lateral View of Brain & Brainstem

PLATE 7.41   BRAIN

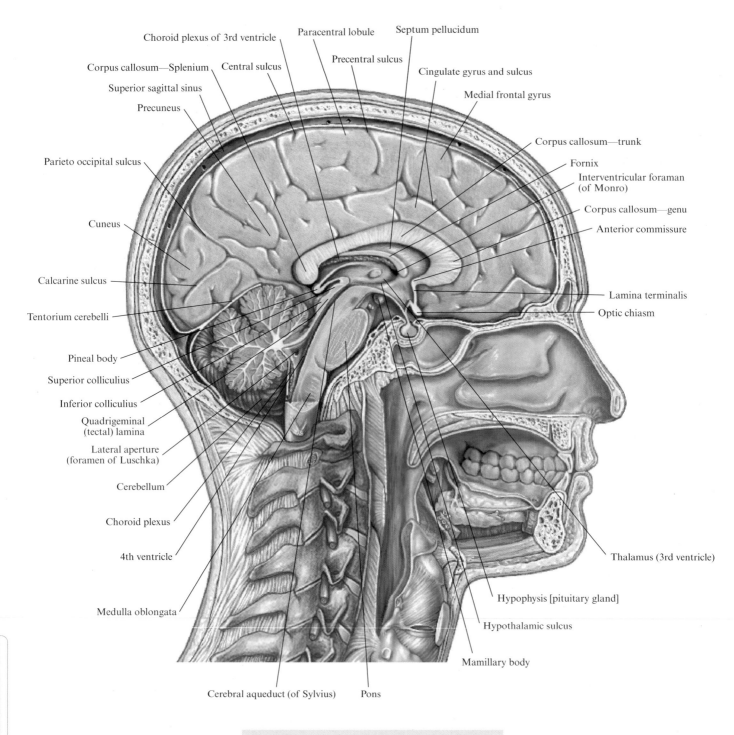

Choroid plexus of 3rd ventricle

Paracentral lobule

Septum pellucidum

Corpus callosum—Splenium

Central sulcus

Precentral sulcus

Superior sagittal sinus

Cingulate gyrus and sulcus

Precuneus

Medial frontal gyrus

Parieto occipital sulcus

Corpus callosum—trunk

Fornix

Interventricular foraman (of Monro)

Corpus callosum—genu

Cuneus

Anterior commissure

Calcarine sulcus

Lamina terminalis

Optic chiasm

Tentorium cerebelli

Pineal body

Superior colliculius

Inferior colliculius

Quadrigeminal (tectal) lamina

Lateral aperture (foramen of Luschka)

Cerebellum

Choroid plexus

Thalamus (3rd ventricle)

4th ventricle

Hypophysis [pituitary gland]

Medulla oblongata

Hypothalamic sulcus

Mamillary body

Cerebral aqueduct (of Sylvius)   Pons

Lateral View with Brain & Brainstem Median Sectioned

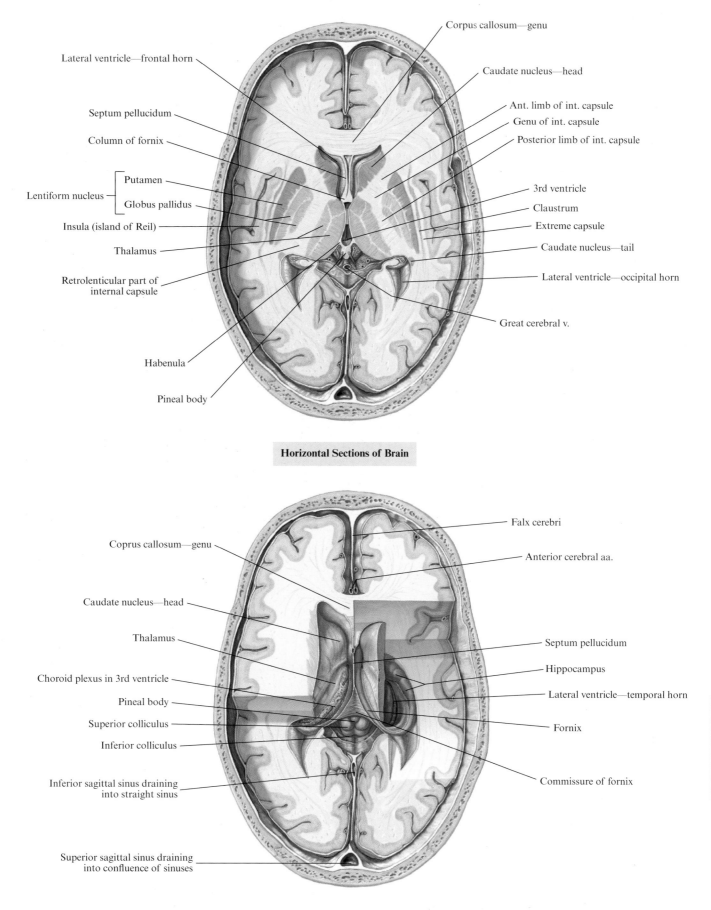

Corpus callosum—genu

Lateral ventricle—frontal horn

Caudate nucleus—head

Septum pellucidum

Ant. limb of int. capsule

Genu of int. capsule

Column of fornix

Posterior limb of int. capsule

Putamen
Lentiform nucleus
Globus pallidus

3rd ventricle

Claustrum

Insula (island of Reil)

Extreme capsule

Thalamus

Caudate nucleus—tail

Retrolenticular part of
internal capsule

Lateral ventricle—occipital horn

Great cerebral v.

Habenula

Pineal body

Horizontal Sections of Brain

Falx cerebri

Coprus callosum—genu

Anterior cerebral aa.

Caudate nucleus—head

Thalamus

Septum pellucidum

Choroid plexus in 3rd ventricle

Hippocampus

Pineal body

Lateral ventricle—temporal horn

Superior colliculus

Fornix

Inferior colliculus

Inferior sagittal sinus draining
into straight sinus

Commissure of fornix

Superior sagittal sinus draining
into confluence of sinuses

PLATE 7.43   LYMPHATICS

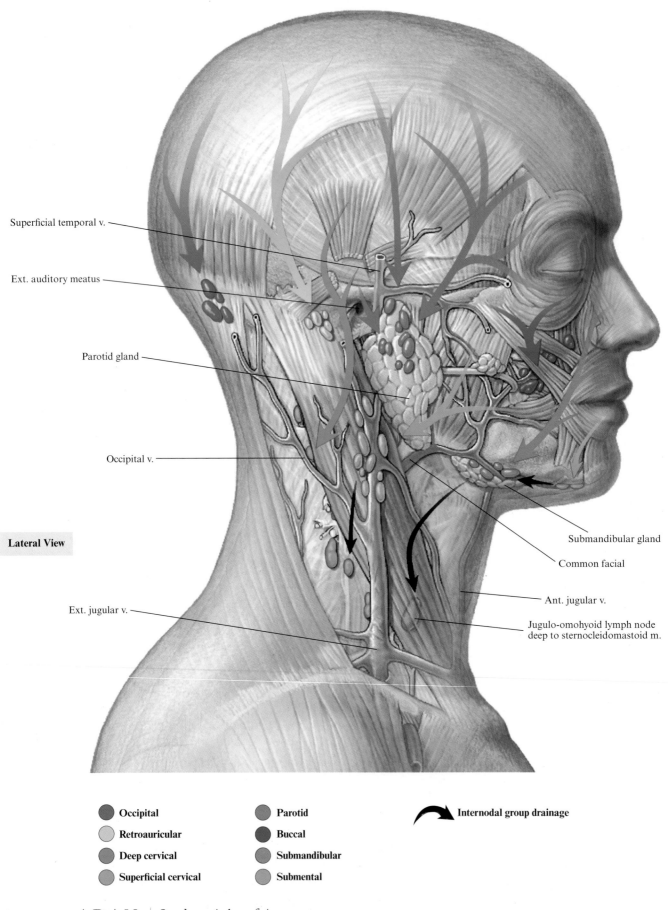

Superficial temporal v.

Ext. auditory meatus

Parotid gland

Occipital v.

Lateral View

Ext. jugular v.

Submandibular gland

Common facial

Ant. jugular v.

Jugulo-omohyoid lymph node
deep to sternocleidomastoid m.

● Occipital   ● Parotid   ⤻ **Internodal group drainage**

○ **Retroauricular**   ● **Buccal**

● **Deep cervical**   ● **Submandibular**

● **Superficial cervical**   ● **Submental**

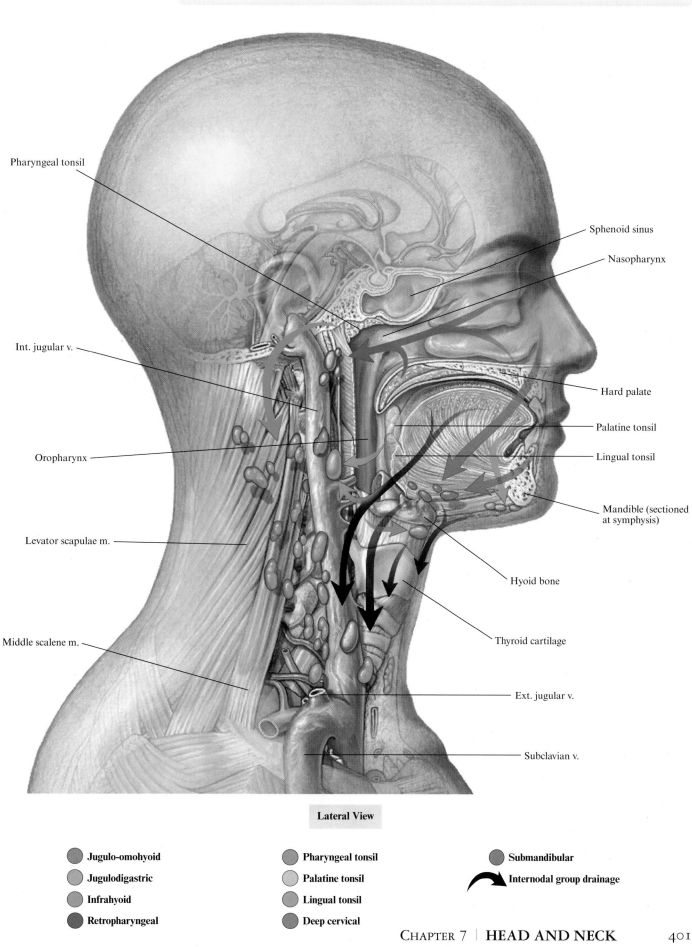

Pharyngeal tonsil

Sphenoid sinus

Nasopharynx

Int. jugular v.

Hard palate

Palatine tonsil

Oropharynx

Lingual tonsil

Mandible (sectioned
at symphysis)

Levator scapulae m.

Hyoid bone

Middle scalene m.

Thyroid cartilage

Ext. jugular v.

Subclavian v.

Lateral View

🔵 **Jugulo-omohyoid**   🔵 **Pharyngeal tonsil**   🔵 **Submandibular**

🔵 **Jugulodigastric**   🔵 **Palatine tonsil**   ⟶ **Internodal group drainage**

🔵 **Infrahyoid**   🔵 **Lingual tonsil**

🔵 **Retropharyngeal**   🔵 **Deep cervical**

PLATE 7.45   LYMPHATICS

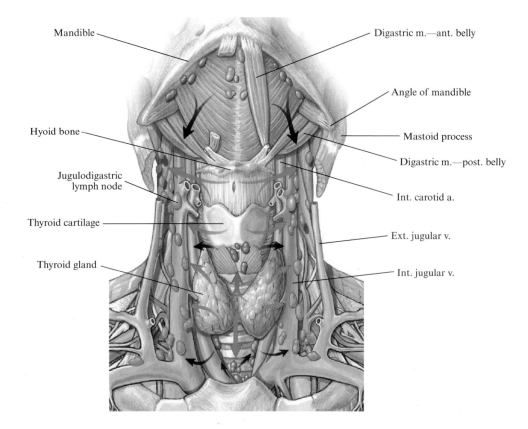

Mandible

Digastric m.—ant. belly

Anterior View of Anterior Triangle of the Neck & Submandibular Regions

Angle of mandible

Mastoid process

Hyoid bone

Digastric m.—post. belly

Jugulodigastric lymph node

Int. carotid a.

Thyroid cartilage

Ext. jugular v.

Thyroid gland

Int. jugular v.

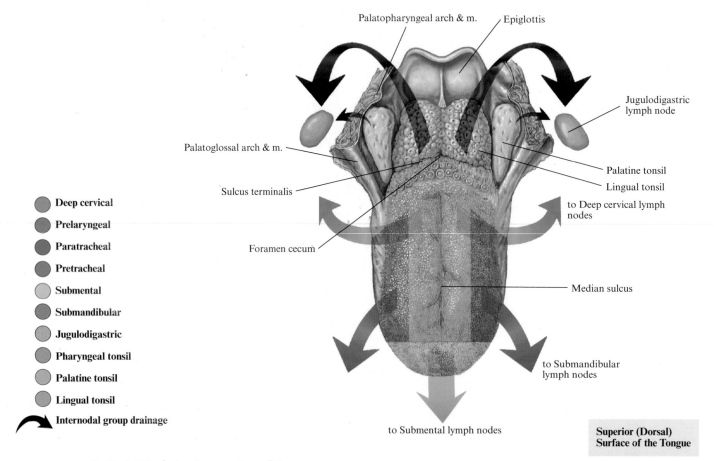

Palatopharyngeal arch & m.   Epiglottis

Jugulodigastric lymph node

Palatoglossal arch & m.

Palatine tonsil

Lingual tonsil

Sulcus terminalis

to Deep cervical lymph nodes

Foramen cecum

Median sulcus

⬤ **Deep cervical**

⬤ **Prelaryngeal**

⬤ **Paratracheal**

⬤ **Pretracheal**

⬤ **Submental**

⬤ **Submandibular**

⬤ **Jugulodigastric**

⬤ **Pharyngeal tonsil**

⬤ **Palatine tonsil**

⬤ **Lingual tonsil**

to Submandibular lymph nodes

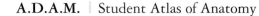 **Internodal group drainage**

to Submental lymph nodes

Superior (Dorsal) Surface of the Tongue

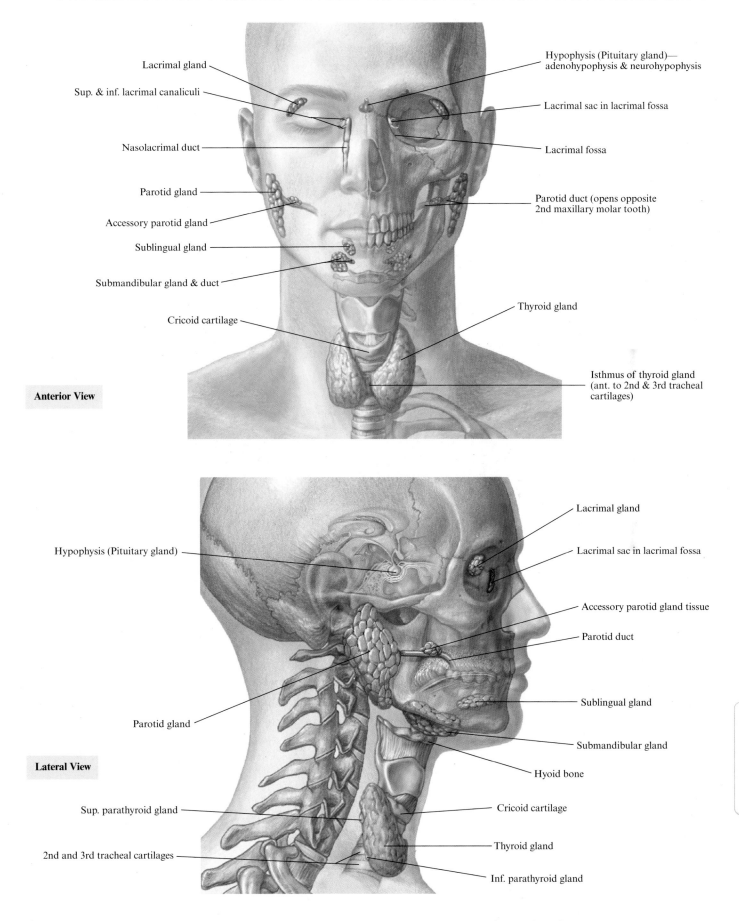

Anterior View

Lacrimal gland

Sup. & inf. lacrimal canaliculi

Nasolacrimal duct

Parotid gland

Accessory parotid gland

Sublingual gland

Submandibular gland & duct

Cricoid cartilage

Hypophysis (Pituitary gland)—adenohypophysis & neurohypophysis

Lacrimal sac in lacrimal fossa

Lacrimal fossa

Parotid duct (opens opposite 2nd maxillary molar tooth)

Thyroid gland

Isthmus of thyroid gland (ant. to 2nd & 3rd tracheal cartilages)

Lateral View

Hypophysis (Pituitary gland)

Parotid gland

Sup. parathyroid gland

2nd and 3rd tracheal cartilages

Lacrimal gland

Lacrimal sac in lacrimal fossa

Accessory parotid gland tissue

Parotid duct

Sublingual gland

Submandibular gland

Hyoid bone

Cricoid cartilage

Thyroid gland

Inf. parathyroid gland

PLATE 7.47   FACE & NECK—SUPERFICIAL

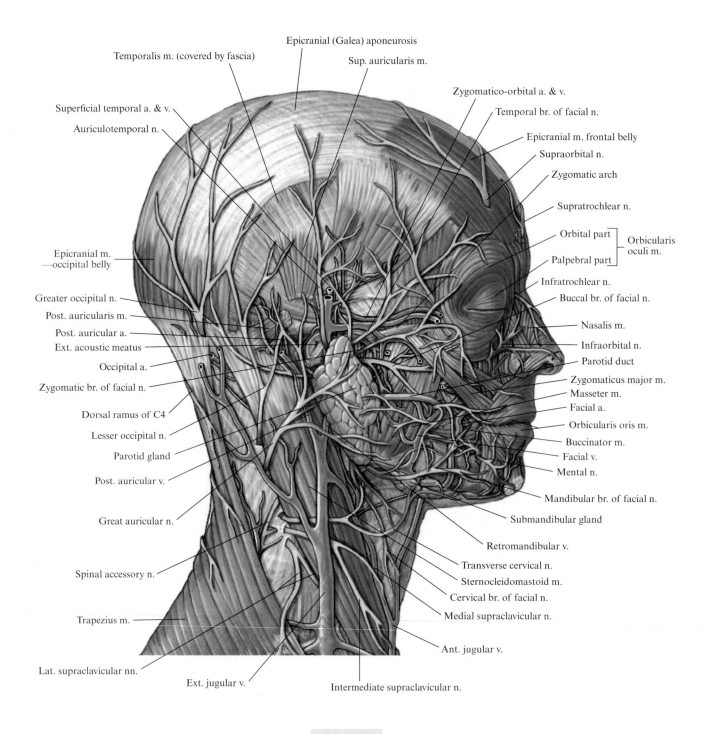

Epicranial (Galea) aponeurosis

Temporalis m. (covered by fascia)

Sup. auricularis m.

Zygomatico-orbital a. & v.

Superficial temporal a. & v.

Temporal br. of facial n.

Auriculotemporal n.

Epicranial m. frontal belly

Supraorbital n.

Zygomatic arch

Supratrochlear n.

Orbital part

Palpebral part

Orbicularis oculi m.

Epicranial m. —occipital belly

Infratrochlear n.

Buccal br. of facial n.

Greater occipital n.

Post. auricularis m.

Nasalis m.

Post. auricular a.

Ext. acoustic meatus

Infraorbital n.

Parotid duct

Occipital a.

Zygomaticus major m.

Zygomatic br. of facial n.

Masseter m.

Facial a.

Dorsal ramus of C4

Orbicularis oris m.

Lesser occipital n.

Buccinator m.

Facial v.

Parotid gland

Mental n.

Post. auricular v.

Mandibular br. of facial n.

Submandibular gland

Great auricular n.

Retromandibular v.

Spinal accessory n.

Transverse cervical n.

Sternocleidomastoid m.

Cervical br. of facial n.

Trapezius m.

Medial supraclavicular n.

Ant. jugular v.

Lat. supraclavicular nn.

Ext. jugular v.

Intermediate supraclavicular n.

Lateral View

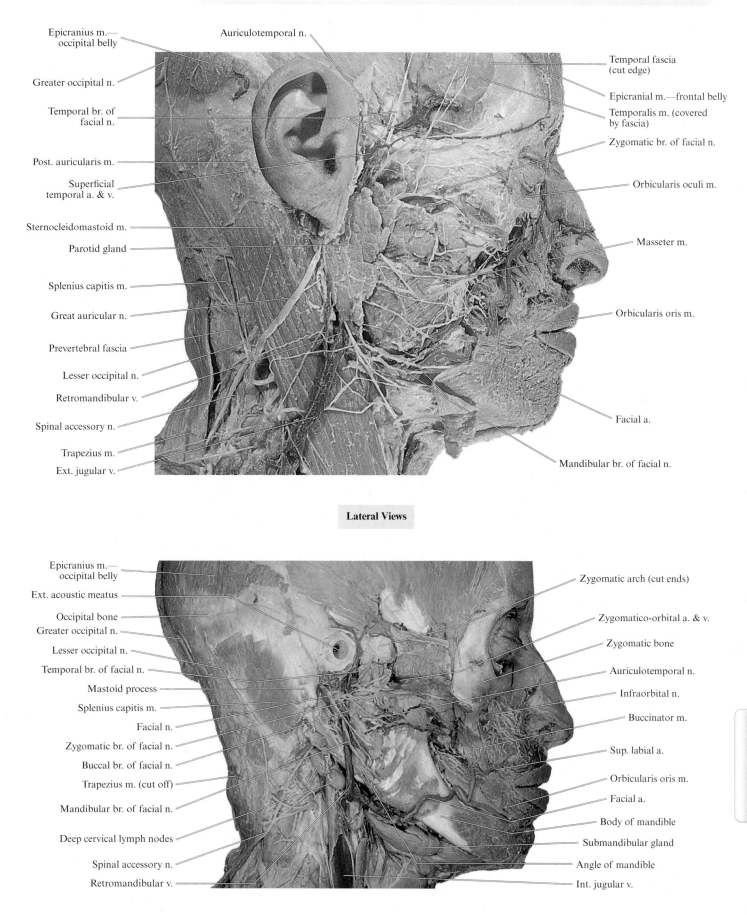

Epicranius m.— occipital belly

Auriculotemporal n.

Temporal fascia (cut edge)

Greater occipital n.

Epicranial m.—frontal belly

Temporal br. of facial n.

Temporalis m. (covered by fascia)

Zygomatic br. of facial n.

Post. auricularis m.

Orbicularis oculi m.

Superficial temporal a. & v.

Sternocleidomastoid m.

Masseter m.

Parotid gland

Splenius capitis m.

Great auricular n.

Orbicularis oris m.

Prevertebral fascia

Lesser occipital n.

Retromandibular v.

Spinal accessory n.

Facial a.

Trapezius m.

Ext. jugular v.

Mandibular br. of facial n.

Lateral Views

Epicranius m.— occipital belly

Zygomatic arch (cut ends)

Ext. acoustic meatus

Zygomatico-orbital a. & v.

Occipital bone

Zygomatic bone

Greater occipital n.

Lesser occipital n.

Auriculotemporal n.

Temporal br. of facial n.

Infraorbital n.

Mastoid process

Buccinator m.

Splenius capitis m.

Facial n.

Sup. labial a.

Zygomatic br. of facial n.

Buccal br. of facial n.

Orbicularis oris m.

Trapezius m. (cut off)

Facial a.

Mandibular br. of facial n.

Body of mandible

Deep cervical lymph nodes

Submandibular gland

Spinal accessory n.

Angle of mandible

Retromandibular v.

Int. jugular v.

PLATE 7.49   NECK—SUPERFICIAL

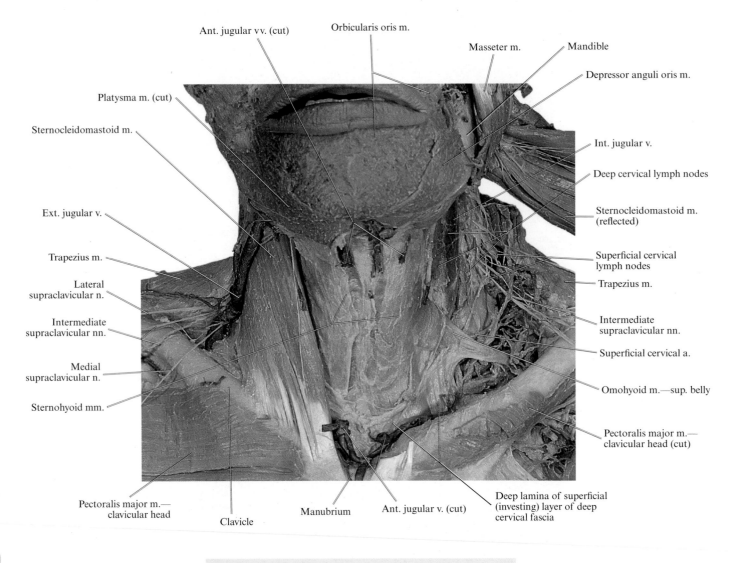

Ant. jugular vv. (cut)

Orbicularis oris m.

Masseter m.

Mandible

Depressor anguli oris m.

Platysma m. (cut)

Sternocleidomastoid m.

Int. jugular v.

Deep cervical lymph nodes

Sternocleidomastoid m. (reflected)

Ext. jugular v.

Superficial cervical lymph nodes

Trapezius m.

Trapezius m.

Lateral supraclavicular n.

Intermediate supraclavicular nn.

Intermediate supraclavicular nn.

Superficial cervical a.

Medial supraclavicular n.

Omohyoid m.—sup. belly

Sternohyoid mm.

Pectoralis major m.— clavicular head (cut)

Pectoralis major m.— clavicular head

Clavicle

Manubrium

Ant. jugular v. (cut)

Deep lamina of superficial (investing) layer of deep cervical fascia

Anterior View of Neck with Deeper Structures Exposed on Left Side

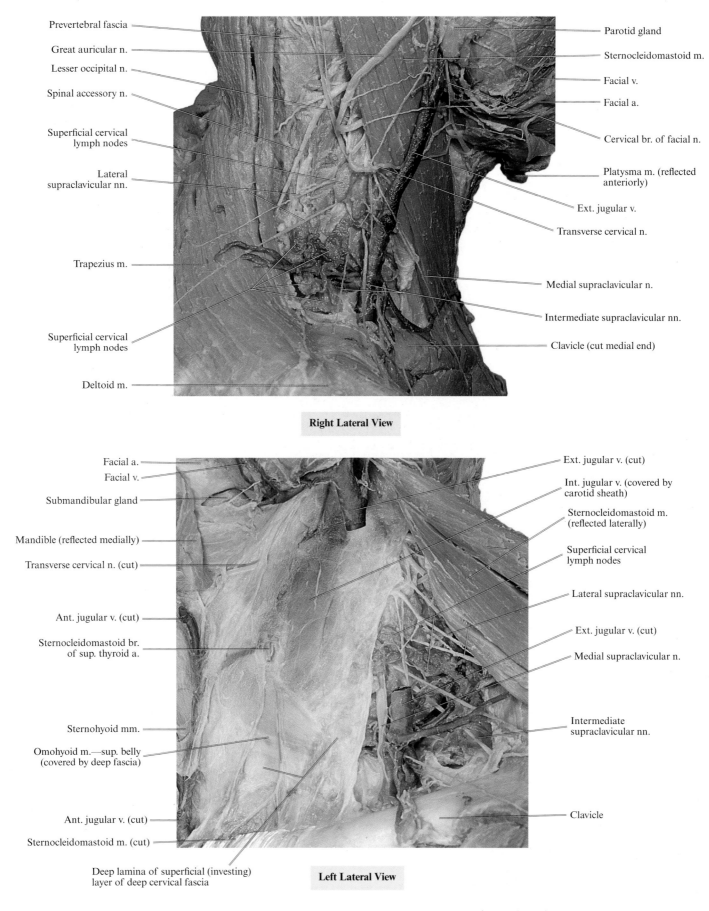

Prevertebral fascia

Great auricular n.

Lesser occipital n.

Spinal accessory n.

Superficial cervical
lymph nodes

Lateral
supraclavicular nn.

Trapezius m.

Superficial cervical
lymph nodes

Deltoid m.

Parotid gland

Sternocleidomastoid m.

Facial v.

Facial a.

Cervical br. of facial n.

Platysma m. (reflected
anteriorly)

Ext. jugular v.

Transverse cervical n.

Medial supraclavicular n.

Intermediate supraclavicular nn.

Clavicle (cut medial end)

Right Lateral View

Facial a.

Facial v.

Submandibular gland

Mandible (reflected medially)

Transverse cervical n. (cut)

Ant. jugular v. (cut)

Sternocleidomastoid br.
of sup. thyroid a.

Sternohyoid mm.

Omohyoid m.—sup. belly
(covered by deep fascia)

Ant. jugular v. (cut)

Sternocleidomastoid m. (cut)

Deep lamina of superficial (investing)
layer of deep cervical fascia

Ext. jugular v. (cut)

Int. jugular v. (covered by
carotid sheath)

Sternocleidomastoid m.
(reflected laterally)

Superficial cervical
lymph nodes

Lateral supraclavicular nn.

Ext. jugular v. (cut)

Medial supraclavicular n.

Intermediate
supraclavicular nn.

Clavicle

Left Lateral View

PLATE 7.51   NECK—LATERAL

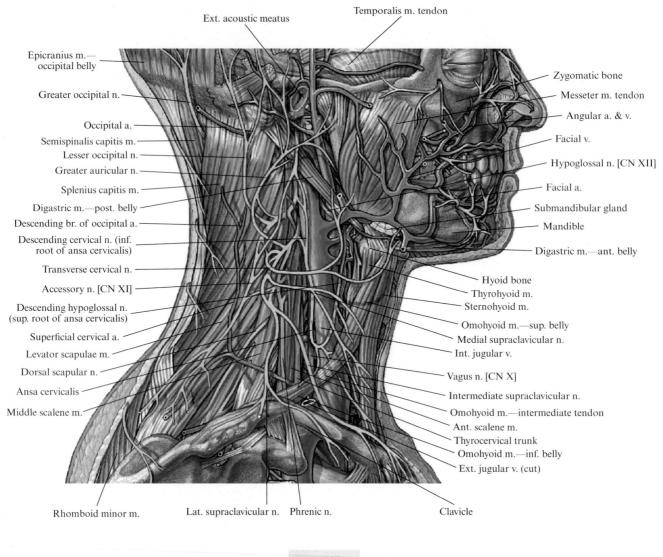

Ext. acoustic meatus

Temporalis m. tendon

Epicranius m.—
occipital belly

Greater occipital n.

Occipital a.

Semispinalis capitis m.

Lesser occipital n.

Greater auricular n.

Splenius capitis m.

Digastric m.—post. belly

Descending br. of occipital a.

Descending cervical n. (inf.
root of ansa cervicalis)

Transverse cervical n.

Accessory n. [CN XI]

Descending hypoglossal n.
(sup. root of ansa cervicalis)

Superficial cervical a.

Levator scapulae m.

Dorsal scapular n.

Ansa cervicalis

Middle scalene m.

Zygomatic bone

Messeter m. tendon

Angular a. & v.

Facial v.

Hypoglossal n. [CN XII]

Facial a.

Submandibular gland

Mandible

Digastric m.—ant. belly

Hyoid bone

Thyrohyoid m.

Sternohyoid m.

Omohyoid m.—sup. belly

Medial supraclavicular n.

Int. jugular v.

Vagus n. [CN X]

Intermediate supraclavicular n.

Omohyoid m.—intermediate tendon

Ant. scalene m.

Thyrocervical trunk

Omohyoid m.—inf. belly

Ext. jugular v. (cut)

Rhomboid minor m.

Lat. supraclavicular n.

Phrenic n.

Clavicle

Lateral View

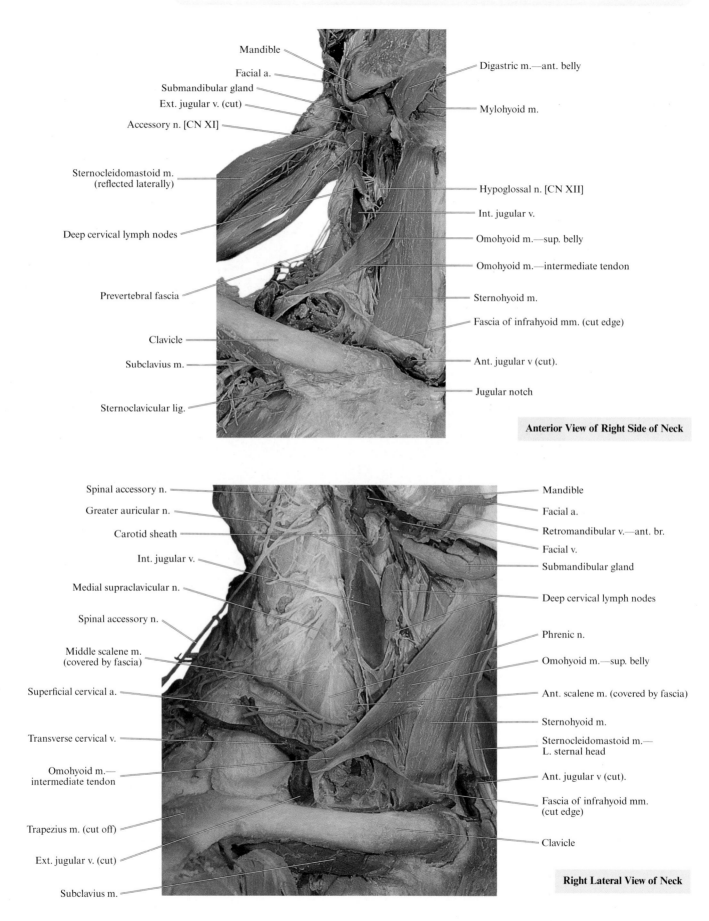

Mandible

Facial a.

Submandibular gland

Ext. jugular v. (cut)

Accessory n. [CN XI]

Sternocleidomastoid m.
(reflected laterally)

Deep cervical lymph nodes

Prevertebral fascia

Clavicle

Subclavius m.

Sternoclavicular lig.

Digastric m.—ant. belly

Mylohyoid m.

Hypoglossal n. [CN XII]

Int. jugular v.

Omohyoid m.—sup. belly

Omohyoid m.—intermediate tendon

Sternohyoid m.

Fascia of infrahyoid mm. (cut edge)

Ant. jugular v (cut).

Jugular notch

Anterior View of Right Side of Neck

Spinal accessory n.

Greater auricular n.

Carotid sheath

Int. jugular v.

Medial supraclavicular n.

Spinal accessory n.

Middle scalene m.
(covered by fascia)

Superficial cervical a.

Transverse cervical v.

Omohyoid m.—
intermediate tendon

Trapezius m. (cut off)

Ext. jugular v. (cut)

Subclavius m.

Mandible

Facial a.

Retromandibular v.—ant. br.

Facial v.

Submandibular gland

Deep cervical lymph nodes

Phrenic n.

Omohyoid m.—sup. belly

Ant. scalene m. (covered by fascia)

Sternohyoid m.

Sternocleidomastoid m.—
L. sternal head

Ant. jugular v (cut).

Fascia of infrahyoid mm.
(cut edge)

Clavicle

Right Lateral View of Neck

PLATE 7.53   NECK—DEEP ANTERIOR

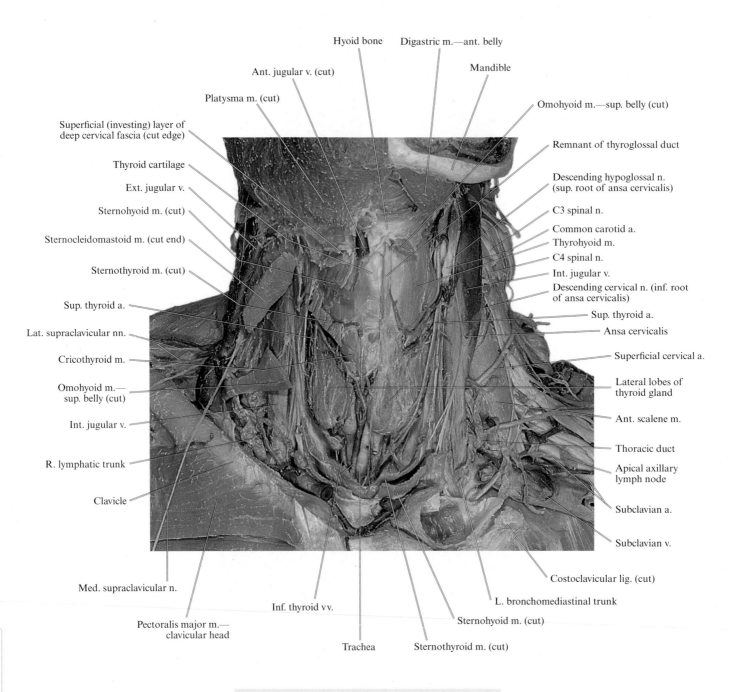

Hyoid bone

Digastric m.—ant. belly

Ant. jugular v. (cut)

Mandible

Platysma m. (cut)

Omohyoid m.—sup. belly (cut)

Superficial (investing) layer of
deep cervical fascia (cut edge)

Remnant of thyroglossal duct

Thyroid cartilage

Descending hypoglossal n.
(sup. root of ansa cervicalis)

Ext. jugular v.

C3 spinal n.

Sternohyoid m. (cut)

Common carotid a.

Thyrohyoid m.

Sternocleidomastoid m. (cut end)

C4 spinal n.

Sternothyroid m. (cut)

Int. jugular v.

Descending cervical n. (inf. root
of ansa cervicalis)

Sup. thyroid a.

Sup. thyroid a.

Lat. supraclavicular nn.

Ansa cervicalis

Cricothyroid m.

Superficial cervical a.

Omohyoid m.—
sup. belly (cut)

Lateral lobes of
thyroid gland

Int. jugular v.

Ant. scalene m.

R. lymphatic trunk

Thoracic duct

Apical axillary
lymph node

Clavicle

Subclavian a.

Subclavian v.

Costoclavicular lig. (cut)

Med. supraclavicular n.

L. bronchomediastinal trunk

Inf. thyroid v v.

Sternohyoid m. (cut)

Pectoralis major m.—
clavicular head

Sternothyroid m. (cut)

Trachea

Anterior View of Neck with Deep Structures on Right Side

A.D.A.M. | Student Atlas of Anatomy

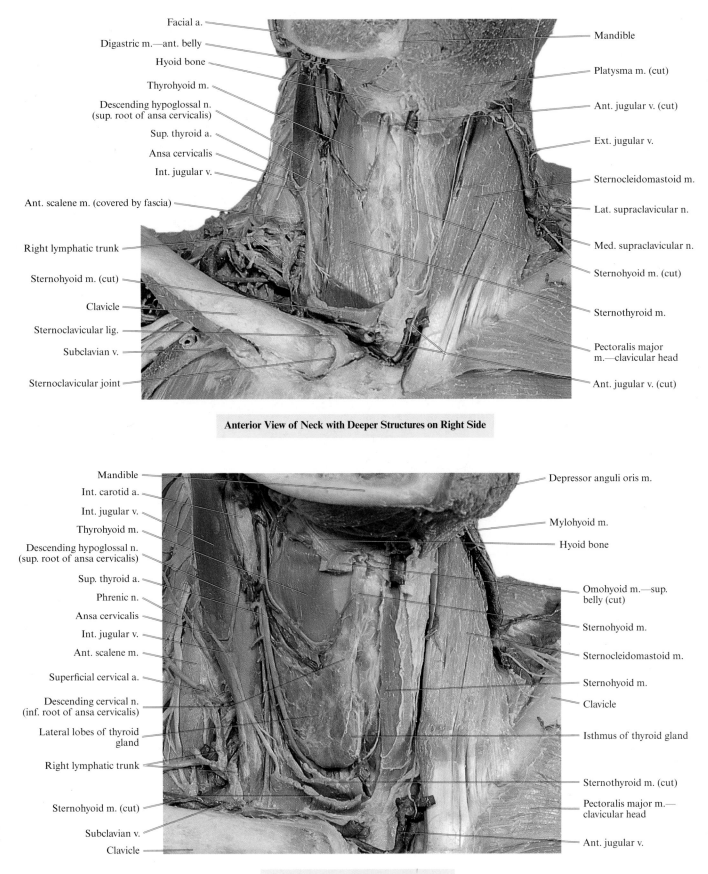

Facial a.

Digastric m.—ant. belly

Hyoid bone

Thyrohyoid m.

Descending hypoglossal n.
(sup. root of ansa cervicalis)

Sup. thyroid a.

Ansa cervicalis

Int. jugular v.

Ant. scalene m. (covered by fascia)

Right lymphatic trunk

Sternohyoid m. (cut)

Clavicle

Sternoclavicular lig.

Subclavian v.

Sternoclavicular joint

Mandible

Platysma m. (cut)

Ant. jugular v. (cut)

Ext. jugular v.

Sternocleidomastoid m.

Lat. supraclavicular n.

Med. supraclavicular n.

Sternohyoid m. (cut)

Sternothyroid m.

Pectoralis major
m.—clavicular head

Ant. jugular v. (cut)

Anterior View of Neck with Deeper Structures on Right Side

Mandible

Int. carotid a.

Int. jugular v.

Thyrohyoid m.

Descending hypoglossal n.
(sup. root of ansa cervicalis)

Sup. thyroid a.

Phrenic n.

Ansa cervicalis

Int. jugular v.

Ant. scalene m.

Superficial cervical a.

Descending cervical n.
(inf. root of ansa cervicalis)

Lateral lobes of thyroid
gland

Right lymphatic trunk

Sternohyoid m. (cut)

Subclavian v.

Clavicle

Depressor anguli oris m.

Mylohyoid m.

Hyoid bone

Omohyoid m.—sup.
belly (cut)

Sternohyoid m.

Sternocleidomastoid m.

Sternohyoid m.

Clavicle

Isthmus of thyroid gland

Sternothyroid m. (cut)

Pectoralis major m.—
clavicular head

Ant. jugular v.

Anterolateral View of Right Side of Neck

PLATE 7.55   NECK—DEEP LATERAL

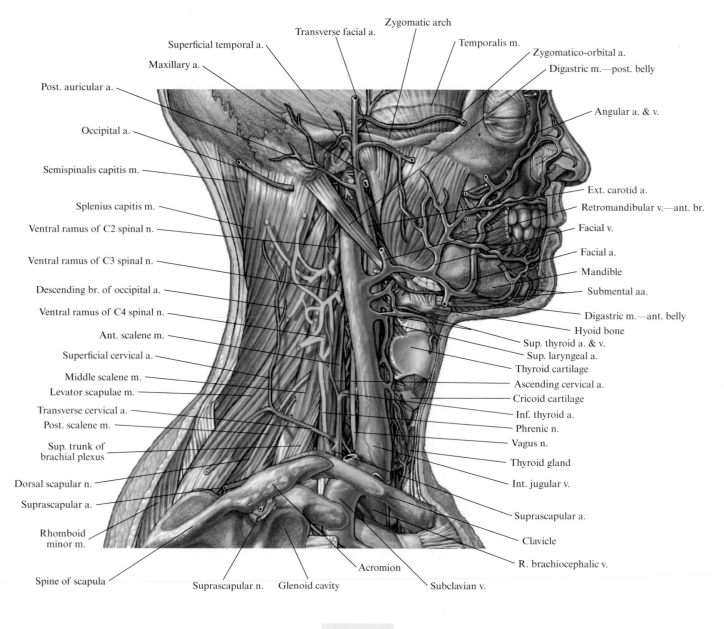

Zygomatic arch

Transverse facial a.

Temporalis m.

Superficial temporal a.

Zygomatico-orbital a.

Maxillary a.

Digastric m.—post. belly

Post. auricular a.

Angular a. & v.

Occipital a.

Semispinalis capitis m.

Ext. carotid a.

Splenius capitis m.

Retromandibular v.—ant. br.

Ventral ramus of C2 spinal n.

Facial v.

Ventral ramus of C3 spinal n.

Facial a.

Mandible

Descending br. of occipital a.

Submental aa.

Ventral ramus of C4 spinal n.

Digastric m.—ant. belly

Ant. scalene m.

Hyoid bone

Superficial cervical a.

Sup. thyroid a. & v.

Sup. laryngeal a.

Middle scalene m.

Thyroid cartilage

Levator scapulae m.

Ascending cervical a.

Transverse cervical a.

Cricoid cartilage

Post. scalene m.

Inf. thyroid a.

Phrenic n.

Sup. trunk of
brachial plexus

Vagus n.

Thyroid gland

Dorsal scapular n.

Int. jugular v.

Suprascapular a.

Rhomboid
minor m.

Suprascapular a.

Clavicle

Spine of scapula

R. brachiocephalic v.

Suprascapular n.   Glenoid cavity

Acromion

Subclavian v.

Lateral View

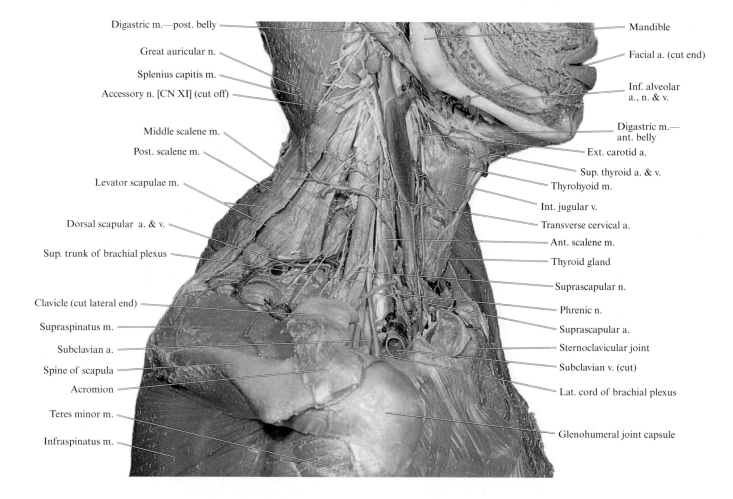

Digastric m.—post. belly

Great auricular n.

Splenius capitis m.

Accessory n. [CN XI] (cut off)

Middle scalene m.

Post. scalene m.

Levator scapulae m.

Dorsal scapular a. & v.

Sup. trunk of brachial plexus

Clavicle (cut lateral end)

Supraspinatus m.

Subclavian a.

Spine of scapula

Acromion

Teres minor m.

Infraspinatus m.

Mandible

Facial a. (cut end)

Inf. alveolar a., n. & v.

Digastric m.—ant. belly

Ext. carotid a.

Sup. thyroid a. & v.

Thyrohyoid m.

Int. jugular v.

Transverse cervical a.

Ant. scalene m.

Thyroid gland

Suprascapular n.

Phrenic n.

Suprascapular a.

Sternoclavicular joint

Subclavian v. (cut)

Lat. cord of brachial plexus

Glenohumeral joint capsule

Lateral View

PLATE 7.57   LARYNX—SUPERFICIAL ANTERIOR

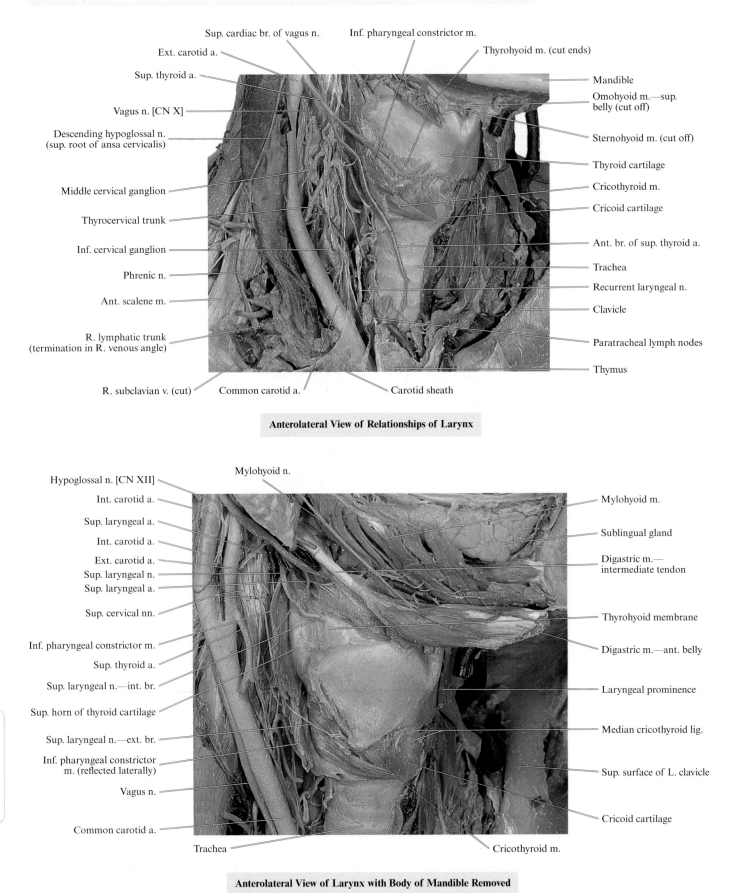

Sup. cardiac br. of vagus n.

Inf. pharyngeal constrictor m.

Thyrohyoid m. (cut ends)

Ext. carotid a.

Sup. thyroid a.

Mandible

Omohyoid m.—sup. belly (cut off)

Vagus n. [CN X]

Sternohyoid m. (cut off)

Descending hypoglossal n. (sup. root of ansa cervicalis)

Thyroid cartilage

Middle cervical ganglion

Cricothyroid m.

Thyrocervical trunk

Cricoid cartilage

Inf. cervical ganglion

Ant. br. of sup. thyroid a.

Phrenic n.

Trachea

Ant. scalene m.

Recurrent laryngeal n.

Clavicle

R. lymphatic trunk (termination in R. venous angle)

Paratracheal lymph nodes

Thymus

R. subclavian v. (cut)

Common carotid a.

Carotid sheath

Anterolateral View of Relationships of Larynx

Hypoglossal n. [CN XII]

Mylohyoid n.

Int. carotid a.

Mylohyoid m.

Sup. laryngeal a.

Sublingual gland

Int. carotid a.

Ext. carotid a.

Digastric m.—intermediate tendon

Sup. laryngeal n.

Sup. laryngeal a.

Sup. cervical nn.

Inf. pharyngeal constrictor m.

Thyrohyoid membrane

Sup. thyroid a.

Digastric m.—ant. belly

Sup. laryngeal n.—int. br.

Sup. horn of thyroid cartilage

Laryngeal prominence

Sup. laryngeal n.—ext. br.

Median cricothyroid lig.

Inf. pharyngeal constrictor m. (reflected laterally)

Vagus n.

Sup. surface of L. clavicle

Common carotid a.

Cricoid cartilage

Trachea

Cricothyroid m.

Anterolateral View of Larynx with Body of Mandible Removed

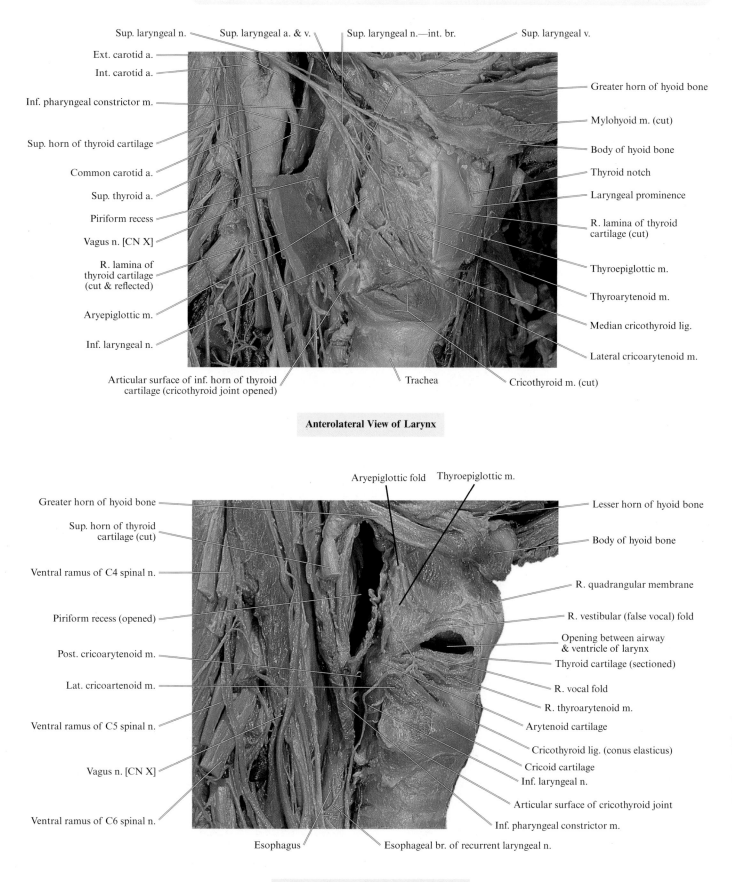

Sup. laryngeal n.   Sup. laryngeal a. & v.   Sup. laryngeal n.—int. br.   Sup. laryngeal v.

Ext. carotid a.

Int. carotid a.

Greater horn of hyoid bone

Inf. pharyngeal constrictor m.

Mylohyoid m. (cut)

Sup. horn of thyroid cartilage

Body of hyoid bone

Common carotid a.

Thyroid notch

Sup. thyroid a.

Laryngeal prominence

Piriform recess

R. lamina of thyroid cartilage (cut)

Vagus n. [CN X]

R. lamina of thyroid cartilage (cut & reflected)

Thyroepiglottic m.

Thyroarytenoid m.

Aryepiglottic m.

Median cricothyroid lig.

Inf. laryngeal n.

Lateral cricoarytenoid m.

Articular surface of inf. horn of thyroid cartilage (cricothyroid joint opened)   Trachea   Cricothyroid m. (cut)

Anterolateral View of Larynx

Aryepiglottic fold   Thyroepiglottic m.

Greater horn of hyoid bone

Lesser horn of hyoid bone

Sup. horn of thyroid cartilage (cut)

Body of hyoid bone

Ventral ramus of C4 spinal n.

R. quadrangular membrane

Piriform recess (opened)

R. vestibular (false vocal) fold

Opening between airway & ventricle of larynx

Post. cricoarytenoid m.

Thyroid cartilage (sectioned)

Lat. cricoartenoid m.

R. vocal fold

R. thyroarytenoid m.

Ventral ramus of C5 spinal n.

Arytenoid cartilage

Cricothyroid lig. (conus elasticus)

Vagus n. [CN X]

Cricoid cartilage

Inf. laryngeal n.

Articular surface of cricothyroid joint

Ventral ramus of C6 spinal n.

Inf. pharyngeal constrictor m.

Esophagus   Esophageal br. of recurrent laryngeal n.

Lateral View of Larynx & R. Vocal Folds

PLATE 7.59   LARYNX—POSTERIOR & SUPERIOR

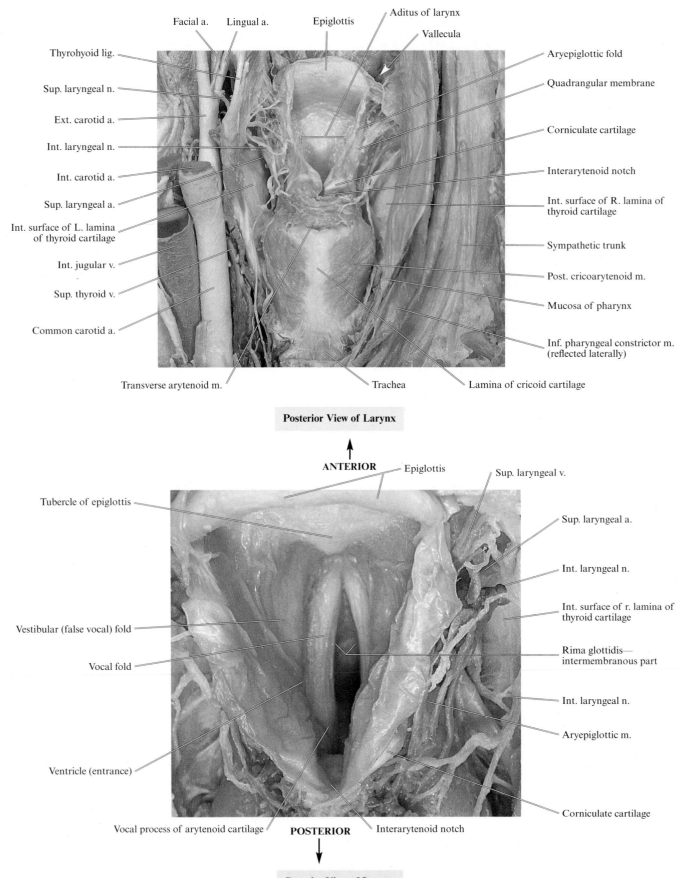

Facial a.   Lingual a.   Epiglottis   Aditus of larynx

Vallecula

Thyrohyoid lig.

Sup. laryngeal n.

Ext. carotid a.

Int. laryngeal n.

Int. carotid a.

Sup. laryngeal a.

Int. surface of L. lamina
of thyroid cartilage

Int. jugular v.

Sup. thyroid v.

Common carotid a.

Aryepiglottic fold

Quadrangular membrane

Corniculate cartilage

Interarytenoid notch

Int. surface of R. lamina of
thyroid cartilage

Sympathetic trunk

Post. cricoarytenoid m.

Mucosa of pharynx

Inf. pharyngeal constrictor m.
(reflected laterally)

Transverse arytenoid m.   Trachea   Lamina of cricoid cartilage

Posterior View of Larynx

↑

ANTERIOR   Epiglottis   Sup. laryngeal v.

Tubercle of epiglottis

Sup. laryngeal a.

Int. laryngeal n.

Int. surface of r. lamina of
thyroid cartilage

Vestibular (false vocal) fold

Rima glottidis—
intermembranous part

Vocal fold

Int. laryngeal n.

Aryepiglottic m.

Ventricle (entrance)

Corniculate cartilage

Vocal process of arytenoid cartilage   **POSTERIOR**   Interarytenoid notch

↓

Superior View of Larynx

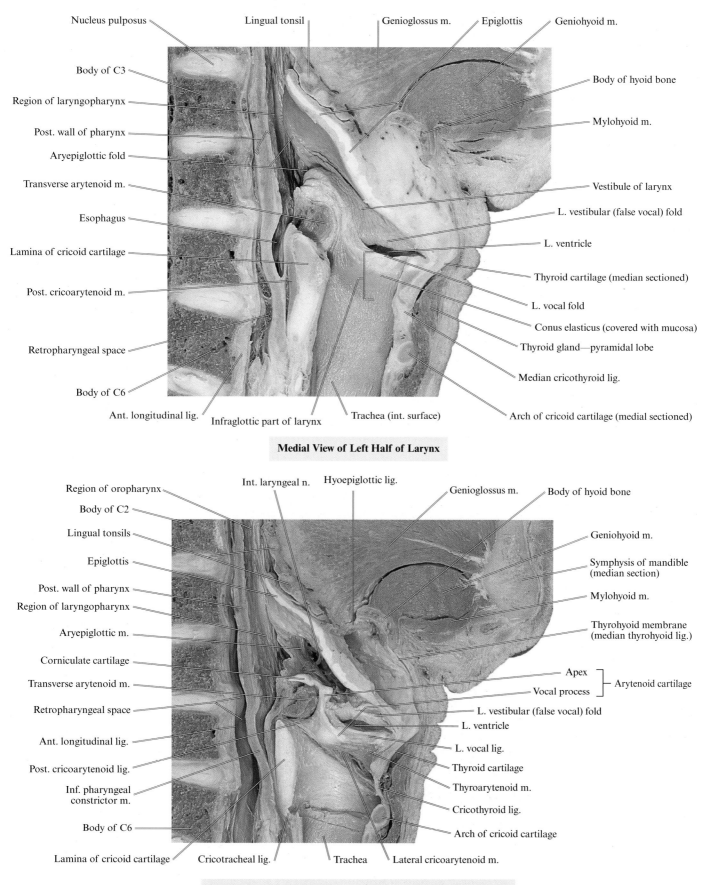

Nucleus pulposus

Lingual tonsil

Genioglossus m.

Epiglottis

Geniohyoid m.

Body of C3

Region of laryngopharynx

Post. wall of pharynx

Aryepiglottic fold

Transverse arytenoid m.

Esophagus

Lamina of cricoid cartilage

Post. cricoarytenoid m.

Retropharyngeal space

Body of C6

Ant. longitudinal lig.

Infraglottic part of larynx

Trachea (int. surface)

Body of hyoid bone

Mylohyoid m.

Vestibule of larynx

L. vestibular (false vocal) fold

L. ventricle

Thyroid cartilage (median sectioned)

L. vocal fold

Conus elasticus (covered with mucosa)

Thyroid gland—pyramidal lobe

Median cricothyroid lig.

Arch of cricoid cartilage (medial sectioned)

Medial View of Left Half of Larynx

Region of oropharynx

Int. laryngeal n.

Hyoepiglottic lig.

Genioglossus m.

Body of hyoid bone

Body of C2

Lingual tonsils

Epiglottis

Post. wall of pharynx

Region of laryngopharynx

Aryepiglottic m.

Corniculate cartilage

Transverse arytenoid m.

Retropharyngeal space

Ant. longitudinal lig.

Post. cricoarytenoid lig.

Inf. pharyngeal constrictor m.

Body of C6

Lamina of cricoid cartilage

Cricotracheal lig.

Trachea

Lateral cricoarytenoid m.

Geniohyoid m.

Symphysis of mandible (median section)

Mylohyoid m.

Thyrohyoid membrane (median thyrohyoid lig.)

Apex

Vocal process

Arytenoid cartilage

L. vestibular (false vocal) fold

L. ventricle

L. vocal lig.

Thyroid cartilage

Thyroarytenoid m.

Cricothyroid lig.

Arch of cricoid cartilage

Medial View of Left Half Larynx with Laryngeal Mucosa Removed

PLATE 7.61   POSTERIOR PHARYNX

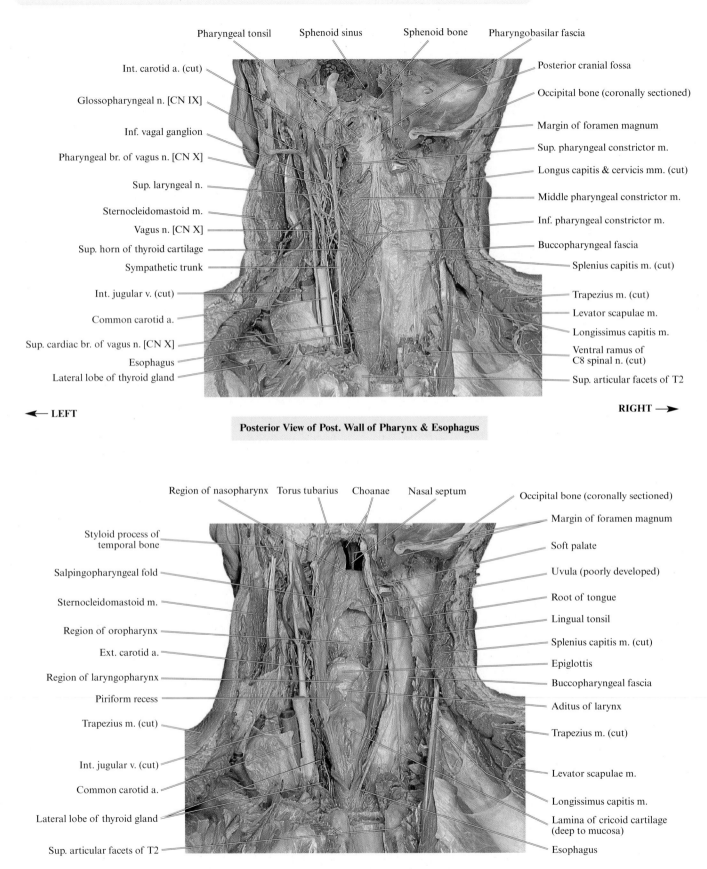

Pharyngeal tonsil   Sphenoid sinus   Sphenoid bone   Pharyngobasilar fascia

Int. carotid a. (cut)

Glossopharyngeal n. [CN IX]

Inf. vagal ganglion

Pharyngeal br. of vagus n. [CN X]

Sup. laryngeal n.

Sternocleidomastoid m.

Vagus n. [CN X]

Sup. horn of thyroid cartilage

Sympathetic trunk

Int. jugular v. (cut)

Common carotid a.

Sup. cardiac br. of vagus n. [CN X]

Esophagus

Lateral lobe of thyroid gland

Posterior cranial fossa

Occipital bone (coronally sectioned)

Margin of foramen magnum

Sup. pharyngeal constrictor m.

Longus capitis & cervicis mm. (cut)

Middle pharyngeal constrictor m.

Inf. pharyngeal constrictor m.

Buccopharyngeal fascia

Splenius capitis m. (cut)

Trapezius m. (cut)

Levator scapulae m.

Longissimus capitis m.

Ventral ramus of
C8 spinal n. (cut)

Sup. articular facets of T2

← LEFT   RIGHT →

Posterior View of Post. Wall of Pharynx & Esophagus

Region of nasopharynx   Torus tubarius   Choanae   Nasal septum

Styloid process of
temporal bone

Salpingopharyngeal fold

Sternocleidomastoid m.

Region of oropharynx

Ext. carotid a.

Region of laryngopharynx

Piriform recess

Trapezius m. (cut)

Int. jugular v. (cut)

Common carotid a.

Lateral lobe of thyroid gland

Sup. articular facets of T2

Occipital bone (coronally sectioned)

Margin of foramen magnum

Soft palate

Uvula (poorly developed)

Root of tongue

Lingual tonsil

Splenius capitis m. (cut)

Epiglottis

Buccopharyngeal fascia

Aditus of larynx

Trapezius m. (cut)

Levator scapulae m.

Longissimus capitis m.

Lamina of cricoid cartilage
(deep to mucosa)

Esophagus

Ant. Wall of Pharynx & Posterior View of Larynx

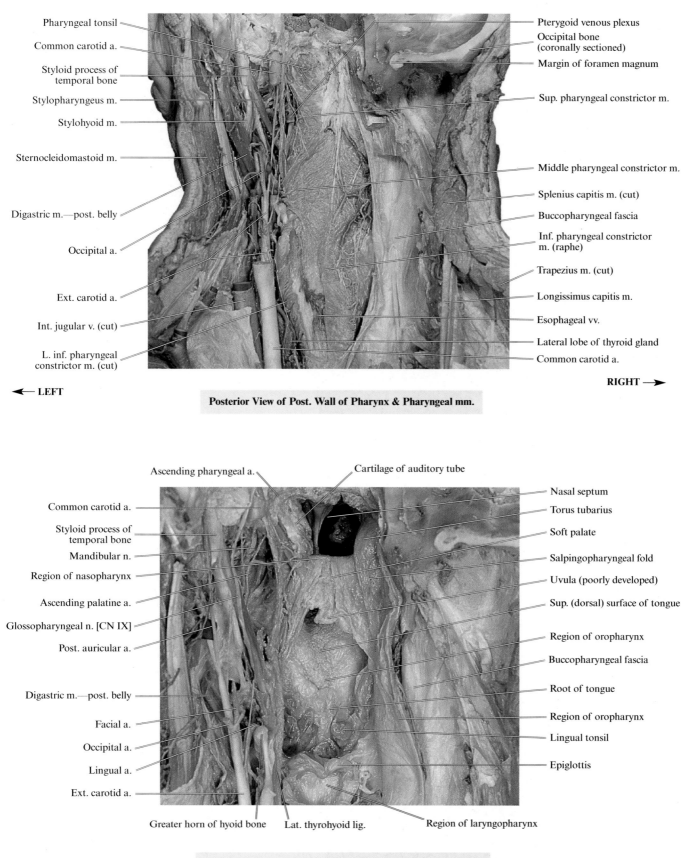

Pharyngeal tonsil

Common carotid a.

Styloid process of
temporal bone

Stylopharyngeus m.

Stylohyoid m.

Sternocleidomastoid m.

Digastric m.—post. belly

Occipital a.

Ext. carotid a.

Int. jugular v. (cut)

L. inf. pharyngeal
constrictor m. (cut)

Pterygoid venous plexus

Occipital bone
(coronally sectioned)

Margin of foramen magnum

Sup. pharyngeal constrictor m.

Middle pharyngeal constrictor m.

Splenius capitis m. (cut)

Buccopharyngeal fascia

Inf. pharyngeal constrictor
m. (raphe)

Trapezius m. (cut)

Longissimus capitis m.

Esophageal vv.

Lateral lobe of thyroid gland

Common carotid a.

← **LEFT**   **RIGHT** →

Posterior View of Post. Wall of Pharynx & Pharyngeal mm.

Ascending pharyngeal a.

Common carotid a.

Styloid process of
temporal bone

Mandibular n.

Region of nasopharynx

Ascending palatine a.

Glossopharyngeal n. [CN IX]

Post. auricular a.

Digastric m.—post. belly

Facial a.

Occipital a.

Lingual a.

Ext. carotid a.

Cartilage of auditory tube

Nasal septum

Torus tubarius

Soft palate

Salpingopharyngeal fold

Uvula (poorly developed)

Sup. (dorsal) surface of tongue

Region of oropharynx

Buccopharyngeal fascia

Root of tongue

Region of oropharynx

Lingual tonsil

Epiglottis

Greater horn of hyoid bone   Lat. thyrohyoid lig.   Region of laryngopharynx

Posterior View of Ant. Wall of Pharynx (Including Soft Palate)

PLATE 7.63   PHARYNX & ORAL CAVITY

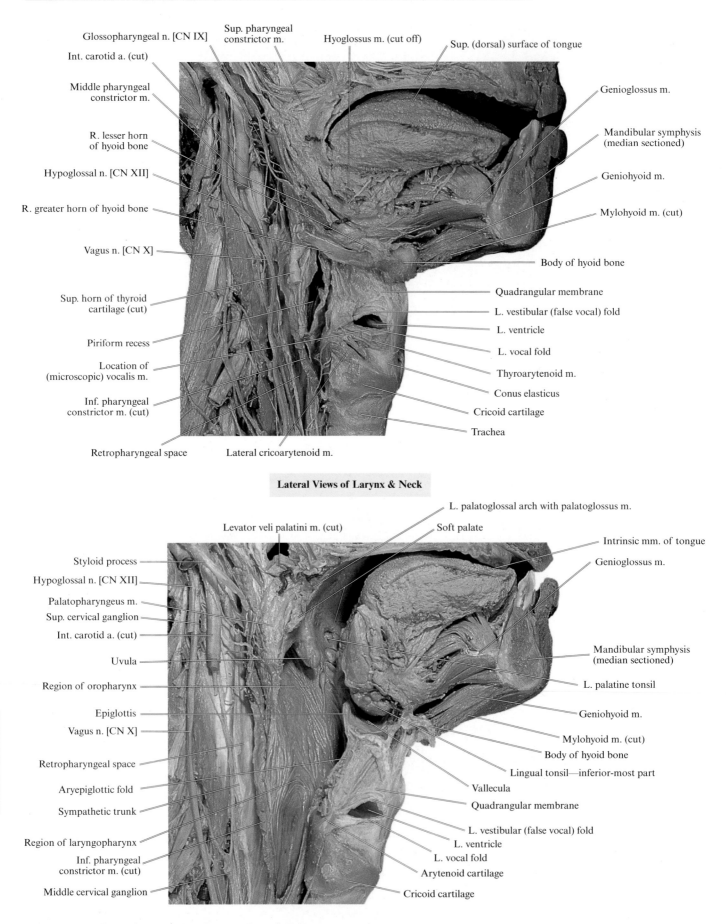

Glossopharyngeal n. [CN IX]
Int. carotid a. (cut)
Middle pharyngeal constrictor m.
R. lesser horn of hyoid bone
Hypoglossal n. [CN XII]
R. greater horn of hyoid bone
Vagus n. [CN X]
Sup. horn of thyroid cartilage (cut)
Piriform recess
Location of (microscopic) vocalis m.
Inf. pharyngeal constrictor m. (cut)
Retropharyngeal space

Sup. pharyngeal constrictor m.
Hyoglossus m. (cut off)
Sup. (dorsal) surface of tongue

Genioglossus m.
Mandibular symphysis (median sectioned)
Geniohyoid m.
Mylohyoid m. (cut)
Body of hyoid bone
Quadrangular membrane
L. vestibular (false vocal) fold
L. ventricle
L. vocal fold
Thyroarytenoid m.
Conus elasticus
Cricoid cartilage
Trachea

Lateral cricoarytenoid m.

Lateral Views of Larynx & Neck

Levator veli palatini m. (cut)
Styloid process
Hypoglossal n. [CN XII]
Palatopharyngeus m.
Sup. cervical ganglion
Int. carotid a. (cut)
Uvula
Region of oropharynx
Epiglottis
Vagus n. [CN X]
Retropharyngeal space
Aryepiglottic fold
Sympathetic trunk
Region of laryngopharynx
Inf. pharyngeal constrictor m. (cut)
Middle cervical ganglion

L. palatoglossal arch with palatoglossus m.
Soft palate
Intrinsic mm. of tongue
Genioglossus m.
Mandibular symphysis (median sectioned)
L. palatine tonsil
Geniohyoid m.
Mylohyoid m. (cut)
Body of hyoid bone
Lingual tonsil—inferior-most part
Vallecula
Quadrangular membrane
L. vestibular (false vocal) fold
L. ventricle
L. vocal fold
Arytenoid cartilage
Cricoid cartilage

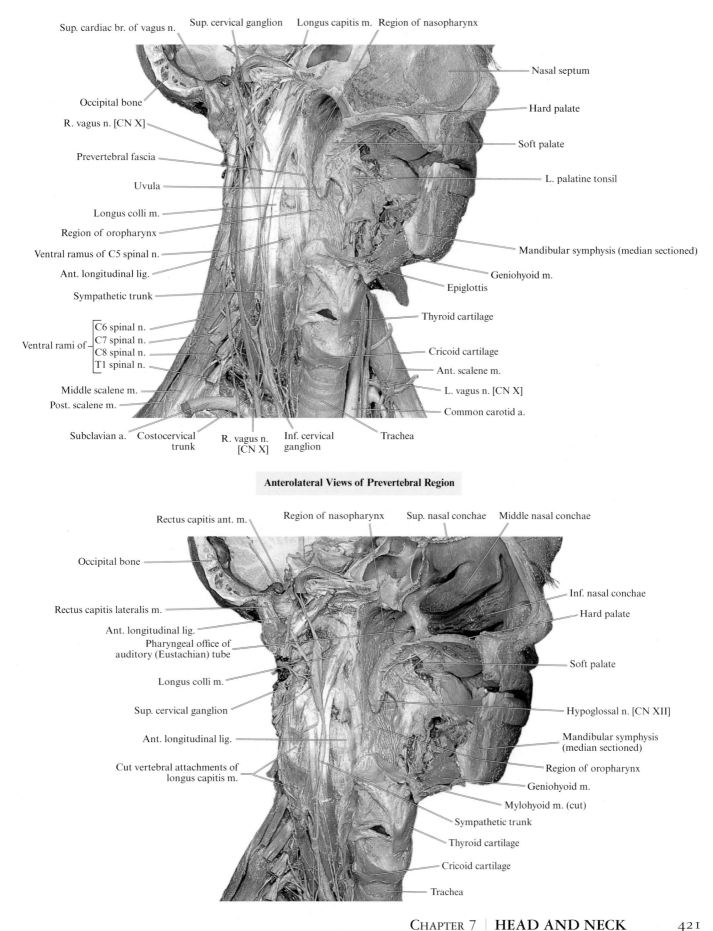

Sup. cardiac br. of vagus n.
Sup. cervical ganglion
Longus capitis m.
Region of nasopharynx

Nasal septum

Occipital bone

Hard palate

R. vagus n. [CN X]

Soft palate

Prevertebral fascia

Uvula

L. palatine tonsil

Longus colli m.

Region of oropharynx

Ventral ramus of C5 spinal n.

Mandibular symphysis (median sectioned)

Ant. longitudinal lig.

Geniohyoid m.

Sympathetic trunk

Epiglottis

Thyroid cartilage

C6 spinal n.
C7 spinal n.
Ventral rami of —
C8 spinal n.
T1 spinal n.

Cricoid cartilage

Ant. scalene m.

Middle scalene m.

L. vagus n. [CN X]

Post. scalene m.

Common carotid a.

Subclavian a.   Costocervical
trunk
R. vagus n.
[CN X]
Inf. cervical
ganglion
Trachea

Anterolateral Views of Prevertebral Region

Rectus capitis ant. m.
Region of nasopharynx
Sup. nasal conchae
Middle nasal conchae

Occipital bone

Rectus capitis lateralis m.

Inf. nasal conchae

Ant. longitudinal lig.

Hard palate

Pharyngeal office of
auditory (Eustachian) tube

Longus colli m.

Soft palate

Sup. cervical ganglion

Ant. longitudinal lig.

Hypoglossal n. [CN XII]

Mandibular symphysis
(median sectioned)

Cut vertebral attachments of
longus capitis m.

Region of oropharynx

Geniohyoid m.

Mylohyoid m. (cut)

Sympathetic trunk

Thyroid cartilage

Cricoid cartilage

Trachea

PLATE 7.65   ORAL CAVITY

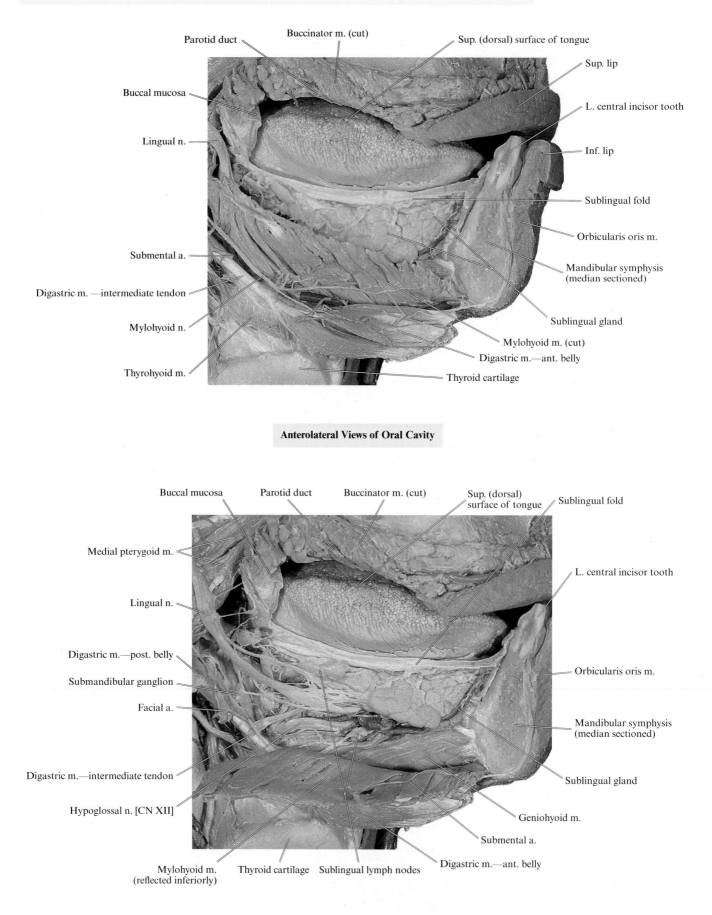

Parotid duct

Buccinator m. (cut)

Sup. (dorsal) surface of tongue

Sup. lip

Buccal mucosa

L. central incisor tooth

Lingual n.

Inf. lip

Submental a.

Sublingual fold

Digastric m. —intermediate tendon

Orbicularis oris m.

Mylohyoid n.

Mandibular symphysis (median sectioned)

Thyrohyoid m.

Sublingual gland

Mylohyoid m. (cut)

Digastric m.—ant. belly

Thyroid cartilage

Anterolateral Views of Oral Cavity

Buccal mucosa

Parotid duct

Buccinator m. (cut)

Sup. (dorsal) surface of tongue

Sublingual fold

Medial pterygoid m.

L. central incisor tooth

Lingual n.

Digastric m.—post. belly

Submandibular ganglion

Orbicularis oris m.

Facial a.

Mandibular symphysis (median sectioned)

Digastric m.—intermediate tendon

Sublingual gland

Hypoglossal n. [CN XII]

Geniohyoid m.

Submental a.

Digastric m.—ant. belly

Mylohyoid m. (reflected inferiorly)

Thyroid cartilage

Sublingual lymph nodes

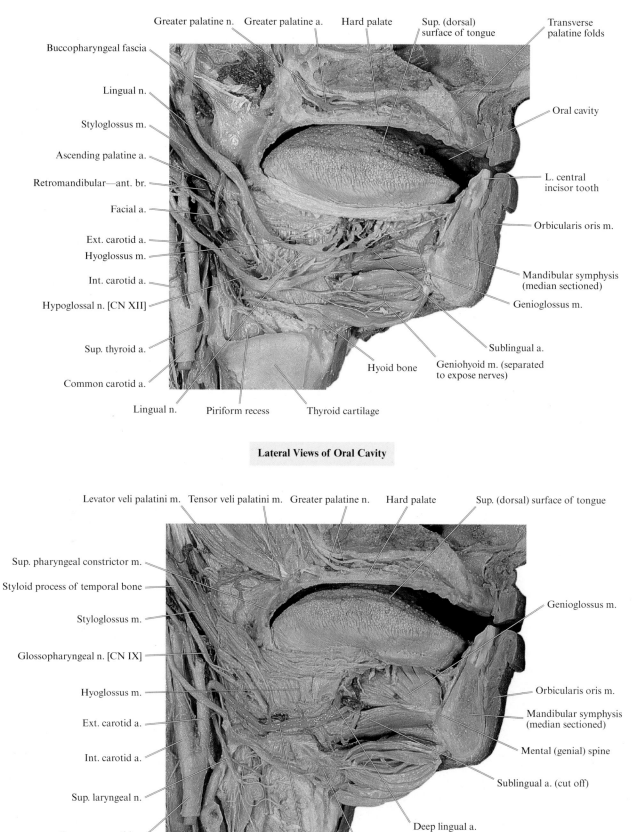

Greater palatine n.   Greater palatine a.   Hard palate   Sup. (dorsal) surface of tongue   Transverse palatine folds

Buccopharyngeal fascia

Lingual n.

Styloglossus m.

Ascending palatine a.

Retromandibular—ant. br.

Facial a.

Ext. carotid a.

Hyoglossus m.

Int. carotid a.

Hypoglossal n. [CN XII]

Sup. thyroid a.

Common carotid a.

Oral cavity

L. central incisor tooth

Orbicularis oris m.

Mandibular symphysis (median sectioned)

Genioglossus m.

Sublingual a.

Geniohyoid m. (separated to expose nerves)

Lingual n.   Piriform recess   Thyroid cartilage

Hyoid bone

Lateral Views of Oral Cavity

Levator veli palatini m.   Tensor veli palatini m.   Greater palatine n.   Hard palate   Sup. (dorsal) surface of tongue

Sup. pharyngeal constrictor m.

Styloid process of temporal bone

Styloglossus m.

Glossopharyngeal n. [CN IX]

Hyoglossus m.

Ext. carotid a.

Int. carotid a.

Sup. laryngeal n.

Common carotid a.

Genioglossus m.

Orbicularis oris m.

Mandibular symphysis (median sectioned)

Mental (genial) spine

Sublingual a. (cut off)

Deep lingual a.

Sup. laryngeal a.   Lingual a.   Hyoid bone

PLATE 7.67   ORAL CAVITY

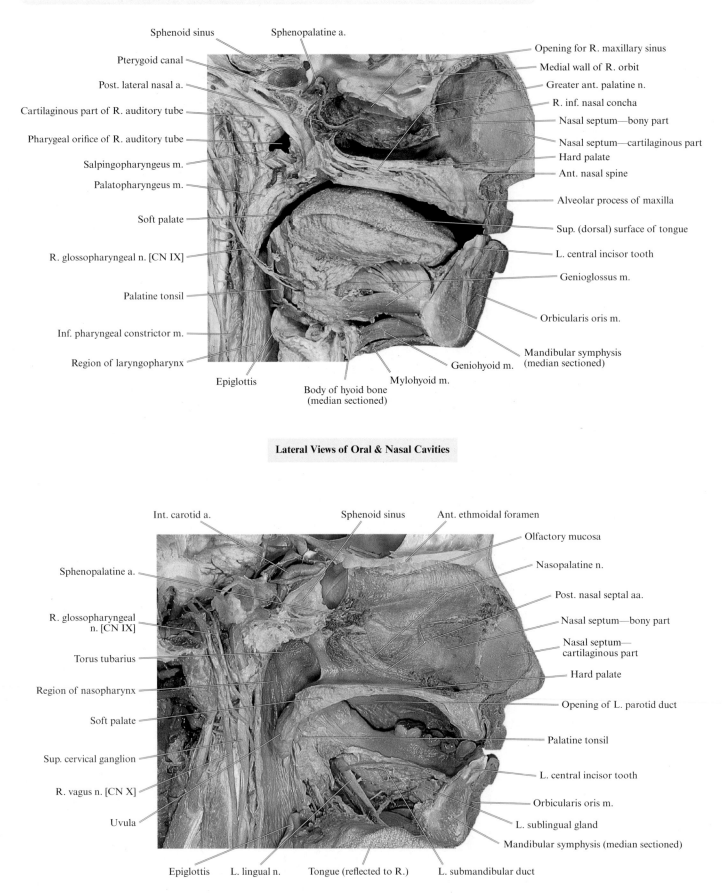

Sphenoid sinus
Sphenopalatine a.
Pterygoid canal
Post. lateral nasal a.
Cartilaginous part of R. auditory tube
Pharygeal orifice of R. auditory tube
Salpingopharyngeus m.
Palatopharyngeus m.
Soft palate
R. glossopharyngeal n. [CN IX]
Palatine tonsil
Inf. pharyngeal constrictor m.
Region of laryngopharynx
Epiglottis
Body of hyoid bone (median sectioned)
Mylohyoid m.
Geniohyoid m.

Opening for R. maxillary sinus
Medial wall of R. orbit
Greater ant. palatine n.
R. inf. nasal concha
Nasal septum—bony part
Nasal septum—cartilaginous part
Hard palate
Ant. nasal spine
Alveolar process of maxilla
Sup. (dorsal) surface of tongue
L. central incisor tooth
Genioglossus m.
Orbicularis oris m.
Mandibular symphysis (median sectioned)

Lateral Views of Oral & Nasal Cavities

Int. carotid a.
Sphenoid sinus
Ant. ethmoidal foramen
Sphenopalatine a.
R. glossopharyngeal n. [CN IX]
Torus tubarius
Region of nasopharynx
Soft palate
Sup. cervical ganglion
R. vagus n. [CN X]
Uvula
Epiglottis
L. lingual n.
Tongue (reflected to R.)
L. submandibular duct

Olfactory mucosa
Nasopalatine n.
Post. nasal septal aa.
Nasal septum—bony part
Nasal septum—cartilaginous part
Hard palate
Opening of L. parotid duct
Palatine tonsil
L. central incisor tooth
Orbicularis oris m.
L. sublingual gland
Mandibular symphysis (median sectioned)

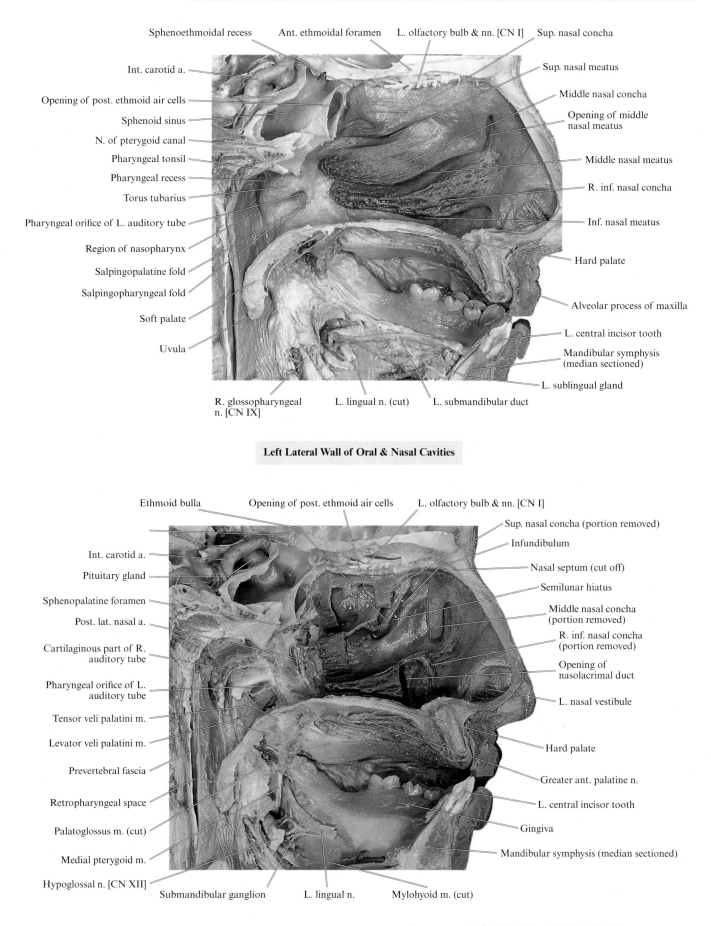

Sphenoethmoidal recess — Ant. ethmoidal foramen — L. olfactory bulb & nn. [CN I] — Sup. nasal concha

Int. carotid a.

Opening of post. ethmoid air cells

Sphenoid sinus

N. of pterygoid canal

Pharyngeal tonsil

Pharyngeal recess

Torus tubarius

Pharyngeal orifice of L. auditory tube

Region of nasopharynx

Salpingopalatine fold

Salpingopharyngeal fold

Soft palate

Uvula

Sup. nasal meatus

Middle nasal concha

Opening of middle nasal meatus

Middle nasal meatus

R. inf. nasal concha

Inf. nasal meatus

Hard palate

Alveolar process of maxilla

L. central incisor tooth

Mandibular symphysis (median sectioned)

L. sublingual gland

R. glossopharyngeal n. [CN IX]   L. lingual n. (cut)   L. submandibular duct

Left Lateral Wall of Oral & Nasal Cavities

Ethmoid bulla — Opening of post. ethmoid air cells — L. olfactory bulb & nn. [CN I]

Int. carotid a.

Pituitary gland

Sphenopalatine foramen

Post. lat. nasal a.

Cartilaginous part of R. auditory tube

Pharyngeal orifice of L. auditory tube

Tensor veli palatini m.

Levator veli palatini m.

Prevertebral fascia

Retropharyngeal space

Palatoglossus m. (cut)

Medial pterygoid m.

Hypoglossal n. [CN XII]

Sup. nasal concha (portion removed)

Infundibulum

Nasal septum (cut off)

Semilunar hiatus

Middle nasal concha (portion removed)

R. inf. nasal concha (portion removed)

Opening of nasolacrimal duct

L. nasal vestibule

Hard palate

Greater ant. palatine n.

L. central incisor tooth

Gingiva

Mandibular symphysis (median sectioned)

Submandibular ganglion   L. lingual n.   Mylohyoid m. (cut)

PLATE 7.69   HEAD & NECK—MEDIAN SECTION

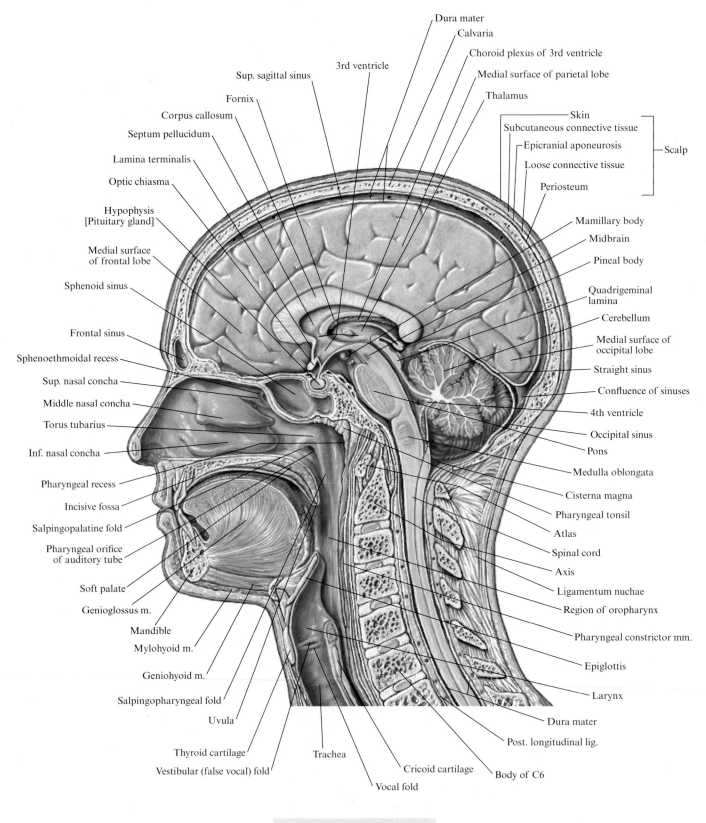

Dura mater
Calvaria
Choroid plexus of 3rd ventricle
Medial surface of parietal lobe
Thalamus
3rd ventricle
Sup. sagittal sinus
Fornix
Corpus callosum
Septum pellucidum
Lamina terminalis
Optic chiasma
Hypophysis [Pituitary gland]
Medial surface of frontal lobe
Sphenoid sinus
Frontal sinus
Sphenoethmoidal recess
Sup. nasal concha
Middle nasal concha
Torus tubarius
Inf. nasal concha
Pharyngeal recess
Incisive fossa
Salpingopalatine fold
Pharyngeal orifice of auditory tube
Soft palate
Genioglossus m.
Mandible
Mylohyoid m.
Geniohyoid m.
Salpingopharyngeal fold
Uvula
Thyroid cartilage
Vestibular (false vocal) fold
Trachea
Vocal fold
Cricoid cartilage
Body of C6

Skin
Subcutaneous connective tissue
Epicranial aponeurosis
Loose connective tissue
Periosteum
Scalp
Mamillary body
Midbrain
Pineal body
Quadrigeminal lamina
Cerebellum
Medial surface of occipital lobe
Straight sinus
Confluence of sinuses
4th ventricle
Occipital sinus
Pons
Medulla oblongata
Cisterna magna
Pharyngeal tonsil
Atlas
Spinal cord
Axis
Ligamentum nuchae
Region of oropharynx
Pharyngeal constrictor mm.
Epiglottis
Larynx
Dura mater
Post. longitudinal lig.

Median Section of Head & Neck

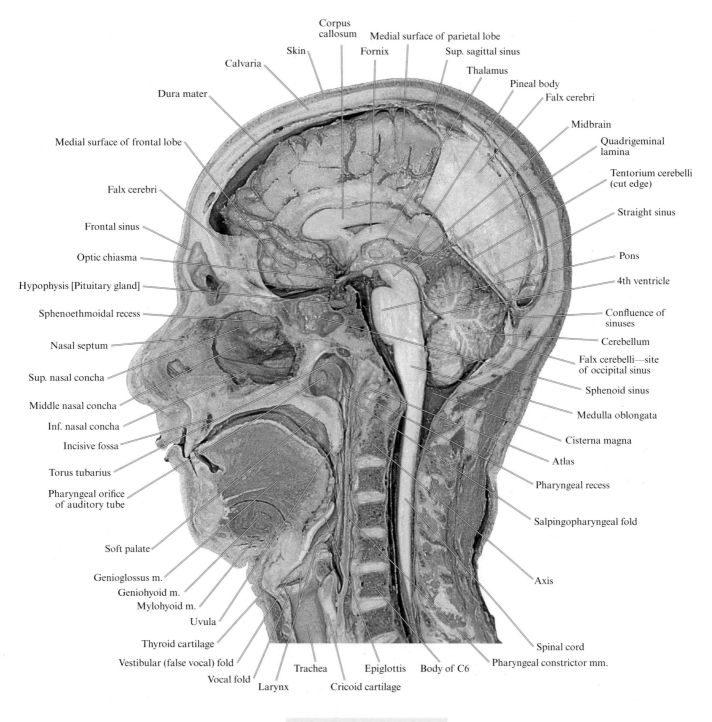

Corpus callosum
Skin
Calvaria
Dura mater
Medial surface of frontal lobe
Falx cerebri
Frontal sinus
Optic chiasma
Hypophysis [Pituitary gland]
Sphenoethmoidal recess
Nasal septum
Sup. nasal concha
Middle nasal concha
Inf. nasal concha
Incisive fossa
Torus tubarius
Pharyngeal orifice of auditory tube
Soft palate
Genioglossus m.
Geniohyoid m.
Mylohyoid m.
Uvula
Thyroid cartilage
Vestibular (false vocal) fold
Vocal fold
Larynx
Trachea
Epiglottis
Cricoid cartilage
Body of C6

Medial surface of parietal lobe
Fornix
Sup. sagittal sinus
Thalamus
Pineal body
Falx cerebri
Midbrain
Quadrigeminal lamina
Tentorium cerebelli (cut edge)
Straight sinus
Pons
4th ventricle
Confluence of sinuses
Cerebellum
Falx cerebelli—site of occipital sinus
Sphenoid sinus
Medulla oblongata
Cisterna magna
Atlas
Pharyngeal recess
Salpingopharyngeal fold
Axis
Spinal cord
Pharyngeal constrictor mm.

Median Section of Head & Neck

PLATE 7.71   ORBIT—SUPERFICIAL

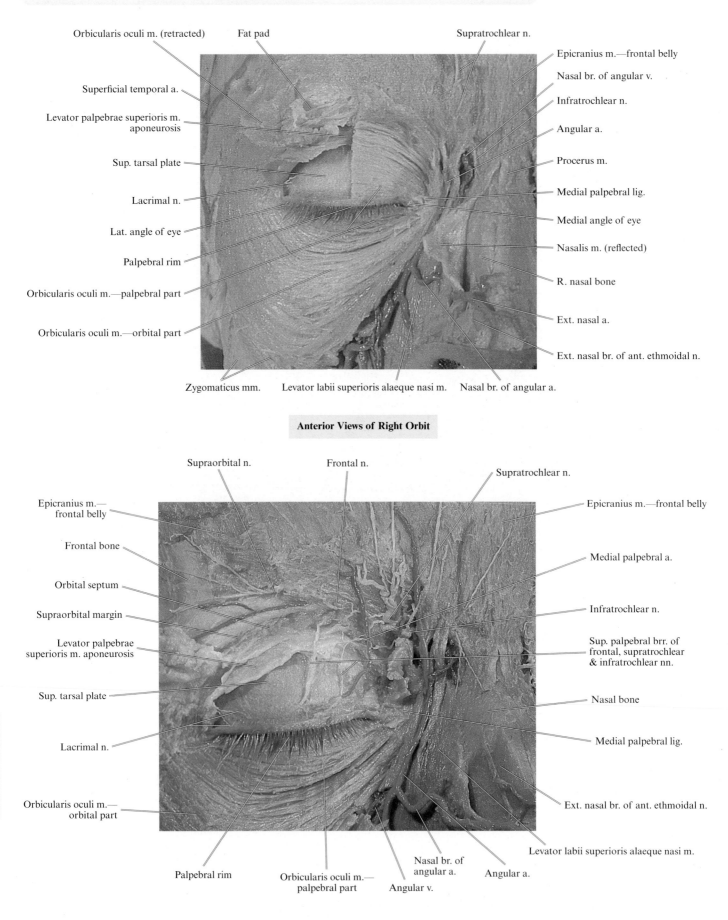

Orbicularis oculi m. (retracted)   Fat pad   Supratrochlear n.

Superficial temporal a.

Levator palpebrae superioris m. aponeurosis

Sup. tarsal plate

Lacrimal n.

Lat. angle of eye

Palpebral rim

Orbicularis oculi m.—palpebral part

Orbicularis oculi m.—orbital part

Epicranius m.—frontal belly

Nasal br. of angular v.

Infratrochlear n.

Angular a.

Procerus m.

Medial palpebral lig.

Medial angle of eye

Nasalis m. (reflected)

R. nasal bone

Ext. nasal a.

Ext. nasal br. of ant. ethmoidal n.

Zygomaticus mm.   Levator labii superioris alaeque nasi m.   Nasal br. of angular a.

Anterior Views of Right Orbit

Supraorbital n.   Frontal n.   Supratrochlear n.

Epicranius m.—frontal belly

Frontal bone

Orbital septum

Supraorbital margin

Levator palpebrae superioris m. aponeurosis

Sup. tarsal plate

Lacrimal n.

Orbicularis oculi m.—orbital part

Epicranius m.—frontal belly

Medial palpebral a.

Infratrochlear n.

Sup. palpebral brr. of frontal, supratrochlear & infratrochlear nn.

Nasal bone

Medial palpebral lig.

Ext. nasal br. of ant. ethmoidal n.

Levator labii superioris alaeque nasi m.

Palpebral rim   Orbicularis oculi m.—palpebral part   Nasal br. of angular a.   Angular v.   Angular a.

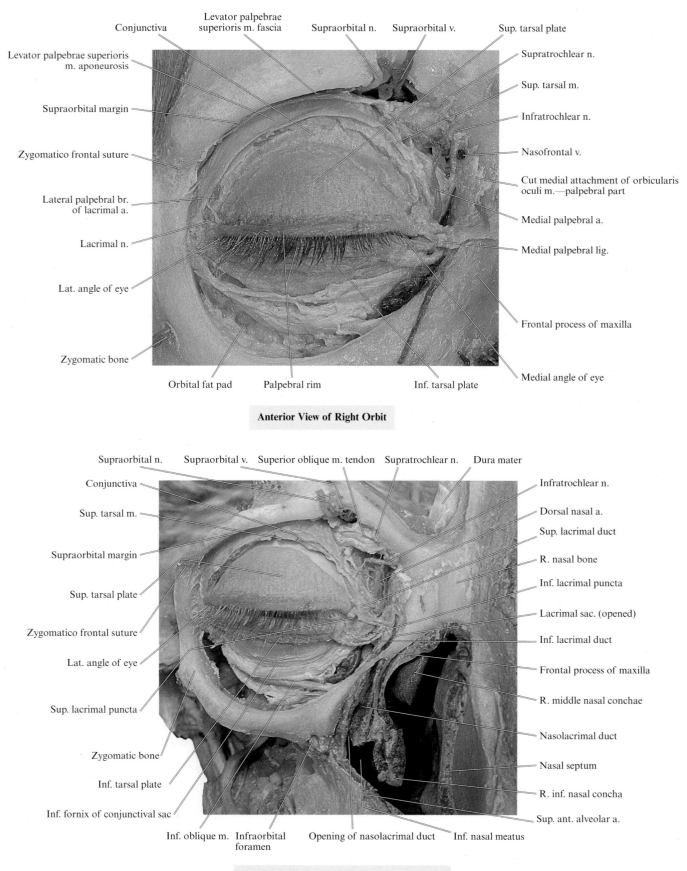

Conjunctiva

Levator palpebrae
superioris m. fascia

Supraorbital n.

Supraorbital v.

Sup. tarsal plate

Levator palpebrae superioris
m. aponeurosis

Supraorbital margin

Zygomatico frontal suture

Lateral palpebral br.
of lacrimal a.

Lacrimal n.

Lat. angle of eye

Zygomatic bone

Orbital fat pad

Palpebral rim

Inf. tarsal plate

Supratrochlear n.

Sup. tarsal m.

Infratrochlear n.

Nasofrontal v.

Cut medial attachment of orbicularis
oculi m.—palpebral part

Medial palpebral a.

Medial palpebral lig.

Frontal process of maxilla

Medial angle of eye

Anterior View of Right Orbit

Supraorbital n.

Supraorbital v.

Superior oblique m. tendon

Supratrochlear n.

Dura mater

Conjunctiva

Sup. tarsal m.

Supraorbital margin

Sup. tarsal plate

Zygomatico frontal suture

Lat. angle of eye

Sup. lacrimal puncta

Zygomatic bone

Inf. tarsal plate

Inf. fornix of conjunctival sac

Inf. oblique m.

Infraorbital
foramen

Opening of nasolacrimal duct

Inf. nasal meatus

Infratrochlear n.

Dorsal nasal a.

Sup. lacrimal duct

R. nasal bone

Inf. lacrimal puncta

Lacrimal sac. (opened)

Inf. lacrimal duct

Frontal process of maxilla

R. middle nasal conchae

Nasolacrimal duct

Nasal septum

R. inf. nasal concha

Sup. ant. alveolar a.

Anterior View of Right Orbit & Nasal Cavity

PLATE 7.73   ORBIT—DEEP

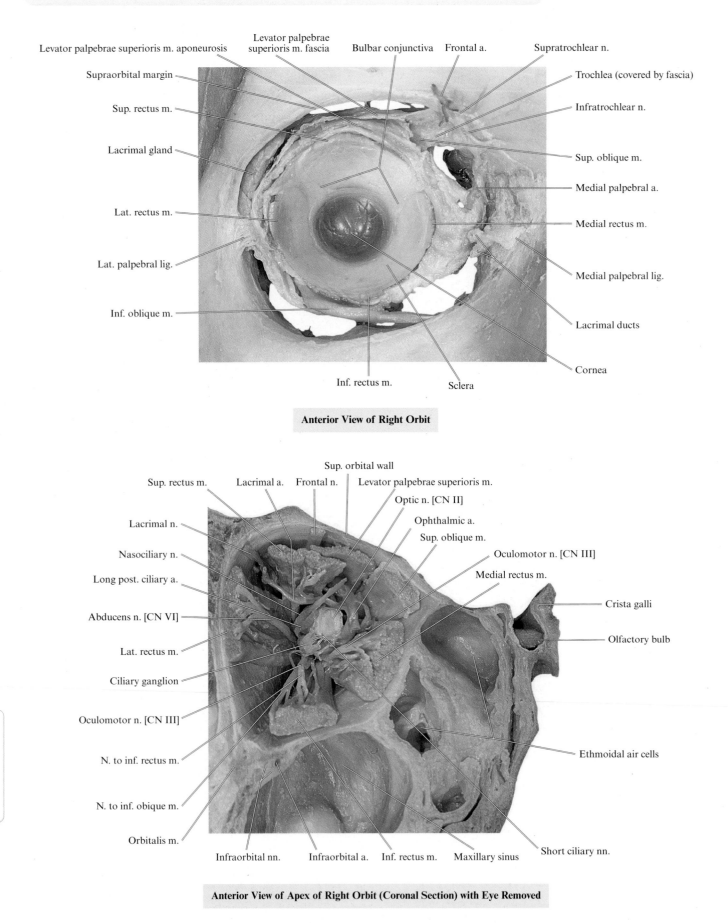

Levator palpebrae superioris m. aponeurosis

Levator palpebrae superioris m. fascia

Bulbar conjunctiva   Frontal a.   Supratrochlear n.

Supraorbital margin

Sup. rectus m.

Lacrimal gland

Lat. rectus m.

Lat. palpebral lig.

Inf. oblique m.

Trochlea (covered by fascia)

Infratrochlear n.

Sup. oblique m.

Medial palpebral a.

Medial rectus m.

Medial palpebral lig.

Lacrimal ducts

Cornea

Inf. rectus m.   Sclera

Anterior View of Right Orbit

Sup. rectus m.   Lacrimal a.   Frontal n.

Sup. orbital wall

Levator palpebrae superioris m.

Optic n. [CN II]

Ophthalmic a.

Sup. oblique m.

Lacrimal n.

Nasociliary n.

Long post. ciliary a.

Abducens n. [CN VI]

Lat. rectus m.

Ciliary ganglion

Oculomotor n. [CN III]

N. to inf. rectus m.

N. to inf. obique m.

Orbitalis m.

Oculomotor n. [CN III]

Medial rectus m.

Crista galli

Olfactory bulb

Ethmoidal air cells

Short ciliary nn.

Infraorbital nn.   Infraorbital a.   Inf. rectus m.   Maxillary sinus

Anterior View of Apex of Right Orbit (Coronal Section) with Eye Removed

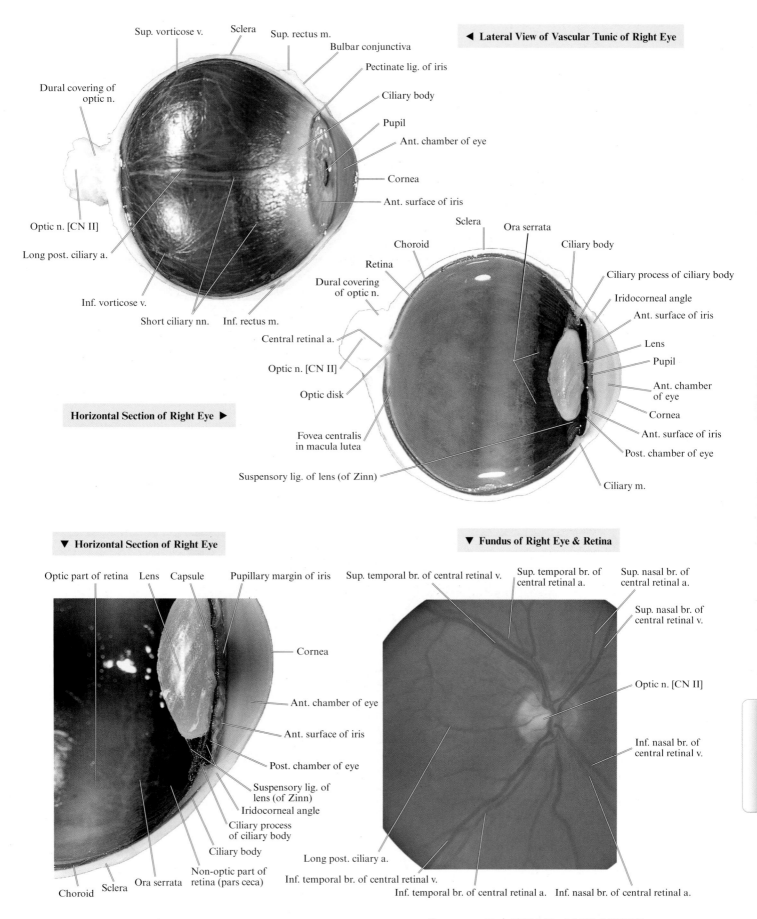

◀ **Lateral View of Vascular Tunic of Right Eye**

Sup. vorticose v.
Sclera
Sup. rectus m.
Bulbar conjunctiva
Pectinate lig. of iris
Ciliary body
Pupil
Ant. chamber of eye
Cornea
Ant. surface of iris

Dural covering of optic n.

Optic n. [CN II]
Long post. ciliary a.

Inf. vorticose v.
Short ciliary nn.   Inf. rectus m.

Horizontal Section of Right Eye ▶

Sclera   Ora serrata
Choroid
Retina
Dural covering of optic n.
Central retinal a.
Optic n. [CN II]
Optic disk
Fovea centralis in macula lutea
Suspensory lig. of lens (of Zinn)

Ciliary body
Ciliary process of ciliary body
Iridocorneal angle
Ant. surface of iris
Lens
Pupil
Ant. chamber of eye
Cornea
Ant. surface of iris
Post. chamber of eye
Ciliary m.

▼ **Horizontal Section of Right Eye**

Optic part of retina   Lens   Capsule   Pupillary margin of iris
Cornea
Ant. chamber of eye
Ant. surface of iris
Post. chamber of eye
Suspensory lig. of lens (of Zinn)
Iridocorneal angle
Ciliary process of ciliary body
Ciliary body
Non-optic part of retina (pars ceca)
Choroid   Sclera   Ora serrata

▼ **Fundus of Right Eye & Retina**

Sup. temporal br. of central retinal v.
Sup. temporal br. of central retinal a.
Sup. nasal br. of central retinal a.
Sup. nasal br. of central retinal v.
Optic n. [CN II]
Inf. nasal br. of central retinal v.
Long post. ciliary a.
Inf. temporal br. of central retinal v.
Inf. temporal br. of central retinal a.   Inf. nasal br. of central retinal a.

PLATE 7.75   ORBIT—LATERAL

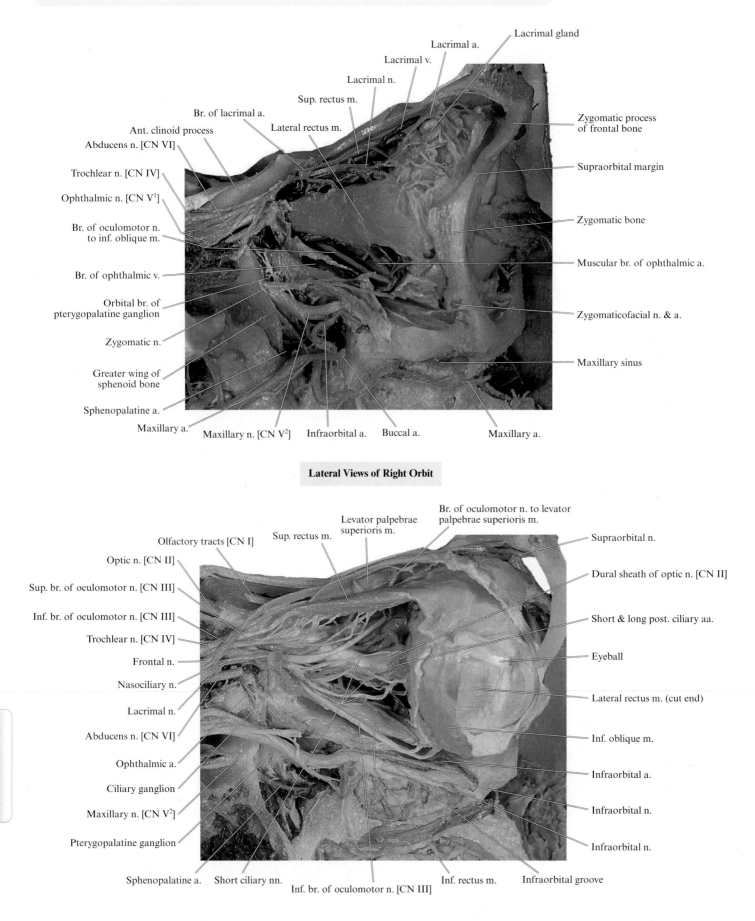

Lacrimal gland

Lacrimal a.

Lacrimal v.

Lacrimal n.

Sup. rectus m.

Br. of lacrimal a.

Lateral rectus m.

Ant. clinoid process

Abducens n. [CN VI]

Trochlear n. [CN IV]

Ophthalmic n. [CN V¹]

Br. of oculomotor n.
to inf. oblique m.

Br. of ophthalmic v.

Orbital br. of
pterygopalatine ganglion

Zygomatic n.

Greater wing of
sphenoid bone

Sphenopalatine a.

Maxillary a.   Maxillary n. [CN V²]   Infraorbital a.   Buccal a.   Maxillary a.

Zygomatic process
of frontal bone

Supraorbital margin

Zygomatic bone

Muscular br. of ophthalmic a.

Zygomaticofacial n. & a.

Maxillary sinus

Lateral Views of Right Orbit

Br. of oculomotor n. to levator
palpebrae superioris m.

Levator palpebrae
superioris m.

Olfactory tracts [CN I]

Sup. rectus m.

Optic n. [CN II]

Sup. br. of oculomotor n. [CN III]

Inf. br. of oculomotor n. [CN III]

Trochlear n. [CN IV]

Frontal n.

Nasociliary n.

Lacrimal n.

Abducens n. [CN VI]

Ophthalmic a.

Ciliary ganglion

Maxillary n. [CN V²]

Pterygopalatine ganglion

Sphenopalatine a.   Short ciliary nn.   Inf. br. of oculomotor n. [CN III]   Inf. rectus m.   Infraorbital groove

Supraorbital n.

Dural sheath of optic n. [CN II]

Short & long post. ciliary aa.

Eyeball

Lateral rectus m. (cut end)

Inf. oblique m.

Infraorbital a.

Infraorbital n.

Infraorbital n.

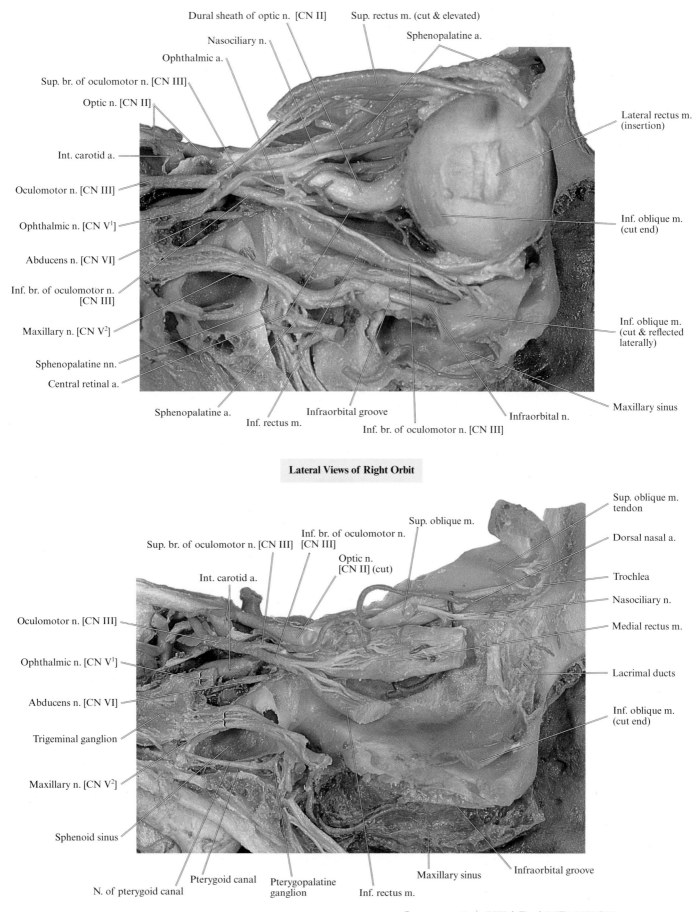

Dural sheath of optic n. [CN II]

Nasociliary n.

Ophthalmic a.

Sup. br. of oculomotor n. [CN III]

Optic n. [CN II]

Int. carotid a.

Oculomotor n. [CN III]

Ophthalmic n. [CN V¹]

Abducens n. [CN VI]

Inf. br. of oculomotor n. [CN III]

Maxillary n. [CN V²]

Sphenopalatine nn.

Central retinal a.

Sphenopalatine a.

Inf. rectus m.

Infraorbital groove

Inf. br. of oculomotor n. [CN III]

Sup. rectus m. (cut & elevated)

Sphenopalatine a.

Lateral rectus m. (insertion)

Inf. oblique m. (cut end)

Inf. oblique m. (cut & reflected laterally)

Maxillary sinus

Infraorbital n.

Lateral Views of Right Orbit

Sup. br. of oculomotor n. [CN III]

Int. carotid a.

Inf. br. of oculomotor n. [CN III]

Optic n. [CN II] (cut)

Sup. oblique m.

Oculomotor n. [CN III]

Ophthalmic n. [CN V¹]

Abducens n. [CN VI]

Trigeminal ganglion

Maxillary n. [CN V²]

Sphenoid sinus

N. of pterygoid canal

Pterygoid canal

Pterygopalatine ganglion

Inf. rectus m.

Maxillary sinus

Infraorbital groove

Sup. oblique m. tendon

Dorsal nasal a.

Trochlea

Nasociliary n.

Medial rectus m.

Lacrimal ducts

Inf. oblique m. (cut end)

PLATE 7.77   ORBIT—SUPERIOR

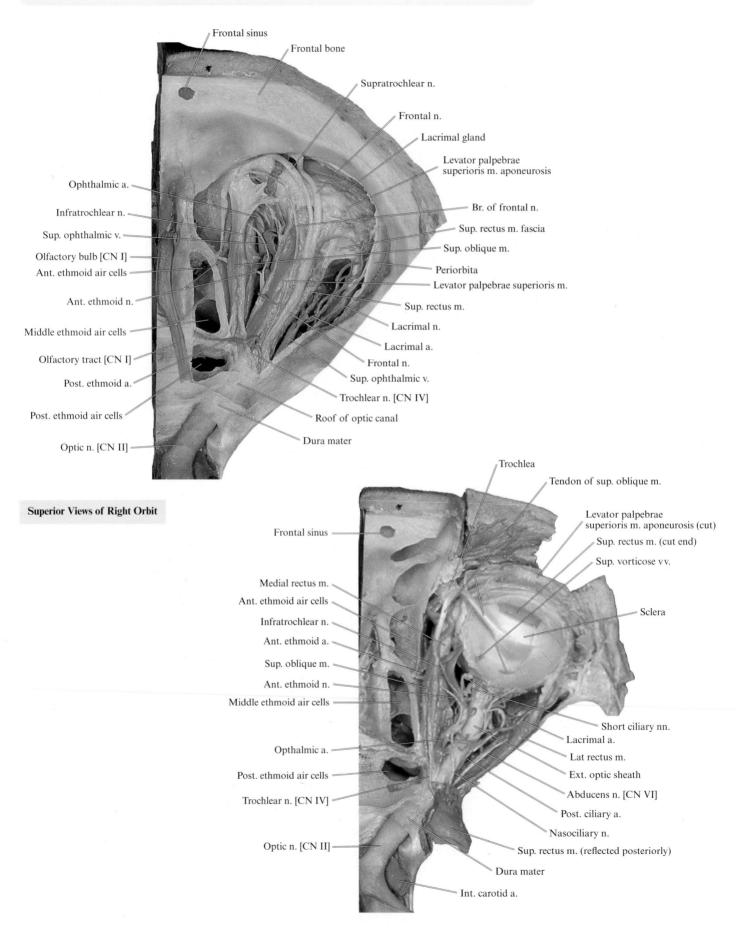

Frontal sinus

Frontal bone

Supratrochlear n.

Frontal n.

Lacrimal gland

Levator palpebrae superioris m. aponeurosis

Ophthalmic a.

Infratrochlear n.

Sup. ophthalmic v.

Olfactory bulb [CN I]

Ant. ethmoid air cells

Ant. ethmoid n.

Middle ethmoid air cells

Olfactory tract [CN I]

Post. ethmoid a.

Post. ethmoid air cells

Optic n. [CN II]

Br. of frontal n.

Sup. rectus m. fascia

Sup. oblique m.

Periorbita

Levator palpebrae superioris m.

Sup. rectus m.

Lacrimal n.

Lacrimal a.

Frontal n.

Sup. ophthalmic v.

Trochlear n. [CN IV]

Roof of optic canal

Dura mater

Superior Views of Right Orbit

Trochlea

Tendon of sup. oblique m.

Levator palpebrae superioris m. aponeurosis (cut)

Sup. rectus m. (cut end)

Sup. vorticose vv.

Frontal sinus

Medial rectus m.

Ant. ethmoid air cells

Infratrochlear n.

Ant. ethmoid a.

Sup. oblique m.

Ant. ethmoid n.

Middle ethmoid air cells

Opthalmic a.

Post. ethmoid air cells

Trochlear n. [CN IV]

Optic n. [CN II]

Sclera

Short ciliary nn.

Lacrimal a.

Lat rectus m.

Ext. optic sheath

Abducens n. [CN VI]

Post. ciliary a.

Nasociliary n.

Sup. rectus m. (reflected posteriorly)

Dura mater

Int. carotid a.

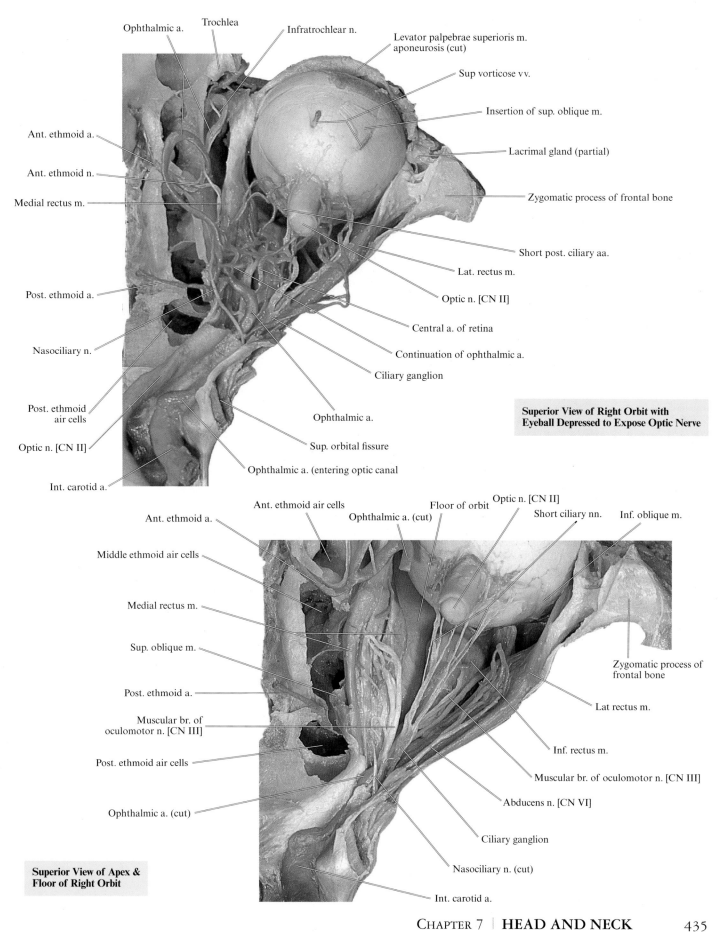

Ophthalmic a.
Trochlea
Infratrochlear n.
Levator palpebrae superioris m.
aponeurosis (cut)
Sup vorticose vv.
Insertion of sup. oblique m.
Lacrimal gland (partial)
Zygomatic process of frontal bone
Short post. ciliary aa.
Lat. rectus m.
Optic n. [CN II]
Central a. of retina
Continuation of ophthalmic a.
Ciliary ganglion
Ophthalmic a.
Sup. orbital fissure
Ophthalmic a. (entering optic canal

Ant. ethmoid a.
Ant. ethmoid n.
Medial rectus m.
Post. ethmoid a.
Nasociliary n.
Post. ethmoid
air cells
Optic n. [CN II]
Int. carotid a.

**Superior View of Right Orbit with
Eyeball Depressed to Expose Optic Nerve**

Ant. ethmoid a.
Middle ethmoid air cells
Medial rectus m.
Sup. oblique m.
Post. ethmoid a.
Muscular br. of
oculomotor n. [CN III]
Post. ethmoid air cells
Ophthalmic a. (cut)

Ant. ethmoid air cells
Ophthalmic a. (cut)
Floor of orbit
Optic n. [CN II]
Short ciliary nn.
Inf. oblique m.
Zygomatic process of
frontal bone
Lat rectus m.
Inf. rectus m.
Muscular br. of oculomotor n. [CN III]
Abducens n. [CN VI]
Ciliary ganglion
Nasociliary n. (cut)
Int. carotid a.

**Superior View of Apex &
Floor of Right Orbit**

PLATE 7.79   INFRATEMPORAL FOSSA

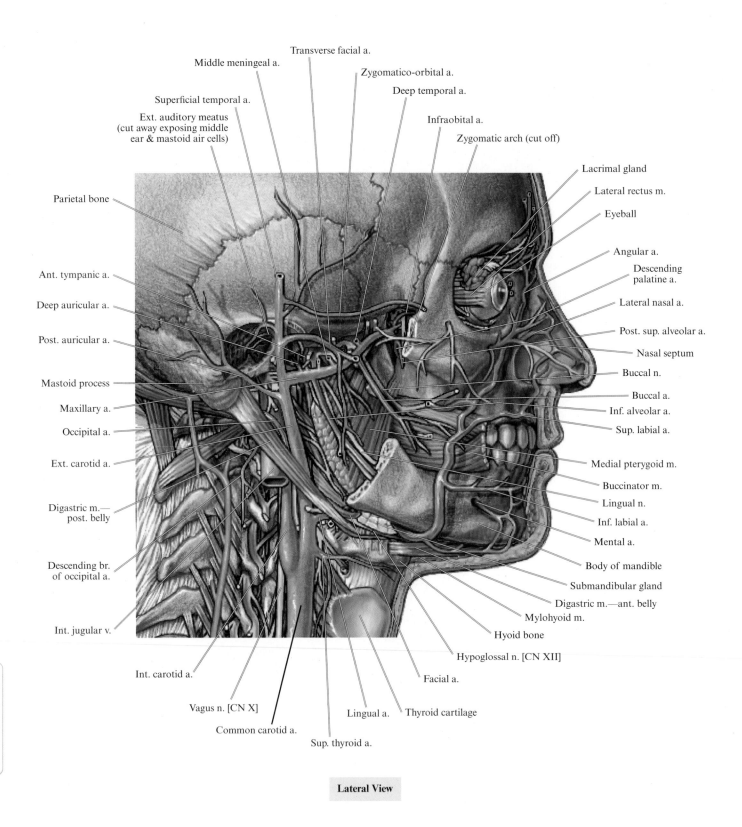

Transverse facial a.

Middle meningeal a.

Zygomatico-orbital a.

Superficial temporal a.

Deep temporal a.

Ext. auditory meatus
(cut away exposing middle
ear & mastoid air cells)

Infraobital a.

Zygomatic arch (cut off)

Lacrimal gland

Parietal bone

Lateral rectus m.

Eyeball

Angular a.

Ant. tympanic a.

Descending
palatine a.

Deep auricular a.

Lateral nasal a.

Post. auricular a.

Post. sup. alveolar a.

Nasal septum

Buccal n.

Mastoid process

Buccal a.

Maxillary a.

Inf. alveolar a.

Occipital a.

Sup. labial a.

Ext. carotid a.

Medial pterygoid m.

Buccinator m.

Digastric m.—
post. belly

Lingual n.

Inf. labial a.

Mental a.

Descending br.
of occipital a.

Body of mandible

Submandibular gland

Digastric m.—ant. belly

Mylohyoid m.

Int. jugular v.

Hyoid bone

Int. carotid a.

Hypoglossal n. [CN XII]

Facial a.

Vagus n. [CN X]

Common carotid a.

Lingual a.

Thyroid cartilage

Sup. thyroid a.

Lateral View

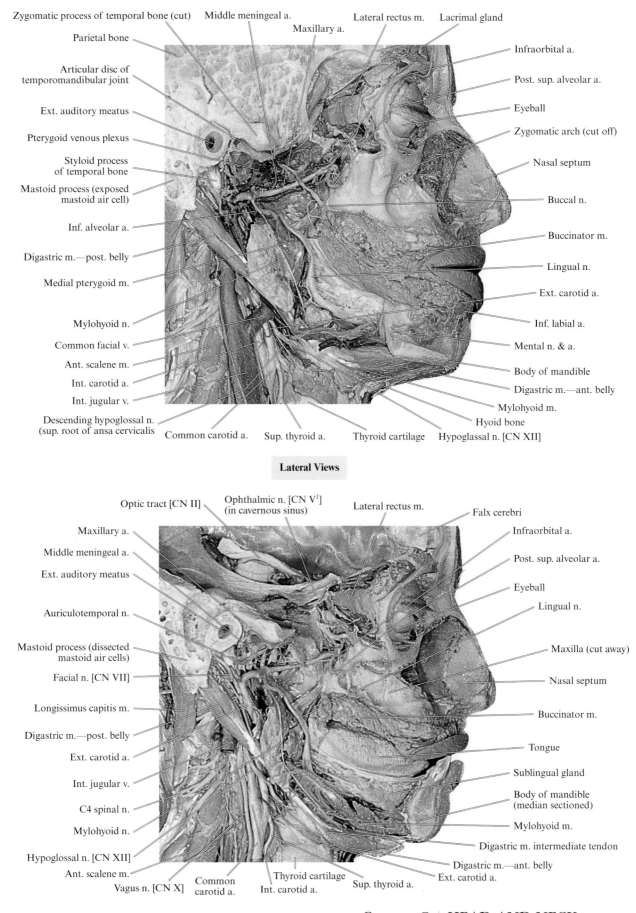

Zygomatic process of temporal bone (cut)
Parietal bone
Articular disc of temporomandibular joint
Ext. auditory meatus
Pterygoid venous plexus
Styloid process of temporal bone
Mastoid process (exposed mastoid air cell)
Inf. alveolar a.
Digastric m.—post. belly
Medial pterygoid m.
Mylohyoid n.
Common facial v.
Ant. scalene m.
Int. carotid a.
Int. jugular v.
Descending hypoglossal n. (sup. root of ansa cervicalis)
Common carotid a.
Sup. thyroid a.
Thyroid cartilage

Middle meningeal a.
Maxillary a.
Lateral rectus m.
Lacrimal gland
Infraorbital a.
Post. sup. alveolar a.
Eyeball
Zygomatic arch (cut off)
Nasal septum
Buccal n.
Buccinator m.
Lingual n.
Ext. carotid a.
Inf. labial a.
Mental n. & a.
Body of mandible
Digastric m.—ant. belly
Mylohyoid m.
Hyoid bone
Hypoglossal n. [CN XII]

Lateral Views

Optic tract [CN II]
Ophthalmic n. [CN V¹] (in cavernous sinus)
Lateral rectus m.
Falx cerebri
Maxillary a.
Infraorbital a.
Middle meningeal a.
Post. sup. alveolar a.
Ext. auditory meatus
Eyeball
Auriculotemporal n.
Lingual n.
Mastoid process (dissected mastoid air cells)
Maxilla (cut away)
Facial n. [CN VII]
Nasal septum
Longissimus capitis m.
Buccinator m.
Digastric m.—post. belly
Tongue
Ext. carotid a.
Sublingual gland
Int. jugular v.
Body of mandible (median sectioned)
C4 spinal n.
Mylohyoid n.
Mylohyoid m.
Hypoglossal n. [CN XII]
Digastric m. intermediate tendon
Ant. scalene m.
Digastric m.—ant. belly
Vagus n. [CN X]
Common carotid a.
Thyroid cartilage
Int. carotid a.
Sup. thyroid a.
Ext. carotid a.

PLATE 7.81   INFRATEMPORAL FOSSA

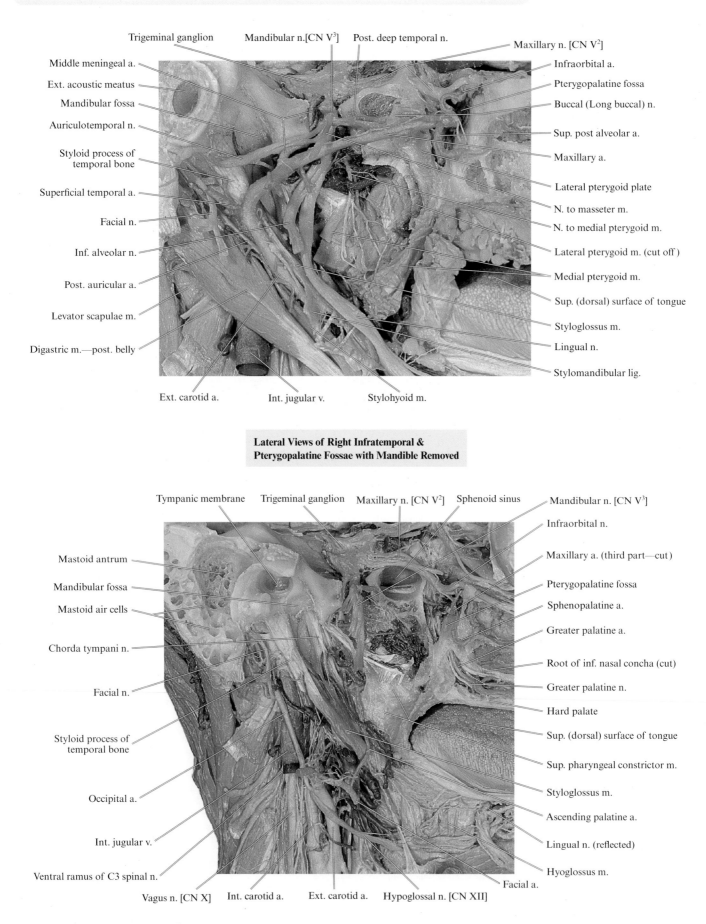

Trigeminal ganglion   Mandibular n.[CN V³]   Post. deep temporal n.   Maxillary n. [CN V²]

Middle meningeal a.   Infraorbital a.

Ext. acoustic meatus   Pterygopalatine fossa

Mandibular fossa   Buccal (Long buccal) n.

Auriculotemporal n.   Sup. post alveolar a.

Styloid process of
temporal bone   Maxillary a.

Superficial temporal a.   Lateral pterygoid plate

Facial n.   N. to masseter m.

Inf. alveolar n.   N. to medial pterygoid m.

Post. auricular a.   Lateral pterygoid m. (cut off)

Levator scapulae m.   Medial pterygoid m.

Digastric m.—post. belly   Sup. (dorsal) surface of tongue

Styloglossus m.

Lingual n.

Stylomandibular lig.

Ext. carotid a.   Int. jugular v.   Stylohyoid m.

**Lateral Views of Right Infratemporal &
Pterygopalatine Fossae with Mandible Removed**

Tympanic membrane   Trigeminal ganglion   Maxillary n. [CN V²]   Sphenoid sinus   Mandibular n. [CN V³]

Infraorbital n.

Mastoid antrum   Maxillary a. (third part—cut)

Mandibular fossa   Pterygopalatine fossa

Mastoid air cells   Sphenopalatine a.

Greater palatine a.

Chorda tympani n.   Root of inf. nasal concha (cut)

Greater palatine n.

Facial n.   Hard palate

Sup. (dorsal) surface of tongue

Styloid process of
temporal bone   Sup. pharyngeal constrictor m.

Styloglossus m.

Occipital a.   Ascending palatine a.

Lingual n. (reflected)

Int. jugular v.   Hyoglossus m.

Ventral ramus of C3 spinal n.   Facial a.

Vagus n. [CN X]   Int. carotid a.   Ext. carotid a.   Hypoglossal n. [CN XII]

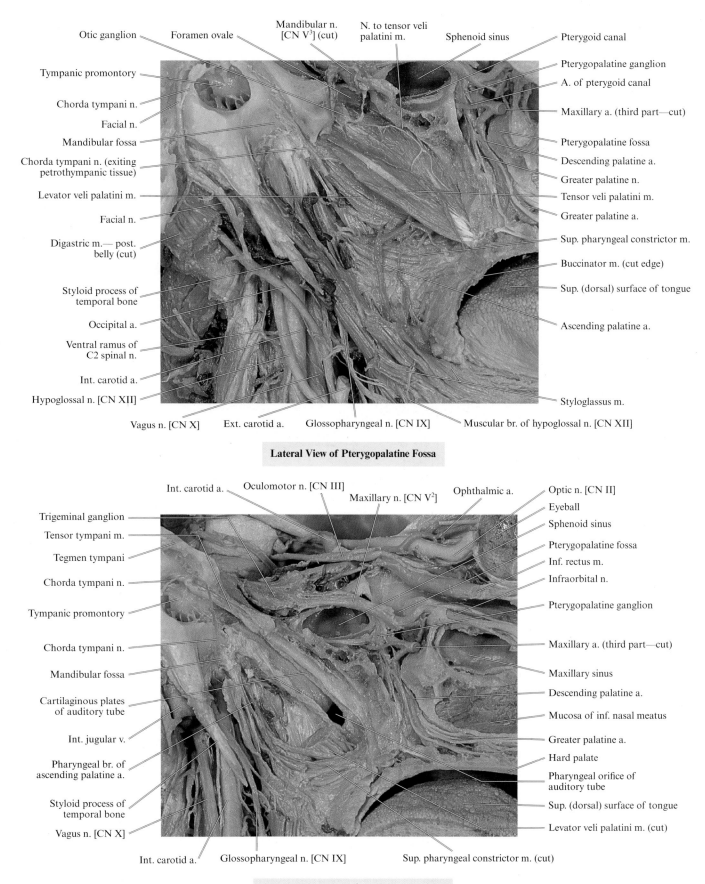

Otic ganglion
Tympanic promontory
Chorda tympani n.
Facial n.
Mandibular fossa
Chorda tympani n. (exiting petrothympanic tissue)
Levator veli palatini m.
Facial n.
Digastric m.— post. belly (cut)
Styloid process of temporal bone
Occipital a.
Ventral ramus of C2 spinal n.
Int. carotid a.
Hypoglossal n. [CN XII]

Mandibular n. [CN V³] (cut)
N. to tensor veli palatini m.
Sphenoid sinus
Pterygoid canal

Pterygopalatine ganglion
A. of pterygoid canal
Maxillary a. (third part—cut)
Pterygopalatine fossa
Descending palatine a.
Greater palatine n.
Tensor veli palatini m.
Greater palatine a.
Sup. pharyngeal constrictor m.
Buccinator m. (cut edge)
Sup. (dorsal) surface of tongue
Ascending palatine a.
Styloglassus m.

Vagus n. [CN X]   Ext. carotid a.   Glossopharyngeal n. [CN IX]   Muscular br. of hypoglossal n. [CN XII]

Lateral View of Pterygopalatine Fossa

Int. carotid a.
Oculomotor n. [CN III]
Maxillary n. [CN V²]
Ophthalmic a.
Optic n. [CN II]

Trigeminal ganglion
Tensor tympani m.
Tegmen tympani
Chorda tympani n.
Tympanic promontory
Chorda tympani n.
Mandibular fossa
Cartilaginous plates of auditory tube
Int. jugular v.
Pharyngeal br. of ascending palatine a.
Styloid process of temporal bone
Vagus n. [CN X]

Eyeball
Sphenoid sinus
Pterygopalatine fossa
Inf. rectus m.
Infraorbital n.
Pterygopalatine ganglion
Maxillary a. (third part—cut)
Maxillary sinus
Descending palatine a.
Mucosa of inf. nasal meatus
Greater palatine a.
Hard palate
Pharyngeal orifice of auditory tube
Sup. (dorsal) surface of tongue
Levator veli palatini m. (cut)

Int. carotid a.   Glossopharyngeal n. [CN IX]   Sup. pharyngeal constrictor m. (cut)

Lateral View of Pharynx & Auditory Tube

PLATE 7.83   PTERYGOPALATINE FOSSA

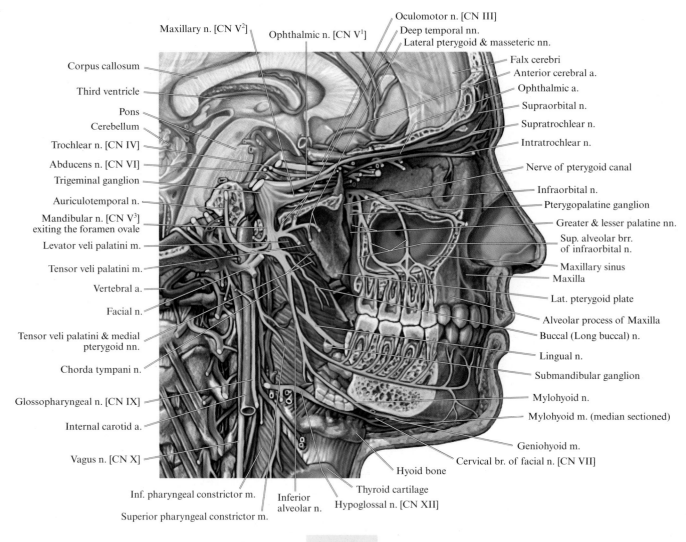

Maxillary n. [CN V²]

Ophthalmic n. [CN V¹]

Oculomotor n. [CN III]

Deep temporal nn.

Lateral pterygoid & masseteric nn.

Corpus callosum

Third ventricle

Pons

Cerebellum

Trochlear n. [CN IV]

Abducens n. [CN VI]

Trigeminal ganglion

Auriculotemporal n.

Mandibular n. [CN V³]
exiting the foramen ovale

Levator veli palatini m.

Tensor veli palatini m.

Vertebral a.

Facial n.

Tensor veli palatini & medial
pterygoid nn.

Chorda tympani n.

Glossopharyngeal n. [CN IX]

Internal carotid a.

Vagus n. [CN X]

Falx cerebri

Anterior cerebral a.

Ophthalmic a.

Supraorbital n.

Supratrochlear n.

Intratrochlear n.

Nerve of pterygoid canal

Infraorbital n.

Pterygopalatine ganglion

Greater & lesser palatine nn.

Sup. alveolar brr.
of infraorbital n.

Maxillary sinus

Maxilla

Lat. pterygoid plate

Alveolar process of Maxilla

Buccal (Long buccal) n.

Lingual n.

Submandibular ganglion

Mylohyoid n.

Mylohyoid m. (median sectioned)

Geniohyoid m.

Cervical br. of facial n. [CN VII]

Inf. pharyngeal constrictor m.

Superior pharyngeal constrictor m.

Inferior
alveolar n.

Hypoglossal n. [CN XII]

Thyroid cartilage

Hyoid bone

Lateral View

Zygomatic process of temporal bone

Squamous part of temporal bone

Sphenosquamosal suture

Infratemporal surface of greater
wing of sphenoid bone

Petrotympanic fissure

Foramen ovale

Foramen spinosum

Spine of sphenoid bone

Temporal bone—petrous part

Foramen venosum (of Vesalius)

Occipital bone—basilar part

Temporal process of zygomatic bone

Frontal process of
zygomatic bone

Roof of orbit

Supraorbital margin

Inf. orbital fissure

Infratemporal surface of maxilla

Infraorbital foramen

Pterygomaxillary fissure

Pterygopalatine fossa

Sphenopalatine fissure

Alveolar process of maxilla

Pyramidal process
of palatine bone

Hard palate

Lat. pterygoid plate

Vomer

Hamulus of med.
pterygoid plate

Right Inferolateral View of Infratemporal & Pterygopalatine Fossae

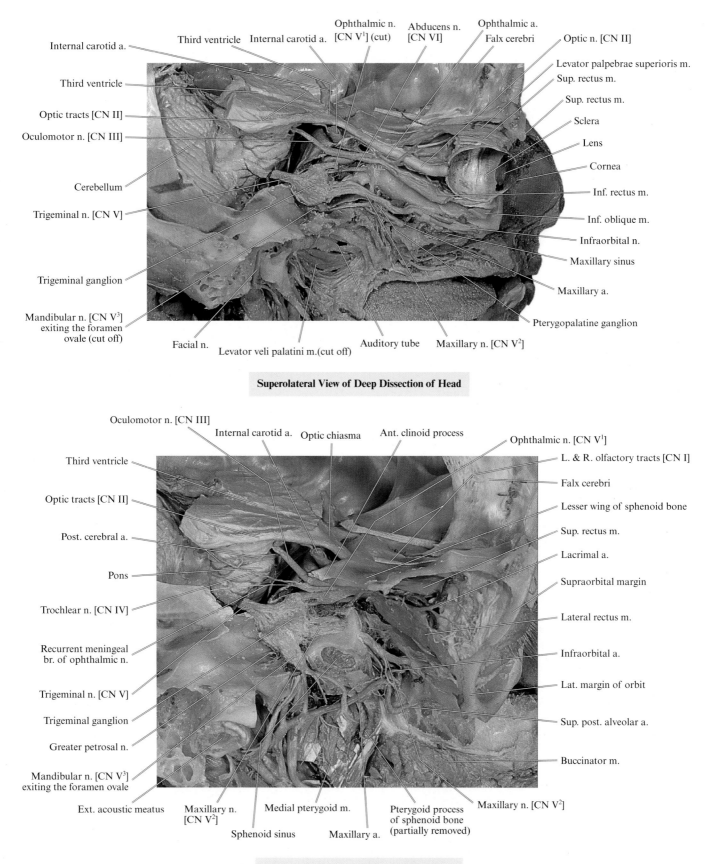

Internal carotid a.
Third ventricle
Optic tracts [CN II]
Oculomotor n. [CN III]
Cerebellum
Trigeminal n. [CN V]
Trigeminal ganglion
Mandibular n. [CN V³] exiting the foramen ovale (cut off)

Third ventricle   Internal carotid a.   Ophthalmic n. [CN V¹] (cut)   Abducens n. [CN VI]   Ophthalmic a.   Falx cerebri   Optic n. [CN II]

Levator palpebrae superioris m.
Sup. rectus m.
Sup. rectus m.
Sclera
Lens
Cornea
Inf. rectus m.
Inf. oblique m.
Infraorbital n.
Maxillary sinus
Maxillary a.
Pterygopalatine ganglion

Facial n.   Levator veli palatini m.(cut off)   Auditory tube   Maxillary n. [CN V²]

Superolateral View of Deep Dissection of Head

Oculomotor n. [CN III]   Internal carotid a.   Optic chiasma   Ant. clinoid process   Ophthalmic n. [CN V¹]

Third ventricle
Optic tracts [CN II]
Post. cerebral a.
Pons
Trochlear n. [CN IV]
Recurrent meningeal br. of ophthalmic n.
Trigeminal n. [CN V]
Trigeminal ganglion
Greater petrosal n.
Mandibular n. [CN V³] exiting the foramen ovale

L. & R. olfactory tracts [CN I]
Falx cerebri
Lesser wing of sphenoid bone
Sup. rectus m.
Lacrimal a.
Supraorbital margin
Lateral rectus m.
Infraorbital a.
Lat. margin of orbit
Sup. post. alveolar a.
Buccinator m.
Maxillary n. [CN V²]

Ext. acoustic meatus   Maxillary n. [CN V²]   Medial pterygoid m.   Pterygoid process of sphenoid bone (partially removed)
Sphenoid sinus   Maxillary a.

Superolateral View of Pterygopalatine Fossa

PLATE 7.85   EAR

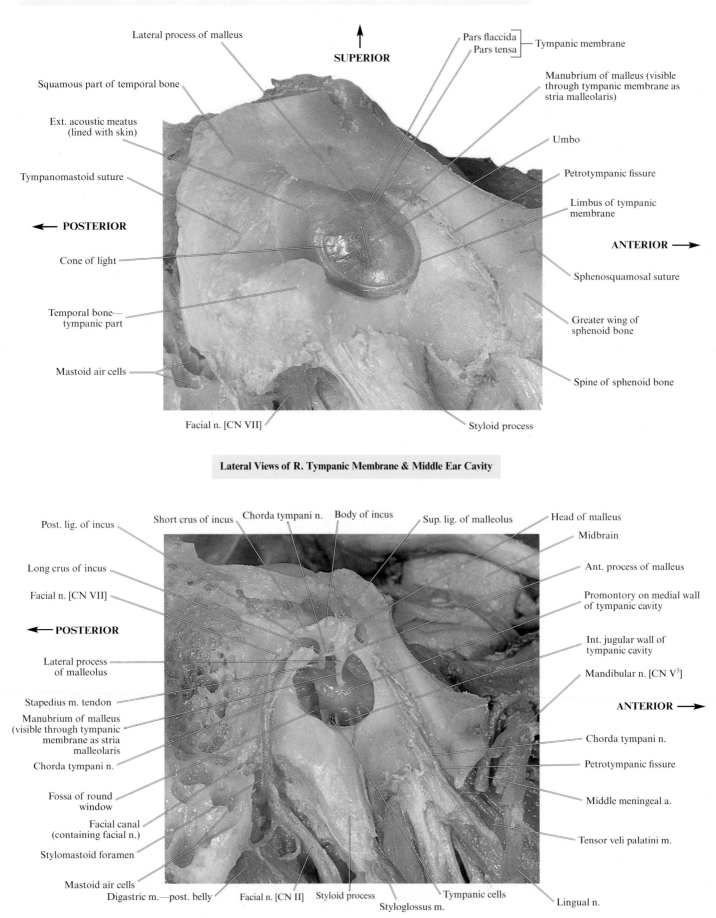

Lateral process of malleus

SUPERIOR

Pars flaccida
Pars tensa ⎤ Tympanic membrane

Squamous part of temporal bone

Manubrium of malleus (visible through tympanic membrane as stria malleolaris)

Ext. acoustic meatus (lined with skin)

Umbo

Tympanomastoid suture

Petrotympanic fissure

Limbus of tympanic membrane

POSTERIOR

ANTERIOR

Cone of light

Sphenosquamosal suture

Temporal bone— tympanic part

Greater wing of sphenoid bone

Mastoid air cells

Spine of sphenoid bone

Facial n. [CN VII]

Styloid process

Lateral Views of R. Tympanic Membrane & Middle Ear Cavity

Post. lig. of incus

Short crus of incus

Chorda tympani n.

Body of incus

Sup. lig. of malleolus

Head of malleus

Midbrain

Long crus of incus

Ant. process of malleus

Facial n. [CN VII]

Promontory on medial wall of tympanic cavity

POSTERIOR

Int. jugular wall of tympanic cavity

Lateral process of malleolus

Mandibular n. [CN V³]

Stapedius m. tendon

ANTERIOR

Manubrium of malleus (visible through tympanic membrane as stria malleolaris

Chorda tympani n.

Chorda tympani n.

Petrotympanic fissure

Fossa of round window

Middle meningeal a.

Facial canal (containing facial n.)

Stylomastoid foramen

Tensor veli palatini m.

Mastoid air cells

Digastric m.—post. belly

Facial n. [CN II]

Styloid process

Styloglossus m.

Tympanic cells

Lingual n.

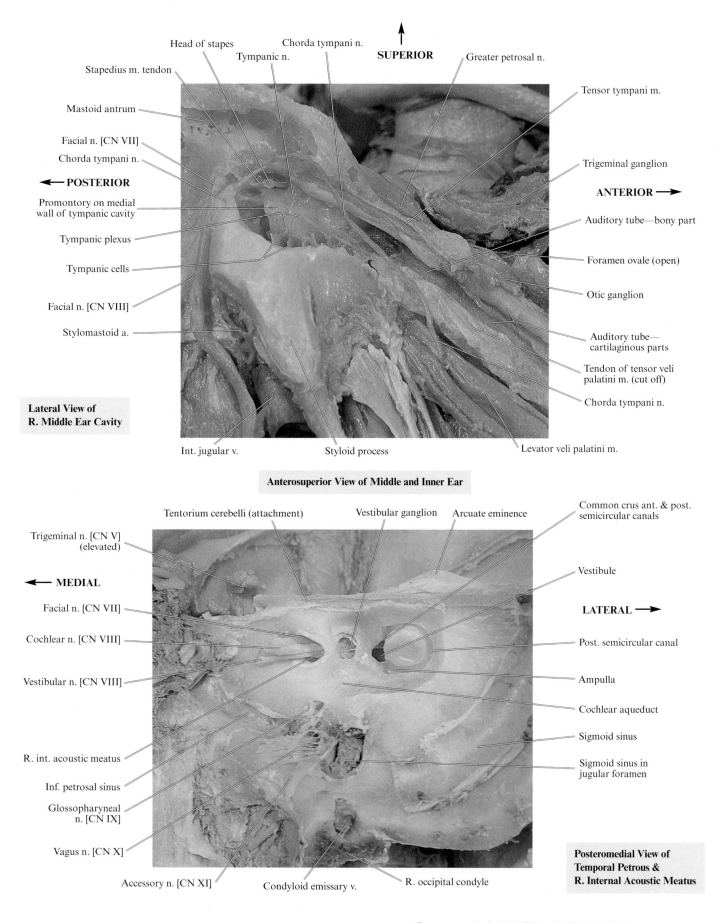

Head of stapes
Chorda tympani n.
Stapedius m. tendon
Tympanic n.
SUPERIOR
Greater petrosal n.
Tensor tympani m.

Mastoid antrum

Facial n. [CN VII]
Chorda tympani n.

Trigeminal ganglion

← **POSTERIOR**

ANTERIOR →

Promontory on medial
wall of tympanic cavity

Auditory tube—bony part

Tympanic plexus

Foramen ovale (open)

Tympanic cells

Otic ganglion

Facial n. [CN VIII]

Auditory tube—
cartilaginous parts

Stylomastoid a.

Tendon of tensor veli
palatini m. (cut off)

Chorda tympani n.

**Lateral View of
R. Middle Ear Cavity**

Int. jugular v.
Styloid process
Levator veli palatini m.

Anterosuperior View of Middle and Inner Ear

Tentorium cerebelli (attachment)
Vestibular ganglion
Arcuate eminence
Common crus ant. & post.
semicircular canals

Trigeminal n. [CN V]
(elevated)

Vestibule

← **MEDIAL**

LATERAL →

Facial n. [CN VII]

Cochlear n. [CN VIII]

Post. semicircular canal

Vestibular n. [CN VIII]

Ampulla

Cochlear aqueduct

R. int. acoustic meatus

Sigmoid sinus

Inf. petrosal sinus

Sigmoid sinus in
jugular foramen

Glossopharyneal
n. [CN IX]

Vagus n. [CN X]

**Posteromedial View of
Temporal Petrous &
R. Internal Acoustic Meatus**

Accessory n. [CN XI]
Condyloid emissary v.
R. occipital condyle

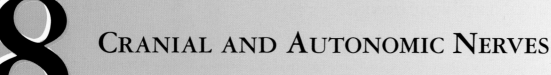

8 CRANIAL AND AUTONOMIC NERVES

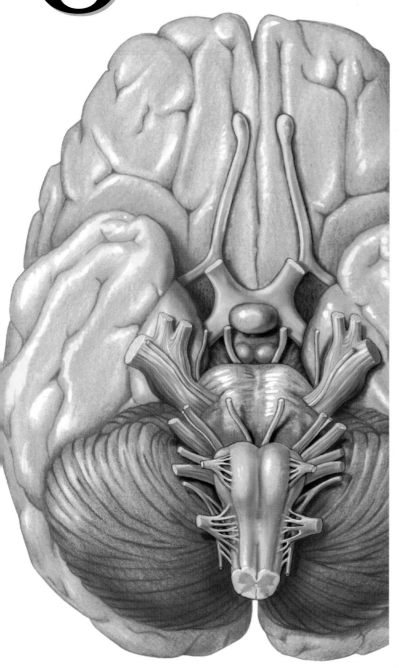

CRANIAL NERVE FUNCTIONS

CRANIAL NERVE ORIGINS

OLFACTORY NERVE–I

OPTIC NERVE–II

OCULOMOTOR NERVE–III

CILIARY GANGLION

TROCHLEAR NERVE–IV

TRIGEMINAL NERVE–V

ABDUCENS NERVE–VI

FACIAL NERVE–VII

PTERYGOPALATINE GANGLION

SUBMANDIBULAR GANGLION

VESTIBULOCOCHLEAR NERVE–VIII

OTIC GANGLION & TASTE NERVE PATHWAYS

GLOSSOPHARYNGEAL NERVE–IX

VAGUS NERVE–X

THORACO-ABDOMINAL SYMPATHETIC NERVES

PELVIC AUTONOMIC NERVES

ACCESSORY NERVE–XI

HYPOGLOSSAL NERVE–XII

CERVICAL PLEXUS

TABLE 8.1   **CRANIAL NERVE FUNCTIONS**

Overview of Cranial Nerves

| Nerve | Efferent or Motor | | Afferent or Sensory | | |
	Striated Muscles	Smooth & Cardiac Muscles & Glands	Skin	Mucous Membranes & Organs	Special Senses
CN I					Olfaction or sensation of smell
CN II					Vision or sight
CN III	Supplies all muscles of eyeball except lat. rectus & sup. oblique mm.	Parasympathetic to ciliary m. (lens) & sphincter pupillae m.		Proprioceptive fibers from eye mm.	
CN IV	Supplies sup. oblique m. of eyeball			Proprioceptive fibers from sup. oblique m.	
CN V	Supplies muscles of mastication, tensor tympani, tensor veli palatini, mylohyoid m. & ant. belly of digastric m.	Carries parasympathetic preganglionic nerve fibers of CN III, VII & IX	Face & ant. part of scalp	Teeth, mucous membrane of mouth, nose & eye, general sensory from anterior two-thirds of tongue	Taste (fibers from chorda tympani) from ant. two-thirds of tongue
CN VI	Supplies lat. rectus m. of eyeball			Proprioceptive fibers from lat. rectus m.	
CN VII	Supplies muscles of facial expression, stapedius m., stylohyoid m., & post. belly of digastric m.	Parasympathetic nervus intermedius; glands of mouth, nose & palate; lacrimal gland; submandibular & sublingual glands	Ext. ear	Proprioceptive fibers from muscles of facial expression	Nervus intermedius, taste from ant. two-thirds of tongue
CN VIII					Hearing & equilibrium
CN IX	Supplies stylopharyngeus m.	Parasympathetic to parotid gland		Internal surface of tympanic membrane, middle ear, auditory tube, upper pharynx & general sensory from tongue (post. one-third)	Taste from post. one-third of tongue
CN X	Supplies muscles of soft palate (except tensor veli palatini m.), pharynx (except stylopharyngeus m.), larynx, & palatoglossus m.	Parasympathetic to organs in neck, thorax & abdomen	Ext. acoustic meatus & tympanic membrane	Organs in neck, thorax & abdomen, general sensory from root of tongue	Taste, epiglottis
CN XI	Supplies sternocleidomastoid & trapezius mm.				
CN XII	Supplies extrinsic & intrinsic mm. of tongue except palatoglossus m.				

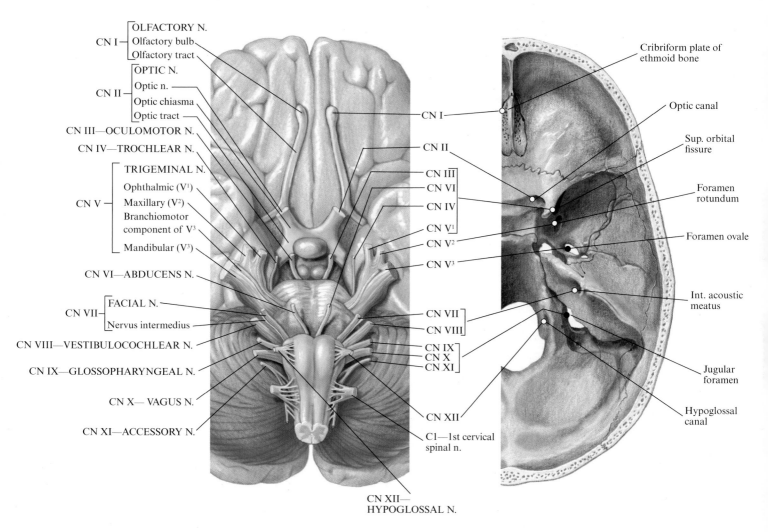

OLFACTORY N.
CN I — Olfactory bulb
Olfactory tract

OPTIC N.
CN II — Optic n.
Optic chiasma
Optic tract

CN III—OCULOMOTOR N.

CN IV—TROCHLEAR N.

TRIGEMINAL N.
Ophthalmic (V^1)
CN V — Maxillary (V^2)
Branchiomotor
component of V^3
Mandibular (V^3)

CN VI—ABDUCENS N.

FACIAL N.
CN VII —
Nervus intermedius

CN VIII—VESTIBULOCOCHLEAR N.

CN IX—GLOSSOPHARYNGEAL N.

CN X— VAGUS N.

CN XI—ACCESSORY N.

CN I

CN II

CN III

CN VI

CN IV

CN V^1

CN V^2

CN V^3

CN VII

CN VIII

CN IX
CN X
CN XI

CN XII

C1—1st cervical
spinal n.

CN XII—
HYPOGLOSSAL N.

Cribriform plate of
ethmoid bone

Optic canal

Sup. orbital
fissure

Foramen
rotundum

Foramen ovale

Int. acoustic
meatus

Jugular
foramen

Hypoglossal
canal

PLATE 8.2   OLFACTORY NERVE—CN I

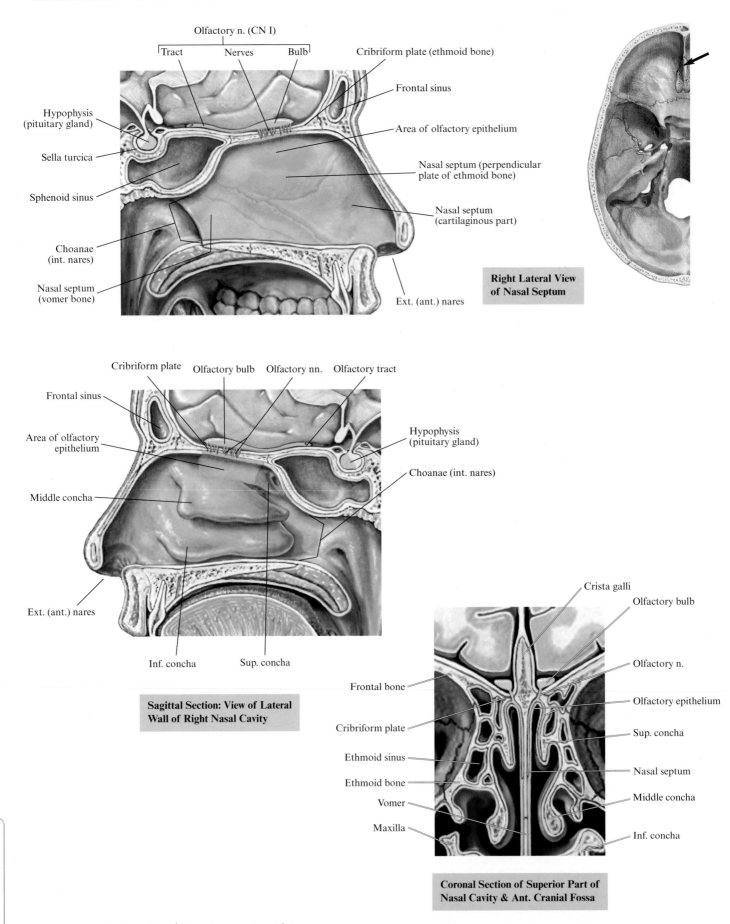

Olfactory n. (CN I)

Tract   Nerves   Bulb

Cribriform plate (ethmoid bone)

Frontal sinus

Hypophysis (pituitary gland)

Area of olfactory epithelium

Sella turcica

Nasal septum (perpendicular plate of ethmoid bone)

Sphenoid sinus

Nasal septum (cartilaginous part)

Choanae (int. nares)

Nasal septum (vomer bone)

Ext. (ant.) nares

Right Lateral View of Nasal Septum

Cribriform plate   Olfactory bulb   Olfactory nn.   Olfactory tract

Frontal sinus

Hypophysis (pituitary gland)

Area of olfactory epithelium

Choanae (int. nares)

Middle concha

Ext. (ant.) nares

Inf. concha   Sup. concha

Sagittal Section: View of Lateral Wall of Right Nasal Cavity

Crista galli

Olfactory bulb

Olfactory n.

Frontal bone

Olfactory epithelium

Cribriform plate

Sup. concha

Ethmoid sinus

Nasal septum

Ethmoid bone

Middle concha

Vomer

Maxilla

Inf. concha

Coronal Section of Superior Part of Nasal Cavity & Ant. Cranial Fossa

A.D.A.M. | Student Atlas of Anatomy

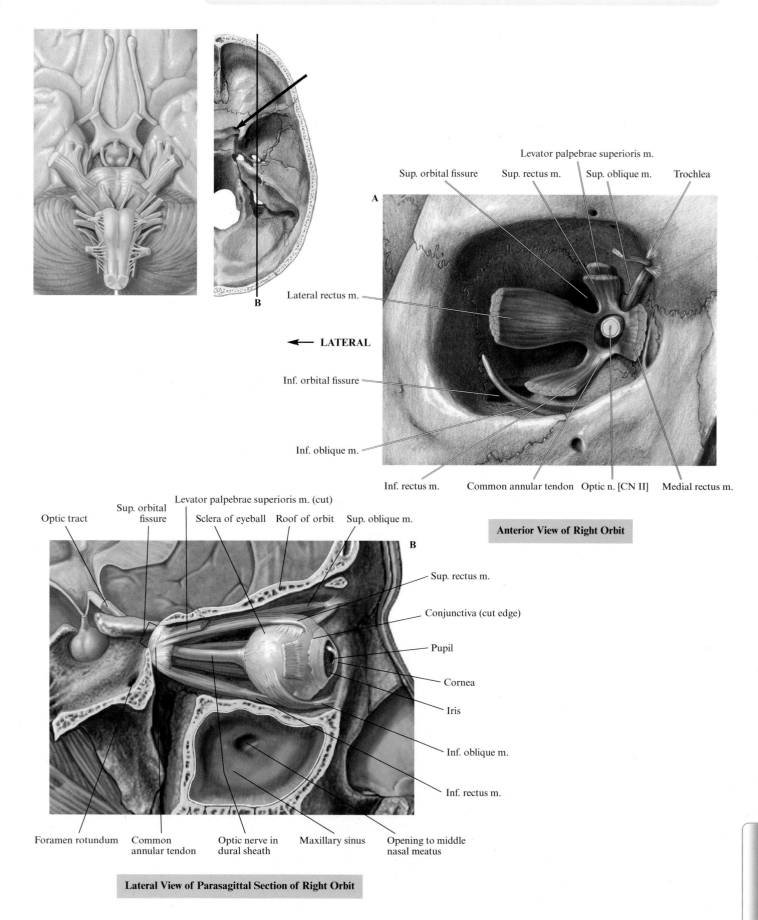

A

Levator palpebrae superioris m.

Sup. orbital fissure   Sup. rectus m.   Sup. oblique m.   Trochlea

Lateral rectus m.

← LATERAL

Inf. orbital fissure

Inf. oblique m.

Inf. rectus m.   Common annular tendon   Optic n. [CN II]   Medial rectus m.

Anterior View of Right Orbit

Optic tract   Sup. orbital fissure   Levator palpebrae superioris m. (cut)   Sclera of eyeball   Roof of orbit   Sup. oblique m.

B

Sup. rectus m.

Conjunctiva (cut edge)

Pupil

Cornea

Iris

Inf. oblique m.

Inf. rectus m.

Foramen rotundum   Common annular tendon   Optic nerve in dural sheath   Maxillary sinus   Opening to middle nasal meatus

Lateral View of Parasagittal Section of Right Orbit

PLATE 8.4   OCULOMOTOR NERVE—CN III

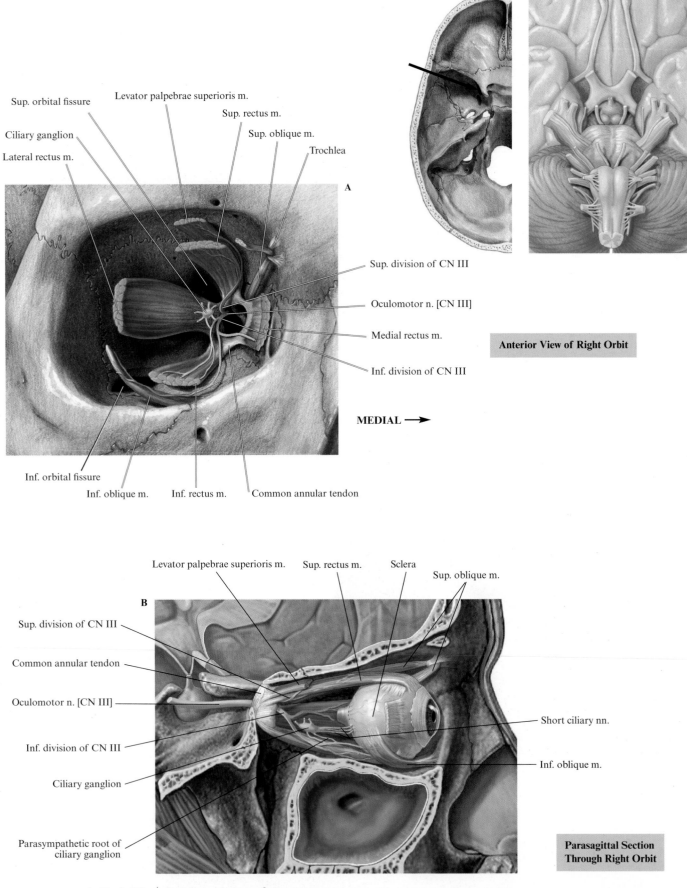

Sup. orbital fissure

Levator palpebrae superioris m.

Sup. rectus m.

Ciliary ganglion

Sup. oblique m.

Lateral rectus m.

Trochlea

A

Sup. division of CN III

Oculomotor n. [CN III]

Medial rectus m.

Inf. division of CN III

Anterior View of Right Orbit

MEDIAL ⟶

Inf. orbital fissure

Inf. oblique m.

Inf. rectus m.

Common annular tendon

Levator palpebrae superioris m.

Sup. rectus m.

Sclera

Sup. oblique m.

B

Sup. division of CN III

Common annular tendon

Oculomotor n. [CN III]

Short ciliary nn.

Inf. division of CN III

Inf. oblique m.

Ciliary ganglion

Parasympathetic root of
ciliary ganglion

**Parasagittal Section
Through Right Orbit**

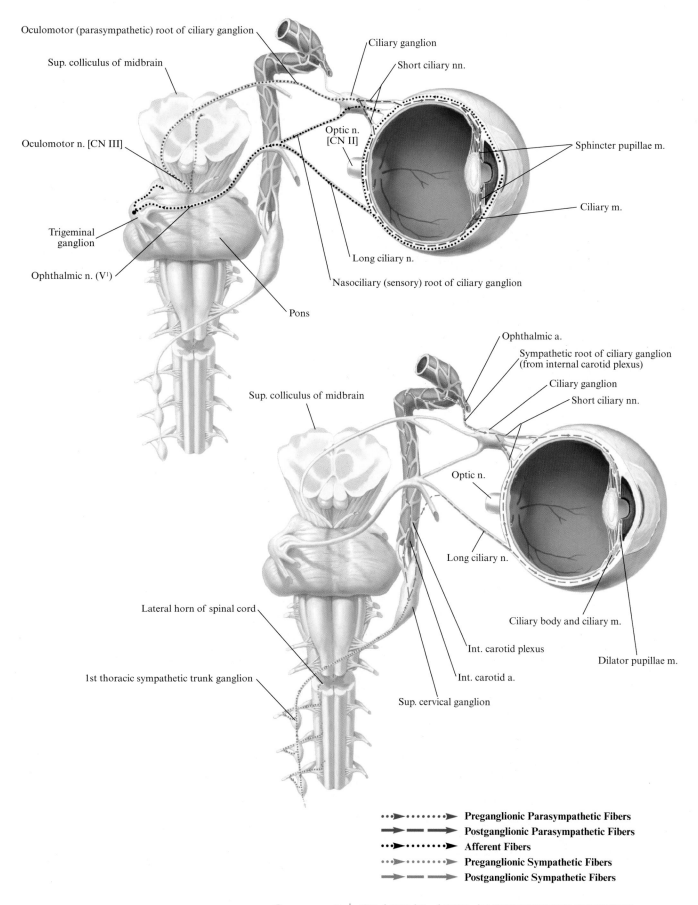

Oculomotor (parasympathetic) root of ciliary ganglion

Sup. colliculus of midbrain

Oculomotor n. [CN III]

Trigeminal ganglion

Ophthalmic n. (V¹)

Pons

Ciliary ganglion

Short ciliary nn.

Optic n. [CN II]

Sphincter pupillae m.

Ciliary m.

Long ciliary n.

Nasociliary (sensory) root of ciliary ganglion

Sup. colliculus of midbrain

Ophthalmic a.

Sympathetic root of ciliary ganglion (from internal carotid plexus)

Ciliary ganglion

Short ciliary nn.

Optic n.

Long ciliary n.

Ciliary body and ciliary m.

Dilator pupillae m.

Lateral horn of spinal cord

Int. carotid plexus

Int. carotid a.

1st thoracic sympathetic trunk ganglion

Sup. cervical ganglion

•••▶•••••••▶   **Preganglionic Parasympathetic Fibers**
━━━ ━ ━ ━━▶   **Postganglionic Parasympathetic Fibers**
•••▶•••••••▶   **Afferent Fibers**
•••▶•••••••▶   **Preganglionic Sympathetic Fibers**
━━━ ━ ━ ━━▶   **Postganglionic Sympathetic Fibers**

PLATE 8.6   TROCHLEAR NERVE—CN IV

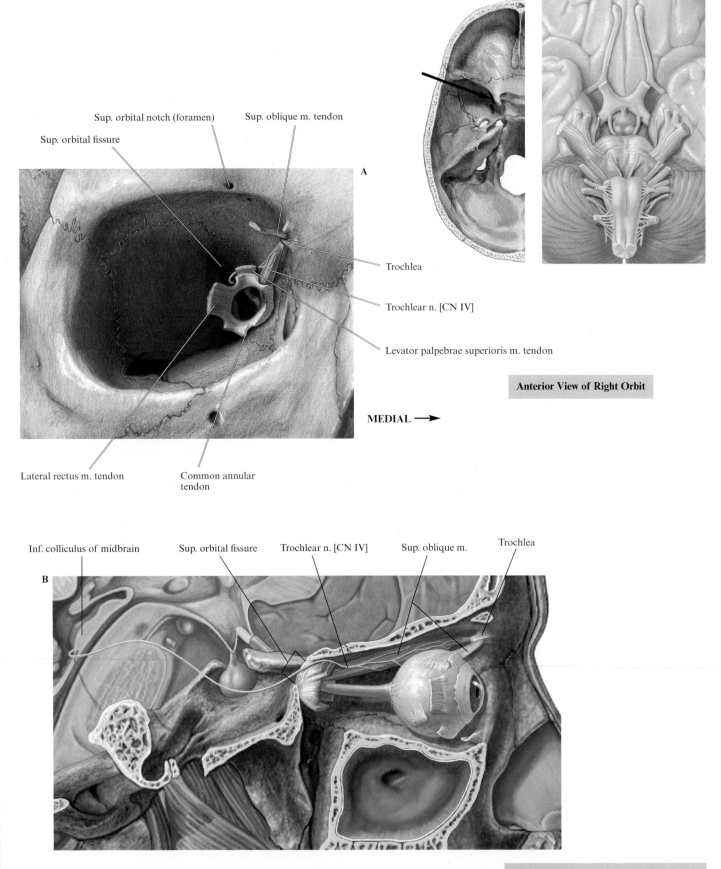

Sup. orbital notch (foramen)

Sup. oblique m. tendon

Sup. orbital fissure

A

Trochlea

Trochlear n. [CN IV]

Levator palpebrae superioris m. tendon

Anterior View of Right Orbit

MEDIAL ➝

Lateral rectus m. tendon

Common annular
tendon

Inf. colliculus of midbrain

Sup. orbital fissure

Trochlear n. [CN IV]

Sup. oblique m.

Trochlea

B

Parasagittal Section Through Right Orbit

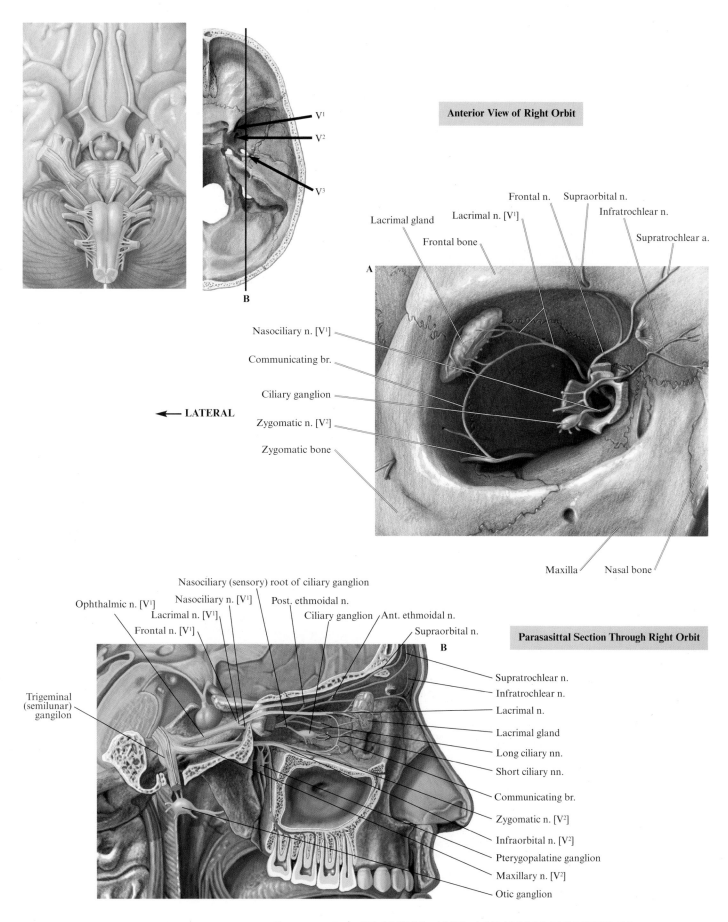

Anterior View of Right Orbit

Frontal n.   Supraorbital n.

Lacrimal n. [V¹]   Infratrochlear n.

Lacrimal gland   Supratrochlear a.

Frontal bone

A

Nasociliary n. [V¹]

Communicating br.

Ciliary ganglion

← **LATERAL**

Zygomatic n. [V²]

Zygomatic bone

Maxilla   Nasal bone

Nasociliary (sensory) root of ciliary ganglion

Ophthalmic n. [V¹]   Nasociliary n. [V¹]   Post. ethmoidal n.

Lacrimal n. [V¹]   Ciliary ganglion   Ant. ethmoidal n.

Frontal n. [V¹]   Supraorbital n.

B

Parasasittal Section Through Right Orbit

Supratrochlear n.

Infratrochlear n.

Trigeminal   Lacrimal n.
(semilunar)
gangilon   Lacrimal gland

Long ciliary nn.

Short ciliary nn.

Communicating br.

Zygomatic n. [V²]

Infraorbital n. [V²]

Pterygopalatine ganglion

Maxillary n. [V²]

Otic ganglion

PLATE 8.8   TRIGEMINAL NERVE—CN V² MAXILLARY DIVISION

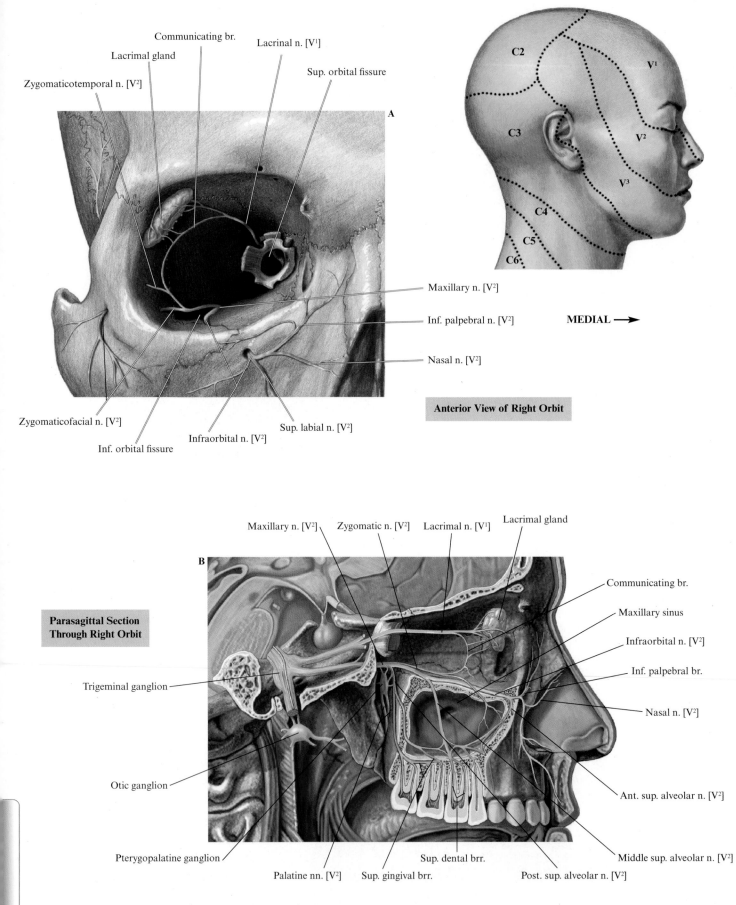

Communicating br.

Lacrimal gland

Lacrinal n. [V¹]

Zygomaticotemporal n. [V²]

Sup. orbital fissure

C2

V¹

C3

V²

V³

C4

C5

C6

A

Maxillary n. [V²]

Inf. palpebral n. [V²]

MEDIAL ⟶

Nasal n. [V²]

Zygomaticofacial n. [V²]

Inf. orbital fissure

Infraorbital n. [V²]

Sup. labial n. [V²]

Anterior View of Right Orbit

Maxillary n. [V²]   Zygomatic n. [V²]   Lacrimal n. [V¹]   Lacrimal gland

B

**Parasagittal Section
Through Right Orbit**

Communicating br.

Maxillary sinus

Infraorbital n. [V²]

Inf. palpebral br.

Trigeminal ganglion

Nasal n. [V²]

Otic ganglion

Ant. sup. alveolar n. [V²]

Pterygopalatine ganglion

Middle sup. alveolar n. [V²]

Palatine nn. [V²]   Sup. gingival brr.   Sup. dental brr.   Post. sup. alveolar n. [V²]

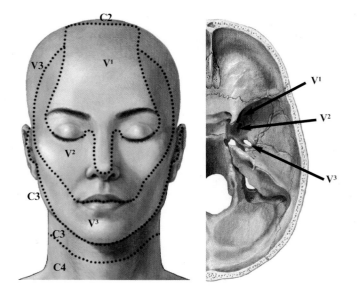

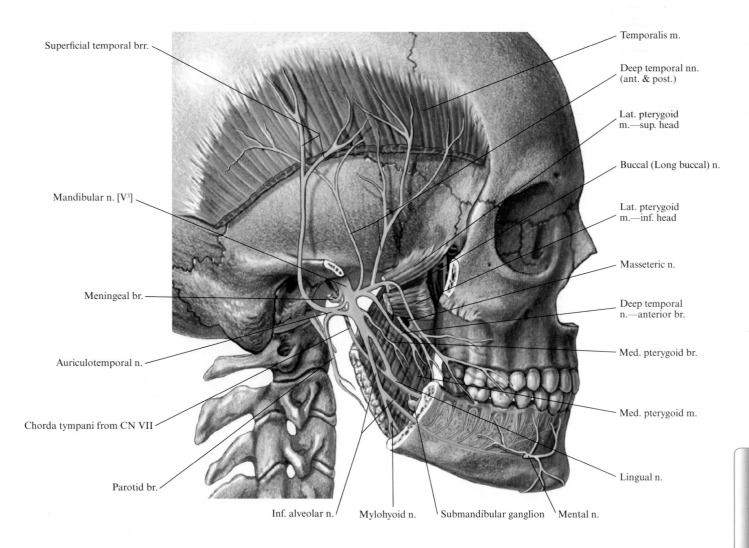

Superficial temporal brr.

Temporalis m.

Deep temporal nn.
(ant. & post.)

Lat. pterygoid
m.—sup. head

Buccal (Long buccal) n.

Mandibular n. [V³]

Lat. pterygoid
m.—inf. head

Meningeal br.

Masseteric n.

Deep temporal
n.—anterior br.

Auriculotemporal n.

Med. pterygoid br.

Med. pterygoid m.

Chorda tympani from CN VII

Lingual n.

Parotid br.

Inf. alveolar n.   Mylohyoid n.   Submandibular ganglion   Mental n.

PLATE 8.10   ABDUCENS NERVE—CN VI

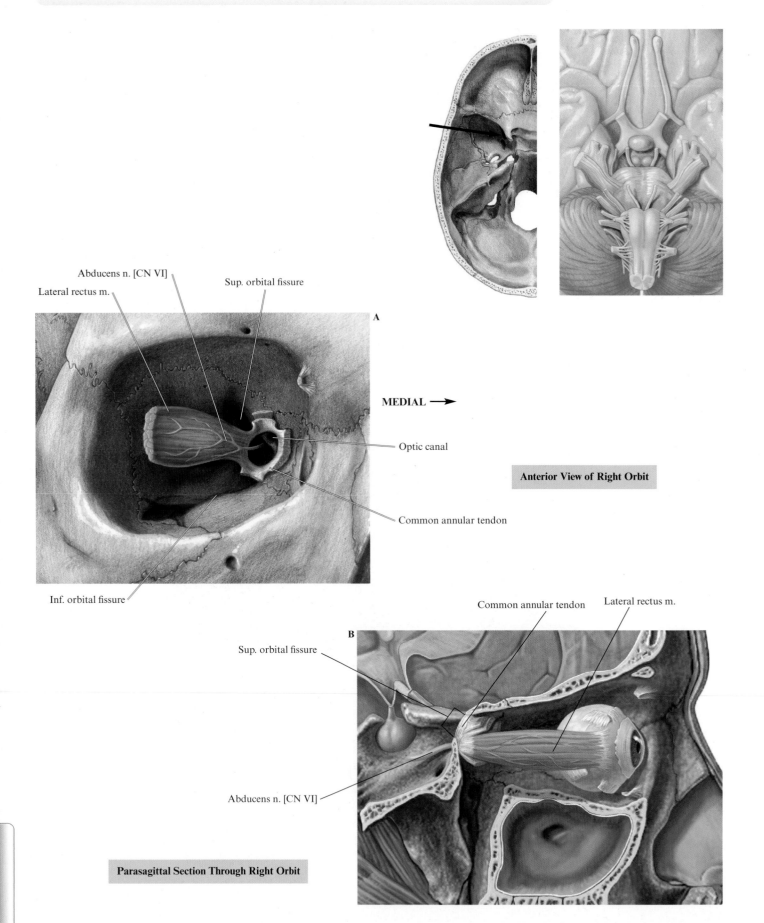

Abducens n. [CN VI]

Sup. orbital fissure

Lateral rectus m.

A

MEDIAL ⟶

Optic canal

Anterior View of Right Orbit

Common annular tendon

Inf. orbital fissure

Common annular tendon   Lateral rectus m.

B

Sup. orbital fissure

Abducens n. [CN VI]

Parasagittal Section Through Right Orbit

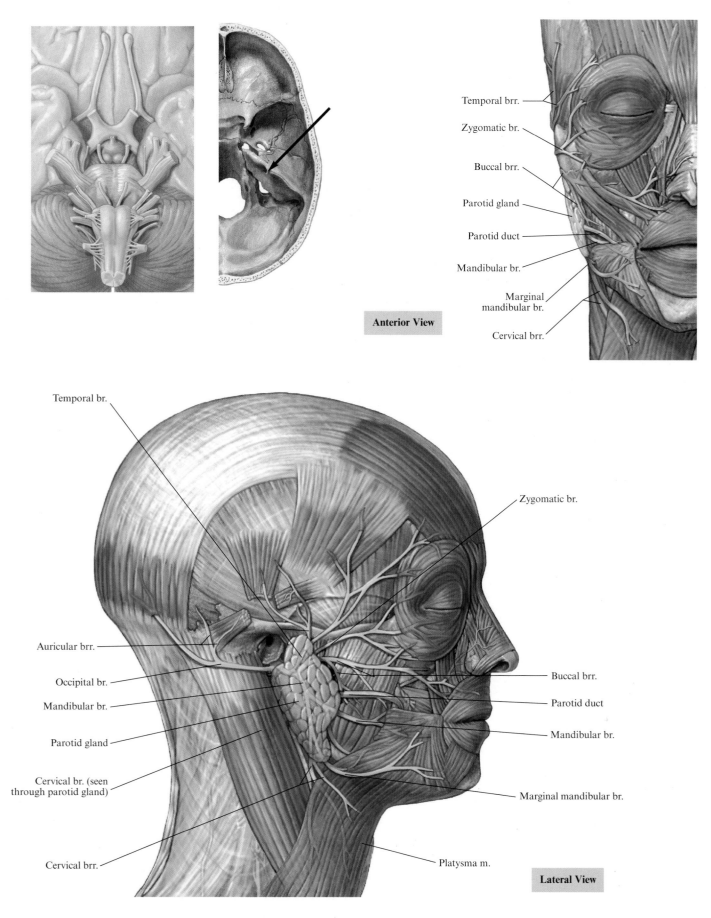

Temporal brr.

Zygomatic br.

Buccal brr.

Parotid gland

Parotid duct

Mandibular br.

Marginal
mandibular br.

Cervical brr.

Anterior View

Temporal br.

Zygomatic br.

Auricular brr.

Occipital br.

Mandibular br.

Parotid gland

Cervical br. (seen
through parotid gland)

Cervical brr.

Buccal brr.

Parotid duct

Mandibular br.

Marginal mandibular br.

Platysma m.

Lateral View

PLATE 8.12   PTERYGOPALATINE GANGLION

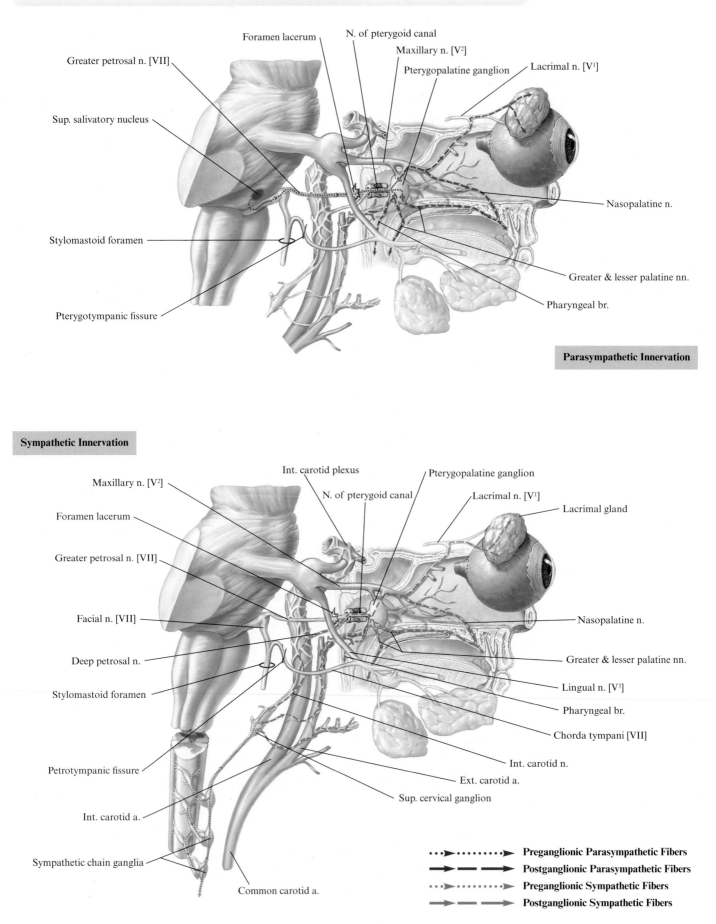

Greater petrosal n. [VII]

Sup. salivatory nucleus

Stylomastoid foramen

Pterygotympanic fissure

Foramen lacerum

N. of pterygoid canal

Maxillary n. [V²]

Pterygopalatine ganglion

Lacrimal n. [V¹]

Nasopalatine n.

Greater & lesser palatine nn.

Pharyngeal br.

Parasympathetic Innervation

Sympathetic Innervation

Maxillary n. [V²]

Foramen lacerum

Greater petrosal n. [VII]

Facial n. [VII]

Deep petrosal n.

Stylomastoid foramen

Petrotympanic fissure

Int. carotid a.

Sympathetic chain ganglia

Common carotid a.

Int. carotid plexus

N. of pterygoid canal

Pterygopalatine ganglion

Lacrimal n. [V¹]

Lacrimal gland

Nasopalatine n.

Greater & lesser palatine nn.

Lingual n. [V³]

Pharyngeal br.

Chorda tympani [VII]

Int. carotid n.

Ext. carotid a.

Sup. cervical ganglion

••••▶••••••••▶   **Preganglionic Parasympathetic Fibers**

▬▬▬▶ ▬ ▬ ▬▶   **Postganglionic Parasympathetic Fibers**

••••▶••••••••••   **Preganglionic Sympathetic Fibers**

▬▬▶ ▬ ▬ ▬▶   **Postganglionic Sympathetic Fibers**

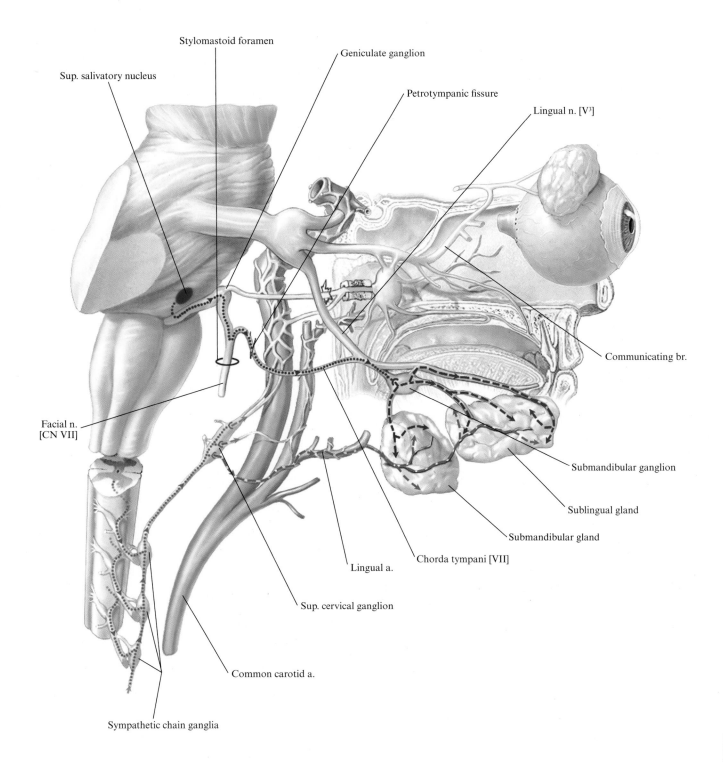

•••▶••••••▶ **Preganglionic Parasympathetic Fibers**
━━━▶━ ━ ━▶ **Postganglionic Parasympathetic Fibers**
•••▶••••••▶ **Preganglionic Sympathetic Fibers**
━━▶━ ━ ━▶ **Postganglionic Sympathetic Fibers**

Stylomastoid foramen

Geniculate ganglion

Petrotympanic fissure

Lingual n. [V³]

Sup. salivatory nucleus

Communicating br.

Facial n.
[CN VII]

Submandibular ganglion

Sublingual gland

Submandibular gland

Chorda tympani [VII]

Lingual a.

Sup. cervical ganglion

Common carotid a.

Sympathetic chain ganglia

PLATE 8.14   VESTIBULOCOCHLEAR NERVE—CN VIII

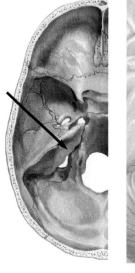
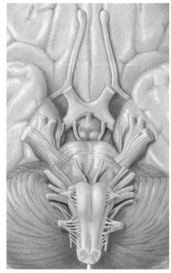

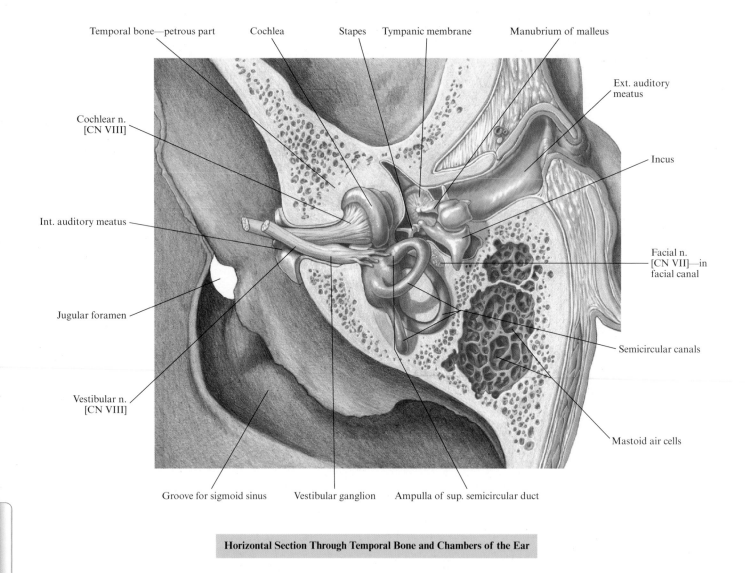

Temporal bone—petrous part   Cochlea   Stapes   Tympanic membrane   Manubrium of malleus

Ext. auditory meatus

Cochlear n. [CN VIII]

Incus

Int. auditory meatus

Facial n. [CN VII]—in facial canal

Jugular foramen

Semicircular canals

Vestibular n. [CN VIII]

Mastoid air cells

Groove for sigmoid sinus   Vestibular ganglion   Ampulla of sup. semicircular duct

Horizontal Section Through Temporal Bone and Chambers of the Ear

```
••••▸••••••••▸   Preganglionic Parasympathetic Fibers
━━━▸━ ━ ━ ━▸   Postganglionic Parasympathetic Fibers
•••▸•••••••••▸   Afferent Fibers
••▸•••••••••▸   Preganglionic Sympathetic Fibers
━━▸ ━ ━ ━ ━▸   Postganglionic Sympathetic Fibers
```

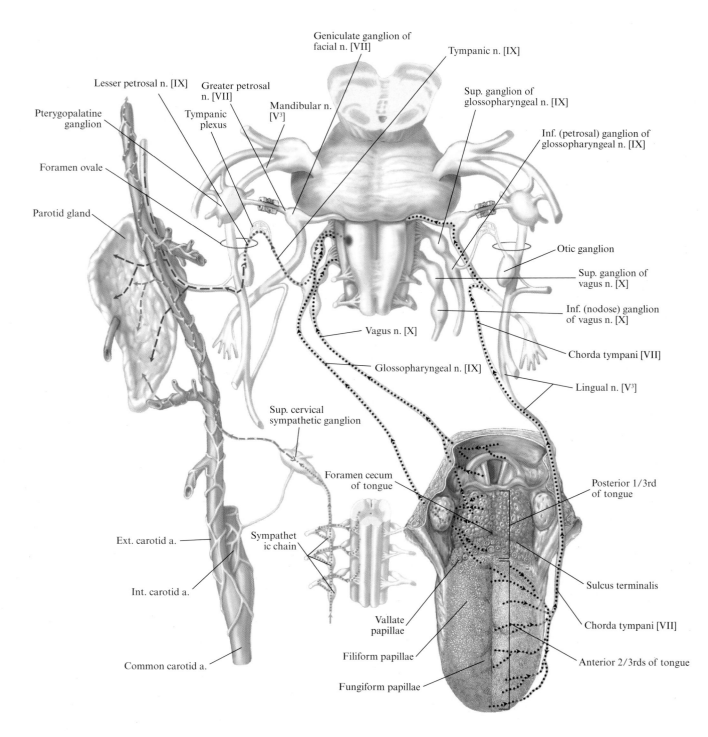

PLATE 8.16 GLOSSOPHARYNGEAL NERVE—CN IX

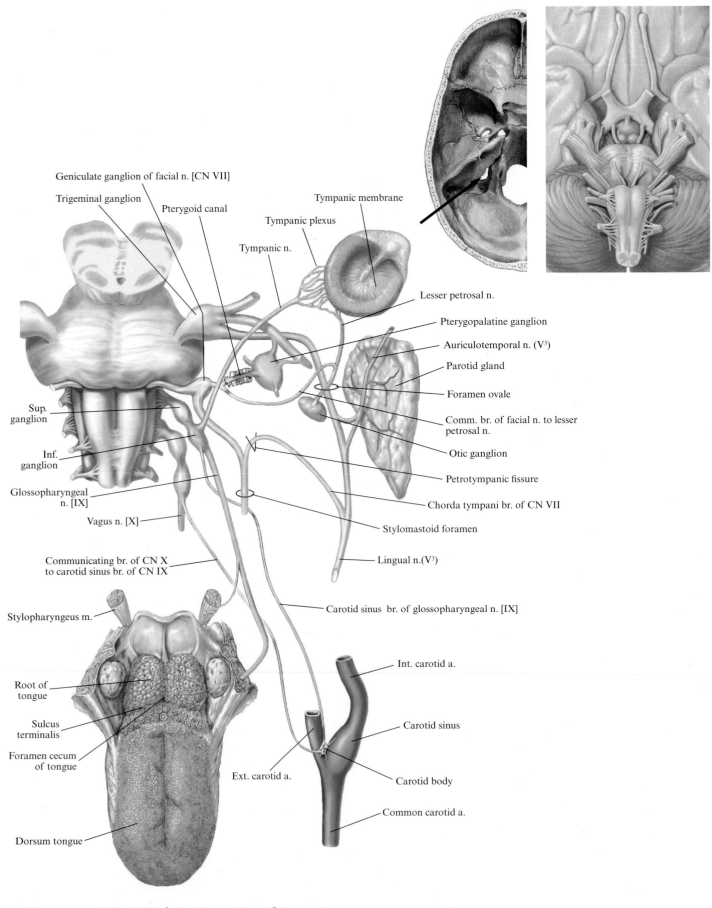

Geniculate ganglion of facial n. [CN VII]

Trigeminal ganglion

Pterygoid canal

Tympanic membrane

Tympanic plexus

Tympanic n.

Lesser petrosal n.

Pterygopalatine ganglion

Auriculotemporal n. (V³)

Parotid gland

Foramen ovale

Comm. br. of facial n. to lesser petrosal n.

Otic ganglion

Petrotympanic fissure

Chorda tympani br. of CN VII

Stylomastoid foramen

Lingual n.(V³)

Sup. ganglion

Inf. ganglion

Glossopharyngeal n. [IX]

Vagus n. [X]

Communicating br. of CN X to carotid sinus br. of CN IX

Carotid sinus br. of glossopharyngeal n. [IX]

Stylopharyngeus m.

Int. carotid a.

Root of tongue

Sulcus terminalis

Foramen cecum of tongue

Carotid sinus

Ext. carotid a.

Carotid body

Common carotid a.

Dorsum tongue

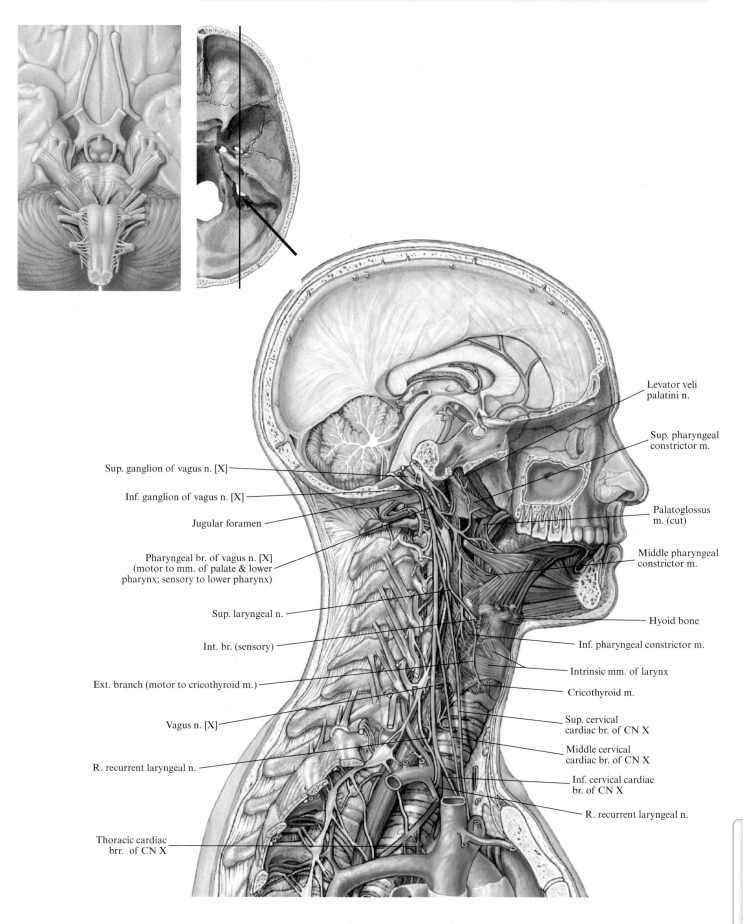

Levator veli
palatini n.

Sup. pharyngeal
constrictor m.

Sup. ganglion of vagus n. [X]

Inf. ganglion of vagus n. [X]

Palatoglossus
m. (cut)

Jugular foramen

Pharyngeal br. of vagus n. [X]
(motor to mm. of palate & lower
pharynx; sensory to lower pharynx)

Middle pharyngeal
constrictor m.

Sup. laryngeal n.

Hyoid bone

Int. br. (sensory)

Inf. pharyngeal constrictor m.

Intrinsic mm. of larynx

Ext. branch (motor to cricothyroid m.)

Cricothyroid m.

Vagus n. [X]

Sup. cervical
cardiac br. of CN X

Middle cervical
cardiac br. of CN X

Inf. cervical cardiac
br. of CN X

R. recurrent laryngeal n.

R. recurrent laryngeal n.

Thoracic cardiac
brr. of CN X

PLATE 8.18   VAGUS NERVE—CN X THORACO-ABDOMINAL BRANCHES

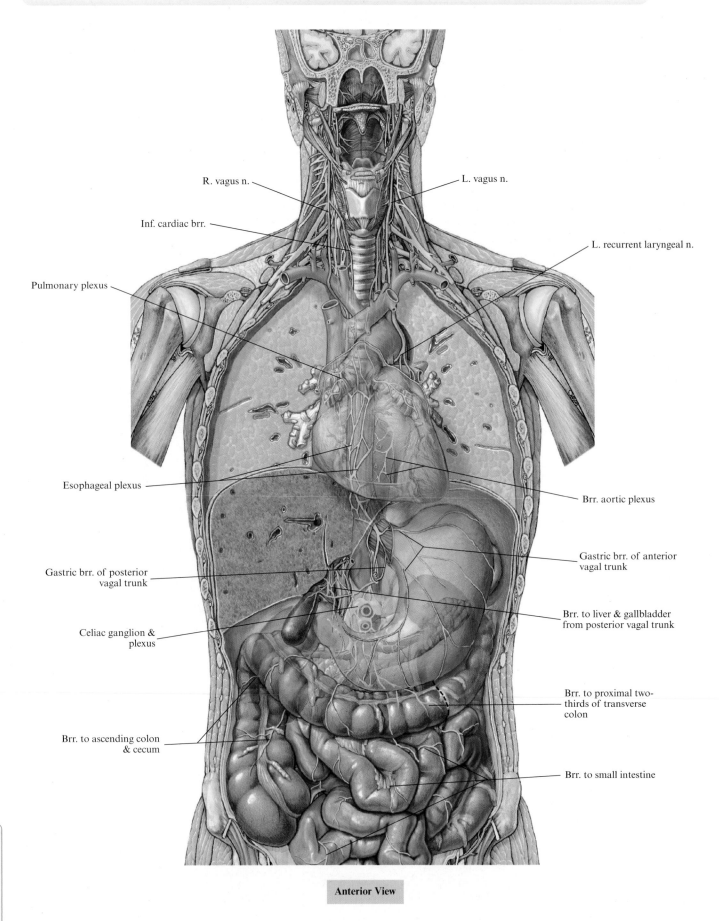

R. vagus n.

L. vagus n.

Inf. cardiac brr.

L. recurrent laryngeal n.

Pulmonary plexus

Esophageal plexus

Brr. aortic plexus

Gastric brr. of anterior vagal trunk

Gastric brr. of posterior vagal trunk

Brr. to liver & gallbladder from posterior vagal trunk

Celiac ganglion & plexus

Brr. to proximal two-thirds of transverse colon

Brr. to ascending colon & cecum

Brr. to small intestine

Anterior View

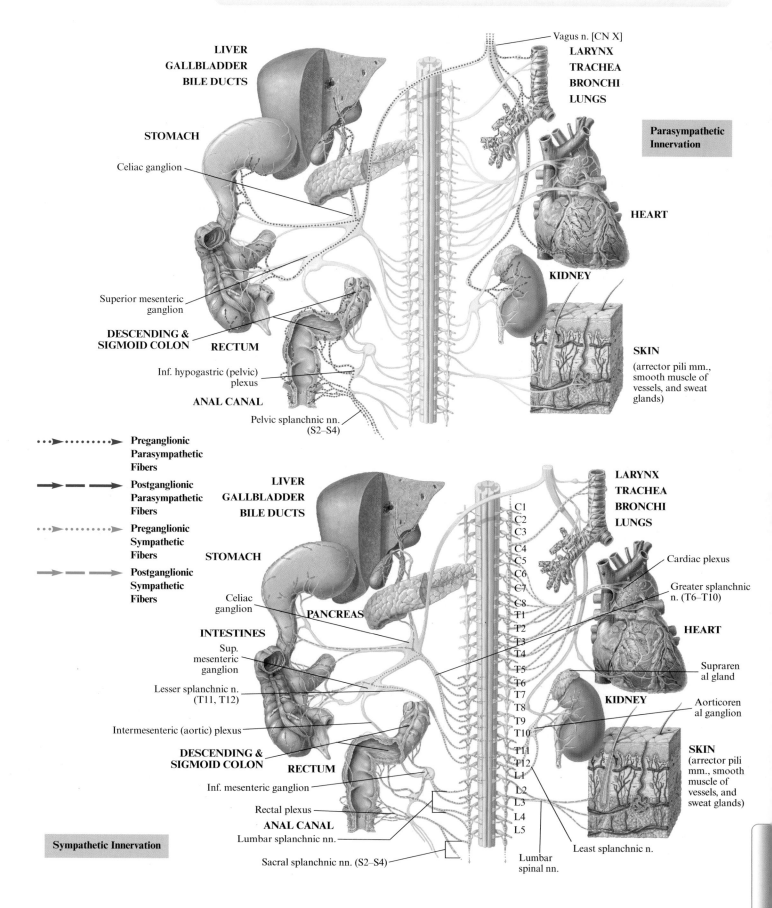

Vagus n. [CN X]

LIVER
GALLBLADDER
BILE DUCTS

LARYNX
TRACHEA
BRONCHI
LUNGS

STOMACH

**Parasympathetic
Innervation**

Celiac ganglion

HEART

KIDNEY

Superior mesenteric
ganglion

DESCENDING &
SIGMOID COLON   RECTUM

SKIN
(arrector pili mm.,
smooth muscle of
vessels, and sweat
glands)

Inf. hypogastric (pelvic)
plexus

ANAL CANAL

Pelvic splanchnic nn.
(S2–S4)

•••▶•••••••▶ **Preganglionic
Parasympathetic
Fibers**

➤ – – – ➤ **Postganglionic
Parasympathetic
Fibers**

•••▶•••••••▶ **Preganglionic
Sympathetic
Fibers**

➤ – – ➤ **Postganglionic
Sympathetic
Fibers**

LIVER
GALLBLADDER
BILE DUCTS

LARYNX
TRACHEA
BRONCHI
LUNGS

C1
C2
C3
C4
C5
C6
C7
C8
T1
T2
T3
T4
T5
T6
T7
T8
T9
T10
T11
T12
L1
L2
L3
L4
L5

Cardiac plexus

Greater splanchnic
n. (T6–T10)

STOMACH

Celiac
ganglion

PANCREAS

HEART

INTESTINES

Supraren
al gland

Sup.
mesenteric
ganglion

Lesser splanchnic n.
(T11, T12)

KIDNEY

Aorticoren
al ganglion

Intermesenteric (aortic) plexus

DESCENDING &
SIGMOID COLON   RECTUM

SKIN
(arrector pili
mm., smooth
muscle of
vessels, and
sweat glands)

Inf. mesenteric ganglion

Rectal plexus

ANAL CANAL

Lumbar splanchnic nn.

Least splanchnic n.

Sacral splanchnic nn. (S2–S4)

Lumbar
spinal nn.

Sympathetic Innervation

CHAPTER 8 | CRANIAL AND AUTONOMIC NERVES   465

PLATE 8.20 PELVIC AUTONOMIC NERVES—FEMALE

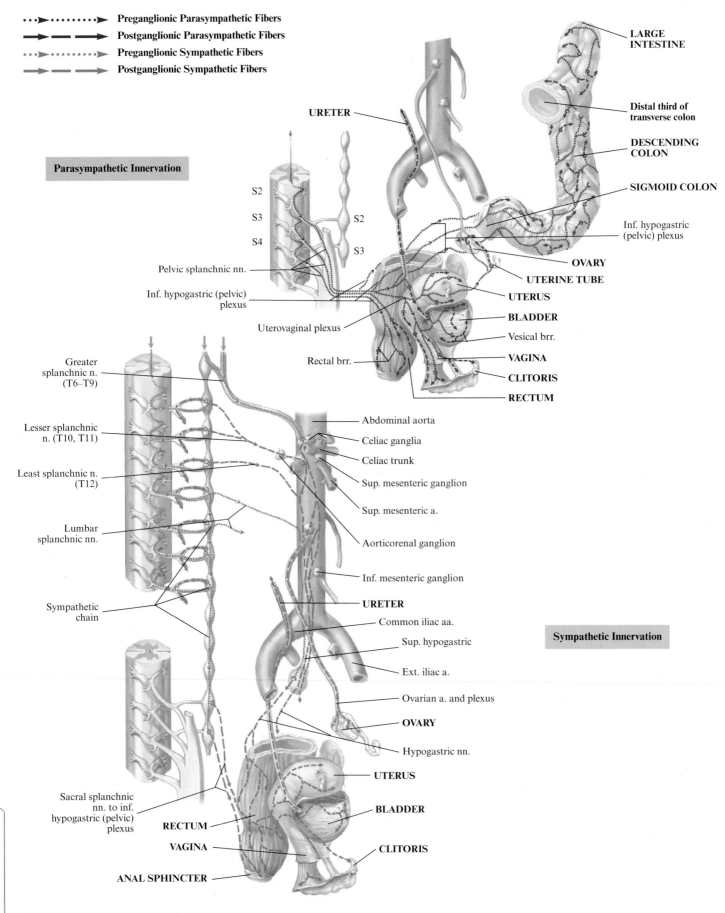

Preganglionic Parasympathetic Fibers
Postganglionic Parasympathetic Fibers
Preganglionic Sympathetic Fibers
Postganglionic Sympathetic Fibers

Parasympathetic Innervation

URETER

LARGE INTESTINE

Distal third of transverse colon

DESCENDING COLON

SIGMOID COLON

Inf. hypogastric (pelvic) plexus

S2
S3
S4

S2

S3

OVARY
UTERINE TUBE
UTERUS
BLADDER
Vesical brr.
VAGINA
CLITORIS
RECTUM

Pelvic splanchnic nn.

Inf. hypogastric (pelvic) plexus

Uterovaginal plexus

Rectal brr.

Greater splanchnic n. (T6–T9)

Lesser splanchnic n. (T10, T11)

Least splanchnic n. (T12)

Lumbar splanchnic nn.

Sympathetic chain

Abdominal aorta
Celiac ganglia
Celiac trunk
Sup. mesenteric ganglion
Sup. mesenteric a.

Aorticorenal ganglion

Inf. mesenteric ganglion

URETER

Common iliac aa.

Sup. hypogastric

Ext. iliac a.

Sympathetic Innervation

Ovarian a. and plexus

OVARY

Hypogastric nn.

UTERUS

BLADDER

Sacral splanchnic nn. to inf. hypogastric (pelvic) plexus

RECTUM

VAGINA

CLITORIS

ANAL SPHINCTER

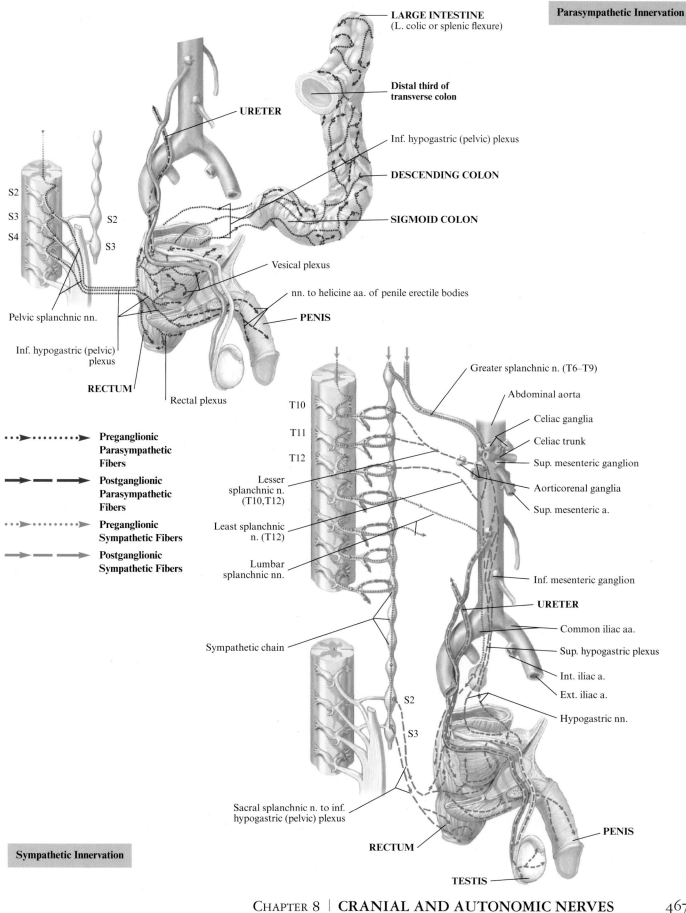

LARGE INTESTINE
(L. colic or splenic flexure)

Distal third of
transverse colon

URETER

Inf. hypogastric (pelvic) plexus

DESCENDING COLON

SIGMOID COLON

Vesical plexus

nn. to helicine aa. of penile erectile bodies

PENIS

S2
S3
S4

S2

S3

Pelvic splanchnic nn.

Inf. hypogastric (pelvic)
plexus

RECTUM

Rectal plexus

••▶••••••▶ Preganglionic
Parasympathetic
Fibers

——————— Postganglionic
Parasympathetic
Fibers

••▶••••••▶ Preganglionic
Sympathetic Fibers

——————— Postganglionic
Sympathetic Fibers

Greater splanchnic n. (T6–T9)

Abdominal aorta

Celiac ganglia

Celiac trunk

Sup. mesenteric ganglion

Aorticorenal ganglia

Sup. mesenteric a.

T10

T11

T12

Lesser
splanchnic n.
(T10,T12)

Least splanchnic
n. (T12)

Lumbar
splanchnic nn.

Inf. mesenteric ganglion

URETER

Common iliac aa.

Sup. hypogastric plexus

Int. iliac a.

Ext. iliac a.

Hypogastric nn.

Sympathetic chain

S2

S3

Sacral splanchnic n. to inf.
hypogastric (pelvic) plexus

PENIS

RECTUM

TESTIS

PLATE 8.22   ACCESSORY NERVE—CN XI

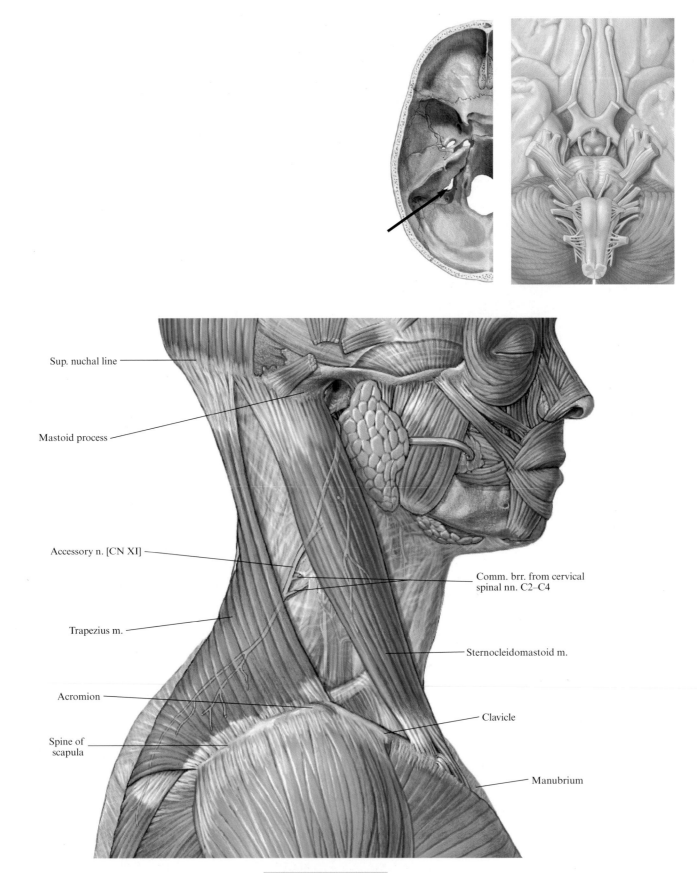

Sup. nuchal line

Mastoid process

Accessory n. [CN XI]

Comm. brr. from cervical
spinal nn. C2–C4

Trapezius m.

Sternocleidomastoid m.

Acromion

Clavicle

Spine of
scapula

Manubrium

Sympathetic Innervation

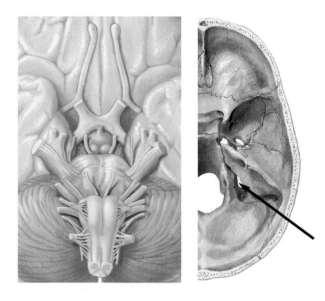

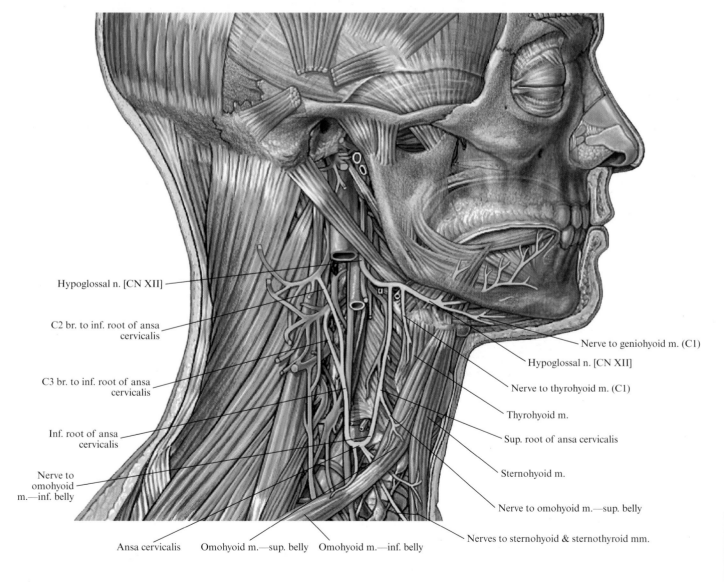

Hypoglossal n. [CN XII]

C2 br. to inf. root of ansa cervicalis

C3 br. to inf. root of ansa cervicalis

Inf. root of ansa cervicalis

Nerve to omohyoid m.—inf. belly

Nerve to geniohyoid m. (C1)

Hypoglossal n. [CN XII]

Nerve to thyrohyoid m. (C1)

Thyrohyoid m.

Sup. root of ansa cervicalis

Sternohyoid m.

Nerve to omohyoid m.—sup. belly

Nerves to sternohyoid & sternothyroid mm.

Ansa cervicalis   Omohyoid m.—sup. belly   Omohyoid m.—inf. belly

PLATE 8.24   CERVICAL PLEXUS

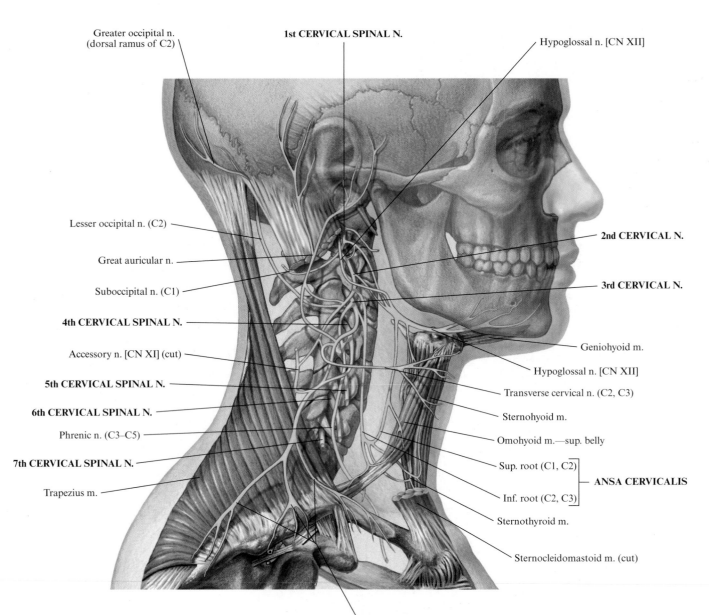

Greater occipital n.
(dorsal ramus of C2)

1st CERVICAL SPINAL N.

Hypoglossal n. [CN XII]

Lesser occipital n. (C2)

2nd CERVICAL N.

Great auricular n.

3rd CERVICAL N.

Suboccipital n. (C1)

4th CERVICAL SPINAL N.

Geniohyoid m.

Accessory n. [CN XI] (cut)

Hypoglossal n. [CN XII]

5th CERVICAL SPINAL N.

Transverse cervical n. (C2, C3)

6th CERVICAL SPINAL N.

Sternohyoid m.

Phrenic n. (C3–C5)

Omohyoid m.—sup. belly

7th CERVICAL SPINAL N.

Sup. root (C1, C2)

ANSA CERVICALIS

Trapezius m.

Inf. root (C2, C3)

Sternothyroid m.

Sternocleidomastoid m. (cut)

Supraclavicular nn. (C3, C4)

A

Abdomen
   abdominal wall muscles, 22–23
   innervation, 465
   peritoneal cavity, 112–117
   posterior wall, 140–143
   regions, 111
   right scapular line, 111
   topography, 110
Abdominal esophagus, 117–120
Abducens nerve (CN VI), 392–393, 396, 430,
      432–435, 440–441
   auricular branch, 457
   buccal branch, 457
   cervical branch, 457
   function, 471
   groove, 362
   mandibular branch, 457
   marginal mandibular branch, 457
   occipital branch, 457
   overview, 446–447, 456–457
   temporal branch, 457
   zygomatic branch, 457
Accessory nerve (CN XI), 60–62, 392, 396,
      443, 470
   function, 471
   overview, 446–447, 468
Accessory pancreatic duct, 123–125
Accessory parotid gland, 403
Acetabular fossa, 259
Acetabulum
   anatomical position, 154–155
   labrum, 153, 205
   lunate surface, 153–154
   notch, 154–155
Achilles tendon (Tendo calcaneus), 210–211,
      215, 261–264, 273
Acoustic meatus
   external, 358, 365, 405, 438, 441–442
   interior, 354, 361, 365, 441, 443, 447
   internal, 360
Acromioclavicular joint, 319
Acromioclavicular ligament, 319
Acromion, 4–6, 58–60, 280, 316–319
Adductor canal, membranous roof, 265
Adductor hiatus, 221, 250–251, 265
Adductor tubercle, 212–214, 221, 269
Ala. *See specific anatomical feature*
Alar fascia, 384–385
Alar folds, 268
Alveolar processes, 352–356
Ampulla
   of ductus deferens, 177, 188–189
   hepatopancreatic (of Vater), 123, 125
   of lactiferous duct, 42, 46–47
   semicircular duct, superior, 443, 460
Anal canal, 158, 180–182, 185–186, 188–191,
      208
   arteries, 206
   innervation, 465
   veins, 207
Anal columns, 162–163, 208
Anal sinus, 163
Anal sphincter, 173

Anal triangle
   female, 151
   male, 150
Anastomotic loops between anterior &
      posterior spinal artery, 34
Anatomical neck, 280–281
Anatomical snuffbox, 278, 330–331
Angiogram, coronary, 85
Angle of scapula. *See* Scapula
Angles. *See specific anatomical feature*
Ankle joint actions, 238
Annular tendon, common, 449–450, 452, 456
Annulus fibrosus, 84, 106, 385
Anorectal (pectinate) line, 162–163, 208
Ansa cervicalis, 314, 385, 408, 410–411, 470
   inferior root, 410–411, 469
   superior root, 408, 410–411, 414, 437, 469
Ansa subclavia, 98, 305, 316
Antebrachial fascia, 289
Anterior triangle, 376
Anus, 150–151, 156, 163, 180, 192–203, 205,
      253
   inferior rectal artery, 196
   levator ani muscle, 192
   perineum (perineal body), central tendon,
      181
Aorticorenal ganglia, 172–173, 465–467
Aortic plexus, 146–147
Apex. *See specific anatomical feature*
Aponeuroses
   bicipital, 289, 320, 322, 324–325, 331
   epicranial, 370–371, 404, 426
   external abdominal oblique, intercrural fibers,
      23, 53
   external abdominal oblique muscle, 23, 42,
      52, 54, 56, 174, 311
   internal abdominal oblique muscle, 23, 55
   levator palpebrae superioris muscle, 428–430,
      434–435
   palmar, 278, 289, 324–325, 336–338
   plantar, 264, 270
   plantar, lateral band, 270
   serratus posterior superior muscle, 317,
      332–333
   transversus abdominis, 23, 44, 56–57
   triangular, 335
Appendicular artery, 132
Appendix
   mesoappendix, 141
   vermiform, 49, 111, 132, 134, 136–138, 178
Arachnoid mater, 19, 35, 41
Arches
   of aorta, 28–29, 49, 78–79, 82–83, 86–92,
      94–95, 98–103
   atlas (C1), 10–11, 27, 62–63
   of azygos vein, 30, 96–98
   carpal venous, dorsal, 335
   costal, 285
   cricoid cartilage, 368–369, 417
   dorsal carpal artery, 334–335
   dorsal venous, 233
   dosal carpal, radial branch, 330
   palatoglossal, 351, 402, 420
   palatopharyngeal, 351, 402

palmar
   deep, 296–297, 340
   superficial, 296, 337–338
pelvic fascia, 160–161
plantar, 230–231
plantar arterial, deep, 270–271
Arcuate eminence, 365, 443
Arcuate line of ilium, 23, 44, 48, 153–155
Areola, 2, 66
Arm
   dermatomes, 300–303
   muscles, 286–287
   muscles, anterior, 288–289
   nerves, cutaneous, 300–303
   nerves, deep, 306–307
   skeleton/muscle attachments, 280–283
   surface anatomy, 278–279
   veins, 298–299
Arrector pili muscles, 465
Arterial arcades, 132–133, 135
Arteries, named
   accessory obturator, 175
   alveolar
      anterior superior, 387
      inferior, 387, 413, 436–437
      interior, 386
      middle superior, 387
      posterior superior, 387, 436–437
      superior anterior, 429
      superior posterior, 438, 441
   angular, 408, 412, 428, 436
   aorta, 28–29, 94–95, 117–121, 134, 138,
      146–147
      abdominal, 28–29, 106–107, 134, 140,
         142–143, 164–165, 170, 172–173, 175,
         178, 206, 230, 466–467
      aortic plexus, 146–147, 170
      arch of, 28–29, 49, 78–79, 82–83, 86–92,
         94–95, 98–103
      ascending, 28–29, 49, 81–82
      grooves for, in lungs, 74–75
      intermesenteric (aortic) plexus, 465
      thoracic, 28–29, 78–80, 94–95, 99
      valve, 84, 86, 90
   arcuate, 144, 230–231, 260
   auricular
      deep, 436
      posterior, 386, 404, 412, 419, 436, 438
   axillary, 28–29, 72–73, 296–297, 305,
      312–315, 318–320, 322–323,
   basilar, 34, 387, 389
   brachial, 296–297, 311–312, 314, 320–327,
      337
   brachiocephalic, 28–29
   buccal, 386–387, 432, 436
   carotid
      common, 28–29, 78–79, 81–82, 99, 296,
         410, 414, 436–437
      external, 386–387, 412–416, 433, 436, 458
      interior, 386–387, 411, 418, 423, 433, 451
      internal, 385, 388–389, 392–393, 440–441
      internal (cerebral part), 393
      plexus, internal, 393
      right common, 28–29, 86, 98–99

Arteries, named—*continued*
  carpal, dorsal, 334–335
  carpal arterial rete, dorsal, 297
  central retinal, 431, 433
  cerebellar
    anterior inferior, 388–389
    posterior inferior, 34, 388–389
    right superior, 387
    superior, 388–389
  cerebral
    anterior, 388–389, 399, 440
    circle (of Willis), 389
    left middle, 387
    middle, 388–389
    middle right, 387
    posterior, 34, 388–389, 441
    posterior right, 387
  cervical
    ascending, 28–29, 98, 312, 386, 412
    deep, 98, 386–387
    left ascending, 34
    left deep, 34
    superficial, 386, 406, 408–412
    transverse, 28–29, 98, 297, 386
  chorioidal, anterior, 389
  ciliary
    long posterior, 430–432
    posterior, 434
    short posterior, 432, 435
  circumflex, 296
  circumflex femoral
    lateral, 230–231, 246
    lateral ascending branch, 231
    lateral descending branch, 231
    medial, 230
  circumflex humeral
    anterior, 296–297, 312–316, 318, 320–323
    posterior, 296–297, 310, 314–320, 332–333
  circumflex iliac
    deep, 29, 48, 142, 230, 246
    superficial, 42, 230, 248–249
  circumflex inguinal, 140
  circumflex scapular, 60, 296–297, 314
  colic
    left, 134, 139, 206
    middle, 121, 134–135, 139
    right, 132, 134–135
  collateral
    middle, 296–297, 323
    radial, 296–297, 323
  common hepatic, 121–123, 125, 129, 132, 146–147
  communicating
    anterior, 387–389
    posterior, 387–389
  coronary
    left, 83, 86
      circumflex branch, 83, 86
      marginal branch, 83, 86
    right, 82–83, 86, 89
      marginal branch, 86
      posterior interventricular branch, 83
  cremasteric, 56
  cystic, 118, 120, 123, 136
  digital, dorsal, 230, 260
  digital dorsal, 297
  digital palmar, common, 296
  dorsalis pedis, 230–231, 260, 272
  dorsalis pollicis, 297, 334, 341

dorsal metacarpal, 297
epigastric, 179
  inferior, 28–29, 44, 48, 57, 164–165, 175, 178, 230, 246, 248–249
  superficial, 248–249
  superior, 28–29, 44–45, 48, 51, 72, 311
esophageal, 78, 122–123
ethmoid, 434–435
facial, 386–387, 404–405, 407–409
  transverse, 386, 412
femoral, 28–29, 42, 174, 230–231, 246–249
  deep, 230–231, 246, 248–249, 255–256
  left, 140
  right, 175
femoral triangle, 248–249
fibular (peroneal), 230–231, 262
frontal, 430
gastric
  left, 120–123, 125, 130, 146–147
  right, 120–122
  short, 120–121
gastroduodenal, 121–123, 132
gastro-omental (gastroepiploic)
  left, 120–121, 129
  right, 114, 118–122, 129, 136
genicular
  anastomoses, 230–321
  descending, 230–231, 246–247, 264–266, 269
  inferior lateral, 230–231, 268
  inferior medial, 230–231, 254, 264, 268
  lateral inferior, 246–247, 260–261, 265
  lateral inguinal, 266
  lateral superior, 246–247, 260–261, 265–266, 269
  medial inferior, 246–247, 260, 265–266, 269
  medial superior, 246–247, 260, 265–266, 269
  middle, 230–231, 269
  superior lateral, 230–231, 268
  superior medial, 230–231, 254, 264, 268
gluteal
  inferior, 185–187, 204–206, 230–231, 251–253
  left inferior, 164–165
  left superior, 164
  right inferior, 164–165, 175
  right superior, 165
  superior, 186–187, 204–206, 230–231, 250–253
gonadal, 123, 146
helicine, nerve to, 467
hepatic
  left, 120–121, 123, 130, 136
  proper, 120–123, 126, 128–130, 136
  right, 120–121, 123, 136
ileal, 132, 134
ileocolic, 132–135
iliac
  common, 29, 134, 164–165, 185, 206, 230
  external, 29, 48, 140, 142–143, 164–165, 182–186, 230
  interior posterior division, 206
  internal, 29, 172, 185, 230, 246, 254, 467
  left external, 187
  left interior, 142, 164, 182–185, 188–189, 209
  right common, 134, 142–143, 164–165, 170, 185, 189

  right interior, 164–165, 170–171, 175, 181, 206
iliolumbar, 29, 206, 230
infraorbital, 386–387, 430, 432, 436–438, 441
intercostal, 28–29, 33, 35, 94–98
  anterior, 33, 44–45, 48
  highest, 28, 386–387
  left posterior, 33
  posterior, 33, 35, 98–99, 386–387
  posterior, dorsal branch, 35
  posterior, lateral cutaneous branch, 33
  posterior, right, 33
  posterior, spinal branch of, 33
interlobar, 144
intermesenteric (aortic) plexus, 465
interosseous
  anterior, 296–297, 327–328, 336–337
  common, 296
  posterior, 296–297, 327–328, 330, 335
  recurrent, 297
interventricular
  anterior, 82, 86, 90
  posterior, 86
jejunal, 132, 134–135
labial
  inferior, 386, 436–437
  left posterior, 165
  posterior, 192, 194, 200
  superior, 386, 405, 436
laryngeal, superior, 412, 414–416, 423
legs, 230–231
lingual, 386, 416, 419, 423, 436, 459
lumbar, 28–29
marginal, left, 86–87
marginal (of Drummond), 134
maxillary, 386–387, 412, 432, 436–439, 441
medial plantar artery, deep branch, 231
meningeal
  anterior, 389
  left middle, 387
  middle, 365, 389, 436–438, 442
mental, 386, 436–437
mesenteric
  inferior, 29, 121–124, 134, 139, 165, 170–171
  superior, 29, 121–125, 132, 134–135
metacarpal, dorsal, 296–297, 334–335
metatarsal, dorsal, 230–231, 272
musculophrenic, 28–29, 97, 105
nasal
  dorsal, 429, 433
  external, 428
  lateral, 436
  posterior lateral, 424
  septal, posterior, 424
obturator, 175, 185–187, 230–231
  left, 164–165, 188–189
  right, 164, 206
occipital, 62–63, 386–387, 408
  descending branch, 408, 412, 436
  meningeal branch, 389
  sternocleidomastoid branch, 386
ophthalmic, 386–387, 430, 432–435
ovarian (testicular), 48, 57, 248, 466
  left, 29, 121, 140, 164, 175, 182–184
  right, 28, 121, 140, 164–165
overview, 28–29
palatine
  ascending, 419, 423, 438–439

descending, 436, 439
  greater, 423, 438–439
palmar digital
  common, 338
  proper, 336, 338
palmar metacarpal, 296, 340–341
palmar rete, 340
palpebral, medial, 428–430
pancreaticoduodenal
  anterior inferior, 121, 132
  anterior superior, 121–122
  inferior, 134
  posterior superior, 122, 132
papillary, anterior, 89–91
perforating, 230–231
pericardiacophrenic, 94–97, 102, 104, 314
perineal, 161, 164–165, 195–198
peroneal, 263
pharyngeal, ascending, 419
phrenic
  inferior, 129
  left inferior, 106–107, 140, 146–147
  right inferior, 106–107, 140–142, 146–147
plantar
  lateral, 230–231, 270–271
  medial, 230–231, 270
  medial, superficial branch, 231
plantar digital, 231, 271
plantar metatarsal, 231, 271
pollicis, dorsal, 335
pontine, 388–389
popliteal, 230–231, 250–251, 255–257, 262–264, 267, 269
princeps pollicis, 296, 340
profunda brachii, 296–297, 314, 316, 320
proper digital, 270–272
  dorsal branch, 334
  to thumb, 297
proper digital palmar, 296
pudendal
  external, 52–53, 230, 248–249
  internal, 198–199
  internal, 160–161, 185–187, 193, 200–201, 204–206, 208
  left internal, 164–165
  right internal, 175
pulmonary
  left, 82–83, 89–90, 94–95
  right, 82–83, 89–90, 96–97
radial, 296–297, 324–328, 330–331, 334
  in anatomical snuffbox, 330–331
  dorsal carpal branch, 297, 330, 335
  palmar carpal branch, 296
  recurrent, 296–297, 324, 326–327
  superficial branch, 340
  superficial palmar branch, 296, 324, 338
radialis indicis, 296–297
radicular, 34–35
rectal
  inferior, 192, 194–202, 205–206, 230
  left inferior, 164–165
  left middle, 164–165
  middle, 206
  superior, 134, 140–141, 164–165, 206
renal, 28–29, 144
  left, 107
  right, 142, 146
  ureteric branch, 144
sacral
  lateral, 206, 230, 246, 254

median, 206
  middle, 29, 189, 230
scapular
  dorsal, 28–29, 60, 296, 332–333, 386
  transverse, 312–313, 315
scrotal
  anterior, 52
  left, 164
  left posterior, 164
  posterior, 193, 197
segmental
  anterior inferior, 144
  inferior, 144
  superior, 144
sigmoid, 134, 139, 141, 206
sphenopalatine, 387, 424, 432–433, 438
spinal
  anastomotic loops between anterior & posterior, 34
  anterior, 34, 388–389
  left posterior, 34
  right posterior, 34–35
splenic, 121–123, 125, 146–147
straight, 132
striate, distal medial (recurrent artery of Heubner), 389
stylomastoid, 443
subclavian, 43–45, 48–51, 72, 296–297, 312–316
  left, 28–29, 94–95, 99–100
  right, 28–29, 96–99
subcostal, 28–29, 34, 44
sublingual, 423
submental, 412, 422
subscapular, 28–29, 296–297, 314
supraorbital, 386–387
suprarenal
  inferior, 144, 146–147
  left superior, 140, 142–143, 146
  middle, 146–147
  right inferior, 142
  right middle, 142
  right superior, 142
suprascapular, 28–29, 297, 312, 314, 332–333, 386, 412–413
supratrochlear, 386–387, 453
supreme intercostal, 28
tarsal, 230
temporal
  superficial, 386, 404–405, 412, 428, 436
temporal
  deep, 436
  superficial, 438
thoracic
  interior, 28–29, 33, 42, 312, 314, 322–323
  internal, 28–29, 44–49, 72, 98, 386
  lateral, 30, 46–47, 296, 312–315, 317, 322–323, 332–333
  lateral, mammary branch, 46–47
  left internal, 81, 87, 94, 102–104
  right internal, 96–97, 102–104
  superior, 314–315
thoracoacromial, 312
thoracoacromial trunk, 28–29, 296
thoracodorsal, 50, 60, 296–297, 314–315, 323
thyrocervical trunk, 28–29, 81, 98, 296, 312, 386, 408, 414
thyroid
  inferior, 28–29, 312, 314, 385–386, 412
  superior, 385–386, 407, 410–415, 423, 436–437

tibial
  anterior, 230–231, 260, 263, 268–269
    lateral malleolar branch, 230–231, 260
    medial malleolar branch, 230, 260
  posterior, 230–231, 262–264, 269–270
  recurrent, anterior, 230–231, 260–261, 265
tympanic, anterior, 436
ulnar, 296, 321, 324–327, 337–341
  deep branch, 296
  deep palmar branch, 326, 340
  dorsal carpal branch, 296–297, 335
  opening for passage of, 289
  palmar carpal branch, 296
  superficial palmar branch, 338
ulnar collateral
  inferior, 296–297, 320, 326
  inferior anterior branch, 320
  inferior posterior branch, 320
  superior, 296–297, 320, 323, 332–333
ulnar recurrent
  anterior, 296, 326–327
  posterior, 296–297, 326–327, 332–333
umbilical, 206, 254
  left, 164–165, 188
  right, 164
upper limb, 296–297
ureteric lumbar branch of, 164
uterine, 165
vaginal, 165
vertebral, 28–29, 385–389
  left, 34, 102
  meningeal branch, 389
  right, 34, 103
vesical
  left inferior, 164
  left superior, 164–165
  right inferior, 206
  right superior, 164, 206
zygomaticofacial, 432
zygomatico-orbital, 386, 404–405, 412, 436
Articular process, inferior, 9
Articular surfaces, 268
Articular tubercle, 356, 359, 365
Aryepiglottic fold, 415–417, 420
Arytenoid cartilage, 368–369, 381, 415, 420
  apex, 417
  articular process, 369
  corniculate process, 369
  muscular process, 368–369
  right, 369
  vocal process, 369, 416–417
Atlantooccipital joint, 27, 348
Atlas (C1), 348–349, 426–427
  anterior arch, 10–11
  anterior tubercle, 9–11
  muscle attachments, 4, 6–7
  posterior arch/tubercle, 10–11, 27, 62–63
  transverse process, 10, 25, 27, 62, 285, 383
Auditory (Eustachian) tube, 365, 441
  bony part, 358, 366, 443
  cartilage, 419
  cartilaginous part, 375, 378, 424–425, 443
  cartilaginous plates, 439
  groove, 359
  pharyngeal orifice, 421, 424–427, 439
Auditory meatus
  external, 349–350, 400, 436–437, 460
  interior, 460
Auscultation, triangle of, 58

Automonic nerves, thoraco-abdominal, 465
Axilla
    axillary fold, anterior, 318–319
    axillary line, anterior, 67
    brachial plexus, 314–315
    fossa, 278, 318
    lymph nodes, 43, 46
    radiograph, 319
    sagittal section, 318–319
    vasculature/nerves, 312–313
Axillary fold, posterior, 318
Axillary line
    anterior, 67
    mid, 67
    posterior, 67
Axis (C2), 348–349, 426–427
    body, 417
    dens, 6–11, 27
    spinous process, 10–11, 27, 62–63

B
Back
    muscles, 24–26
Bases. *See specific anatomical feature*
Basilic hiatus, 299–300
Belly. *See specific anatomical feature*
Bicipital groove, medial, 279
Bile ducts
    common, 121, 123–126, 128
    innervation, 465
Bladder. *See* Urinary bladder
Body
    of ischium, 155
    of penis, 2, 150, 174, 177, 193, 195, 205
    of pubis, 154–155, 199, 201, 258–259
    of sphenoid bone, 362–364, 393
    of uterus, 178, 180–184
Bones. *See also specific bones*
    capitata, 282–283, 328, 340–342, 344–345
    carpals, 282–283, 295, 328, 344 (*See also specific bones*)
    cuboid, 214–215, 227, 274–275
    cuneiform, 214–215
        intermediate/medial, 275
        lateral, 227, 274
        medial, 225, 271
        medial/intermediate/lateral, 274
    ethmoid, 352, 354, 357, 448
        cribriform plate, 361, 364, 447–448
        orbital plate, 364
        perpendicular plate, 354, 364, 448
    lunate, 282–283, 328–329, 344–345
    metacarpals, 283, 295, 328, 344–345
        1st, 328–329
        2nd, 330–331
        2nd, base, 289, 291
        3rd, base, 291
        5th, 340–341
        body/head, 345
    metatarsals, 214–215, 225, 227, 275
        1st, 211, 260, 264, 271–272, 274
        2nd, 273
        5th, 272
        5th, base, 223, 227
        5th, tuberosity, 211, 214, 223, 270–271, 274–275
        tuberosity, 210
    nasal, 348–349, 352, 356–357, 359, 364
    navicular, 214–215, 225, 271, 274–275
    occipital, 348–349, 354–357, 359, 361
        base, 359, 383

basilar part, 366, 440
    coronal section, 418–419
parietal, 348–349, 352, 354–357, 359
pisiform, 282–283, 328–329, 337, 341–342, 344–345
scaphoid, 282–283, 328–329, 335, 341, 343–345
sesamoid, 215, 274–275, 329, 345
of skull (*See* Cranium)
trapezium, 282–283, 295, 327–329, 341–345
trapezoid, 282, 328, 344–345
triquetral, 282–283, 328–329, 341, 344–345
vomer, 352, 354, 359, 364, 366, 440, 448
Borders. *See specific anatomical feature*
Brachial plexus, 38–39, 97–100, 103, 305
    anterior divisions, 305
    axilla, 314–315
    inferior trunk, 305–306, 314
    lateral cord, 305–306, 314–315, 413
    medial cord, 305–306, 314
    middle trunk, 305–306, 313–314
    posterior cord, 305–306
    posterior divisions, 305
    superior trunk, 305–307, 314, 323, 412–413
    thyrocervical trunk, 314
    trunks, 316
    upper trunk, 312–313
Brachiocephalic trunk, 28–29, 78–79, 98–99, 296–297
Brain
    angular gyrus, 397
    anterior commissure, 398
    arteries, 388
    caudate nucleus, head/tail, 399
    central sulcus, 397–398
    cerebellum, 396–398, 426–427, 440–441
    cerebral peduncle, 396
    choroid plexus, 398
    claustrum, 399
    confluence of sinuses, 361, 391–393, 399, 426–427
    corpus callosum, 426–427, 440
        genu, 398–399
        splenium, 398
        trunk, 398
    cuneus, 398
    extreme capsule, 399
    falx cerebri, 391–392, 399, 427, 437, 440–441
    fornix, 398–399
    frontal poles, 396–397
    globus pallidus, 399
    gray matter, 19, 35
    gyri
        cingulate, 398
        inferior frontal, 397
        inferior temporal, 397
        medial frontal, 398
        middle frontal, 397
        middle temporal, 397
        postcentral, 397
        precentral, 397
        superior frontal, 397
        superior temporal, 397
        supramarginal, 397
    habenula, 399
    inferior colliculus, 398–399
    inferior parietal lobule, 397
    insula (island of Reil), 399
    interior capsule
        anterior limb, 399

genu, 399
    posterior limb, 399
interventricular foramen (of Monro), 398
lamina terminalis, 398
lateral aperture (foramen of Luschka), 398
lentiform nucleus, 399
lobes
    frontal, 396–397, 426–427
    occipital, 397, 426
    parietal, 397, 426–427
    temporal, 396–397
longitudinal fissure, 396
mamillary bodies, 396, 398, 426
menages, 19, 35
midbrain, 426–427, 442
    inferior colliculus of, 452
    superior colliculus, 451
occipital poles, 396–397
olive, 396–397
optic chiasma, 426, 441
paracentral lobule, 398
pineal body, 398–399
pons, 396–398, 426–427, 440–441, 451
precuneus, 398
preoccipital notch, 397
putamen, 399
quadrigeminal (tectal) lamina, 398
septum pellucidum, 398–399
sinuses
    inferior sagittal sinus/straight sinus, 399
    occipital, 427
    superior sagittal, 398
    superior sagittal sinus/confluence of sinuses, 399
sulci
    calcarine, 397–398
    cingulate, 398
    inferior frontal, 397
    inferior temporal, 397
    intraparietal, 397
    lateral, 397
    lunate, 397
    olfactory, 396
    parieto-occipital, 397–398
    postcentral, 397
    precentral, 397–398
    superior frontal, 397
    superior temporal, 397
superior colliculus, 398–399
superior parietal lobule, 397
temporal poles, 397
tentorium cerebelli, 398
topography, 396–399
trigeminal ganglion, 396
ventricles
    3rd, 399, 426, 440–441
    3rd, choroid plexus, 398–399, 426
    4th, 398, 426–427
    lateral, 399
white matter, 19, 35
Brainstem arteries, 388
Breasts, 42, 46–47, 101
Bregma, 349, 356
Bronchi, 76, 79, 94–100, 102. *See also* Lungs
Bronchomediastinal trunk left, 410
Bronchopulmonary (hilar) lymph nodes, 78–79
Buccal mucosa, 422
Buccopharyngeal fascia, 384–385, 418–419, 423
Bulb. *See specific anatomical feature*

Bulbar conjunctiva, 430–431
Bulb of penis. *See* Penis, bulb
Bulbourethral gland (of Cowper), 157, 160,
        193, 197, 199, 201
Bursa(e)
    deep infrapatellar, 268
    flexor pollicis longus tendon radial, 339
    infrapatellar (subtendinosus), deep, 267
    olecranon synovial, 328
    omental
        lesser sac, 112–113, 136, 141
        splenic recess, 129
        superior recess, 112
    pes anserinus, synovial, 263
    subcutaneous infrapatellar, 263, 268
    subcutaneous prepatellar, 268
    subdeltoid synovial, 312, 316–318
    suprapatellar, 247
    suprapatellar synovial, 268
    synovial, 263, 267
    trochanteric, 246–247
    ulnar, for flexor tendons, 338

C

Calcaneus, 214–215, 271, 273–275
    anterior tubercle, 215
    body, 274
    fibular (peroneal) trochlea, 274
    flexor hallucis longus muscle, groove, 215
    lateral process, 274
    medial process, 274
    sustentaculum tali, 274–275
    tarsal sinus, 274
    tuberosity, 210–211, 215, 273–275
    tuberosity, lateral process, 270, 274
Calvaria, 426–427
Canals. *See specific anatomical feature*
Canine teeth, 351, 364, 366–367
Capitulum, 280, 328–329
Capsule. *See specific anatomical feature*
Cardiac plexus, 465
Carotid arteries. *See* Arteries, named
Carotid body, 462
Carotid canal, 359, 361, 366
    overview, 358
    roof irregular erosion, 365
Carotid sheath, 385, 409, 414
Carotid sinus, 462
Carotid sulcus, 362–363
Carotid triangle, 376
Carpal region, 278
Carpometacarpal joints
    actions, 304
    of thumb, 343
Cartilages
    arytenoid (*See* Arytenoid cartilage)
    corniculate, 368–369, 381, 416–417
    cricoid (*See* Cricoid cartilage)
    thyroid (*See* Thyroid cartilage)
    trachea, 368, 375, 379, 381
Cauda equina, 34, 41
Cavernous sinus, 391–393
Cavity. *See specific anatomical feature*
Cecum, 111, 115–116, 132–134
Celiac ganglia, 122–123, 140, 142, 146–147
Celiac trunk, 28–29, 106–107, 121–124, 140,
        142–143
Cerebellum, 396–398, 426–427, 440–441
Cerebral aqueduct (of Sylvius), 398
Cervical fascia, deep superficial (investing)
        layer, 371, 384–385, 406–407, 410

Cervical ganglion
    inferior, 414, 421
    middle, 98, 414, 420
    superior, 420–421, 424, 451, 458–459
    superior sympathetic, 461
Cervical nerves, 103
Cervical pleura cupola (dome), 314
Cervical plexus, 395, 470
Cervical vertebrae
    articular processes, superior/inferrior,
        10–11
    bifurcated spinous process, 11
    C1 (*See* Atlas (C1))
    C2 (*See* Axis (C2))
    C3 body, 11, 417
    C4
        dorsal ramus, 395, 404
        transverse process, 26, 285
    C5
        body, 385
        dorsal ramus, 395
        transverse process, 8, 10
    C6
        body, 417
        carotid tubercle, 8–11, 348–349
        dorsal ramus, 395
        spinous process, 285
        transverse process, 8–11, 34
    C7 (Vertebra prominens), 3, 8, 70,
        348–349
        body, 10–11
        spinous process, 9, 11, 25, 285
        transverse process, 9
    inferior articular facet, 10–11
    intervertebral foramen, 10–11
    overview, 8–11
    pedicle, 10
    transverse foramen, 10–11
    transverse process, anterior/posterior
        tubercle, 10–11
Cervix, 180–184. *See also* Uterus
Chest, rotator cuff muscles, 316–317
Chiasma, optic, 393, 396, 398, 427
Chiasmatic groove, 361–362
Choanae (interior nares), 358–359, 363, 366,
        418, 448
Chordae tendineae, 90–91
Ciliary body, 431, 451
Ciliary ganglion, 430, 432, 435, 450–451
    nasociliary (sensory) root, 451, 453
    oculomotor (parasympathetic) root, 451
    parasympathetic root, 450
    sympathetic root, 451
Cisterna chyli, 106
Cisterna magna, 426–427
Clavicle, 278, 280–281, 313, 348–349
    costoclavicular ligament, 18
    left superior surface, 414
    ligament attachments, 18
    muscle attachments, 5–6, 42
    radiograph, 101
Clinoid process
    anterior, 354, 361–362, 432, 441
    posterior, 354, 361–363
Clitoris
    anatomical position, 151, 167, 173–174, 198,
        200
    crus, 161, 192, 194, 196, 198, 200
    deep artery, 202
    deep dorsal vein, opening for, 157
    dorsal artery, left, 165

dorsal nerve, 171, 200
prepuce, 151, 174
suspensory ligament, 190, 198
Clivus, 361–362
Coccygeal cornua, 154–155
Coccyx, 150–151,180–184, 212
    muscle attachments, 4–6
    nerve plexi, 243
    overview, 8, 18, 41, 150–151, 154–159,
        162
Cochlea, 460
Cochlear aqueduct, 443
Colon
    ascending, 113, 115–116, 118, 133–134,
        136–137, 139, 178
    descending, 113, 116, 134, 136–139, 141,
        innervation, 465
    transverse, 112, 114–116, 118–120, 136–137,
        139,
    transverse, distal third of, 172–173
Common annular tendon, 449–450, 452, 456
Common hepatic duct, 120, 122–125, 128,
        130, 136
Concha(e)
    of ear (*See* Ears)
    nasal (*See* Nasal conchae)
Condylar canal & fossa, 359
Condylar foramen, 361
Condylar fossa/canal, 358, 360
Condyles. *See specific anatomical feature*
Condyloid emissary vein, 443
Confluence of sinuses, 361, 391–393, 399,
        426–427
Conjoint tendon (falx inguinalis), 23, 54–57
Conus arteriosus, 81–82, 86–87, 89, 101
Conus elasticus, 417, 420
Conus medullaris, 34
Coracoid process. *See* Scapula
Cords. *See specific anatomical feature*
Cornea, 350, 430–431, 441, 449. *See also* Eyes
Corniculate cartilage, 368–369, 381, 416–417
Coronal suture, 348–349, 356
Coronary sinus, 83, 87–88, 90–91
Coronoid fossa, 280, 328
Coronoid process, 356
Corpora cavernosa, 156
Corpus callosum, 398–399, 426–427, 440
Corpus cavernosum, 191, 197, 199
Corpus spongiosum, 156, 160–161
Costal arch, 285, 311
Costal cartilages, 4–5, 18, 45, 48, 68
Costal margins, 2, 4–8, 45, 66, 68
Costal parietal pleura, 48–49, 80, 97
Costal pleura, 45, 103
Costal visceral pleura, 80
Costocervical trunk, 28–29, 99, 386–387
Costochondral articulation, 17–18, 21
Costodiaphragmatic recess, 48, 68–70, 72, 96,
        104–105
Cranial fossa
    anterior, 354, 361, 387, 391
    anterior floor, 353
    foramina/fissures/canals, 360
    middle, 354, 361–363, 387, 391
    posterior, 354, 361, 387, 391, 418
Cranial nerves. *See also specific nerves*
    foramina/fissures/canals, 358, 360
    functions, 446–447, 471
    otic ganglion/taste pathways, 461
    pterygopalatine ganglion, 458
    submandibular ganglion, 459

Cranium
    foramina/fissures/canals, 358, 360
    mandible, 367
    muscle attachments, 352, 354, 357, 359, 366
    orbital/nasal walls, 364
    palate/pharyngeal region, 366
    radiograph, 353, 355
    temporal bone, 365
    topography, 352–354
Cremasteric fascia, 191
Crest. *See specific anatomical feature*
Cribriform fascia, 52–53
Cribriform plates/foramina, 354, 358, 360
Cricoarytenoid joints, 368
Cricoid cartilage, 367–368, 412, 414–415
    arch, 368–369, 417
    lamina, 368–369, 381, 416–418
Cricothyroid joint, 368
    articular capsule, 381
    articular surface, 415
    capsule, 369
    fibrous capsule, 380
Crista galli, 353–354, 361, 364, 430, 448
Crista terminalis, 88, 91
Cruciate ligament, anterior, 266–268
Crus
    of clitoris, 161, 192, 194, 196, 198, 200
    of diaphragm, 106–107, 140, 142–143
    of penis, 160, 177, 193, 195, 197, 199
Cubital fossa, 278–279
Cubital lymph nodes, 308
Cystic duct, 123–126, 128, 136

D

Dartos tunic, 191
Deep infrapatellar bursa, 268
Deltoid tuberosity, 280
Deltopectoral sulcus, 278
Deltopectoral triangle, 2, 66, 278, 299
Deltopectoral triangle, hiatus, 42
Dermatomes
    arm, 300–303
    females, 169
    forearm, 300–303
    head, 394–395
    leg, 234–237
    males, 168
    neck, 394–395
    overview, 36
    shoulder, 300–303
    upper limb, 300–303
Descending aorta. *See Arteries, named*
Diaphragm, 48–49, 79, 93–95, 104–107, 117, 130–131, 146–147
    central tendon, 104–107
    costal portion, 106
    crus, 106–107, 123, 140, 142–143, 146–147
Diaphragmatic parietal pleura, 48, 104
Digastric fossae, 367
Digital extensor tendon, 334
Distal interphalangeal joint (DIP), 343
Dorsalis indicis artery, 334, 341
Dorsalis pedis vein venous rete, 232
Dorsal mesogastrium, 129, 136
Dorsum sellae, 361–362
Ducts, ductules. *See specific anatomical feature*
Ductus deferens, 48, 57, 164, 166, 175, 188–189
Duodenojejunal flexure, 122–124, 129, 139, 141

Duodenum, 68, 118–125, 129–136, 141
Dura mater, 19, 34–35, 41, 429
Dura sac, termination of, 41

E

Ears
    acoustic meatus
        external, 356, 358, 438
        internal, 354, 361, 365,
    ampulla, 443
    antihelix, 350
    antitragus, 350
    auditory (eustachian) tube, 365, 441
        bony part, 358, 366, 443
        cartilaginous part, 375, 378, 424–425, 443
        cartilaginous plates, 439
        pharyngeal orifice, 421, 424–427, 439
    auditory meatus
        external, 349–350, 400, 436–437, 460
        interior, 460
    common crus anterior/posterior, 443
    concha, 350
    cone of light, 442
    crura of antihelix, 350
    foramina/fissures/canals, 358, 360
    helix, 350
    intertragic incisure, 350
    lobule, 350
    mastoid antrum, 443
    occipital condyle, 443
    ossicles, 369
    otic ganglion, 439, 443, 453–454, 461–462
    round window fossa, 442
    scaphoid fossa, 350
    semicircular canals, 443, 460
    semicircular duct, superior, ampulla of, 460
    styloid process, 442–443
    topography, 349–350, 442–443
    tragus, 350
    triangular fossa, 350
    tympanic membrane, 438, 442, 460, 462
        limbus, 442
        pars flaccida, 442
        pars tensa, 442
    umbo, 442
    vestibule, 443
Ejaculatory ducts, 160
Elbow, radiograph, 329
Elbow joint
    actions, 304
    collateral veins, 298–299
    overview, 328
Eminencies
    arcuate, 365, 443
    hypothenar, 278–279
    iliopubic, 152–155, 212, 258
    intercondylar, 212–213, 267, 269
    intertubercular, 215
    thenar, 278–279
Epicardium (serous), 80–81
Epicondyles. *See specific anatomical feature*
Epididymis, 175, 177, 191
Epidural space, 41
Epiglottis, 351, 368–369, 416–421
Erector spinae muscle group
    iliocostalis, 24, 26
    longissimus , 24, 26
    spinalis, 24, 26
Esophageal hiatus, 106–107
Esophageal plexus, 100, 114, 117, 134, 464

Esophagus, 78–80, 94–107, 136, 146–147, 375, 377, 384–385,
    abdominal, 117–120
    groove for, in lungs, 74–75, 92
Ethmoid air cells, 425, 434–435
Ethmoidal air cells, 430
Ethmoidal artery
    anterior, 389
Ethmoidal foramen, posterior, 358
Ethmoid bulla, 425
Ethmoid foramen
    anterior, 358, 360–361, 424–425
    posterior, 360–361
    posterior/anterior, 364
Ethmoid sinus, 353, 448
Extensor (dorsal) expansions, 272, 330, 334–335
Extensor retinaculum, 334
    inferior, 260–261, 264, 272
    superior, 260–261, 264, 272
Extensor tendon, 334
Eyes
    anterior chamber, 431
    bulbar conjunctiva covering sclera, 350
    capsule, 431
    choroid, 431
    ciliary body, 431
    ciliary body/ciliary process, 431
    conjunctiva, 429, 449
    conjunctival sac, inferior fornix of, 429
    cornea, 350, 430–431, 441, 449
    eyeball, 432, 436–437, 439, 449
    foramina/fissures/canals, 358, 360
    infraorbital groove, 364, 432–433
    iridocorneal angle, 431
    iris, 350, 449
        anterior surface, 431
        pectinate ligament, 431
        pupillary margin, 431
    lacrimal lake/lacrimal caruncle, 350
    lacrimal papilla/puncta
        inferior, 350
        superior, 350
    lateral angle, 428–429
    lens, 431, 441
    macula lutea, fovea centralis in, 431
    medial angle, 428–429
    muscles of, 373
    optic disk, 431
    ora serrata, 431
    orbit
        deep, 430
        floor, 435
        lateral margin, 441
        roof, 355, 361, 440, 449
        superficial, 428–429
    orbital fissures
        inferior, 352, 358, 364, 440, 449–450
        superior, 352–353, 358, 360, 362–364, 449–450,
    orbital margins
        superior, 353
    orbital notch (foramen), superior, 452
    orbital wall, superior, 430
    overview, 431
    palpebrae conjunctiva/tarsal glands, inferior, 350
    plica semilunaris, 350
    posterior chamber, 431
    pupil, 350, 431, 449
        ciliary muscle, 451

dilator muscle, 451
 sphincter muscle, 451
retina, 431
 central artery, 435
 non-optic part of (pars ceca), 431
 optic part of, 431
sclera, 350, 430–431, 434, 441, 450
supraorbital margin, 440–441
suspensory ligament (of Zinn), lens, 431
topography, 350

F

Face
 foramina/fissures/canals, 358, 360
 topography, 350, 404–405
Facets. *See specific anatomical feature*
Facial canal, 442, 460
Facial hiatus, 360
Facial nerve (CN VII), 392, 396, 405, 437–443,
  458, 460
 buccal branch, 404–405
 cervical branch, 404, 407, 440
 chorda tympani, 455, 458–459, 461–462
 communicating branch to lesser petrosal
  nerve, 462
 functions, 471
 geniculate ganglion, 461–462
 mandibular branch, 404–405
 overview, 446–447
 temporal branch, 404–405
 zygomatic branch, 404–405
False (minor) pelvis, 153
Falx cerebelli, 393
Falx cerebri, 393, 427, 437
Fascia
 abdominal wall, deep, 36, 42, 53, 190–191
 abdominal wall, superficial
  fatty layer (Camper's), 190–191
  membranous layer (Scarpa's), 52, 160,
   190–191
 cervical
  deep, 371
  superficial, 384–385
 deltopectoral, 299
 endothoracic, 48
 geniohyoid, 384
 iliac, 48
 of infrahyoid muscle, 385
 levator palpebrae superioris muscle,
  429–430
 obturator, 160–161, 186
 pectoral, 46–47
 pelvic, tendinous arch, 160–161
 perineal (Gallaudet's), deep, 192–195
 popliteal, 267
 pretracheal, 384–385
 prevertebral, 384–385, 405, 407, 409, 421,
  425
 rectal, 163, 190–191
 renal, 142, 146
 spermatic
  external, 42, 44, 53–55, 191
  internal, 55–57, 191
 superficial perineal (Colles'), 190–191
 temporal, 405
 thoracolumbar, 3, 50–51, 58–59, 61,
  285, 310
 transversalis, 23, 44, 48, 56–57, 114
 uterovaginal, 190
 vesical, 190–191
 visceral, 171

Fascia lata, 52, 174, 193, 248–249
Fasciculi, transverse, 270, 289
Femoral calcar, 259
Femoral sheath, 43–44, 53–54, 246
Femoral triangle, 248–249
Femur, 213–215, 258–260, 268–269
 articular surface of medial condyle, 268
 greater trochanter, 150–152, 210–213,
  246–247
 head, 212–213, 259
 head, ligament of, 153
 inferior articular surface, 260
 intertrochanteric crest, 213
 lateral condyle, 214–215, 261, 267–269
 lateral epicondyle, 212–215, 225, 268
 lesser trochanter, 152, 212–213
 medial condyle, 212–215, 266–267
 neck, 212–213, 259
 pectineal line, 213, 258–259
 popliteal plane, 266
 shaft, 212
 trochanter, 257
Fibrous digital flexor sheath, 339
Fibula, 212–215, 261–263, 275
 apex, 215
 head, 210, 212–215, 260–261
 head, posterior ligament, 266
 medial crest, 215
 neck, 212, 214
Fibular collateral ligament, 260, 265–268
Fibular (peroneal) retinaculum
 inferior, 223, 261, 270
 superior, 223, 261, 270, 273
Fibular (peroneal) trochlea, 215, 274
Fingers
 distal interphalangeal joint capsule, 335
 distal phalanx of 1st digit, 223
 dorsal expansion, 291
 extensor expansions, 293
 index finger (2nd digit), 278–279
 joint capsule, 343
 little finger (5th digit), 278–279
 lymphatic drainage, 308
 middle finger (3rd digit), 278–279
 phalanges, 215
  base, 291, 295
  base/body/head, 344
  bases, 295
  extensor expansions, 295
  extensor tendon insertion, 335
  middle bodies, 289
  promixal/medial/distal, 337
  promxial/distal, 331
  proximal, 329
  proximal/distal, 330
  proximal/medial/distal, 274, 282–283,
   335, 344
  radiographs, 345
 proximal interphalangeal joint capsule, 335
 ring finger (4th digit), 278–279
 thumb (1st digit) pollex, 278–279
Fissures. *See specific anatomical feature*
Flexor retinaculum (transverse carpal
  ligament), 289, 295, 324, 327, 338–339
Folds
 alar, 268
 palatine, transverse, 423
 rectal, 163, 180–181, 208
 stomach rugae, 130
 umbilical
  left medial, 188–189

 medial, 48–49, 115–116, 178, 206
 median, 115–116, 178, 189
Foliate papillae, 351
Foot
 articular capsule, 272–273, 319
 cutaneous nerve, 240
 distal phalanges, 225, 227
 dorsal surface, 210–211, 272
 lateral malleolus, 275
 ligaments/tendons, 273
 medial malleolus, 275
 muscles, intrinsic, 226–227
 nerves
  intermediate dorsal cutaneous, 240
  lateral dorsal cutaneous, 234, 237
  medial dorsal cutaneous, 240
 phalanges, 214
  1st distal, 275
  1st distal, base/tuberosity, 274
  1st proximal base/body/head, 274
  proximal/medial/distal, 275
 plantar surface, 210–211
 pleural lumbrical muscles, 270–271
 proximal phalanges, 227
 radiographs, 275
 skeleton, 274
 sole, 270–271
 tarsal plate, superior, 428–429
 tarsal sinus, 275
Foramen
 cecum, 351, 360, 402
 lacerum, 358–361, 366, 458
 magnum, 354, 361, 366
 ovale, 90, 358–362, 366, 439–441, 443, 447,
  461–462
 rotundum, 353, 360, 362–363, 447, 449
 spinosum, 358–362, 366, 440
 venosum (of Vesalius), 440
Forearm
 anterior, 327
 anterior, superficial, 324–325
 dermatomes, 300–303
 flexor muscle, 278
 lateral, 330–331
 medial, 336–337
 muscles, 288–293
 nerves, cutaneous, 300–303
 nerves, deep, 306–307
 veins, 298–299
Fornix. *See specific anatomical feature*
Fossa. *See specific anatomical feature*
Fossa ovalis, 88, 91
Frontal bone, 348–349, 352–357
 orbital part, 361, 364
 orbital surface, 352
 zygomatic process, 364, 432, 435
Frontal sinus, 353–355

G

Gait cycle, 229–230
Gallbladder, 68, 70, 117–120, 122–125
 fundus of, 126–127
 innervation, 465
Ganglia
 celiac, 122–123, 146–147, 464–467
 cervical (*See* Cervical ganglion)
 ciliary (*See* Ciliary ganglion)
 geniculate, 459
 glossopharyngeal nerve (CN IX),
  461–462
 impar, 239, 243

Ganglia—*continued*
  mesenteric
    inferior, 140, 172–173, 465–467
    superior, 147, 172–173, 465–467
  otic, 439, 443, 453–454, 461–462
  pterygopalatine, 432–433, 439–441
  renal plexus, 147
  stellate, 79, 94–96, 98–100, 102
  submandibular, 422, 425, 440, 455, 459
  sympathetic, 40, 102
  sympathetic chain, 458–459
  thoracic sympathetic trunk, 94–97
  vestibular, 443, 460
Gastropancreatic fold, 120, 129, 141
Genicular anastomoses, 230–231
Gingiva, 425
Glabella, 348–350, 352, 356
Glands
  bulbourethral (of Cowper), 160, 193
  head, 403
  lacrimal, 403, 434–437
  mammary, 42, 46–47, 101
  neck, 403
  palpebrae conjunctiva/tarsal, inferior, 350
  parathyroid
    inferior, 403
    superior, 403
  parotid, 400, 403–405, 407, 457, 461–462
  pituitary (*See* Hypophysis (pituitary gland))
  prostate, 48, 160, 177, 188–189
  sublingual, 403, 414, 422, 424, 437, 459
  submandibular, 400, 403–405, 407–409, 436,
    459
  suprarenal, 140, 142–143, 146–147
    left, 111, 142–143, 146–147
    right, 140, 142–143, 146
  thymus, 72–73, 95, 97, 414
  thyroid (*See* Thyroid gland)
  vestibular, greater, 196
Glandular lobe, 46–47
Glenohumeral joint
  actions, 304
  capsule, 316, 318, 320–321, 413
Glenoid cavity, 412
Glenoid fossa, 318–319
Glenoid labrum, 318–319
Glossoepiglottic fold, 351
Glossopharyngeal nerve (CN IX), 392, 396,
    418–420, 461
  carotid sinus branch, 462
  functions, 471
  inferior (petrosal) ganglion, 461–462
  overview, 446–447, 462
  right, 424–425
  superior ganglion, 461–462
  vagus nerve communicating branch to, 462
Gluteal fold (sulcus), 210–211
Gluteal line
  anterior, 153, 219, 252–253
  inferior, 153
  posterior, 153, 219, 253
Gluteal region overview, 253–254
Gluteal tuberosity, 213, 219, 258
Gray ramus communicantes, 40–41, 96–97, 243
Greater omentum, 112, 114–119, 248
Grooves. *See specific anatomical feature*
Gyrus, gyri. *See under* Brain

H
Hamate, 282–283, 328–329,
  hook (hamulus), 295, 342, 344–345

Hand
  1st dorsal interosseous muscle, 278
  bones of, 344
  cross section, 341
  dorsal surface, 278–279
  dorsal venous rete, 298–299
  dorsum, 335
  dorsum, superficial, 334
  hypothenar eminence, 278–279
  intertendinous connections, 291
  lateral, 330–331
  ligaments/tendons, 342–343
  lymphatic drainage, 308
  medial, 336–337
  metacarpal bones, 282
  muscles, intrinsic, 294–295
  palm, deep, 340
  palm, intermediate, 339
  palm, superficial, 338
  palmar surface, 278–279
  phalanges proximal/medial/distal, 282
  radiograph, 345
  thenar eminence, 278–279
Hard palate, 378, 401, 421, 423–425, 438–440
Haustra coli, 114, 118, 136–137
Head
  apex, 212–213
  arteries, deep, 387
  arteries, superficial, 386
  cervical fascial planes, 384–385
  dermatomes/cutaneous innervation,
    394–395
  glands, 403
  infratemporal fossa, 436–439
  lymph system, 400–402
  median section, 426–427
  muscle attachments, 366–369
  muscles, superficial, 370–371
  pterygopalatine fossa, 440–441
  topography, 348–351, 404
  veins
    deep, 391
    dural/cavernous sinuses, 392–393
    superficial, 390
Heart, 88
  acute margin, 82
  apex, 81–83, 86–87, 90–91
  arteries, 86
  atria, 80, 82–84, 89
    left, 90
    right, 88, 91, 96–97
  atrioventricular (tricuspid) valve, right, 84,
    88–89
  auricles, 82, 86–91
  coronary angiogram, 85
  cross section, 80
  innervation, 465
  membranous septum, 88
  obtuse margin, 82
  radiograph, 101
  systole/diastole, 84
  valves
    auscultation location, 71
    cusps, 91
    left atrioventricular (bicuspid), 84, 90
    location, 71
    systole/diastole, 84
  veins, 87
  ventricles, 80–83, 86–87, 90–91, 95
Hepatic ducts, 123
Hepatopancreatic ampulla (of Vater), 123, 125

Hilum. *See specific anatomical organ*
Hip joint, 212
  actions, 238
  articular capsule, 153
  overview, 258
  radiograph, 259
Hippocampus, 399
Horns. *See specific anatomical feature*
Humerus, 280, 282–283, 315, 319, 322–324,
    329
  anatomical neck, 319
  body, 289, 316–317
  deltoid tuberosity, 281, 287
  greater tubercle, 6, 280–281
    crest, 285, 316
    inferior facet, 287
    middle facet, 287
  head, 280–281, 289, 318–320
  infraglenoid tubercle, 280
  intertubercular groove, 280, 289, 319
    lateral lip, 285
    medial lip, 280
  lateral epicondyle, 278–283, 326, 328–329
  lateral supracondylar ridge, 280–283, 291
  lesser tubercle, 4, 280, 319
    crest, 280, 287
  medial epicondyle, 278–283, 324–326, 329
  medial supracondylar ridge, 280–283
  scapular notch, 280
  surgical neck, 280–281, 316, 319
Hyoid, 368, 375, 378–379,
  body, 368–369, 380, 424
  greater horn, 368–369, 380–381
  lesser horn, 368–369, 380–381
  muscles, 376–377
Hypogastric (pelvic) plexus, inferior, 170–173,
    182–184
Hypoglossal canal, 354, 358, 360–361, 447
Hypoglossal nerve (CN XII), 392, 408–409,
    420–423, 470
  descending, 408, 410–411, 414, 437
  functions, 471
  muscular branch, 439
  overview, 446–447, 469
Hypophyseal fossa (sella turcica), 354–355,
    361–362,
Hypophysis (pituitary gland), 393, 396, 398,
    425–427
Hypothalamic sulcus, 398
Hypothenar eminence, 278–279

I
Ileum, 114–116, 132–137, 139, 154–155
Iliac crest, 210–213, 258
  muscle attachments, 4, 6–7, 22, 43
  tubercle of, 5–7, 22, 150–155, 204, 212, 258
Iliac fossa, 152, 154–155,
Iliac spines
  anterior inferior, 8, 152–155, 258–259
  anterior superior, 2, 5, 8, 42–44, 111,
    246–248
  muscle attachments, 4–5
  posterior inferior, 5–7, 18, 152–155,
    252–253
  posterior superior, 3, 5–7, 18, 60–61, 258
Iliopubic eminence, 152–155, 212, 258
Iliotibial tract, 50–51, 246–249, 254–257
Ilium, 219
  ala, 213, 258
  body, 154–155, 212–213, 258–259
  gluteal surface, 204

Incisive canals, 358, 364
Incisive fossa/canals, 358, 366, 426–427
Incisor teeth, 351, 364, 366–367, 422–425
Incus, 369, 460
    body, 442
    long crus of, 442
    posterior ligament, 442
    short crus of, 442
Infraglenoid tubercle, 280
Infraorbital foramen, 352, 356, 364, 429, 440
Infraorbital notch/foramen, 358
Infrapatellar fat pad, 267–268
Infrapatellar (subtendinosus) bursa, deep, 267
Infraspinous fossa, 287
Infundibulum
    nasal cavity, 425
    of heart (See conus arteriosus)
    of uterine tube, 182–184
Inguinal fold, left, 150–151
Inguinal ring
    deep, 48–49, 56–57
    superficial, 23, 42, 52–53, 174
Interarytenoid notch, 416
Interatrial septum, 88
Intercavernosus septum, 198
Intercavernous sinuses, 392–393
Intercondylar eminence, 212–213, 215, 267, 269
Intercondylar fossa, 213, 215
Intercondylar groove (of humerus), 280
Intercondylar line, 213, 215
Intercostal membranes, external, 20–21, 50,
    322–323
Intermaxillary suture, 366
Intermuscular groove (white line of Hilton),
    163, 208
Intermuscular septum
    anterior, 263
    medial, 255–256, 323
    posterior, 263
Intermuscular septum, lateral, 255, 323
Interosseous membrane
    (lower limb), 214–215, 268, 272
    (upper limb), 282–283, 327–328
Intersphincteric space, 163
Interspinous plane, 110
Intertendinous connections, 334
Intertransversarius muscle, 61–62
Intertrochanteric crest, 258–259
Intertrochanteric line, 212, 258
Intertubercular eminence, 215
Intertubercular groove floor, 285
Intervertebral discs, 33, 103
    anulus fibrosus, 12, 19
    lumbar vertebrae, 19
    nucleus pulposus, 12, 19, 106, 385, 417
    thoracic vertebrae, 14
Intervertebral foramen, 9–10, 33
Ischial spine, 18, 153–158, 162
Ischial tuberosity, 18, 150–158, 162, 192–204
Ischioanal fossa, 48, 160–161, 208
Ischiopubic ramus, 157
Ischium, 155, 212–213, 258–259

J

Jejunum, 114–116, 118, 120–125
Joints
    acromioclavicular, 319
    actions, 238
    ankle, actions, 238
    atlantooccipital, 27, 348
    capsule, 334, 337, 342

carpometacarpal, 304, 343
cricoarytenoid, 368
cricothyroid (See Cricothyroid joint)
elbow (See Elbow joint)
glenohumeral (See Glenohumeral joint)
hip (See Hip joint)
knee (See Knee joint)
manubriosternal, 18
metacarpophalangeal, 335, 343
metatarsophalangeal, 238
overview, 19
proximal interphalangeal (PIP), 343
radiocarpal, 304
radioulnar, 304
sacroiliac (See Sacroiliac joint)
shoulder, 332–333
sternoclavicular, 18, 411, 413
subtalar, 238
talocrural, 238
temporomandibular, 349–350, 437
tibiofibular, 212, 214, 266
wrist, 328
xiphisternal, 18
zygapophyseal, 19
Jugular foramen, 354, 358, 391, 443, 447, 460,
    463
Jugular fossa, 358–360, 366
Jugular lymph trunk, 78
Jugular (suprasternal) notch, 2, 4, 66, 68, 348,
    409

K

Kidneys. See also under Renal
    anatomical position, 69–70, 139–141, 143,
        146–147
    capsule, 144
    hilum, 144
    inferior pole, 144
    innervation, 465
    lateral margin, 144
    major calyx, 144–145
    medial margin, 144
    minor calyces, 144–145
    overview/vasculature, 144
    peritoneal fat, 121–125, 129
    renal column, 144
    renal papilla, 144
    renal pyramids, 144
    superior pole, 144
    urogram, 145
    veins, 30, 32
Knee
    radiographs, 269
Knee joint
    actions, 238
    articular capsule, 247, 266
    fibrous capsule, 267
    overview, 267–268
    synovial capsule, 254, 267
    transverse ligament, 267–268

L

Labial commissure, posterior, 174
Labium majus, 151, 161, 176
Labium majus (cut edge), 174
Labium minus, 161, 174, 192, 194, 200, 202
Labium minus, 196, 198
Labrum of acetabulum, 153
Labyrinthine artery (internal acoustic artery),
    388–389
Lacrimal artery, 429–430, 432, 434, 441

Lacrimal bone, 352, 356–357, 364
Lacrimal canaliculi, superior/inferior, 403
Lacrimal duct, inferior, 429
Lacrimal ducts, 430, 433
Lacrimal ducts, 429
Lacrimal fossa, 403
Lacrimal gland, 403, 434–437
Lacrimal nerve, 428–430, 453–454,
Lacrimal puncta, 429
Lacrimal sac, 364, 403, 429
Lacrimal vein, 432
Lactiferous ducts, 47
Lambdoid suture, 348–349, 354–356
Lamina terminalis, 426
Large intestine, 172–173
    arteriograph, 135
    colic/splenic flexure, 130, 133–134, 172
    innervation, 465
    overview, 136
    portal vasculature, 138
    ultrasound, 137
    vasculature, 134, 139
Laryngeal prominence, 368, 381, 414–415
Laryngopharynx region, 417–420, 424
Larynx, 426
    aditus, 416, 418
    bones of, 368–369
    infraglottic part, 417
    innervation, 465
    intrinsic muscles, 463
    lateral wall, 417
    left ventricle, 417, 420
    left vestibular (false vocal) fold, 417, 420
    left vocal fold, 417, 420
    left vocal ligament, 417
    muscle attachments, 368–369
    muscles, 379–381
    posterior/superior view, 416
    quadrangular membrane, right, 415
    rima glottidis intermembranous part, 416
    ventricle (entrance), 416
    vestibular (false vocal) fold, 426–427
    vestibular (false vocal) fold, right, 415
    vestibule, 417
    vocal fold, 426–427
    vocal fold, right, 415
Lateral bands, 335
Lateral bicipital groove, 278
Lateral mammary vein, 46
Lateral meniscus, 266–268
Leg
    arteries, 230–231
    cross section, 263
    deep fascia, 245
    dermatomes/cutaneous nerves, 234–237
    lymphatics, superficial, 244
    muscles
        anterior/lateral, 222–223
        posterior, 224–225
    nerves, deep, 240–241
    posterior view/popliteal fossa, 262
    veins, superficial, 233
Levator veli palatini nerve, 463
Ligaments
    annular, 76, 328
    anococcygeal, 156, 190–195, 205
    arcuate
        lateral, 106–107
        medial, 106–107
        popliteal, 262, 266
    pubic, 157–159, 162, 198, 200–203

Ligaments—*continued*
  bifurcate, 273
    calcaneocuboid part, 272–273
    calcaneonavicular part, 273
  calcaneocuboid, dorsal, 273
  calcaneofibular, 273
  capitotriquetral, 340, 342
  carpal arcuate, dorsal, 343
  carpal dorsal, 331
  carpometacarpal, dorsal, 335, 343
  collateral, 272, 334, 337, 342
    distal, 334
    distal radial, 335
    distal ulnar, 335
    interphalangeal, 273
    lateral, 272
    metatarsophalangeal, 273
  coronary, 112, 117, 126–129
  costoclavicular, 18, 410
  cricoarytenoid, posterior, 417
  cricothyroid (conus elasticus), 368–369, 381, 414–415, 417
  cricotracheal, 417
  cruciate, posterior, 266–268
  cuboideonavicular, dorsal, 273
  cuneocuboid, dorsal, 272
  cuneonavicular, dorsal, 272–273
  deltoid, 264, 270–273
  denticulate, 19
  digital fibrous flexor sheath cruciate, 338
  digital retinacular, 334
  falciform, 48, 117, 124
  fibular collateral, 260, 265–268
  gastrosplenic (gastrolienal), 129, 136, 141
  glenohumeral, inferior, 318
  hepatoduodenal, 118–119, 126, 141
  hepatogastric, 118–119, 141
  hepatorenal, 141
  hyoepiglottic, 417
  iliofemoral, 152, 246–247, 258
  ilioinguinal, 54–55
  iliolumbar, 18, 152
  inguinal, 23, 42–44, 52–57, 150–151, 242, 246, 248–249
  interchondral, 18
  interspinous, 19, 61, 153
  ischiofemoral, 152, 258
  lacunar, 248
  of liver (*See* Liver)
  longitudinal
    anterior, 33, 35, 103–104, 106–107,
    posterior, 19, 33, 35, 103
  meniscofemoral
    anterior, 267
    posterior, 266–267
  metacarpal
    deep transverse, 339–340, 342
    superficial, 289
    superficial transverse, 338
  metatarsal
    dorsal, 272
    superficial transverse, 270
  palmar, 342
  palmar carpal, 289, 324–325, 336, 338
  palmar carpometacarpal, 342
  palmar radiocarpal, 328, 339–340, 342
  palmar radioulnar, 342
  palmar ulnocarpal, 328, 339–340, 342
  palpebral, 430
    medial, 428–429

  patellar, 210, 212, 217, 246–247, 254, 260–261
  perineal, transverse, 157, 159, 199–201
  phrenicocolic, 129
  pisohamate, 289, 342
  pisometacarpal, 289, 342
  plantar, long, 271, 273
  plantar calcaneocuboid, 273
  plantar calcaneonavicular (spring), 271, 273
  popliteal, oblique, 262, 266
  pubofemoral, 153, 247, 258
  puboprostatic
    lateral, 195, 199
    right, 160
  pubovesical, left lateral, 161
  radial collateral, 328, 339–340, 342–343
  radiate sternocostal, 18
  radiocapitate, 342
  radiocarpal, dorsal, 328, 335, 343
  radioscapholunate, 342
  radiotriquetral, 342
  radioulnar, dorsal, 328, 335, 343
  sacrococcygeal, posterior, 18
  sacroiliac
    anterior, 152–153, 247
    posterior, 18, 152–153, 252–253
  sacrospinous, 18, 152–153, 204, 250–252
  sacrotuberous, 18, 150–153, 250–253, 258
  sacrum, attachments, 18
  splenorenal (lienorenal), 113, 129, 136
  sternoclavicular, 409, 411
  sternum, attachments, 18
  stylohyoid, 368, 375, 379
  stylomandibular, 438
  supraspinous, 19, 152–153
  suspensory
    of breast, 46–47
    of clitoris, 190, 198
    of ovaries, 178
    of penis, 42–43, 170, 188, 191
  talocalcaneal, 273
  talofibular, 272–273
  talonavicular, dorsal, 273
  tarsometatarsal, dorsal, 272–273
  thyroepiglottic, 368, 380–381
  thyrohyoid, 416
    lateral, 368, 381, 419
    medial, 368, 381, 417
  tibial collateral, 246–247, 260, 262, 264–268
  tibiofibular
    anterior, 272–273
    posterior, 273
  tibionavicular, 273
  tibiotalar
    anterior, 273
    posterior, 273
  transverse acetabular, 153
  transverse carpal (*See* Flexor retinaculum (transverse carpal ligament))
  ulnar collateral, 328, 340, 342–343
  umbilical
    medial, 164-165, 178–179
    median (urachus), 164–165, 176–178
  vocal, 369, 380
Ligamentum
  arteriosum, 82, 86, 89–90, 94, 100, 102
  flavum, 18–19, 35
  nuchae, 3, 25–26, 60, 285, 384–385, 426
  venosum, 126–127
Linea alba, 2, 23, 42–44, 72–73, 174, 178, 190–191

Linea aspera, 213, 221
Lingual tonsils/lingual follicles, 351, 401–402, 417–420
Lingula, 367
Lips
  commissure, 350
  inferior, 350, 422
  superior, 350, 422
  superior tubercle, 350
Liver
  anatomical position, 68–70, 112–113, 130, 132–134
  anatomical/surgical divisions, 126–127
  bed, 129
  caudate lobe, 123, 126–127
  colic (hepatic) flexure, right, 118, 130, 133–134, 137–139
  colic impression, 126–128
  coronary ligament, 112, 117, 126–129
  diaphragmatic surface, 126–127
  duodenal impression, 126–128
  esophageal impression, 127–128
  falciform ligament/round ligament, 68, 117, 124, 126–129
  innervation, 465
  lobes, 114–115, 117–119, 126–128
  peritoneal ligaments, 128
  renal impression, 126–128
  triangular ligament, 69, 126–127, 141
Lower limb surface anatomy, 209–210
Lumbar plexus, 242
Lumbar triangle, 58
Lumbar vertebrae
  accessory process, 15
  articular process, superior/inferior, 15, 19
  body, 15
  intervertebral disc, 19
  intervertebral foramen, 19
  L1 spinous process, 281
  L2 spinous process, 26
  L3
    body, 8
    spinous process, 5, 9
    transverse process, 5, 7, 9
  lamina of vertebral arch, 15
  mamillary process, 15
  pedicle, 15, 19
  spinous process, 15, 19
  transverse process, 15, 18–19, 135
Lumbosacral trunk, 186–187, 239–243
Lumbosacral trunk, 189
Lunate, 282–283, 328–329, 344–345
Lungs
  anatomical position, 100, 111, 118, 123, 146
  apex, 69, 74–75
  areas
    esophageal, 74–75
    for thymus & mediastinal fatty tissue, 74–75
    for trachea, 74–75
  bronchus, left inferior lobe, 79
  cardiac notch, 68, 72, 74, 81
  cross section, 80
  cupula of pleura over apex, 68, 70
  fissures
    horizontal, 68–70, 72, 74
    oblique, 68–70, 72–75
  grooves
    for arch of aorta, 74
    for azygous vein, 74–75
    for descending aorta, 74–75

for esophagus, 74–75, 92
  for left subclavian artery, 74–75
  for right brachiocephalic vein, 74–75
  for superior vena cava, 74–75
hilum, 74–75
innervation, 465
lingula, 74–75
lingular division, 76–77
lobes
  inferior, 68–70, 72–75, 78, 111
  middle, 69–70, 72, 74–75
  segments, 76–77, 92
  superior, 68–70, 72–75
mediastinal surface, 74
overview, 74–75
pulmonary artery/vein, 75
pulmonary ligament, 74–75
pulmonary lymph nodes, 74
Lymphatic trunk right, 410, 414
Lymphatic vessels, 46, 244–245
Lymph nodes
apical, 46
apical axillary, 410
axillary, 43, 46
brachial, 308–309
bronchomediastinal lymph trunk, left, 78
bronchomediastinal trunk, right, 78
bronchus, left main, 78–79
buccal, 400
cecal, 133
central axillary, 308–309
cervical, 385
  deep, 309, 400–402, 405–406, 409
  scalene, inferior deep, 46, 78
  superficial, 400, 406–407
facial drainage, common, 400
hepatic, 123
ileocolic, 133
iliac
  common, 140
  external, 182–184, 188–189
  inferior, 183–184
  interior, 182, 188
  right common, 175
  right external, 175
  right interior, 175
infrahyoid, 401
inguinal, deep, 174–175, 244, 249
inguinal, highest deep, 174
inguinal, superficial, 52
  distal group, 174, 244
  horizontal group, 174
  proximal group, 174, 244
  vertical group, 174
internodal group drainage, 401
intestinal trunk, 106
jugulodigastric, 401–402
jugulo-omohyoid, 400–401
lateral, 46
lateral aortic, 175
lumbar, 140
lumbar trunks, 106
mediastinal, posterior, 98, 105
mesenteric, 133, 146–147
occipital, 400
pancreaticoduodenal, 123
para-aortic, 146–147
pararectal, 175
parasternal, 46, 309
paratracheal, 46, 402, 414
parotid, 400

pectoral, 46, 308–309
popliteal, 245
preaortic, 175
prelaryngeal, 402
presymphyseal, 175
pretracheal, 402
promontory (middle sacral), 175
pulmonary, 78
renal, 147
retroauricular, 400
retropharyngeal, 401
sacral, 175
segmental bronchus, 78
subclavian, 46, 308–309
subclavian trunk, 78
sublingual, 422
submandibular, 400–402
submental, 400, 402
subscapular, 308
superior tracheobronchial, 99
supraclavicular, 308–309
tracheal, 78
tracheobronchial (carinal), inferior, 78–79
Lymph system
femoral triangle, 248–249
head/neck, 400–402
jugular trunk, 78
leg, lymphatic system, 244–245
lymphatic trunk, right, 309, 411
small intestines, 133
superficial, 174, 308
thigh, posterior, 250–251
thoracic, 105
trachea/bronchi/lungs, 78
upper limb, 308–309

M
Males
bony pelvis, 154
dermatomes/cutaneous nerves, 168
pelvic arteries, 164
pelvic autonomic nerves, 172, 467
pelvic contents, 188–189
pelvic muscles, 160
pelvic veins, 166
perineum, 193, 195, 197, 199, 201, 203
peritoneal fasciae/spaces, 191
topography, 150
urogenital tract, 177
Malleolus, 442
lateral, 210–211, 214–215, 233, 270–273
lateral, rete of, 231
medial, 210–211, 214–215, 233, 270–273
medial, rete of, 230
Malleus, 369
anterior process, 442
head, 442
lateral process, 442
manubrium, 442, 460
Mammary glands, 42, 46–47, 101
Mandible, 352, 357, 367
alveolar process, 367
angle, 352–355, 359, 366–367
body, 354–356, 367
condylar process, 366–367
coronoid process, 367
mental (genial) spines, 367
muscle attachments, 367
neck, 366–367
ramus, 348–349, 352–354, 356, 367
symphysis, 417

Mandibular canal, 358
Mandibular foramen, 367
Mandibular fossa, 359, 365, 438–439
Mandibular notch, 356, 367
Mandibular symphysis, 354–355, 384, 420–425
Manubriosternal joint, 18
Manubrium, 4–5, 18, 68, 72–73, 316
Mastoid air cells, 438, 442, 460
Mastoid antrum, 438
Mastoid canaliculus, 358
Mastoid foramen, 358, 360–361, 365
Mastoid process, 26, 348–349, 352–353, 356,
  364–365
Maxilla, 352, 354, 357, 359, 364
alveolar process, 424–425, 440
frontal process, 356, 364, 429
infratemporal surface, 440
palatine process, 359, 364, 366
zygomatic process, 366
Maxillary sinus, 353, 355, 432–433
McBurney's point, 111
Meatus
acoustic
  external, 358, 365,
  interior, 354, 361, 441, 443, 447
  internal, 360
auditory, 349–350, 400, 436–437, 460
nasal
  anterior, 358
  inferior, 364, 425, 429, 439
  middle, 358, 364, 425, 449
  superior, 358, 364, 425
urethral, 150–151, 156, 174, 194
Median (midsagittal) plane, 66–67, 110–111
Median sulcus, 351, 402
Median umbilical ligament/fold, 178
Mediastinal parietal pericardium, 93
Mediastinal parietal pleura, 48, 93, 104
Mediastinal visceral pleura, 80
Mediastinum, 80, 93–97
Medulla oblongata, 396–398, 426–427
Meniscus, medial, 266–268
Mental foramen, 352, 356, 358
Mental (genial) spine, 423
Mental protuberance, 348–350, 352–353,
  356
Mental tubercle, 352
Mentolabial sulcus, 350
Mesenteric ganglion
inferior, 140, 172–173, 465–467
superior, 147, 172–173, 465–467
Mesentery, 116, 129–130, 132–133, 136, 139,
  141
Mesoappendix, 141
Mesocolons
sigmoid, 141, 180–181
transverse, 112, 129–130, 134, 141
Metacarpophalangeal joints, 335, 343
Metatarsophalangeal joints, 238
Midaxillary line, 67
Midclavicular line, 66, 110
Midinguinal line, 110–111
Midscapular line, 67
Molar teeth, 366–367
Mons pubis, 151, 196, 198, 200
Mouth. *See* Oral cavity
Muscles, named
abdominal oblique
  external, 22–23, 42–45, 50, 54
  internal, 22–23, 43–44, 50–51, 54
abdominal wall, 22–23

Muscles, named—*continued*
abductor digiti minimi (of foot), 226–227, 261, 270–272,
abductor digiti minimi (of hand), 294–295, 334–335
abductor hallucis, 226–227, 264
abductor pollicis brevis, 294–295, 324–325, 338, 341
abductor pollicis longus, 279, 282–283, 327, 330–331
  attachments, 282–283
  Compartment I, 334
  tendons (Compartment I), 341, 334–335
adductor, 210
adductor brevis, 196, 212–213, 220, 247–249, 255–256
adductor hallucis, 270–271
  oblique head, 227, 271
  overview, 226
  transverse head, 227, 271
adductor longus, 211–213, 220–221, 246, 248–249
adductor magnus, 211, 221, 246–248, 250–252,
  attachments, 212–213, 215
  overview, 220
  tendon, 247, 250–251, 255–256, 262, 268
adductor pollicis, 326, 330–331, 336–338, 341
  oblique head, 339–340
  overview, 294
  transverse head, 339–340
adductor pollicis brevis, 336–337
anal sphincter
  external, 156, 159, 162–163, 192–203,
  internal, 162–163
anconeus, 278–279, 286
arrector pili, 465
articularis genus, 212, 247, 255–256, 264, 268
aryepiglottic, 381, 415–417
arytenoids
  oblique, 380–381
  overview, 380
  transverse, 380–381, 416–417
  attachments, 368–369
auricularis
  anterior, 370
  posterior, 370, 404–405
  superior, 370, 404
axillary, 313
biceps brachii, 278–279, 325, 328, 331
  attachments, 280, 282
  common belly, 320
  long head, 280–281, 289, 311–313
  long head tendon, 318–319
  overview, 288
  short head, 280, 289, 311–313, 315, 319–320, 322, 324
  short head tendon, 318
  tendon, 43, 289, 322, 328
biceps femoris, 152, 210–214, 246, 266–267
  attachments, 212–214
  lateral head, 266
  long head, 219, 250–252, 254–257
  long head tendon, 258, 262, 266
  overview, 218
  short head, 219, 250–251, 254–257
  tendon, 260–261, 265
brachialis, 280–281, 289, 321, 323–326,
  attachments, 280–282
  overview, 288

brachioradialis, 291, 320–328
  attachments, 280–283
  overview, 290
  tendon, 278, 327, 338–339
buccinator, 404–405, 422, 436–437, 439, 441
  attachments, 352, 357, 367
bulbospongiosus, 156, 159–161, 175
chest, rotator cuff, 316–317
ciliary, 431, 451
coccygeus, 158–159, 162–163
common extensor, tendons, 280, 282
common flexor, tendons, 280–281, 326
  attachments, 280–282
constrictor
  inferior, 378
  middle, 378
  superior, 378
coracobrachialis, 280, 288, 305, 313–315
cremaster, 22–23, 43, 54–57
cricoartenoid, lateral, 415
cricoarytenoid
  lateral, 380–381, 415, 417, 420
  attachments, 368–369
  overview, 380
  posterior, 368–369, 380–381, 415–417
cricothyroid, 375, 379–381, 410, 414–415, 463
  attachments, 368–369
  innervation, 463
  overview, 380
deltoid, 2–3, 42–44, 58–60, 278–281, 287
  attachments, 280–281
  overview, 286
depressor anguli oris, 352, 370–371, 406, 411
depressor labii inferioris, 352, 370–371
digastric
  anterior belly, 376–377, 402, 408–414
  attachments, 359, 367
  intermediate tendon, 414, 422, 437
  intermediate tendon/fibrous loop, 376–377
  overview, 376
  posterior belly, 376–377, 402, 408, 412–413
epicranial
  attachments, 357
  frontal belly, 370–371, 404–405, 428
  occipital belly, 370, 404–405, 408
erector spinae, 40, 60–61, 178, 310, 332
extensor carpi radialis brevis, 278, 280, 282–283, 291, 327, 330
  attachments, 280, 282–283
  Compartment II, 334–335
  overview, 290
  tendon, 331, 341
extensor carpi radialis longus, 278, 280, 282–283, 291, 327, 330
  attachments, 280, 282–283
  Compartment II, 334–335
  overview, 290
  tendon, 331, 338–339
  tendon (Compartment II), 341
extensor carpi ulnaris, 279–280, 282–283, 327, 330, 336–337
  attachments, 282–283
  Compartment VI, 334
  overview, 290
  tendon, 334, 341
extensor digiti minimi, 280, 293, 327

  overview, 292
  tendon, 334–335, 341
extensor digitorum, 278–280, 291, 327–328, 330, 332–333
  attachments, 283
  common, tendons, 282–283
  Compartment IV, 334
  overview, 290
  tendon 1 Compartment IV, 341
  tendons, 278–279, 331
  tendons 3–5, 341
  tendons Compartment IV, 334–335
extensor digitorum brevis, 261, 272
extensor digitorum longus, 210, 214, 246, 260–261, 263, 265
  attachments, 214
  tendon, 210, 260–261, 272
  tendon sheaths, 272
extensor hallucis brevis, 260–261, 272
extensor hallucis digitorum longus, 222
extensor hallucis longus, 214, 223, 260, 263
  attachments, 214
  overview, 222
  tendon, 210, 223, 260–261, 264, 272–273
  tendon sheath, 272
extensor indicis, 282–283, 293
  attachments, 283
  Compartment IV, 334–335
  overview, 292
  tendon Compartment IV, 341
extensor pollicis brevis, 279, 282–283, 327, 330–331
  attachments, 283
  Compartment I, 334
  overview, 292–293
  tendon, 278, 331, 334–335, 341
extensor pollicis longus, 282–283, 293, 327, 330–331
  attachments, 283
  Compartment III, 334
  overview, 292
  tendon, 278–279, 331, 341
femoral triangle, 248–249
fibularis (peroneus) brevis, 214, 223, 260–263
  attachments, 214
  overview, 222
  tendon, 261, 273
fibularis (peroneus) longus, 214, 223, 246–247, 254, 260–263
  attachments, 214–215
  overview, 222
  tendon, 223, 270–273
  tendon groove, 274
fibularis (peroneus) tertius, 210, 214, 223
  attachments, 214
  overview, 222
  tendon, 260–261, 272
flexor carpi radialis, 279–281, 289, 320, 322–326, 336
  attachments, 282
  overview, 288
  tendon, 278, 325–327, 330–331, 338–340
  tendon, synovial sheath, 338
  tendon sheath, 339
  tendon synovial sheath, 338
flexor carpi ulnaris, 280–283, 320–321, 336–338
  attachments, 282–283
  humeral head, 282–283, 326

overview, 288
    tendon, 278–279, 327, 341
flexor digiti minimi, 271, 295, 338–339
flexor digiti minimi brevis, 226–227, 273, 294
flexor digitorum brevis, 226–227, 270
flexor digitorum longus, 215, 224–225, 262–264, 273
    tendon, 227, 271, 273
    tendons, 211
    tendons, flexor sheaths, 270
flexor digitorum profundus, 282–283, 290–291, 337
    tendons, 295, 339, 341
flexor digitorum superficialis, 278, 282, 324–327, 336–337
    humeroulnar head, 280–281, 289, 324–325
    overview, 288
    radial head, 289, 324–325
    tendons, 338–339, 341
    tendon to digit V, 337
flexor hallucis brevis, 226–227, 264, 270–271
flexor hallucis longus, 215, 225, 262–264, 273
    attachments, 215
    groove for, 215
    overview, 224
    tendon, 270–271, 273
    tendon, flexor sheath, 270–271
    tendon groove, 274
flexor pollicis brevis, 294–295, 324, 336–339, 341
flexor pollicis longus, 326–328, 337
    attachments, 282
    overview, 290
    tendon, 324, 338–339, 341
    tendon radial bursa, 339
gastrocnemius, 213, 264–265
    attachments, 213, 215
    lateral head, 210, 213, 215, 250–251, 254, 266–268
    medial head, 210–211, 213, 215, 250–251, 262–263,
    overview, 224
    sagittal section, 264
gemellus
    inferior, 204, 213, 218, 243, 250–253
    superior, 204, 213, 218, 243, 250–253
genioglossus, 375, 377, 379, 417, 420, 423–424, 426–427
    attachments, 354, 367–368
    overview, 374
geniohyoid, 375, 377, 379, 417, 420–424, 426–427, 440, 470
    attachments, 367–369
    nerve to, 469
    overview, 376
gluteus maximus, 3, 58, 192–196, 210–211, 217, 219, 253–254
    attachments, 213
    gluteal fascia, 217
    overview, 218
gluteus medius, 210–211, 213, 219, 246–247, 250–254
    attachments, 213
    gluteal fascia, 217
    overview, 218
gluteus minimus, 212–213, 219, 246–247, 250–253
    overview, 218

gracilis, 211–212, 214, 221, 246–252, 254–257
    attachments, 212, 214
    overview, 220
    tendon, 210–211, 254, 265–267
hyoglossus, 368, 374–375, 377, 379, 420, 423, 438
hypothenar, 336
iliacus, 178, 185–189, 212, 216, 242
iliococcygeus, 158–159, 162–163
iliocostalis, 7, 24, 26, 51, 60–61, 310, 332–333
    aponeurosis, 317
    attachments, 7
iliocostalis cervicis, 24, 26
iliocostalis lumborum, 24, 26
iliocostalis thoracis, 24, 26
iliopsoas, 212–213, 216, 246, 248–249
    attachments, 212–213
    tendon, 242
iliotibial tract, 212, 214
infrahyoid, 384–385, 409
infraspinatus, 50, 58, 281, 286–287, 310, 317
intercostal, 40, 43–45, 48, 50–51, 60–61
    external, 20–21, 33, 43, 45, 48, 50
    innermost, 20, 33, 44, 48, 51
    internal, 20–21, 33, 44–45, 48–49, 51
interosseous (of foot), 226, 272–273,
interosseous (of hand), 294–295, 328, 330–331, 334–335
intertransversarius, 61–62
ischiocavernosus, 156, 159–161, 192–198, 200–202
latissimus dorsi, 3, 44, 58–59, 278–280, 285, 310, 318
    attachments, 5–6, 280
    overview, 284
    tendon, 322–323
levator anguli oris, 352
levator ani, 158–164, 185–188
levatores costarum brevis, 7, 20, 61
levatores costarum longus, 7, 20, 61
levator labii superioris, 352, 370–371
levator labii superioris alaeque nasi, 352, 428
levator palpebrae superioris, 373, 428–430, 432
levator scapulae, 281, 284–285, 317, 332–333, 385
levator veli palatini, 359, 366, 374–375, 420, 425,
longissimus, 7, 24, 26, 60–61,
longissimus capitis, 24, 26, 359, 418–419, 437
longissimus cervicis, 24, 26
longissimus thoracis, 24, 26, 317
longitudinal, inferior, 375
longus capitis, 359, 382–383, 385, 418, 421
longus cervicis, 418
longus colli, 95, 97, 100, 102, 382–383, 385, 421
lumbricalis, 227, 295, 327
    1st, 338–339, 341
    2nd, 339
    3rd, 339, 341
    4th, 339
    overview, 226, 294
masseter, 370–371, 404–406, 408
    attachments, 352, 357, 359, 367
    nerve to, 438
    overview, 372

mentalis, 352, 370–371
multifidus, 24–25, 61, 63
musculus uvulae, 359, 366, 374
mylohyoid, 375–377, 411, 414–415, 420–422
    attachments, 354, 367–368
    overview, 376
nasalis, 370–371, 404, 428
obliquus capitis inferior, 27, 62–63
obliquus capitis superior, 27, 63, 359
obturator externus, 195, 197, 200, 202, 212, 220, 247
obturator internus, 186, 202–208, 213, 250–252
    attachments, 213
    fascia, 203
    membrane, 48, 160, 162–163
    nerve to, 204, 243, 250–252
    overview, 218
    tendon, 204
omohyoid, 305, 311, 316, 385
    attachments, 368
    inferior belly, 317, 332–333, 376–377, 408
    inferior belly, nerve to, 469
    intermediate tendon, 408–409
    intermediate tendon, fascial loop, 376–377
    overview, 377
    superior belly, 376–377, 406–411, 414, 469–470
    superior belly, nerve to, 469
opponens digiti minimi, 294, 337–339, 341
opponens pollicis, 294, 324, 326, 328
opponens pollicis brevis, 339
orbicularis oculi, 405, 428
    attachments, 352
    orbital part, 370–371, 404, 428
    palpebral part, 370–371, 404, 428–429
orbicularis oris, 370–371, 422–424
palatoglossus, 374–375, 420, 463
palatopharyngeus, 351, 374–375, 402, 424
palmar interosseous, 294–295, 339–341
palmaris brevis, 324–325, 337–338
palmaris longus, 280–281, 289, 320–327, 336
    overview, 288
    tendon, 278–279, 325, 337–338
papillary, posterior, 89–91
pectineus, 196, 212–213, 246–249, 257
    attachments, 212–213
    nerve to, 239–240
    overview, 220
pectoralis major, 2, 5, 42, 45, 285, 318–320
    abdominal head, 285, 311
    attachments, 5, 280
    clavicular head, 285, 311, 406, 410–411
    overview, 284
    sternocostal head, 285, 311
pectoralis minor, 5, 43, 50, 280, 285, 311, 315
    attachments, 5, 280
    overview, 284
perineal, 201
    deep transverse, 157, 159, 198–199, 201
    superficial transverse, 156, 159, 194–197
pharyngeal, 378–379
pharyngeal constrictor, 426–427
    inferior, 375, 385, 414–418, 420, 424, 440, 463
    attachments, 368–369
    cricopharyngeal portion, 379
    left, 419

Muscles, named
  pharyngeal constrictor—*continued*
    raphe, 419
    thyropharyngeal portion, 379
    middle, 368–369, 375, 379, 418–420, 463
    right inferior, 378
    right middle, 378
    right superior, 378
    superior, 375, 379, 418–420, 423, 438–440, 463
      attachments, 354, 359, 366–367
  piriformis, 162–163, 185–189, 207, 247
    attachments, 212
    nerve to, 243
    overview, 218
  plantar interosseous, 226–227, 271
  plantaris, 213, 215, 250–251, 262–263, 265–268
    attachments, 213, 215
    overview, 224
    tendon, 262–263
  platysma, 36, 370–371, 406–407457
    attachments, 352, 357
  popliteus, 213, 215, 225, 262, 265–266, 268
    attachments, 213, 215
    overview, 224
    tendon, 266–267
  procerus, 371, 428
  pronator quadratus, 282, 288–289, 339–340
  pronator teres, 282–283, 289, 328, 337
    attachments, 280, 282–283
    humeral head, 280–281, 324
    overview, 288
  psoas major, 106–107, 142–143, 175, 212, 239
  psoas minor, 140, 178, 212, 239, 242
    attachments, 212
    overview, 216
    tendon, 186–187
  pterygoids
    lateral, 438
      attachments, 354, 357, 359, 366–367
      inferior head, 455
      overview, 372
      superior head, 455
    medial, 376, 422, 425, 436–438, 441, 455
      attachments, 354, 359, 366–367
      nerve to, 438
      overview, 372
  pubococcygeus, 158–159, 162–163
  puboprostatic, 203
  puborectalis, 158–159, 162–163, 186
  quadratus femoris, 204–206, 212–213, 247, 252–253
    attachments, 212–213
    nerve to, 243
    overview, 218
  quadratus lumborum, 22, 106–107, 239, 242
  quadratus plantae, 226–227, 264, 271
  quadriceps femoris, 210, 212, 214, 216–217, 250–251
  radius extensor pollicis longus, groove, 328
  rectus (extrinsic muscles of eyeball)
    inferior, 373, 435, 439, 441, 449–450
    lateral, 373, 432–437, 441, 449–450
    medial, 373, 430, 433–435, 449–450
  rectus abdominis, 178
    anatomical position, 22–23, 43–45, 51, 56, 73
    attachments, 5, 43
    tendinous inscription in, 2, 43–45

rectus capitis anterior, 359, 421
rectus capitis lateralis, 359, 421
rectus capitis posterior major, 27, 62–63, 359
rectus capitis posterior minor, 27, 63, 359
rectus femoris, 210, 212–213, 217, 248–249, 265
  attachments, 212–213
  overview, 216
  tendon, 152–153, 217, 258
rhomboid major, 6, 40, 60, 281, 285, 310
  attachments, 6, 281
  overview, 284
rhomboid minor, 6, 60, 281, 285, 310, 408, 412
  attachments, 6, 281
  overview, 284
risorius, 370–371
rotator cuff, 316–317
rotatores, 24–25, 61
salpingopharyngeus, 378, 424
sartorius, 210–214, 217, 246, 248–249, 264–267
  attachments, 212–214
  overview, 216
  tendons, 210–211, 254
scalenes
  anterior, 100, 102–103, 312–315, 370, 376, 408–414
  overview, 382
  middle, 305, 314, 382–383, 385, 401, 408–409, 421
  posterior, 50, 61–62, 382–383, 385, 412–413, 421
semimembranosus, 213, 215, 219, 250–252, 254–257
  attachments, 213, 215
  overview, 218
  tendon, 262, 265–266
semispinalis, 7, 24–25
semispinalis capitis, 24, 58, 60–63, 310, 408, 412
  attachments, 359
semispinalis cervicis, 24, 62–63
semispinalis thoracis, 24, 61
semitendinosus, 211–214, 250–252, 262, 264
  attachments, 212–213
  overview, 218
  tendons, 211, 254, 266–267
septal (medial) papillary, 89
serratus anterior, 5, 42–44, 50, 278, 310–312, 321–323
  attachments, 5, 280
  overview, 284
serratus posterior inferior, 20, 50, 60, 310
  attachments, 7
serratus posterior superior, 20, 50, 60, 310
  aponeurosis, 317, 332–333
  attachments, 7
skeletal attachments, 4–7
soleus, 210–211, 215, 260–265, 268
  attachments, 215
  overview, 224
sphincter urethrae, 157, 159–161, 199
spinalis, 7, 26, 60–61, 310, 332–333
spinalis capitis, 24
spinalis cervicis, 24, 60–62
spinalis thoracis, 24, 26, 317
spinous cervicis, 26
splenius capitis, 24–25, 62, 316, 370, 385, 412–413

attachments, 359
overview, 382
splenius cervicis, 24–25, 332–333, 383
  overview, 382
stapedius, 369, 442–443
sternocleidomastoid, 2–3, 310–311, 348–349, 370–371, 376, 468
  attachments, 352, 357, 359
  clavicular head, 382–383
  sternal head, 382–383
sternohyoid, 311, 376–377, 385, 406–411, 414, 469–470
  attachments, 368
  nerves to, 469
  overview, 377
sternothyroid, 103, 376–377, 385, 410–411, 470
  attachments, 368
  nerves to, 469
  overview, 377
styloglossus, 374–375, 377, 379, 423, 438–439, 442
stylohyoid, 368, 376–377, 419, 438
stylopharyngeus, 378–379, 419, 462
subclavius, 43, 95, 97, 284–285, 305, 311, 409
subcostal, 20–21
suboccipital, 27
subscapularis, 60, 280, 312–316, 320–321
  attachments, 280
  overview, 286
  tendon, 318
superficialis, 338
superior oblique, of eye, 373, 430, 433–435, 449–450, 452
  insertion, 435
  tendon, 429, 433–434, 452
superior rectus, 373, 430–434, 441, 449–450
supinator, 282–283, 321, 323–328, 337
  attachments, 282–283
  overview, 292
supraspinatus, 280–281, 310, 312–314, 316–321
  attachments, 280–281
  overview, 286–287
tarsal, 429
temporalis, 370–371, 404–405, 412, 455
  attachments, 352, 354, 357, 359, 366–367
  overview, 372
  tendon, 408
temporoparietalis, 370
tensor fascia latae, 210, 213, 217, 246–249
  attachments, 213
  overview, 216
tensor tympani, 366, 369, 439, 443
tensor veli palatini, 375, 378, 423, 425, 439–440, 442
  attachments, 359, 366
  nerve to, 439
  overview, 374
  tendon, 443
teres major, 58–61, 278–281, 287, 310, 315–318
  attachments, 280–281
  overview, 286
teres minor, 50, 58, 281, 287, 310, 317–320, 332, 413
  attachments, 281
  overview, 286
thenar, 341
thigh

anterior, 246–247
    cross section, 255–256
    medial/lateral, 254
    overview, 257
    posterior, 250–251
thoracic wall, 20–21
thyroarytenoid, 369, 380, 415, 417, 420
thyroepiglottic, 415
thyrohyoid, 376–377, 408, 410–411, 413–414,
    422
    attachments, 368
    nerve to, 469
    overview, 377
tibialis anterior, 210, 214–215, 254, 260–261
    attachments, 214–215
    overview, 222
    tendon, 210–211, 264, 272–273
    tendon sheath, 272
tibialis posterior, 215, 225, 262–263, 266
    attachments, 215
    groove for, 215
    overview, 224
    tendon, 211, 270–271, 273
trachealis, 381
transversus abdominis, 22–23, 43–45, 61,
    185–187
transversus thoracis, 20–21, 48–49, 72, 104
trapezius, 3, 5–6, 42–44, 58–60, 281, 285,
    321–323, 370, 409, 468,
    attachments, 5–6, 281, 357, 359
    overview, 284
triceps brachii, 50, 58–59, 281
    attachments, 280–281, 283
    lateral head, 278–279, 281, 287, 321, 326
    lateral head tendon, 333
    long head, 278–281, 287, 310, 317–326,
    332–333
    medial head, 281–283, 287, 320–326, 333
    overview, 286
    tendon, 282–283
vastus intermedius, 212–213, 217, 246, 255–256
    attachments, 212–213
    overview, 216
    tendon, 268
vastus lateralis, 210–213, 217, 246–252
    attachments, 212–213
    overview, 216
    tendon, 217
vastus medialis, 210–213, 216–217, 246–247
    attachments, 212–213
    tendon, 217
vocalis, 369, 380, 420
zygomaticus, 428
zygomaticus major, 352, 357, 370–371, 404
zygomaticus minor, 352, 357, 370–371
Muscular triangle, 376
Mylohyoid groove, 367
Mylohyoid line, 367

N

Nares, external (anterior), 448
Nasal artery posterior lateral, 425
Nasal cavity, 421, 425
Nasal conchae
    inferior, 364, 421, 426–427, 438, 448
    middle, 364, 366, 421, 425, 427, 448
    right inferior, 424–425, 429
    right middle, 429
    superior, 364, 366, 421, 425–427, 448
Nasal meatus
    anterior, 358

inferior, 364, 425, 429, 439
middle, 358, 364, 425, 449
superior, 358, 364, 425
Nasal nerve, 454
Nasal septum, 364, 418–419, 429
    bony part, 424
    cartilaginous part, 424, 448
Nasal spines
    anterior, 348–349, 352, 356, 364, 424
    posterior, 366
Nasal vestibule, 425
Nasolacrimal canal, 358
Nasolacrimal duct, 403, 425, 429
Nasopharynx, 393, 401, 418, 421, 424–425
Natal cleft, 3
Neck
    arteries, deep, 387
    arteries, superficial, 386
    brachial plexus, 305
    cervical fascial planes, 384–385
    dermatomes/cutaneous innervation,
    394–395
    glands, 403
    lymph system, 400–402
    median section, 426–427
    topography, 348–349, 404
Nerves
    postganglionic parasympathetic fibers, 173
    postganglionic sympathetic fibers, 173
    preganglionic parasympathetic fibers, 173
    preganglionic sympathetic fibers, 173
Nerves, named
    alveolar
        anterior superior, 454
        inferior, 391, 413, 438, 440, 455
        middle superior, 454
        posterior superior, 454
    anococcygeal, 168–169, 243
    antebrachial cutaneous
        lateral, 300–303, 322, 324, 327, 330–331
        medial, 300–302, 305, 314–315, 322–324,
        331
        posterior, 302–303, 330–331, 333
    articular recurrent, 240
    auricular
        great, 395, 404–405, 407, 413, 470
        greater, 37, 58, 62, 395, 408–409
    auriculotemporal, 394–395, 404–405,
        437–438, 440, 455, 462
    axillary, 305–307, 310, 312–323
        quadrangular space transmitting, 332–333
    brachial cutaneous
        lateral, 36–37, 300, 302–303
        medial, 300–303, 305–306, 312, 322, 324
    brachial plexus, 305 (See also Brachial
        plexus)
    buccal (long buccal), 394–395, 436–438, 440,
        455
    cardiac
        superior, 81
        thoracic sympathetic, 97
    carotid, interior, 458
    carotid plexus, interior, 451, 458
    cervical
        descending, 408, 410–411
        superior, 414
        transverse, 36, 62, 394–395, 404, 407–408
    chorda tympani, 438–440, 442–443
    ciliary
        long, 451, 453
        short, 430–432, 434–435, 450–451, 453

cluneal
    inferior, 38, 168–169, 193, 204, 236–237
    medial, 37, 58, 168–169, 193
    middle, 236
    superior, 37–38, 58–59, 236–237
cochlear, 443, 460
cranial (See Cranial nerves; specific cranial
    nerves)
cutaneous, 240–241, 250, 322
    anterior, intermediate branch, 237
    perforating, 243
digital, dorsal, 234, 237, 240–241
digital plantar, common, 241
ethmoidal, 428, 434–435, 453
dorsal scapular, 61–62, 305, 307, 408
femoral, 43–44, 53, 142, 186, 239–243, 246,
    248–249, 257
    anterior cutaneous branch, 53, 248
    cutaneous branch, 239
    muscular branch, 239–241, 246, 257
    right, 175, 189
femoral cutaneous
    anterior, 52, 168, 234
        intermediate branch, 235
        medial branch, 235
    anterior intermediate branch, 234
    anterior medial branch, 234
    lateral, 36–37, 168–169, 185, 234, 236–237
    posterior, 168–169, 204–205, 235–237,
        240–241, 250–252
    posterior medial branch, 235
    posterior perineal branch, 193, 236
    posterior perineal branch of, 204
femoral triangle, 248–249
fibular (peroneal)
    common, 236–237, 240–241, 247,
        250–251, 265–268
    deep, 234, 237, 240–241, 260–261
    superficial, 234, 237, 240–241, 260–261,
        272
frontal, 428, 430, 432, 434, 453
genitofemoral, 36, 38–39, 107, 142–143,
    168–169, 175, 239–240, 242
    anterior cutaneous branch, 36
    femoral branch, 36, 142–143, 234,
        239–240, 248–249
    genital branch, 36, 55, 142–143, 234,
        239–240, 242
    left, 140
gluteal
    inferior, 204–205, 241, 243, 250–253
    superior, 204, 241, 243, 250–252
gluteal region, 253–254
hypogastric, 170–173, 188–189, 466–467
hypogastric plexus, superior, 142, 170–173,
    467
iliohypogastric, 36–39, 43–44, 168–169,
    239–240
    anterior cutaneous branch, 53, 174, 234
    lateral cutaneous branch, 36, 38–39,
        168–169, 236–237
ilioinguinal, 38–39, 43–44, 168–169,
    239–240, 246
infraorbital, 394–395, 430, 438–441, 453–454
infratrochlear, 394–395, 404, 428–430, 453
intercostal, 38–40, 43–45, 51, 96–99, 239
    anterior cutaneous branch, 38–40, 44,
        46–47
    anterior muscular branch, 44–45
    lateral cutaneous branch, 38–39, 42, 44,
        46–47, 50–51

Nerves, named—*continued*
  intercostobrachial, 37, 300–302, 312, 321–322
  interosseous
    anterior, 306, 326–327
    posterior, 306–307, 327, 335
  intratrochlear, 440
  labial
    anterior, 169
    posterior, 169, 171, 192, 194, 235
    superior, 454
  laryngeal
    inferior, 415
    interior, 416–417
    left recurrent, 79, 94, 99–100, 102–103, 464
    recurrent, 414–415
    right recurrent, 100, 316, 385, 463
    superior, 414–416, 418, 423, 463
  lingual, 422–425, 436–438, 458–459, 461–462
  lumbar, 34
  lumbar plexus, 242
  lumbrosacral/coccygeal plexi, 239
  mandibular, 396, 419, 438–442, 455, 461
  masseteric, 440, 455
  maxillary, 393, 396, 438–441, 453–454, 458
  median, 305–307, 312–315, 337–339
    opening for passage of, 289
    palmar branch, 300–301, 326, 338–339
    palmar branch, superficial, 336–337
    palmar digital, common, 306–307, 338–339
    recurrent branch, 338
    thenar branch, 336–337
  mental, 394–395, 404, 437, 455
  mesenteric ganglion
    inferior, 140, 172–173, 465–467
    superior, 147, 172–173, 465–467
  musculocutaneous, 305–307, 312–315, 318–324, 326
  mylohyoid, 414, 422, 437, 440, 455
  nasociliary, 430, 432–435, 453
  nasopalatine, 424, 458
  obturator, 168, 185–187, 205, 239–243
    anterior division, 247–249
    cutaneous branch, 168–169, 234, 235, 236
    muscular branch, 246–247
  occipital, 37, 58, 62–63, 395
    greater, 37, 58, 60, 395, 404–405, 408
    lesser, 37, 58, 395, 404–405, 407–408
  ophthalmic, 393, 432–433, 440–441, 453
  ovarian plexus, right, 171
  ovarian (testicular) plexus, 173, 466
  palatine, 454
    greater, 423, 438–440
    greater anterior, 424–425
    greater/lesser, 458
    lesser, 440
  palmar digital
    common, 306–308, 339–341
    proper, 306, 336, 338
  pectoral
    lateral, 38–39, 43, 305–306
    medial, 38–39, 43, 305–306
  pelvic, 170–173
  perineal, 170–171, 195
  petrosal
    deep, 458
    greater, 360, 365, 441, 443, 458, 461
    lesser, 360, 365, 461–462

  phrenic, 72–73, 81, 94–97, 100, 102–106, 305–306
  plantar
    lateral, 240–241, 264, 270–271, 273
    medial, 240–241, 264, 270
  plantar digital, 270
  proper digital, 270–271
  pterygoid, 440
  pudendal, 160, 170–171, 204–205, 243, 250
    interior, 160–161, 166–167, 204–205, 250–252
  radial, 305–307, 316–320, 323–324, 332–333
    deep, 306–307, 326, 328
    deep branch, 324
    dorsal digital branch, 302–303
    spiral groove, 281, 287
    superficial branch, 300–303, 306–307, 321, 323, 324–327, 330–331, 338–339
  rectal, 168–171, 194–197, 201–202, 205, 243
  renal plexus (ganglion), 147
  sacral, 182, 185–189, 243
  sacral/cocccygeal plexi, 243
  sacral plexus, 170
  saphenous, 234–235, 254–256, 262–267
    genital branch, 240
    infrapatellar branch, 234–235, 246–247
    intrapatellar branch, 264
    medial calcaneal branch, 236
    medial crural branch, 235–236
  sciatic, 204–205, 239–241, 250–253, 255–257
  scrotal
    anterior, 168
    posterior, 168, 170, 193, 197
  sphenopalatine, 433
  spinal cord, 35–40 (*See also* Spinal nerves)
  splanchnic, 172
    greater, 40, 94–97, 117, 172–173, 465–467
    least, 106, 172–173, 466–467
    lesser, 106, 172–173, 465–467
    lumbar, 172–173, 465–467
    pelvic, 170–173, 188–189, 243, 465–467
    right greater, 104
    sacral, 170, 172–173, 465–467
  subcostal, 36–39, 44, 107, 168–169, 242
    anterior cutaneous branch, 36, 168–169, 234
    lateral cutaneous branch, 37–39, 168–169, 234, 237
  suboccipital, 63, 470
  subscapular
    lower, 305
    upper, 305
  supraclavicular, 36, 300, 302–303, 394–395, 470
    intermediate, 404, 406–408
    lateral, 37, 58, 404, 406–408, 410–411
    medial, 404, 406–411
  supraorbital, 394–395, 428–429, 440
  suprascapular, 305, 312–313, 323, 412–413
  supratrochlear, 394–395, 428–430, 434
  sural, 233, 236–237, 241, 263
    lateral cutaneous, 234, 237, 241, 254, 257, 263, 265
    medial cutaneous, 233, 236–237, 250–251, 262–263
  temporal
    deep, 440, 455
    posterior deep, 438
  testicular plexus, right, 170
  thigh, 257
    anterior, 246–247

    cross section, 255–256
    medial/lateral, 254
    posterior, 250–251
  thoracic, 34, 98, 103
    long, 43, 50, 305–307, 317
  thoracodorsal, 60, 305–307, 313
  tibial, 240–241, 250–251, 262–264, 270
    medial calcaneal branch, 235
    muscular branch, 240
  tympanic, 443, 461–462
  tympanic plexus, 443
  ulnar, 305–307, 318, 320–327, 332–333, 338–341
    common palmar digital, 306
    common palmar digital branch, 338
    deep branch, 338
    deep palmar branch, 306, 340
    dorsal branch, 301–302, 336–340
    dorsal cutaneous branch, 306
    dorsal digital branch, 302
    palmar branch, 300–301, 338
    palmar cutaneous branch, 306
    superficial branch, 338–340
  upper limb
    deep, 306–307
    superficial, 300–303
  ureteric plexus, right, 170–171
  uterovaginal plexus, 173, 466
  zygomatic, 432, 453–454
  zygomaticofacial, 394–395, 454
  zygomaticotemporal, 394–395, 454
Nervus intermedius, 396
Nipple, 2, 42, 46–47, 66
Nose
  ala, 350
  anterior (external) naris (nostril), 350
  apex, 350
  dorsum, 350
  foramina/fissures/canals, 358
  nasal septum, 350
  nasolabial sulcus, 350
  topography, 350
Nuchal line
  inferior, 6–7, 62–63, 348, 359
  superior, 62–63, 285, 348, 359, 383, 468
Nucleus pulposus, 12, 19, 106, 385, 417
Nutrient foramen, 215

O

Oblique cord, 328
Oblique line, 368
Obturator canal, 153, 203
Obturator foramen, 18, 152, 154–155, 159
Obturator membrane, 153, 161, 193
Occipital condyle, 356, 359
Occipital crest, 359, 361
Occipital protuberance
  external, 3, 62–63, 348–349, 354–356
  interior, 361
Occipital sinus, 391, 426
Occipital triangle, 376
Oculomotor nerve (CN III), 392–393, 430, 439–441, 451
  branch to inferior oblique muscle, 432
  branch to levator palpebrae superioris muscle, 432
  functions, 471
  inferior branch, 432–433
  inferior division, 450
  muscular branch, 435
  overview, 446–447, 450

superior branch, 432–433
superior division, 450
Olecranon, 278–279, 325, 328–329
Olecranon fossa, 281, 329
Olecranon synovial bursa, 328
Olfactory bulb, 430, 434, 448
Olfactory bulb/nerves, 425
Olfactory bulb/tract, 396
Olfactory epithelium, 448
Olfactory mucosa, 424
Olfactory nerve (CN I)
    functions, 471
    overview, 425, 446–448
    tracts, 396, 432
Olfactory tracts, 441, 448
Omental bursa
    lesser sac, 112–113, 136, 141
    splenic recess, 129
    superior recess, 112
Omental (epiploic) appendages, 114–116, 136, 178–181
Omental (epiploic) foramen, 112, 120, 130
Omentum, lesser, 112, 114, 117–119, 126, 129
Optic canal, 361, 363–364, 447, 456
    overview, 358, 360
    roof, 434
Optic chiasma, 393, 396, 398, 427
Optic nerve (CN II), 392, 396, 430–435, 441, 451
    dural sheath, 431–433, 449
    functions, 471
    overview, 446–447, 449
    right, 424
    tract, 437
Optic sheath, external, 434
Optic tracts, 441, 449
Oral cavity, 351, 420–424
Orbitalis muscle, 430
Orbital septum, 428
Oropharynx, 401
    posterior wall, 351
    region of, 417–421, 426
Os coccygis (coccyx), 155
Ostium of ureter, 160–161, 194
Otic ganglion, 439, 453–454, 461–462
Ovaries, 165, 173, 180–184, 190
    ligament of, 178
    right, 178–179
    suspensory ligament, 178

P

Palate
    hard, 378, 423–425, 438–440
    region, 366
    soft, 374–375, 378, 418–421
Palatine bone, 359
    horizontal plate, 364, 366
    orbital process, 364
    perpendicular plate, 364
    pyramidal process, 440
Palatine canal, 358–359
Palatine folds, transverse, 423
Palatine foramina, 358–359, 366
Palatine process, 354–355
Palatine suture, median, 359
Palatine tonsil, 351, 401–402, 420–421, 424
Palatomaxillary suture, 366
Palmar arch
    deep, 296–297, 340
    superficial, 296, 337–338
Palpebral rim, 428–429

Pancreas
    anatomical position, 120–122, 129
    body, 122–123, 132, 138
    head, 122–123
    innervation, 465
    tail, 122–123
    uncinate process, 123
Pancreatic duct, main, 123–125
Parahippocampal gyrus uncus, 396
Parasternal line, 66
Paravertebral line, 67, 111
Paravertebral structures, 98–99
Parietal costal pleura, 99, 104
Parietal layer, 191
Parietal pericardium, 81–82, 92–95, 100
    fibrous, 81, 93, 96–97
    serous, 80, 92
Parietal peritoneum, 112–114, 190–191
Parietal pleura, 95, 111
Parotid duct, 403–404, 422, 424, 457
Parotid gland, 400, 403–405, 461–462
Patella, 210–212, 246–247, 260–261, 268–269
Patellar retinaculum
    lateral, 246, 260, 265, 267
    medial, 246, 254, 264, 267
Pelvic contents
    female, 178–185
    male, 188–189
Pelvic diaphragm, 48, 158, 163, 179, 182
    fascia, inferior, 191
    inferior fascia, 190–191, 193, 202
Pelvic fascia tendinous arch, 208
Pelvic nerves
    female, 171, 173, 466
    male, 172, 467
    plexus, 170–171, 173
Pelvis
    autonomic nerves, 466–467
    false (minor), 153
    muscles, 156–158
    true (major), 153
    wall muscles, 163
Penis, 210
    body, 2, 150, 177, 195, 205
    bulb, 160, 177, 193, 197, 199
    cavernous nerve, 170
    crus, 160, 177, 193, 195, 197, 199
    deep artery, 199
    deep dorsal veins, 157, 188, 203
    deep fascia (Buck's), 53, 156, 191, 197
    dorsal artery/vein, 43, 52, 157, 164, 166
    dorsal nerve, 36, 168, 170, 201
    fundiform ligament, 52, 174
    glans, 2, 150, 174
    innervation, 467
    overview, 172
    seminal vesicle, right, 177
    spermatic cord, right, 199
    superficial dorsal vein, 52
    superficial fascia (dartos fascia), 191
    suspensory ligament, 42–43, 170, 188, 191
    tunica albuginea, 191
Pericardial cavity, 80, 92, 95
Pericardial reflection, 83, 88
Pericardial sac, 79
Pericardial sinuses, 83, 89–92
Pericardium, 68, 91, 93, 96–97, 102, 104–105
Perineal body, 156, 158, 180, 200–203
Perineal pouch
    deep, 160–161, 192
    superficial, 160–161, 190–192

Perineal raphe, 150, 174
Perineum 180, 193, 201
    female, 192, 194, 196, 198, 200, 202
    males, 193, 195, 197, 199, 201, 203
    overview, 150–151
Periorbita, 434
Periosteum, 426
Perirenal fat, 140, 142–143, 146–147, 175
Peritoneal cavity, 112–117
Peritoneal reflection, 69
Peritoneum, 48–49, 248
Peroneal. *See* Fibular (Peroneal)
Perpendicular plate, 352–353
Pes anserinus, 211, 254, 263, 268
Pes anserinus, 263
Petrosal sinus
    inferior, 361, 391–393, 443
    superior, 361, 392–393
Petrotympanic fissure, 358, 440, 458–459, 462
Phalanx/phalanges. *See* Fingers; Foot
Pharyngeal recess, 425–427
Pharyngeal tonsil, 401–402, 418–419, 425–426
Pharyngeal tubercle, 359
Pharyngobasilar fascia, 418
Pharynx
    innervation, 463
    mucosa, 416
    posterior wall, 417
    topography, 420
Philtrum, 350
Phrenicoesophageal membrane, 79
Pia mater, 19, 34–35, 41
Pineal body, 426–427
Piriform aperture (anterior nasal aperture), 352, 358
Piriform recess, 415, 418, 420, 423
Pituitary gland. *See* Hypophysis (pituitary gland)
Pleural cavity, 80
Pleural reflection, 68–70
Pons. *See under* Brain
Popliteal fossa, 211
Popliteal plane, 215
Popliteal surface, 213
Posterior superior iliac spine. *See* Iliac spines
Premolar teeth, 366–367
Prostate gland, 48, 160, 177, 188–189
Prostatic utricle, 160
Prostatic venous plexus, 166, 170
Proximal interphalangeal joint (PIP), 343
Pterygoid fossa, 359, 363
Pterygoid hamulus, 362–364, 366
Pterygoid notch, 362–363
Pterygoid plates
    lateral, 359, 364, 366, 438, 440
    medial, 359, 364, 366
    medial hamulus, 440
Pterygoid process, 363
    lateral plate, 362, 363
    medial/lateral plates, 354
    medial plate, 362, 363
Pterygoid (vidian) canal, 363, 424, 433, 439, 462
    artery, 439
    nerve, 425, 433, 440, 458
    overview, 358
Pterygomaxillary fissure, 358, 440
Pterygopalatine fossa, 363, 438–441
Pterygopalatine ganglion, 432–433, 453–454, 458, 461–462
Pterygopalatine sulcus, 363

Pubic crest, 2, 150–155, 212, 221, 258
Pubic ramus
    inferior, 150–156, 158, 221, 258
    superior, 152–155, 258–259
Pubic symphysis, 4–5, 150–153, 156–158,
        176–177, 258–259
Pubic tubercle, 2, 5, 150–155, 212, 257–259
Pubis
    body, 154–155, 258–259
    pectineal line, 153–155, 212, 258
Pudendal canal (Alcock's), 160–161, 192–193,
        206–208
Pudendal structures, 204–205
Pulmonary trunk, 82, 89–92, 95
Pulmonic valve, 84, 89
Pyloric canal, 130–131
Pyloric sphincter, 122, 124, 129–131, 138

Q
Quadrangular membrane, 416, 420
Quadrangular space, 316
Quadrigeminal lamina, 426–427

R
Radial fossa, 280, 328–329
Radial tuberosity, 280, 328–329
Radiocarpal joint, 304
Radioulnar joint, 304
Radius, 280–281, 327–330, 339–340, 342–345
    body, 282–283, 289
    distal end, 291
    dorsal tubercle, 282–283, 335
    grooves for
        abductor pollicis longus muscle, 328
        extensor carpi radialis brevis muscle, 328
        extensor carpi radialis longus muscle,
            328
        extensor digitorum muscle tendons,
            282–283
        extensor indicis muscle tendons, 282–283
        extensor pollicis brevis muscle, 328
        extensor pollicis longus brevis muscle
            tendon, 282–283
        extensors carpiradialis muscle tendons,
            282
        extensors carpi radialis muscle tendons,
            283
    head, 280–283
    head, articular circumference, 328–329
    interosseous crest, 282–283
    neck, 280–283, 328–329
    radial tuberosity, 289
    styloid process, 278, 282–283, 328–329, 344
    tubercle, 344
Ramus, rami. See specific anatomical feature
Ramus communicans, 98
Rectal nerve plexus, 170–171
Rectal plexus, 172, 465, 467
Rectosigmoid junction, 208
Rectouterine pouch (of Douglas), 112, 178,
        180–181, 190
Rectovesical fold, 48–49
Rectovesical pouch, 191
Rectum, 134, 136–138, 159, 172–173, 178–181,
        208
    arteries, 206
    innervation, 465
    rectal folds, 163
        inferior, 208
        inferior transverse, 180
        middle, 163, 208

    middle transverse, 180–181
        superior, 208
        superior transverse, 180
    rectal plexus, superior, 138
    veins, 207
Rectus line, left lateral, 110
Rectus sheath, 23, 42–43, 45, 48
Renal cortex, 142–144
Renal medulla, 142–144
Renal nerve plexus (ganglion), 147
Renal pelvis, 121, 144–145
Renal sinus, 144
Retromammary space, 47
Retropharyngeal space, 384–385, 417, 420, 425
Retropubic space (of Retzius), 180–181,
        190–191
Retrosternal fat pads, 94, 96
Ribs. See also Thoracic cage
    1st, 17, 94–97, 100–103
    2nd, 26, 98
    3rd, 17
    4th, 97
    6th, 17
    8th, 17
    9th, angle, 6–7
    angle, 21, 26
    costal groove, 17
    costochondral articulation, 17–18, 21
    cross section, 80
    head, 17
    muscle attachments, 4–7
    neck, 17, 104
    overview, 8–9, 17
    posterior angle, 17
    tubercle, 17
Rima glottidis, 416
Rotator cuff muscles, 316–317
Round ligament of liver. See Liver

S
Sacral vertebrae, 8–9
Sacroiliac joint, 154–155, 212–213, 258–259
Sacrum, 16, 176, 189, 204–205
    apex, 16
    arteries, 29
    articular process, superior, 16
    auricular surface, 16
    base, 16
    iliolumbar ligament, 18
    ligament attachments, 18
    muscle attachments, 4, 6–7
    nerve plexi, 170, 186–187, 243
    pelvic aperture, superior, 16
    promontory, 16, 112, 152–155, 258–259
    sacral canal, 16, 154–155
    sacral cornua, 154–155
    sacral crests, 16, 18
        lateral/median, 16, 18
        median, 154–155, 258, 285
    sacral foramina
        anterior, 16, 152, 258–259
        posterior, 8, 152, 258
    sacral hiatus, 16, 154
    sacral horns, 16
    sacral tuberosity, 16
    transverse line, 16
    veins, 32
    wings (ala), 9, 16, 154–155, 212, 258–259
Sagittal sinus
    inferior, 391, 393
    superior, 391–393, 426

Sagittal suture, 348, 353, 359
Salivatory nucleus, superior, 458–459
Salpingopalatine fold, 425–426
Salpingopharyngeal fold, 418–419, 425–427
Saphenous hiatus, falciform edge, 42, 52
Scalene tubercle, 383
Scalp, 426
Scapula, 40, 104, 280
    angles
        inferior, 3, 5–6, 67, 281, 319
        superior, 3, 6, 281, 285, 319
    arterial rete, 297
    coracoid process, 4–5, 43, 280, 305, 319,
        321–323
    infraglenoid tubercle, 281, 287
    infraspinous fossa, 281
    lateral (axillary) border, 281, 287, 319
    lateral border, 6
    medial (vertebral) border, 3–6, 281, 285,
        319
    muscle attachments, 4
    neck, 281
    notch, 281
    spine, 3, 5–6, 279, 281, 285, 287, 310, 317,
        332–333, 412–413, 468
    superior border, 281, 319
    supraglenoid tubercle, 281, 289
    supraspinous fossa, 281, 287
Sciatic foramen
    greater, 18, 152–153, 162
    lesser, 18, 152–153, 243
Sciatic notch
    greater, 18, 153–155, 258–259
    lesser, 153, 155
Scrotal raphe, 150
Scrotum, 2, 150, 193, 195, 205, 210
Segmental innervation, 238
Sella turcica (hypophyseal fossa), 354–355,
        361–362, 448
Semilunar hiatus, 425
Semilunar line, 2, 23, 44–45, 48
Seminal colliculus, 160
Seminal vesicles, 48, 177, 188–189, 191
Septal band, heart, 89
Septomarginal (moderator) band, heart, 89
Septum pellucidum, 426
Shoulder
    brachial plexus, 305
    coronal section, 318–319
    dermatomes, 300–303
    joint capsule, 332–333
    muscles, 285–287
    muscles, anterior, 311
    muscles, posterior, 310
    nerves, cutaneous, 300–303
    nerves, deep, 306–307
    radiograph, 319
    rotator cuff muscles, 316–317
    sagittal section, 279
    skeleton/muscle attachments, 280–283
    surface anatomy, 278–279
    veins, 298–299
Sigmoid colon, 134, 136–137, 139, 178–181,
        207–208
    innervation, 465
Sigmoid mesocolon, 141, 180–181
Sigmoid sinus, 361, 391–393, 443, 460
Skeleton/muscle attachments, 212–215
Skin, 426–427, 465
Small intestines. See also Ileum; Jejunum
    arteriograph, 135

innervation, 465
overview, 130–133
radiograph, 131
Soft palate, 351, 375, 418–421, 424–427
muscles, 374–375, 378
Soleal line, 215
Spermatic cord, 23, 174
spermatic fascia, external, 193
Sphenoethmoidal recess, 358, 364, 425–427
Sphenoid bone, 352, 354, 357, 366, 418
base, 359
body, 362–364, 393
greater wing, 349, 352, 356, 361–362, 432, 442
cerebral surface, 362–363
infratemporal surface, 363, 366, 440
orbital surface, 352–353, 363–364
temporal surface, 362–363
lesser wing, 353, 361–364, 441
optic canal, 362
pterygoid hamulus, right, 362
pterygoid process, 362, 441
spine, 362–363, 440, 442
topography, 362–363
Sphenoid crest, 363
Sphenoid sinus, 354–355, 363–364, 393, 433, 438–439
Sphenopalatine fissure, 440
Sphenopalatine foramen, 358, 364, 425
Sphenoparietal sinus, 393
Sphenoperital sinus, 392
Sphenosquamosal suture, 366, 440, 442
Spina ischiadica, 155
Spinal cord, 384–385, 396–397, 426–427
anterior border, 93
cross section, 104
lateral horn, 451
nerves, 35–40
overview, 41
vasculature, 34–35
Spinal nerves
C2 ventral ramus, 412, 439
C3 ventral ramus, 412, 438
C4, 437
C4 ventral ramus, 412, 415
C5 ventral ramus, 415, 421
C6 ventral ramus, 415, 426–427
C7 ventral rami, 421
C8 ventral ramus, 418, 421
cervical, 385, 468, 470
cervical plexus, 395, 470
dorsal rami, 40–41
lateral cutaneous branch, 37, 59
medial cutaneous branch, 37, 40, 58–59
lumbar, 41, 465
T2 superior articular facets, 418
ventral rami, 40
anterior cutaneous branches, 36
lateral cutaneous branches, 36–37, 40, 58
ventral root, 396
Spine
articular processes, superior, 9, 154–155
ligament attachments, 19
muscle attachments, 4–7
overview, 8–9
Spleen, 113, 115, 117–125, 134
hilum of, 122
Squamous suture, 356
Stapes, 369, 443, 460
Stellate ganglion, 79, 94–96, 98–100, 102
Sternal line, 66

Sternoclavicular joint, 18, 411, 413
Sternum, 285, 312–313
angle, 2, 5, 8, 18, 68, 72–73, 93
body, 4–5, 8, 18, 68, 93, 280, 316
costal notch, 18
costochondral articulation, 18
cross section, 80, 104
head, left sternal, 409
interchondral ligament, 18
ligament attachments, 18
muscle attachments, 4
radiate sternocostal ligament, 18
sternal angle, 2, 5, 8, 18
sternoclavicular joint, 18, 411, 413
xiphisternal joint, 18
xiphoid process, 2, 4, 18, 68, 93
Stomach
anatomical position, 68, 112–113, 121, 132
body, 114–115, 117–120, 130
cardiac part, 118, 130
fundus, 114–115, 117–120, 130–131
greater curvature, 117–118, 130–131
innervation, 465
lesser curvature, 118–119, 131
overview, 118–121
pylorus, 111, 114–115, 118, 120, 130–131
radiograph, 101
rugae (folds), 130
Straight sinus, 391–393, 426–427
Stria malleolaris, 442
Stylomastoid foramen, 358–359, 366, 458–459
Subarachnoid space, 35, 41
Subcostal plane, 66, 68, 110
Subcutaneous connective tissue, 426
Subcutaneous infrapatellar bursa, 263, 268
Subcutaneous prepatellar bursa, 268
Subdeltoid synovial bursa, 312, 316–318
Sublingual fold, 422
Sublingual gland, 403, 424–425, 459
Submandibular ducts, 424–425
Submandibular fossa, 367
Submandibular ganglion, 422, 425, 455, 459
Submandibular gland, 400, 403–405, 407–409, 459
Submandibular triangle, 376
Submental triangle, 376
Suboccipital muscles, 27
Suboccipital triangle, 61
Subtalar joints, 238
Sulcus tali, 274
Sulcus terminalis, 402, 461–462
Superior laryngeal nerve branch, 415
Superior thoracic aperture, 102
Supraclavicular fossa, 278, 348–349
Supraclavicular triangle, 376
Supracondylar line, 213–215
Supracondylar ridge, 212
Supraorbital foramen, 364
Supraorbital margin, 428–430, 432
Supraorbital notch/foramen, 348, 352, 358
Suprapatellar bursa, 247
Suprapatellar synovial bursa, 268
Suprarenal glands, 140, 142–143, 146–147, 465
Suprasternal space, 384
Supraventricular crest, heart, 89
Sustentaculum tali (calcaneus). See Calcaneus
Sympathetic chain, 172–173, 461, 467
Sympathetic chain ganglia, 458–459
Sympathetic ganglion, 40, 102
Sympathetic trunk, 94–95, 97, 102, 182–187, 416, 418

1st thoracic ganglion, 451
cervical ganglion, middle, 305
lumbar portion, 239
pelvic portion, 239, 243
Synovial bursa, 263, 267

T
Talocrural joint, 238
Talus, 214
articular surface, 272–273
flexor hallucis longus muscle tendon groove, 274
head, 215, 227, 271, 274–275
lateral tubercle, 274
medial tubercle, 274
neck, 274
posterior lateral tubercle (posterior process), 274–275
sulcus tali, 274
trochlea, 214
tuberosity, 274
Tarsal plate, inferior, 429
Tarsal sinus, 274–275
Tarsometatarsal joint line (of Lisfranc), 274–275
Taste pathways, 461
Teeth
canine, 351, 364, 366–367
incisor, 351, 364, 366–367, 422–425
molar, 366–367
premolar, 366–367
Tegmen tympani, 439
Temporal bone, 348–349, 352, 354, 357, 359, 366
canal, 387
facial hiatus, 365
groove for sigmoid sinus, 365
mastoid part, 365
mastoid process, 350
petrous part, 353, 356, 361, 365, 440, 460
squamous part, 356, 365, 440, 442
styloid process, 365, 418–419, 423, 437–439
styloid process sheath, 365
topography, 365
trigeminal impression, 365
tympanic part, 365–366, 442
zygomatic process, 437, 440
Temporal fossa, 352, 359
Temporomandibular joint, 349–350, 437
Tendons. See under muscles, named: specific muscles
Tenia coli, 114–116, 118, 130, 134, 139, 178
Tentorium cerebelli, 393, 427, 443
Terminal sulcus, 351
Testis, 2, 23, 53, 55, 164, 177
Thalamus, 398–399, 426–427
Thenar eminence, 278–279
Thigh
cross section, 255–256
hamstring muscles posterior compartment, 210–211
muscles, anterior, 216–217
muscles, gluteal/posterior, 218–219
muscles, medial, 220–221
topography, 257
anterior, 246–247
cross section, 255–256
medial/lateral, 254
posterior, 250–251
Thoracic aperture, superior, 103

Thoracic cage. *See also* Ribs
  enervation, 36
  muscle attachments, 4–7
  muscles, named, 20–21
  overview, 8–9
Thoracic duct, 78–80, 94–95, 102, 104, 410
Thoracic sympathetic trunk ganglion, 94–97
Thoracic vertebrae
  articular process, inferior/superior, 12–14
  intervertebral discs
    anulus fibrosus, 12
    nucleus pulposus, 12
  intervertebral foramen, 12, 14
  lamina of vertebral arch, 12–14
  mamillary process, 14
  overview, 8, 12–14
  pedicle, 12–14, 34
  spinous process, 12–14
  superior costal facet, 12
  T1, 280
    articular process, superior, 12
    body, 12
    spinous process, 3, 26, 69, 281
  T3
    body, 49
    spinous process, 12
  T4 spinous process, 25, 285
  T5
    articular process, superior/inferior, 12
    spinous process, 33
    transverse process, 33
    transverse section, 40
    vertebral notch, superior/inferior, 12
  T6 spinous process, 33
  T7 spinous process, 285
  T8
    body, 12–13
    spinous process, 281
  T12, 280
    spinous process, 3, 5–7, 25, 285, 385
  transverse costal facet, 12–13
  transverse process, 12–14
  vertebral notch, inferior/superior, 12–14
Thoraco-abdominal autonomic nerves, 465
Thoracoacromial arterial trunk, 28–29, 296, 314
Thumb
  carpometacarpal joint, 340, 343
  carpometacarpal joint actions, 304
  cephalic vein, 299
  common palmar digital nerves, 338
  metacarpophalangeal joint, 343
  proper digital arteries, 340–341
  proper palmar digital arteries, 336–338
  proper palmar digital nerves, 336–338
  proper palmar digital veins, 336–337
Thyrocervical arterial trunk, 28–29, 296, 312, 386
Thyroglossal duct, 410
Thyrohyoid membrane, 375, 378–379, 414, 417
Thyroid cartilage, 368, 375, 379, 381, 401–402, 414–415
  inferior horn, 368, 381
    articular surface, 415
  lamina, 368–369, 415
    interior surface, 416
  superior horn, 368–369, 381, 414–415, 420
Thyroid gland, 72–73, 81, 402–403, 412–413
  isthmus, 384, 403, 411
  lateral lobes, 410–411, 418–419
  pyramidal lobe, 417

Thyroid notch, 381, 415
Tibia, 212–215, 260–261, 263, 268–269
  anterior border, 210–211
  head, apex of, 214
  interosseous border, 215
  interosseous membrane, 268
  lateral condyle, 212–215, 217, 266–269
  medial condyle, 214, 217, 219, 221, 268–269
  medial/lateral condyles, 212
  medial surface, 264–265
  soleal line, 213
  tuberosity, 210, 214, 246–247, 265, 268
Tibiocalcaneal ligament, 273
Tibiofibular joint
  distal, 214
  proximal, 212, 266
Tongue, 378, 424, 437
  anterior 2/3rds of, 461
  apex, 351
  body, 351
  dorsum, 462
  foramen cecum, 461–462
  inferior longitudinal muscle, 375, 378–379
  intrinsic muscles, 420
  muscles, 374–375, 378–379, 420
  papillae
    filiform, 351, 461
    foliate, 351
    fungiform, 351, 461
    lingual, 351
    vallate (circumvallate), 351, 461
  posterior 1/3rd, 461
  root, 351, 418–419, 462
  superior (dorsal) surface, 419–420, 422–424, 438–439
  topography, 351
Tonsillar fossa, 351
Torus tubarius, 418–419, 424–427
Trachea, 76–79, 81, 94, 96–99, 377, 384–385, 410
  cartilages, 368, 375, 379, 381
  innervation, 465
  interior surface, 417
  ring, 381
Transpyloric plane, 66, 68, 110–111
Transtubercular plane, 110–111
Transversalis fascia, 44, 48
Transverse colon, 114–116, 118, 133–134, 136–137
Transverse lines, 154
Transverse mesocolon, 112, 129–130, 134, 141
Transverse sinus, 391–393
Transverse tarsal joint line (talocalcaneocuboideonavicular) (of Shepard), 274–275
Transverse venous sinus groove, 361
Triangle of auscultation, 58, 310
Triangular aponeuroses, 335
Triangular space, 316
Trigeminal nerve (CN V), 392, 397, 441, 443
  communicating branch, 453–454
  functions, 471
  mandibular division, 455
  maxillary division, 454
  medial pterygoid branch, 455
  meningeal branch, 455
  motor root, 396
  ophthalmic division, 453
  overview, 446–447
  palpebral branch, inferior, 454
  parotid branch, 455

sensory root, 396
  superficial temporal branch, 455
  superior dental branch, 454
  superior gingival branch, 454
Trigeminal (semilunar) ganglion, 433, 438–441, 443, 451, 453–454, 462
Trigone, 160–161, 194
Trochanteric bursa, 246–247
Trochanteric fossa, 213, 258–259
Trochlea (of humerus), 280, 328–329
Trochlea (of superior oblique m.), 430, 433–435, 449–450
Trochlea (of talus), 274
Trochlear nerve (CN IV), 393, 432, 440–441
  functions, 471
  overview, 446–447, 452
True (major) pelvis, 153
Tubercle
  iliac crest, 5–7, 22, 150–155, 204, 206, 212, 258
  scaphoid bone, 344–345
Tuberculum sellae, 362–363
Tunica vaginalis, 191
Tympanic canaliculus, 358–359
Tympanic cavity
  interior jugular wall, 442
  medial wall, promontory, 442–443
Tympanic cells, 442–443
Tympanic membrane, 438, 442, 460, 462
  limbus, 442
  pars flaccida, 442
  pars tensa, 442
Tympanic nerve plexus, 443, 461–462
Tympanic promontory, 439
Tympanomastoid suture, 442

U
Ulna, 280–281, 327–329, 342–345
  body, 282–283, 289
  coronoid process, 280, 328, 329
  groove for extensor carpi ulnaris muscle tendon, 282–283
  head, 282–283, 289, 328
  interosseous crest, 282–283
  olecranon, 278–279, 325, 328–329
  posterior (subcutaneous) border, 282–283
  proximal end, 291
  radial notch, 328
  styloid process, 279, 282–283, 336–337
  subcutaneous border, 279
Ulnar bursa for flexor tendons, 338–339
Ulnar tuberosity, 280, 289, 328
Umbilical folds
  lateral, 48–49, 178–179
  left medial, 188–189
  medial, 48–49, 115–116, 178, 206
  median, 115–116, 178, 189
Umbilical plane, 110–111
Umbilicus, 2, 38, 42, 48, 111, 150–151
Upper limb
  arteries, 296–297
  brachial plexus, 305
  dermatomes, 300–303
  lymph system, 308–309
  nerves, cutaneous, 300–303
  nerves, deep, 306–307
  skeleton/muscle attachments, 280–283
  surface anatomy, 278–279
  veins, 298–299
Ureters, 139–146, 160, 164–167, 176–177
  nerve plexus, 170–171

ostia, 160–161, 194
  right, 170–171, 175–178, 189, 206
Urethra, 157–160, 176–177, 180–181
  bulb, 160
  crest, 160
  membranous part, 193
  spongy part, 193
Urethral meatus, 150–151, 156, 174, 194
Urinary bladder, 48, 112, 134, 145, 160–161, 173, 175–184
Urogenital diaphragm, 48, 156–158, 161, 170–171
  inferior fascia (perineal memebrane), 156, 159, 190–199
  sphincter urethrae muscle, 198, 200
Urogenital triangle
  female, 151
  male, 150
Urorectal fascia (of Denonvilliers), 191
Uterine tube, 190
Uterine tubes, 167, 173, 176, 178–181
Uterosacral fold, 178–179
Uterovaginal autonomic nerve plexus, 171
Uterovaginal fascia, 190
Uterovaginal nerve plexus, 173, 466
Uterovaginal venous plexus, 167
Uterus, 112, 165, 171, 173, 176, 190
  body, 178, 180–184
  broad ligament, 178–179
  cervix, 180–184
  fundus, 178–184
  round ligament, 176, 178–179, 182, 192
Uvula, 351, 418–421, 424–427

V

Vagina, 173, 176, 180
  anterior fornix, 180–181
  labium minus, 198
  opening, 151, 156–159, 161
  posterior fornix, 180–181
  vestibular bulb, 161, 194, 196, 198
  vestibule, 151, 174, 180–181, 196
Vaginalis testis, 191
Vagus nerve (CN X), 79, 81, 94–100, 392, 408, 414–415, 443, 461
  branches
    aortic plexus, 464
    to ascending colon/cecum, 464
    cardiac, inferior, 464
    cardiac, inferior cervical, 463
    cardiac, middle cervical, 463
    cardiac, right, 96–97
    cardiac, superior, 414, 418, 421
    cardiac, superior cervical, 463
    communicating, to carotid sinus branch of CN IX, 462
    craniocervical, 463
    external, motor to cricothyroid muscle, 463
    gastric, 464
    interior (sensory), 463
    pharyngeal, 418, 463
    posterior trunk, to liver/gallbladder, 464
    to proximal transverse colon, 464
    to small intestine, 464
    thoracic cardiac, 463
    thoraco-abdominal, 464
  functions, 471
  inferior (nodose) ganglion, 461, 463
  overview, 446–447

  posterior trunk, 122–123, 140, 142–143, 146–147
  pulmonary plexus, 464
  right, 96–97, 305, 314, 316, 421, 424, 464
  superior ganglion, 461, 463
  vagal ganglion, inferior, 418
  vagal trunk, anterior, 120, 122–123, 130, 140, 146
Vallecula, 351, 416, 420
Veins
  deep, 391
  dural/cavernous sinuses, 392–393
  overview, 30–32
  superficial, 390
Veins, named
  angular, 390, 408, 412, 428
  antebrachial, median, 299
  anterior cardiac, 82, 84, 87
  arcuate, 144
  atrium, oblique of left, 90
  auricular, posterior, 390, 404
  axillary, 30, 72–73, 298–299
  azygos, 30–33, 83, 87, 96, 100, 102–104
    arch, 30, 96–98
  basilar plexus, 392
  basilic, 278, 298–299, 322–324
  basivertebral, 33, 35
  brachial (vena comitans), 30–31, 298–299, 318
  brachiocephalic, 312, 412
    left, 32, 72, 81–83, 102
    right, 30–32, 72, 78, 82–83, 89, 96–97
  buccal, 390
  cardiac
    great, 82, 84, 87, 90
    middle, 83, 87
    small, 84, 87
  carpal venous, dorsal arch, 335
  central retinal
    inferior nasal branch, 431
    inferior temporal branch, 431
    superior nasal branch, 431
    superior temporal branch, 431
  cephalic, 42, 298–299, 323
  cerebral
    great (of Galen), 391–393, 399
    inferior, 392
    superior, 393
  cervical
    deep, 30, 391
    superficial, 42, 298, 390
    superior, 391
    transverse, 31, 60, 298, 390–391, 409
  circumflex femoral, 246
  circumflex humeral
    anterior, 298–299, 316, 320–321
    posterior, 298–299, 316–320
  circumflex iliac
    deep, 31, 175
    superficial, 42, 52, 232–233
  circumflex scapular, 60, 298, 310, 317
  colic, 138
    left, 125, 138
    middle, 138
    right, 138
  costoaxillary, 298
  cremasteric, 56
  cubital, median, 278, 299, 325
  cystic, 118, 123, 136, 138
  dorsal digital, 233
  dorsalis pedis, 232, 260

  dorsal metatarsal, 233
  dural/cavernous sinuses, 392–393
  emissary, 390
  epigastric
    inferior, 30–31, 44, 48, 164–167
    superficial, 233
    superior, 30, 44–45, 48, 51, 72, 311
  esophageal, 122–123, 419
  facial, 390–391, 404, 407–409, 412
    common, 390–391, 437
    deep, 390–391
    transverse, 390
  femoral, 30–31, 174, 232, 246–249, 255–257
    deep, 232, 246, 255–256
    left, 140
  femoral cutaneous, 233
  femoral triangle, 248–249
  fibular (peroneal), 232, 262
  gastric
    left, 120, 123–125, 130
    right, 138
    short, 121, 124, 138
  gastro-omental (gastroepiploic)
    left, 121, 129
    right, 114, 118, 124, 129, 136, 138
  genicular, 232–233, 264
    descending, 232, 246–247, 264–266
    inferior lateral, 232, 268
    inferior medial, 232, 254, 264, 268
    lateral inferior, 246–247, 265
    lateral inguinal, 266
    lateral superior, 246–247, 261, 265–266
    medial inferior, 246–247, 265–266
    medial superior, 246–247, 265–266
    middle, 232
    superior lateral, 232, 268
    superior medial, 232, 254, 264, 268
  gluteal
    inferior, 166–167, 204–205, 207, 232, 250–251
    superior, 166, 204–205, 232, 250–253
  gluteal region, 253–254
  gonadal
    left, 32, 123, 146
    right, 32
  hemiazygos, 32–33, 94–95, 104,
    accessory, 32–33, 94–95
  hepatic, 30, 128–129, 146–147
  ileocolic, 138
  iliac
    common, 31–32, 138, 207, 232, 246
    external, 31, 138, 140, 166–167, 232–233, 246
    internal, 31, 166–167, 183–184, 207, 232
  iliolumbar, 32
  infraorbital, 390
  intercapitular, 298–299
  intercostals, 30–33, 43–44, 94–97, 117, 119
    anterior, 33, 48
    highest, 30, 391
    posterior, 30, 33, 96
    posterior, dorsal branch, 33
    posterior, lateral cutaneous branch, 33
    superior, 30, 32, 96–98
  interosseous
    anterior, 298, 327–328
    posterior, 298, 327–328, 335
  intervertebral, 33, 35
  intestinal, 138
  jugular
    anterior, 30–31, 42, 385, 400

Veins, named
 jugular—*continued*
  external, 30–31, 42–43, 72, 385, 390–391, 400
  internal, 30–31, 72–73, 78, 102, 309, 390–391, 401–402, 436–439
 labial
  inferior, 390
  posterior, 167
  superior, 390–391
 laryngeal, superior, 415–416
 lumbar, 30–32
 maxillary, 390
 mesenteric
  inferior, 121–125, 138–139, 166–167, 207
  superior, 121–125, 129, 138, 141
 metacarpal, dorsal, 298
 musculophrenic, 30–31, 97
 nasofrontal, 429
 obturator, 166–167, 254
 occipital, 390–391, 400
 ophthalmic, 391, 432, 434
 ovarian, 167
 palmar digital, 298–299, 336
 palmar superficial, 299
 pampiniform plexus, 57, 166, 175
 pancreaticoduodenal
  anterior inferior, 138
  anterior superior, 138
 paraumbilical, 48, 124
 perforating/anastomosing, 232–233, 250–251
 pericardiacophrenic, 81, 94–96, 102, 104
 perineal superficial, 161
 peroneal, 263
 phrenic
  inferior, 32, 138, 140–142
 pial plexus, 34–35
 plantar
  lateral, 232, 270
  medial, 232, 270
  network, 232–233
 plexus, posterior internal, 33, 35
 popliteal, 232, 250–251, 267
 portal, 120–121, 123–126, 129
 profunda brachii, 298–299, 316, 320
 proper digital, 270–271
 proper dorsal digital, 298–299
 prostatic plexus, 166, 170
 pterygoid plexus, 391, 419, 437
 pudendal, 52, 232–233
 pulmonary
  left, 82, 83, 90–92, 94–95, 100, 102
  right, 82, 83, 88, 90, 96–97, 100, 102
 radial, 298–299, 327–328, 338, 341
 rectal
  inferior, 166–167, 192, 194–195
  interior, 207
  middle, 166–167, 207
  perimuscular plexus, 207
  superior, 138, 141, 166–167, 207
 rectal plexus, 163, 167, 207–208
  communication, interior/external, 207
  external, 163, 207–208
 rectosigmoid, 138
 renal, 144
  left, 30, 32, 142–143, 146–147
  right, 30, 32, 142, 146

 retromandibular, 391, 404–405
  anterior branch, 390, 409, 412, 423
  posterior branch, 390
 sacral
  lateral, 207, 254
  middle, 32, 138, 175, 207
 saphenous
  accessory, 174, 233
  great, 30–31, 52–54, 232–233, 244, 248–249, 265–268
  small, 232–233, 236, 250–251, 265
 scapular
  dorsal, 60, 298, 316–317, 332–333, 413
  transverse, 312–313
 scrotal
  left, 164
  left posterior, 164
  posterior, 166
 sigmoid, 138–139, 141, 207
 spinal posterior, 35
 splenic, 122–125, 138
 subclavian, 43, 72, 298–299, 322, 390
  left, 72, 94–95
  right, 30–31, 97
 subcostal, 30–32, 44
 subscapular, 30, 298–299
 superior vorticose, 435
 supraorbital, 429
 suprarenal, 32, 140, 146–147
 suprascapular, 30–31, 298, 312, 332–333, 390
 supreme (highest), 30, 32, 391
 temporal, superficial, 390, 400, 404–405
 testicular, 48, 248
 thigh
  anterior, 246–247
  cross section, 255–256
  medial/lateral, 254
  overview, 257
  posterior, 250–251
 thoracic
  internal, 31–33, 44–49, 81–82, 103–104,
  lateral, 30, 298, 312–313
  superficial, 298
 thoracoacromial, 30, 298
 thoracodorsal, 60, 298–299
 thoracoepigastric, 42, 46–47, 52
 thymic, 32, 82, 87
 thyroid
  inferior, 32, 72, 103, 385
  superior, 385, 412–413, 416
 tibial
  anterior, 246–247, 260, 263, 266, 268
  posterior, 232, 262–263
 tibialis anterior, 232
 tibial recurrent, anterior, 265
 ulnar, 289, 298–299, 327
 ulnar collateral, 323, 332–333
 ulnar recurrent, 332–333
 upper limb, 298–299
 uterine, 167, 207
 uterovaginal plexus, 167
 vaginal, 167, 207
 vena cava
  inferior, 30–32, 82–83, 96, 118–123, 126, 129–130, 140–143, 207
  superior, 30–32, 81–83, 87–89, 96–97
 ventricular posterior, 83
 vertebral, 30–32, 385, 391

  left, 82, 87
  right, 103
 vesical
  inferior, 166
  superior, 166–167, 207
 vesical plexus, 166–167, 170–172, 467
 vorticose
  inferior, 431
  superior, 431, 434
 zygomaticoorbital, 404–405
Vena caval foramen, 106–107
Vena digiti minimi, 299
Venae comitantes, 33
Ventral division of S2, 243
Vermiform appendix, 49, 111, 136–138, 178
Vertebrae
 cervical (*See* Cervical vertebrae)
 column, 79
 intercostal, 95
 ligament attachments, 19
 lumbar (*See* Lumbar vertebrae)
 muscle attachments, 4–7
 paravertebral structures, 98–99
 sacral (*See* Sacral vertebrae)
 spinous process, 35
 thoracic (*See* Thoracic vertebrae)
Vertebral venous plexus, 391
Vertebra prominens. *See under* Cervical vertebrae
Vertebrocostal trigone, 106–107
Vesical venous plexus, 166–167, 170–172, 467
Vesicouterine pouch, 112, 178–181, 190
Vestibular (false vocal) fold, 416
Vestibular ganglion, 443, 460
Vestibular gland, greater, 196
Vestibulocochlear nerve (CN VIII), 392, 396, 443, 460
 functions, 471
 overview, 446–447, 460
Visceral layer, 191
Visceral pericardium, 81, 93
Visceral peritoneum, 113, 190–191, 208
Vocal fold, 416

W
White ramus communicans, 40–41, 96–97, 102
Wrist
 bones of, 344
 cross section, 341
 joint, 328
 radiograph, 329, 345

X
Xiphisternal joint, 18
Xiphoid process, 2, 4, 18, 68, 93

Z
Zona orbicularis, 152, 258
Zygapophyseal joint, 19
Zygomatic arch, 348–349, 356, 404–405, 412, 436–437
Zygomatic bone, 348–349, 352–353, 356–357, 359, 432
 frontal process, 440
 orbital surface, 364
 temporal process, 440
Zygomaticofacial foramen, 352, 356, 358
Zygomatico frontal suture, 429
Zygomatic process, 352–353, 356, 365